COVER PHOTO

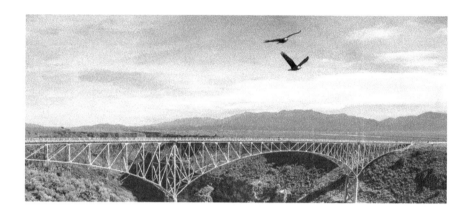

The cover picture is the Rio Grande Gorge Bridge, in Taos, NM. The Gorge Bridge is the seventh highest bridge in the United States, and eighty-second highest in the world. The bridge can be crossed on foot or by car. The Taos Gorge Bridge crosses the canyon created by the Rio Grande River, five hundred sixty-five feet below. The Rio Grande Gorge spans fifty miles, running northwest to southeast; and in parts of the gorge, the canyon walls reach eight hundred feet high.

The cover photo symbolizes the purpose of the book. The eagle is a symbol of vision. Two eagles fly over the Rio Grande Gorge toward Taos Mountain—symbolizing crossing the great divide in medicine, from old ways to new ways. The eagles symbolize new visions in chronic disease and flying to new heights, to conquer chronic disease and extend longevity.

THE
ORIGIN *of*
DISEASE
The War Within

Carolyn Merchant, JD
&
Christopher Merchant, MD

authorHOUSE®

AuthorHouse™
1663 Liberty Drive
Bloomington, IN 47403
www.authorhouse.com
Phone: 1 (800) 839-8640

Published by AuthorHouse 10/11/2018

ISBN: 978-1-5462-5981-7 (sc)
ISBN: 978-1-5462-5980-0 (hc)
ISBN: 978-1-5462-5979-4 (e)

Library of Congress Control Number: 2018910710

Print information available on the last page.

This book is printed on acid-free paper.

DEDICATION

Thank you to my long-time paralegal and friend, Anna Garcia, for her dedication and immense help and assistance during the writing of this book. Thank you to my family and friends, especially Clair, Patrick, Brittie, Crede, Ivan, Dana, and Marie, who have supported our effort to write this book, and who have listened to us discuss these issues for so many decades.

We thank our family, friends, patients, and clients, for their patience and encouragement in writing this book. Thank you to all who gave permission to incorporate knowledge gained from their cases, in this book. A special thanks to Brittie Janson Perez, for her years of effort researching and documenting her remarkable family.

THE ORIGIN OF DISEASE: *THE WAR WITHIN*

CONTENTS

PROLOGUE

<u>Thoughts From A Chinese Parable</u>

One day the emperor summoned to his palace the most famous doctor in all of China and asked the healer a question: "Who is the greatest doctor in our land?" No fool this emperor, for here he was, face-to-face with the most famous doctor in his country, but clearly he, the emperor, was able to make the distinction between fame and greatness. So he had asked a very subtle question, perhaps with the hope of tricking the doctor. But the doctor was no fool, either, and he answered as follows:

"I see people at death's door, in their most dire moments. I operate on them, I draw blood from them. Occasionally I bring them back from the brink of death. And I am the most famous doctor in all of China."

At this, the emperor nodded.

"But I have an older brother," the doctor continued, "and my older brother sees people who are not quite as sick. He sees the earliest forms of their illnesses. He is able to intervene before they knock at death's door, and he saves far more people than I. And he is famous in my village."

Again, the emperor nodded.

"But I have an older brother still, older than he," the doctor added, "and he sees the conditions in our country that make our people sick. He changes these conditions before the people become ill. He has saved millions of lives."

The emperor cocked an eyebrow as the doctor paused.

"And this man, the oldest of my brothers, is well known in my family," the doctor finally said. "So I ask you, Emperor, to tell me: Who is the greatest doctor in all of China?"

At this, the emperor merely smiled and nodded.

The Heart of the Matter
Peter Salgo, MD

CHAPTER 1

THE REBEL WITHIN

Christopher Merchant, MD

Dr. Merchant was born to a long line of social revolutionaries. Critical thinking and voicing opinions, even unpopular opinions, were core values in the lives of his ancestors. His ancestors were intelligent, and spoke out for what was right, at risk to their careers and even at risk to their lives. Dr. Merchant's experiences growing up made clear to him he too had an obligation to speak out for what was right, and fight for justice. His destiny was to be an outspoken rebel, to speak the truth, to speak on behalf of others, and to think beyond what was known. It was his destiny to be a revolutionary in medicine.

Family lore reports Dr. Merchant's distant collateral relatives included Pope Pius IV, Saint Charles Borromeo, seven cardinals, and five Renaissance painters and sculptors named Crespi, whose art is displayed in museums and churches in Europe. Saint Charles Borromeo worked helping the poor with stomach disorders, and became the Patron Saint of Stomach Disorders. At the end of Saint Charles Borromeo's life, contrary to the wishes of his family, he donated his wealth to those in need. At Dr. Merchant's first job, in the South Valley, he was an outspoken rebel on behalf of patients with stomach disorders, caused by drinking contaminated water, which changed the course of his career.

Vincenzo Crespi IV, was born in Ceriana, Italy, in 1808. At the age of fourteen, Vincenzo was tricked into joining a Capuchin monastery. At a gathering of the town for confession, with the travelling friar, the friar verbally condemned Vincenzo to hell for playing billiards, in front of the entire town. Vincenzo was distraught over the public condemnation and humiliation, and fearful of being condemned to hell. After several days

1

of torment, the travelling friar convinced Vincenzo he had no hope of salvation and was destined to be condemned to hell, unless he joined the monastery. The friar likely targeted Vincenzo because he was an intelligent and advanced student, of the kind sought after by the Capuchin monasteries.

When Vincenzo Crespi, IV, joined the monastery, he was required to abandon all worldly possessions, and any contact with family was prohibited, for the rest of his life. The monks in the monastery were brutal to young initiates. Vincenzo was required to keep his head down, and never look up into the face of his superiors, for the first year. If initiates violated monastery rules, they were subject to severe discipline, and various forms of starvation and humiliation. Vincenzo once flogged himself for hours, in his solitary room, as he was directed to do by his superiors. He was taught it was a sin to talk to Protestants, all Protestants were evil, and even talking to a Protestant could lead to condemnation to hell. Vincenzo wanted to leave the monastery many times, but saw the consequences to others who expressed a desire to leave or tried to leave. He feared if he let it be known he wanted to leave, his life could become even more difficult. He feared if he fled and was captured, he would be imprisoned, in the basement of the Vatican. On one of his last travels as a monk, Vincenzo met a family of Protestants, and was surprised at how hospitable, gracious and giving they were.

Vincenzo Crespi, IV, lived in the monastery for twenty years, and became a Doctor of Divinity and master of many languages. Near the end of his time in the monastery, Vincenzo collaborated with the underground press, to write and publish articles critical of the Catholic Church. The articles were published and distributed at night, in secret; and exposed beliefs and practices of the church, which he thought were hypocritical. In 1843, Vincenzo planned his escape to Switzerland, on a night when one of his articles would be published and distributed. As he fled, he heard the senior monks discovering his writings in the underground press and expressing outrage. Vincenzo moved from Switzerland to England, and taught French and Italian at the Royal Court of Queen Victoria and Prince Albert. In 1847, Vincenzo met and married Marie Guillon, a Protestant.

In 1853, Vincenzo collaborated with the Reverend Girolamo Volpe, to write <u>Memoirs of an Ex-Capuchin</u>. The Rev. Girolamo Volpe wrote to Vincenzo, stating he wished to document Vincenzo Crespi's remarkable life.[1] Vincenzo humbly agreed, hoping the book would spread the light of the gospel, by exposing the prejudices of the Catholic Church and the pretentiousness of holiness. The book demonstrates Vincenzo's extensive and highly educated vocabulary, and uses many words no longer in common usage. At the end of <u>Memoirs of an Ex-Capuchin</u>, Vincenzo said:

> *We have written dispassionately, incited alone by the love of truth, and urged by a strong desire, which struggled imperiously, to make known to men truths which we felt they ought to know. Feeling this strong necessity to communicate these facts to the world, woe to us [who] had the fear of human wrath, by whom so ever, or in what manner so ever, manifested, induced us to remain silent. Id @ 403.*

Vincenzo and his wife Marie had eight children, four of whom lived to adulthood. In 1854, three of his children died in the cholera epidemic, in London. Vincenzo, his wife, and their oldest child, moved to Cheltenham, where Vincenzo taught French and Italian, at the University of Cheltenham. Another son Edward was born, and died of scarlet fever, in infancy. Vincenzo and Marie had three more children, in 1855, 1856, and 1862. In 1869, the family moved to Richmond, Virginia, where Vincenzo worked as a Professor of Languages at Richmond schools. Vincenzo's youngest child, Albert Vincent Guillon Crespi, was the father of Chris Merchant's grandmother, Clelia Delia Crespi. Vincenzo deeply loved his wife and family, and his final wish for his children was:

> *[They] not be hampered by the credulity which made him a victim of the Capuchins, and be privileged to labour in the cause of truth.*

<u>Memoirs of an Ex-Capuchin Monk</u> has been restored and preserved, as part of a project aimed at historic preservation of old and important rare

---

[1] Girolamo Volpe (Vincenzo Crespi, IV). 1853. <u>Memoirs of an Ex-Capuchin</u>.

books; and is now available on Amazon. Vincenzo's picture, while living in Richmond, Virginia, shows he wore the same glasses Dr. Merchant has worn, for more than twenty years.

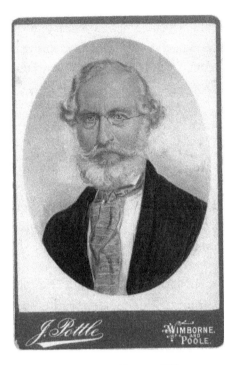

Vincenzo Crespi, IV
Approximately, 1870

In writing <u>Memoirs of an Ex-Capuchin</u>, Vincenzo Crespi, IV, wanted to expose prejudice and hypocrisy in the Catholic Church, and felt an obligation to speak the truth. We feel compelled to write <u>THE ORIGIN OF DISEASE: The War Within</u>, to speak the truth about chronic disease, and expose the biases and false assumptions, inherent in the medical system, which stand in the way of diagnosis and treatment of chronic disease and important new discoveries. The medical system needs new ways of thinking, and a new vision, to conquer chronic disease. We cannot let fear keep us silent, and must report truths which others deserve to know. It is our obligation to write the book—it is your choice whether to act on the knowledge.

Dr. Merchant's collateral ancestors, through his grandfather, Crede Haskins Calhoun, include John C. Calhoun, a controversial political figure early in United States history. John C. Calhoun served as a United States Congressman, a United States Senator, Secretary of State, Secretary of War, and Vice-President of the United States. He was Crede Calhoun's great, great, great, grandfather. Crede H. Calhoun publicly denied his relationship to John C. Calhoun, because he did not approve of the fact John C. Calhoun owned slaves. Crede H. Calhoun was raised by his grandparents, who were part of the Underground Railroad, and helped slaves escape to Canada.

Crede H. Calhoun was Dr. Merchant's grandfather, the father of Dr. Merchant's mother, Clelia Calhoun. Crede Calhoun left home in Indiana, at age nineteen, to seek adventure and opportunity as a reporter, in Panama. He worked for two years as a postal clerk, in Miraflores, before returning to the United States to get a graduate degree in journalism. He returned to Panama, in 1911, and worked as a reporter for the Panama Star & Herald. He wrote many short stories, and articles reporting on the building of the Panama Canal. He worked with Colonel Gorgas to eradicate malaria and yellow fever, in Panama, to stop the deaths of thousands of workers who were building the Panama Canal. Crede Calhoun also contracted malaria, and the quinine treatment for malaria permanently impaired his hearing.

Crede H. Calhoun was appointed the first Director of Posts and the first Chief of Civil Affairs, and served as the Chief of the Division for Civil Affairs and Director of Posts for the Panama Canal Zone, from 1916-1947. He oversaw all functions not related to the actual operation of the Panama Canal, including the Postal service, Customs, Police, Fire, Immigration, Licensing and Registration, Civil Defense, Canal Zone schools, and libraries. Crede, his wife Clelia Delia Crespi Calhoun, and their infant daughter Peggy, were passengers on the first ship to traverse the Panama Canal.

While serving as Chief of Civil Affairs and Director of Posts, Crede Calhoun greeted Charles Lindbergh's Spirit of St. Louis flight to Panama, on February 6, 1929; which was the first air mail delivery from the United States to Panama. Thereafter, Crede Calhoun and Charles Lindbergh became friends.

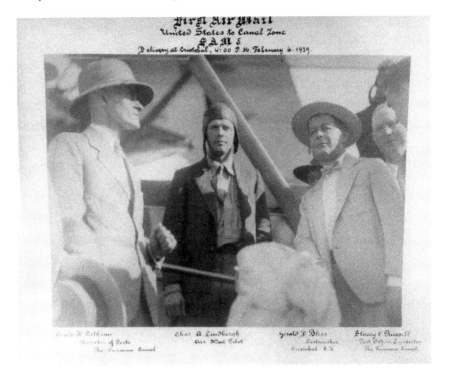

CALHOUN & LINDBERGH
First mail delivery to Panama
February 6, 1929, 4:00 p.m., Cristobel, Panama.
Crede Calhoun, left; Charles Lindbergh, second from left.

Crede Calhoun continued to work as a reporter, writing articles for the New York Herald Tribune, the New York Times, and Newsweek. He interviewed many dignitaries and public figures, including King Edward of England, when he was Duke of Winsor; Charles Lindbergh, when he made the first flight to Panama; author George Bernard Shaw; and Albert Einstein. He had "stringers" throughout Latin America, who provided him news stories. After retiring as Chief of Civil Affairs, he became the New York Times Latin American Bureau Chief. In 1953, he was awarded the Maria Moors Cabot Prize, awarded annually by Columbia University for journalistic excellence, for his work in Latin America. He was awarded the Order of Vasco Nunez de Balboa, the highest honor then awarded by the Republic of Panama, similar to a Medal of Honor in the United States. Many of his writings are preserved at the University of Wyoming, School of Journalism.

Crede Calhoun was fluent in five languages. During World War II, he served as a spy for the United States. He concealed his fluency in German, to enable him to listen to German conversations, and obtain valuable information directly and through his "stringers". He overheard Germans discuss war plans; learned of impending enemy attacks against ships in the Caribbean; and was instrumental in capturing an important German spy. He wrote an article for the New York Times, about an impending attack, which outraged President Franklin Roosevelt. President Roosevelt pressured the New York Times not to publish the article, which was not published until after President Roosevelt died.

Crede H. Calhoun and his wife Clelia Delia Crespi Calhoun had five children. The third child was Clelia Calhoun Merchant, who was Dr. Merchant's mother. Clelia Delia Calhoun was exceptionally intelligent, and devoted her life to her husband and five children. Crede and Clelia Calhoun raised their children to have and demonstrate democratic values, and concern for others. Crede Calhoun died, in 1972, at the age of ninety-three.

Brittmarie Janson Perez, known as Brittie, was born in Sweden and raised in Panama. Brittie is the oldest of ten children, and her mother Peggy was the oldest child of Crede H. Calhoun and Clelia Delia Crespi Calhoun. Brittie was Clelia Calhoun Merchant's niece, and Chris Merchant's cousin. Peggy, Clelia, and Brittie had very similar persona. All were intelligent, outspoken, and engaged in advocacy for just causes. Brittie became an outspoken critic of the military dictatorships of generals Omar Torrijos and Manuel Noriega, who seized power in Panama, in 1968. She risked her freedom and her life to help write, publish, and circulate a clandestine weekly newspaper, El Grito, created and distributed entirely by women, to expose the abuse of power and corruption, in Torrijos' and Noriega's military dictatorships. The El Grito was printed in the middle of the night, on a noisy mimeograph machine, in a secret room built by the editor, to avoid detection by the military gorillas. Brittie and her family had to flee Panama to avoid persecution. After fleeing, Brittie was tried *in absentia*, and declared "provisionally" not guilty, *in absentia*. She was later pardoned by the next administration.

Brittie and her family fled to Albuquerque, where Dr. Merchant and his wife Carolyn lived, and the population has deep Spanish roots. Brittie continued to research and write articles on authoritarianism and corruption, which she has demonstrated go hand-in-hand. At the University of New Mexico, Brittie earned a Master's Degree in Anthropology. She studied the adaptation and protests against repressive regimes, and for her Master's thesis, interviewed Cuban people impacted by the dictatorship of Fidel Castro. She later earned a Ph.D., in anthropology, at the University of Texas. Her Ph.D. thesis, "The Process of Political Protest in Panama: 1968-1989", traced twenty years of protests against corruption and repression, by the military dictatorships of Omar Torrijos and Manuel Noriega. She is also the author of "En nuestras propia voces: 1968-1989 (Spanish language version) and "Golpes y tratados: piezas para el rompecabezas de nuestra historia". Brittie's collection of research and writings, consisting of thirty-five linear feet of documents, clippings, audio recordings, and artifacts, are preserved as part of the Benson Latin American Collection of rare books and manuscripts, at the University of Texas.[2] Brittie was the keynote speaker at a seminar on Latin America, at the University of Reno; and her dissertation has frequently been cited, in books about the military dictatorships, in Panama. She continues today researching and writing about government corruption.

Brittie fled Panama to avoid persecution for writing and distributing articles that exposed the abuse of power and corruption, by the military dictatorships, in Panama—just as Vincenzo Crespi, IV, fled the monastery, in 1843, to avoid persecution by the Catholic Church, for writing and distributing articles critical of the Catholic Church. Brittie followed the Calhoun family tradition of being an outspoken rebel, even at risk to her own freedom and her own life. Brittie is very proud of Chris and Carolyn, who she believes are fearless; and have bravely carried out the family tradition of speaking out for what is right and what will help others, even when the topic is unpopular or controversial. Once an outspoken rebel, always an outspoken rebel! Brittie, Chris and Carolyn carry on the family tradition of speaking the truth to help others.

---

[2] Brittmarie Janson Perez Collection on Panama. Benson Latin American Collection, University of Texas Libraries, the University of Texas at Austin. Doi: https://legacy. lib.utexas.edu/taro/utlac/00191.html.

Colonel Charles Albert Phelps Hatfield was Dr. Merchant's great grandfather on his father's side. Colonel Hatfield was born in Alabama, in 1850, and was a West Point graduate, class of 1872. His uncle and mentor was General Charles Edward Phelps, a Brigadier General during the Civil War, who was awarded the Congressional Medal of Honor for heroism at the Battle of Spotsylvania Courthouse. General Phelps graduated from Princeton and Harvard Law School; and after his military service, became a lawyer, judge and congressman from Vermont. Colonel Hatfield corresponded with General Phelps frequently, during his military career.

Colonel Hatfield served in the 4th, 8th and 13th Calvary. He led his cavalry unit throughout the southwestern United States, in Texas, Arizona and New Mexico, in the late 1880's and early 1900's. He served in the Indian Wars and the Geronimo Campaign; and received a Silver Star, for his bravery during the 1886 attack on Geronimo, in the Santa Cruz Mountains. On April 9, 1891, he and twelve of the men in his command received medals for meritorious acts or conduct in service to the country. Colonel Hatfield later became a controversial figure for actions he had taken during the Geronimo Campaign.

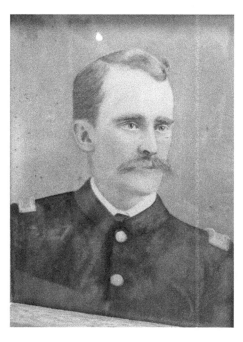

Charles Albert Phelps Hatfield, 1872

"Harper's Weekly" magazine sent Frederic Remington to the Southwest, to document the Geronimo campaign. In 1888, Remington joined Colonel Hatfield's cavalry unit, and they became friends. Colonel Hatfield was the commander of the cavalry unit, and a renowned horseman. Both men were from military families, both were excellent horseman, and both were talented artists. Colonel Hatfield kept a diary and sketch book during his time in New Mexico and Arizona, and drew elaborate pen and ink sketches of his encampments and his surroundings. Colonel Hatfield and Frederic Remington likely sketched together in their tent, during down time at encampments.

Remington decided to change his mission to documenting the "Soldiers of the Southwest". "Harper's Weekly" had a promotional campaign for Remington's art that said, "he draws what he knows, he knows what he draws". Colonel Hatfield was a tall, handsome, and imposing figure, who looked dashing on a horse. He became a frequent model for Remington's art and "Harper's Weekly" magazine covers. Colonel Hatfield can be recognized in some of Remington's most well-known paintings and sculptures, by comparing the Remington works to Colonel Hatfield's 1872 picture, from his West Point graduation. Colonel Hatfield can also be recognized by his hat, his horse, and his mustache; and in some paintings, he was leading the charge, full speed, shooting a rifle.

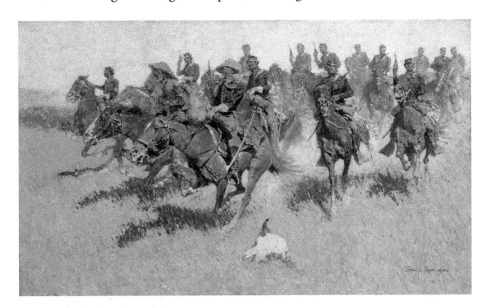

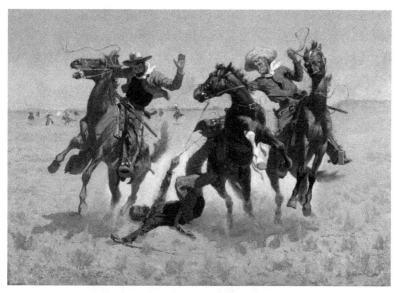

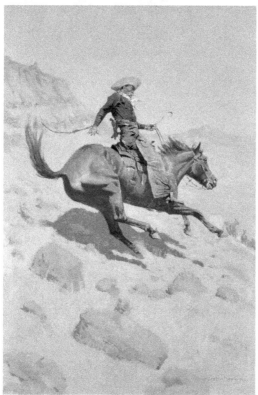

The Geronimo Campaign, Frederic Remington

Carolyn Merchant, JD & Christopher Merchant, MD

Colonel Hatfield was the model for the Bronco Buster, the original of which was given to President Theodore Roosevelt, and sits in the oval office. Dr. Merchant has a small replica of the Bronco Buster, in his office.

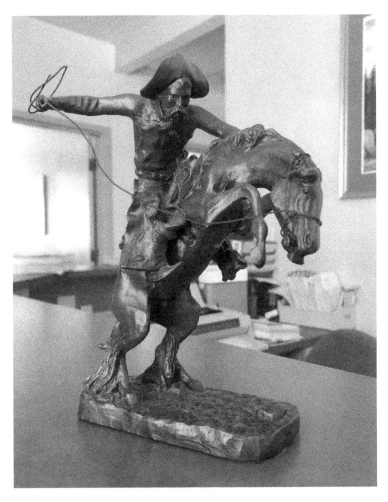

Small Replica Bronco Buster

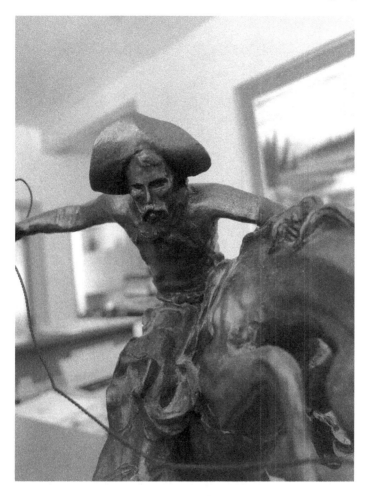

The Bronco Buster, Frederic Remington

Colonel Hatfield served during the Spanish American War, in Cuba and the Philippines. His last assignment was Commandant, at Ft. Myers Virginia. The Remington statute, the "Cowboy", was Remington's only full-size public art, which was commissioned while Colonel Hatfield was stationed at Ft. Myer's Virginia. By history, Colonel Hatfield traveled from Ft. Myers, Virginia, to Philadelphia, to pose with his horse, at the exact spot where the statute stands. The "Cowboy" still stands in Fairmont Park, in Philadelphia.

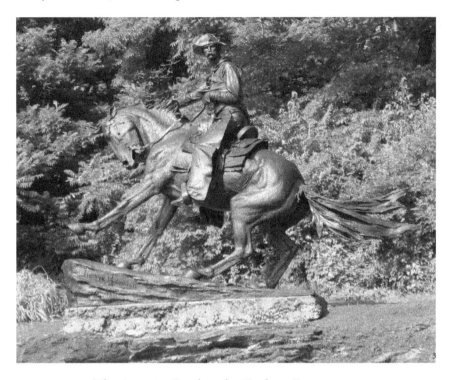

The Arizona Cowboy, by Frederic Remington
Fairmont Park, Philadelphia, Pennsylvania

Colonel Hatfield lost his only son, Albert B. Hatfield, in military service, in Panama, in 1910, at the age of twenty-eight. Colonel Hatfield retired from the Army, due to age, in 1914, after forty-six years of military service. He returned to military service, during World War I, and was recommended for promotion to Brigadier General and Major General, before his second retirement.

Colonel Hatfield died in Ft. Myers Virginia, in 1931, at the age of eighty. Christopher Merchant was born in Ft. Myers, Virginia, in 1948. Dr. Merchant bears a striking resemblance to Colonel Hatfield, but for Colonel Hatfield had blonde hair and blue eyes, and Dr. Merchant has brown hair and brown eyes. Dr. Merchant had a mustache similar to Colonel Hatfield for many years, which made the resemblance even stronger.

---

[3] Martin C, photographer. 2010. Cowboy (1908). Courtesy Association for Public Art.

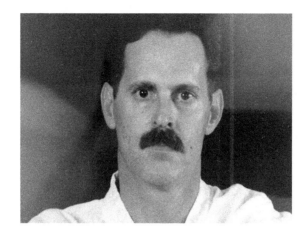

Dr. Christopher Merchant
Approximately 1990

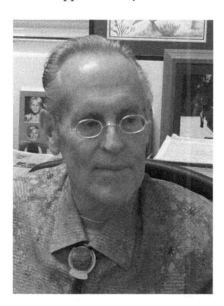

Dr. Christopher Merchant, 2016

Colonel Hatfield had two children, Albert B. Hatfield, born in 1881, and Helen Hatfield, born in 1888. Albert B. Hatfield died in military service, in 1910, and is buried at Arlington Cemetery. Colonel Hatfield's daughter, Helen Hatfield, was Dr. Merchant's grandmother, the mother of Dr. Merchant's father. Berkeley Thorne (Budd) Merchant, Dr. Merchant's grandfather, was a West Point graduate, class of 1905. Budd Merchant's first assignment after

West Point was Ft. Myers Virginia, where he met and married Helen Hatfield. The marriage of Helen Hatfield to Berkeley (Budd) Merchant was reported in the New York Times Society Pages.

Budd Merchant was a tall, handsome, and charming figure. He was a superb horseman, and an accomplished sabreur. Budd Merchant served in the 13th Calvary, as did Colonel Hatfield; and Budd Merchant's father was also a decorated Army officer. Budd Merchant became the Dean of Military Instructors in horsemanship; and was one of the forward looking and outspoken Army officers who advocated for the Army to move away from horses, toward armored warfare. He participated in the Pershing Punitive Expedition, of 1916-1917, seeking to locate and capture Pancho Villa; before being deployed to World War I, to take charge of the Veterinary Corps A.E.F. In 1919, he was awarded the Army Distinguished Service Medal, for his service evacuating sick and wounded animals, during World War I.[4] He led the United States Olympic Equestrian Team, in Antwerp, Belgium, in 1920. He retired from the Army, in 1934, after suffering a heart attack, which was a bitter disappointment to him. Had he remained in the Army, he would have likely gained distinction as a leader in the transformation of the military to armored warfare, during World War II. Budd Merchant was disappointed he could not participate in World War II, but was glad to be represented by his son, Marvin Merchant, Dr. Merchant's father. He started a second successful career in finance.

Budd Merchant and Helen Hatfield had one son, Marvin Merchant, known as "Pat" Merchant, who was born in 1916. Budd Merchant and Helen Hatfield Merchant divorced when Pat Merchant was a toddler, at a time when divorce was rare. Helen Hatfield left Budd Merchant, with plans to marry a man in Philadelphia; and shortly after the divorce, the man died in the Spanish Flu epidemic that struck Philadelphia, in the summer of 1918. Helen returned to Charlottesville, with her son Pat, and never remarried, before her death, in 1974.

In 1925, Budd Merchant married his second wife, Willamete Berenice Wyeth, a Washington socialite, who had a trust fund from her grandfather. Budd and

---

[4] War Department, General Orders No. 108 (1919).

Berenice adopted a daughter, Bernice Wyeth Bull. After Willamete Berenice died, in 1940, her uncle challenged the right of the adopted daughter to inherit the trust, in court, because she was not a natural born child. The court ruled an adopted daughter did not have a right to the inheritance, and the substantial inheritance passed to her uncle and his children.[5]

Budd married his third wife, Alice Coughlin, who was a wealthy Midwest heiress. Alice had volunteered for the Red Cross, during World War I; and met and fell in love with Budd Merchant, in Europe. After she returned to the United States, from World War I, she moved to Washington D.C., and stayed in contact with Budd. Alice had a trust fund, which was a life-estate with a vested remainder in the Red Cross. Upon her death, her entire inheritance was donated to the Red Cross. When Budd Merchant died, in 1952, Alice Coughlin wrote a testament, which describes the thinking and the culture in Dr. Merchant's family. Her words ring true in the years since and today:

> *We live in deeds, not years:*
> *In thoughts, not breaths:*
> *In feelings, not in figures on a dial.*
> *He lives most who thinks most, feels the noblest, acts the best.*
> *Requiesat in peace.*

Chris Merchant's father, Marvin (Pat) Merchant, grew up the only child of divorced parents, and lived with his mother Helen. His father Budd was an authoritarian presence, who dictated major decisions, and was otherwise dismissive of him. Pat went to high school at Lawrenceville, a boarding school in New Jersey, where he was a football star. He was given a new Model-T at age sixteen, and spoke of the joy and adventure driving across the country, in his Model-T, with a friend. Pat wanted to go to college at Princeton; but his father did not give him a choice. Budd demanded Pat go to West Point, as Budd, Budd's father, and Helen's father had done.

In 1940, Pat Merchant became a third generation West Point graduate. In his West Point graduation yearbook, the 1940 Howitzer, he was described as "the man who never lost an argument and never intends to"; a man who "put

---

[5] <u>Wyeth v. Merchant</u>, 34 F. Supp. 785 (W.D. Mo. 1940).

his original stamp on us all"; and a man with a vibrant personality, quick wit, ready smile, and infectious laugh. His first assignment after graduation was in Panama, where a large military presence protected the Panama Canal, during World War II.

Clelia Calhoun Merchant, Chris Merchant's mother, was born in Panama, in 1920, the third of five children. She lived a privileged life, as the daughter of a top government official, in the Canal Zone Administration. She was highly intelligent, and read at an early age. She spoke only Spanish until she went to elementary school, where she learned English. Clelia, her older sister Peggy, and her niece Brittie, attended high school at Notre Dame de Sion, an elite boarding school, in Costa Rica. Notre Dame de Sion was run by French nuns, and taught entirely in French. Clelia graduated from high school at sixteen; and went to Smith College, where she made straight A's. After graduation, she returned home to Panama, and worked in naval intelligence, in the Canal Zone, until she met and married Pat Merchant.

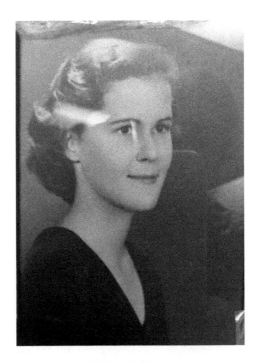

Clelia Calhoun
Approximately 1940

Pat Merchant was a dashing and engaging young military officer. Clelia was an intelligent, engaging, dynamic, and beautiful, Panamanian aristocrat. They met, fell in love, and married on Columbus Day, 1942. Pat was a conservative Republican Military Officer and Clelia an opinionated and outspoken liberal Democrat, from a liberal family with a tradition of speaking out for liberal causes. The conservative man who gave orders met the independent, liberal, and outspoken woman; and it was forever more a clash of wills between authority and privilege, and between conservative and liberal points of view.

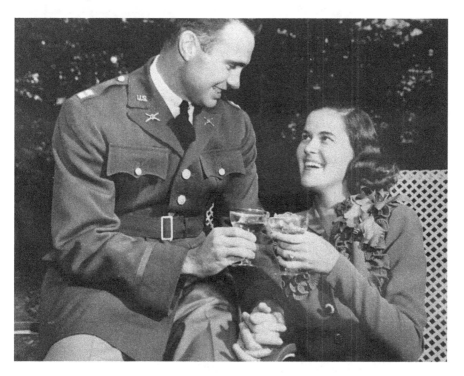

Pat and Clelia Merchant
Wedding Day, October 12, 1942

Crede Ellen, Pat and Clelia's first child, was born in Panama, in July 1944, where Clelia waited with her family until Pat returned from World War II. When Pat returned from World War II, Pat and Clelia had two more children, Berkeley Thorne, in 1946; and Christopher Calhoun Hatfield Merchant, in 1948. Clelia Merchant dedicated her life to her husband

and children. As a military wife, Clelia Merchant was alone when she had their first child, and endured extended time alone. She had to move the family every two years, to follow Pat's career. Each move required uprooting herself and her children, finding new friends, and sending her children to a new school. When stationed in Pennsylvania, she suffered a brain aneurysm, which caused her to be separated from the family for six months. She ultimately fully recovered.

Clelia Merchant was charming, engaging in conversation, and a gracious hostess. She loved interesting conversation, political debate, and loud dinner parties. Clelia Merchant's opinions and political views were inconsistent with most military officers, and most military wives. Clelia's policy was to separate her guests at her huge dining room table, because she believed separating couples encouraged conversation, getting to know one another, and even better and louder debates over dinner. She loved cooking, and prided herself on healthy ingredients, special recipes, and the proper presentation of food. (The family compared her to Julia Child.) Dr. Merchant loved his mother's cooking, which gained him much favor with his mother.

Pat and Clelia valued education, and had high expectations for their children. Clelia encouraged her children to be creative, have original thoughts, express opinions, and think outside the box. She encouraged and demonstrated verbalizing opinions and speaking out for what was right. She instilled in her children the desire to learn, to think critically, to have concern for others, to speak for others, and to think beyond current knowledge. As a young child, Chris loved reading and would carry a book in his pocket to read in the grocery story lines, which also gained him favor with his mother.

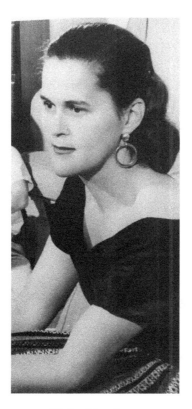

Clelia Merchant
Approximately, 1952

Colonel Pat Merchant served in World War II and Vietnam. In World War II, Pat fought with General Patton, and served with distinction. He was a commander in anti-aircraft artillery; and in July 1944, led troops in battle, in the Ardennes Forrest. The battle continued through the end of the Battle of the Bulge, on January 25, 1945. Pat was one of the people sitting in folding chairs, at the Trinity cite, at White Sands, New Mexico, when the first atomic bomb exploded.

From 1945 to 1948, Colonel Merchant served at the Civil Affairs Department, of the War Department Special Staff, and from 1949-1950 he was assigned to the Office of the Under Secretary of the Army. He graduated from the Command and General Staff College in 1951, and was sent to Portugal to work with the Military Advisory Assistance Group. He graduated from the Armed Forces Staff College, in 1955, and served on its staff and faculty, until 1958. He was the commanding officer in the Ryukyu Islands Support Group, in 1962; deputy commander of the 30th Artillery Brigade, from 1962-1963; and served on the staff and faculty of the Command & General Staff College, at Ft. Leavenworth, Kansas, until 1965. He commanded the 6th Missile Battalion, 6th Artillery, in Philadelphia; and became Deputy Commander of the 9th Logistical Command, supporting operations in Vietnam. On his last assignment, at Headquarters, Commander in Chief, Pacific, in Honolulu, Hawaii, he served as Deputy to General Westmoreland; and he sat beside General Westmoreland when Westmoreland testified before Congress. Colonel Merchant should have been promoted to general during the Vietnam War, but his outspoken criticism of military support services, causing unnecessary deaths of soldiers from equipment failures, likely delayed his promotion. He was offered the opportunity to become a general prior to his retirement, if he agreed to a transfer to South Korea and be separated from his family for another year, but he declined.

Colonel Merchant served twenty-nine years in the Army, and retired in 1968. During his career, Pat Merchant earned the Belgian Fourragere, the Bronze Star, the Legion of Merit, and the Army Commendation Medal for meritorious service as the Director of the Department of Command, at the Army Command General Staff College. He retired to the Charlottesville, Virginia countryside, where he was raised and where his mother Helen still lived. In retirement, Pat developed lung cancer, likely from exposure to the first atomic bomb explosion. He survived, after having one lung removed.

Clelia was proud to be multilingual, and enjoyed volunteering as a Spanish interpreter, for the courts in Charlottesville. She would laugh and tell stories about her experiences in life and at arraignments; and how Spanish speaking defendants would ask in Spanish for her as their lawyer. She loved to find opportunities to speak Spanish; and enjoyed New Mexico, where Spanish is often spoken, although she said New Mexico Spanish was not the same as the Spanish in South America. Clelia died, in 1997; and Pat Merchant died, in 1999. Pat and Clelia, and their military ancestors, are buried at Arlington Cemetery.

Christopher Merchant was sick when he left the hospital, after his birth; and had to be taken back to the hospital. When Chris was three, while in route to Portugal, he got pneumonia, which led to another hospitalization, in London; and he thereafter developed asthma. He grew up living with asthma, allergy testing, allergy shots and emergency room visits for asthma attacks. Doctors told him he might not live past twenty, which warnings of an early demise did not lend itself to great caution in life. He says now he would have been more careful if he knew he would live so long. Asthma shaped his view of life, and created a desire to understand his own illness, medicine, and disease.

Chris had the personality of a youngest child, both charming and mischievous. He had the behavior of a youngest child who was sleep deprived, from asthma. Chris was four when his family was living in Portugal, and his older brother and sister were already in elementary school. Chris was bored at home alone, so he was sent to a Portuguese kindergarten, where only Portuguese was spoken. He quickly learned to speak Portuguese and became a rebel in school. He had a speech impediment as a young child, and would punch kids on the playground if they teased him about how he spoke. His classmates stopped teasing him, and began to imitate his speech impediment, in Portuguese, to the distress of their parents.

In middle school, Chris lived in Okinawa. He started teenage rebellion, and was lucky no one discovered the perpetrator of his antics was the commander's son. He moved from Okinawa, to Leavenworth, Kansas, where he went to Immaculata High School. At Immaculata High School he was a leader in student government and captain of the football team. He suffered two knee injuries playing football, and had two knee surgeries, while still in high school. At the start of his senior year, his father was transferred to Hawaii, and his mother stayed behind in Leavenworth, to allow Chris to finish high school. Chris graduated from high school as the co-Valedictorian.

In the summer before college, Chris lived in Hawaii with his parents. The Commander's house was on the beach, and he learned to surf right outside the door. He worked as a teamster, moving furniture, offices, and safes, and learned the meaning of hard physical labor. On Christmas vacation during his sophomore year in college, he and his brother surfed at Makaha

Beach; and Chris almost drowned, saving his brother from drowning in a dangerous riptide.

Chris was accepted to Dartmouth College, with the intent he would play football. After his pre-football physical examination, the football coach asked Chris to get another knee surgery, as a condition of playing football; and Chris decided to give up football. He started college at Dartmouth interested in everything, not knowing his major interest. He started taking liberal arts courses, and considered majoring in political science and anthropology. Several other family members were anthropologists, and one was the curator of the Frick Museum, in New York City.

Chris dropped-out of college after his sophomore year, still unsure of his major. When he dropped-out, Pat was in the process of retiring from the Army, and Pat and Clelia were moving back to Virginia. His parents said if he was not going to attend college, he had to get a job to support himself. Chris returned to Hawaii and camped on the beach with a friend, surfing, living off the land, and even fighting a wild pig with a small knife, for food. He had time to meditate, take a time-out from the constant push forward with his education, and find his purpose in life. He rekindled his desire to understand disease and longevity, and decided he wanted to be a family doctor.

When Chris returned to Dartmouth, an all-male school, he went to Vassar for one semester, an all-female school, under a Dartmouth-Vassar exchange program. At Vassar, he was one of only seven men in a women's dormitory, housing one-hundred twenty women. He learned to better understand and interact well with women; and he met and dated Meryl Streep. He returned to Dartmouth in September, intending to complete his degree in political science and complete all the prerequisites for medical school. He worked hard and was able to finish all the medical school prerequisites, in two years; but for, stayed one additional semester after graduation, to finish a class in organic chemistry.

Chris came of age in the turbulent sixties and early seventies. His generation was filled with rebellion, idealism, and a desire for social justice. At Dartmouth, Chris participated in sit-ins, demonstrations, and occupations of buildings. He demonstrated for women's rights and civil rights; and is proud to say he participated in the first March on Washington. He was tear-gassed during the March on Washington, and learned from that experience not to stand in the front row at demonstrations. He demonstrated against the Vietnam War, at the same time his father was working as Deputy to General Westmoreland and fighting in the Vietnam War.

When he graduated from Dartmouth, Chris believed the graduating seniors had agreed to donate the money for caps and gowns, to buy medical supplies for refugees from Vietnam. Chris and two others were the only graduates who attended the graduation ceremony without a cap and gown. Chris wore a Hawaiian shirt; one friend brought his dog; and one friend wore a dress, to protest the lack of women at Dartmouth. The other graduates had donated the money *and* paid for caps and gowns.

Chris was accepted to medical school, at the University of Virginia, on the strength of his vocabulary and general knowledge. He earned a ninety-nine percent on the vocabulary and general knowledge portion of the entrance examination for medical school. The average score in his medical school class on vocabulary and general knowledge was twenty-nine percent. On the first day of medical school, Chris was the rebel with long hair, wearing a t-shirt. The other new medical students were wearing Armani suits.

In medical school, Chris quickly recognized the dichotomy between the memorizers and the thinkers. The memorizers wanted the professors to tell them what they needed to know. Chris was willing to question and challenge professors and think beyond what was taught. He asked difficult and probing questions, which were not always well received. He asked professors how to resolve conflicts between information given by different professors—some would roll their eyes, while others admitted he had a point but offered no explanation. He wanted to know the causes and cures for chronic disease, and how to extend life—not just how to name diseases and treat symptoms. He asked what *caused* chronic disease, and was told we don't know, no one knows, keep studying. Chris demonstrated occasional flashes of genius; which others started to notice after he excelled at the laboratory cases in pathology, which required students to identify tissue and organs in a pot. In pathology, he began to think about the origin of disease, when he observed generalized fungus in patients who died of many different chronic diseases.

In medical school Chris was outspoken in his criticism of the Dean. He criticized the Dean over the lack of training and supervision during the newly imposed clinical rotations at a Veteran's Hospital, more than sixty miles from the medical school. He and five others sued the Dean, for adding remote Veteran's Hospital sites to the clinical training program. The Dean called them all into his office and demanded they drop the lawsuit, or "he would ruin them". Four chose to give up right away, and did not have to do a clinical rotation at the remote Veteran's Hospital. Chris and one friend agreed to drop the lawsuit; however, refused the "fix" offered by the Dean, and accepted the clinical rotation to the Veteran's Hospital. As Chris feared, the Veteran's Hospital was staffed with doctors ill-equipped to teach medical students. The attending would ask Chris what to do. Chris would then call his friend and ask what to do, and report back to the attending with the answer.

The Dean retaliated against Chris, causing him not to match when residency positions were assigned. The Dean told Chris he knew he was mad, but he had saved a spot for him in Family Practice, at the University of Virginia. The Dean said he knew Chris was smart, but needed "political re-education" and "training in diplomacy". Chris was not interested in staying at the University of Virginia, for "political re-education" and "training in diplomacy"; and began a search for matches in Family Practice. He found an opening in the Family Practice residency program, at the University of New Mexico.

Dr. Merchant's destiny was to come to New Mexico, which only happened because of his inherent desire to speak out for justice for others and his demand for better training and supervision of medical students. He moved to New Mexico, in July 1976, to train in Family Practice. During his third year of residency, he served as a Chief Resident in Family Practice and the President of the House Staff. Dr. Merchant's life and way of being brought him to New Mexico, where his great grandfather served in the Army, and whom he strongly resembled.

In New Mexico, the eagle chose Dr. Merchant as his spirit animal. The eagle is a symbol of vision. Eagles would appear when Chris was around, sometimes

26

as many as a dozen eagles flying overhead. When a dying tree in the front yard needed to be cut down, outside his home-office window, we asked an artist friend to carve the tree. Out from the inside of the dying tree appeared an eagle!

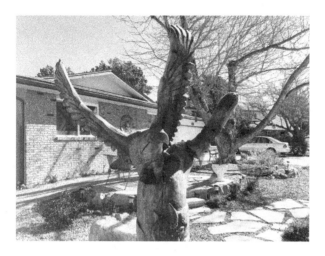

Tree From Front

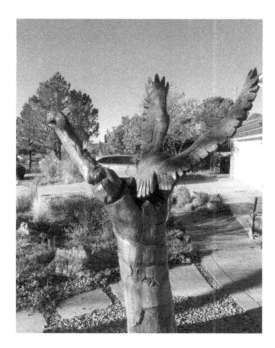

Tree From Back
Tree carving outside Dr. Merchant's home office

Dr. Merchant was born to a long line of social revolutionaries, leaders, and dignitaries, who were outspoken in service to the cause of truth, even at the risk to their career or their life. His ancestors set high standards, and sacrificed to speak the truth and expose hypocrisy. Dr. Merchant's destiny was to question, critically analyze, think beyond what was known, to rebel, and to speak out for justice. He is a social and medical revolutionary, and visionary thinker, who has dedicated his career to finding creative solutions for difficult medical problems; and to understanding the origins of chronic disease. Dr. Merchant carries on his family tradition, by publishing <u>The ORIGIN of DISEASE: *The War Within*</u>, challenging the medical system to re-think what they know; to re-think the diagnosis and treatment of chronic disease; and to shape a new vision for medical practice and medical research.

> *You cannot be afraid to speak up and speak out for what you believe. You have to have courage, raw courage.*

John Lewis

Carolyn Merchant, JD

Carolyn Merchant, was born in 1950, the second child of John and Esther Nies. She was raised in St. Louis, Missouri, the "Show Me State". Fifty-percent of the population in St. Louis is German, and German culture and ways of being dominated St. Louis culture. Carolyn learned from an early age the value of common sense, a trait valued and expected in Missouri. She had a "show-me" way of thinking, was independent, cooperative, helpful, and kind; and brought the spirit of St. Louis to Chris' life. Unlike Chris, Carolyn lived in the same house for the first eighteen years of her life, and went to the same school, with the same classmates, from kindergarten through high school, many of whom went to the same college. Carolyn, like her own mother Esther, was independent enough to move away from her lifetime home, to a place she did not know, to a place she knew no one, to follow her career and dreams of adventure. Carolyn was in many ways like Chris' mother Clelia—both Capricorns, both intelligent and outspoken, and both strong and independent.

John was born, in 1892, the son of a St. Louis saloon owner. His ancestors arrived to St. Louis in the mid-nineteenth century, via a boat from New Orleans. John was born in an age of two-dimensional thinking, before cars and indoor plumbing. He recalled going to the St. Louis World's Fair as a child, when the ice cream cone was invented. John's family lost three young children in one year, two in the diphtheria epidemic, and one in a fall from a high chair. John's father fell down the stairs in the dark, at age thirty-six, and died after suffering at home, in agony, for three days. John was six, and his younger brother was four, when their father died. His mother Agnes remarried and had five more children. John's loss of his father at an early age and the remarriage of his mother lead to a lack of parental supervision, and lack of a father-figure as a role model. John dropped out of school in the eighth grade, and later educated himself by taking college courses in business and finance. John's mother died when he was twenty, in 1912, the year Esther was born.

John worked in the coal and coke business for most of his work life. He started selling stokers, which was a device to keep house heating systems filled with coal. He later worked as a coal broker, and an entrepreneur. John's life was significantly impacted by the Great Depression, which left him with a depression era frugality for the rest of his life. His belief was banks and savings were a one-way street—you put money in, but you do not take it out. He wore the same blue pinstripe suit for fifty years.

Carolyn's mother Esther was born, in 1912, on a chicken farm, in Broken Arrow, Oklahoma. Esther's mother was the oldest of nine children. Esther was the second of six children and oldest girl. Esther was beautiful, smart, and very good at doing mathematics in her head. She played the violin, and church and faith were central to her life. She was loving and kind, and loved and admired by all who knew her.

Esther's father was tragically killed in a flaming car accident, when she was fourteen. He suffered extensive burns, and died after three days of agony. Her youngest sibling was still a toddler, and as the oldest girl, Esther had the responsibility to help her mother with the younger siblings and in supporting the family. The family moved to Tulsa, where her mother worked as a seamstress to support the family. After Esther graduated from high school, she worked one year at Krebs, and turned over her entire paycheck to help her mother support the family. She wanted more in her life than working at Krebs; and in Tulsa, she had no opportunities for a future. It was the Dust Bowl and the Great Depression. Men in Broken Arrow and Tulsa were out of work and standing in food lines.

Esther moved away from her family and home, to seek a higher education and better opportunity, five hundred miles away, alone, to a place where she knew no one, to become a nurse. She earned her degree as a registered nurse, at Lutheran Hospital, in St. Louis, in 1934. John met Esther when he was visiting a sick business partner, and Esther was working as the business partner's home healthcare nurse.

John and Esther married, in March 1937. They moved into their new house on a cul-de-sac, built by the husband of John's cousin Agnes, on the night of their marriage. John and Esther lived in the same house for the rest of their lives. John was fifty-eight and Esther was thirty-eight, when Carolyn was born. The household spanned four generations, and six decades. John and Esther had been married thirty-five years when John died, in 1972. Esther died in 1994.

Five years before Carolyn was born, John was diagnosed with diabetes. Esther became his caretaker-nurse, and gave him insulin shots multiple times a day. Each time she gave John a shot, he would act out passive-aggressively, toward Esther or Carolyn. As John aged and his illness got worse, so did his temperament and his insensitive behavior toward others. John was unpredictable, and could switch from praise and encouragement to acting out and being passive aggressive, or intentionally embarrassing, without warning. Carolyn never knew what to expect, from one encounter to the next. It was hard for Carolyn to watch how John treated Esther, and his lack of empathy for others. Carolyn learned by example how not to behave, when she saw the emotional pain John caused others. The unpredictable responses and turmoil John created helped Carolyn develop a strong emotional intelligence, resilience, and the skills to survive difficult situations and difficult people. She grew into a rebel!

Esther was ahead of her time in parenting style. She had a saying for almost every situation, which condensed the parenting wisdom of her time. She encouraged Carolyn to think for herself, use common sense, and have independence. Esther did not set rigid rules or restrictions. She would tell Carolyn to think for herself; and advised she would let Carolyn know when she was not happy. If Esther was not happy, the consequences were less freedom. Carolyn was taught if you can do it for yourself—just do it! She was taught when someone asks you to do something, you do it! If someone asks you for a favor, you do it! Esther had great intelligence, religious faith, and common sense at her core, which sustained her throughout her life and many life challenges.

Carolyn saw Esther as a saint and savior, and a role model. She admired how Esther lived with the challenges of her life, with dignity and grace, setting an example for how to cope with difficult people and difficult circumstances. She lived with admirable kindness, and an attitude of being helpful, no matter how difficult the situation. Carolyn admired Esther's strength and perseverance. Esther did what she had to do, what she could do, and made the best of any difficult situation. She lived strong and gracious her whole life, including twenty-two years as a widow, when her independence bloomed.

Carolyn's only sister was ten years older, and eleven years ahead of her in school. Carolyn's sister left for college when she was six, leaving Carolyn as an only child at home. The ten-year age difference between Carolyn and her sister gave Carolyn the personality of an oldest child—conscientious, confident, and a hard worker. Being an only child after the age of six caused Carolyn to develop the personality of an only child—creative, self-reliant, confident, and a little adult. Being the youngest child in the family caused Carolyn to develop the personality of a youngest child—funny, and rebellious. Carolyn is very funny, and her humor has provided much entertainment and laughter to Dr. Merchant, over the years.

As the only child at home, Carolyn did all the chores, because that is what kids did. She made her bed every day. She did the dishes by hand, after every meal; the laundry; and the ironing, including sheets and pillowcases, napkins and clothes. She mowed an acre of zoysia grass year-round, including picking up all the clippings and taking the clippings to a compost pile. Carolyn sewed her own clothes during school vacations. She did not resent doing chores; and at times enjoyed chores, because it was something to do and she enjoyed being helpful. Carolyn also learned not to ever tell her mother she was bored, unless she wanted to hear the response, which was always more chores. Carolyn started piano lessons at age six, which continued for seven years. She practiced the piano every day after school, which greatly pleased her parents. Her parents would even ask her to play the piano when their friends visited.

Carolyn grew up as what would now be called a "free-range" kid. Outside was always Carolyn's favorite place to be—outside and out of view, particularly out of the view of her father. Whenever Carolyn finished her chores, she would go outside to play, hanging out at the neighborhood swing set or playing kid games like riding bicycles, playing hide and seek, roller skating, board games, card games, and sledding at a kids' gathering place when it snowed. She and her best friend Steve, a neighbor who was six months older, were almost inseparable as children. The families in their neighborhood moved in when the houses were newly built, as John and Esther had done; and their children were already grown. Carolyn and Steve were two of the very few younger children in the neighborhood. When Steve was not available, Carolyn would visit neighbors on her cul-de-sac, one-by-one, chat like a little adult, and frequently be offered fresh cookies. She walked home from school with friends, every day, from kindergarten until she got her first car.

John retired the first time when Carolyn was in kindergarten. Five years later, a business partner died and he had to return to work to manage the business. He continued working for several years running a machinist business, that manufactured parts needed to make beer. John sold the business and retired permanently when Carolyn was a teenager. From that point until his death, he was at home, and spent most of his time on the living room couch. John's constant presence at home added to Carolyn's desire to be outside, away from his watchful eye.

John and Esther loved flowers, particularly orchids and roses. John built a greenhouse, which allowed them to have hundreds of orchids; and orchid blooms in the house all year round. Both John and Esther were active in flower societies, and displayed their orchids and roses, winning awards for the flowers and Esther's flower arrangements. Esther made orchid corsages for high school boys, to give to their prom dates. John and Esther spent many days at Shaw's Garden, because of their flower activities and friendship with the Director of Shaw's Garden. Carolyn, alone or with Steve, spent many days freely roaming and exploring Shaw's Garden, in a way that would not be allowed today. Carolyn acquired a love of flowers, that later developed into a common bond with Chris; and was an independent and free spirit, starting at an early age.

Church attendance was a persistent point of contention between John and Esther, and between Carolyn and Esther. Carolyn never understood John's complete and total resistance to any church attendance, and any church activity. Esther faithfully attended the Lutheran church, every week—John refused, under any circumstances, to attend church, even when Carolyn had the lead role in a church play. Esther insisted Carolyn attend Sunday school and church every Sunday. She would always say, "If you want to go out on Saturday night, you can get up on Sunday morning and go to church." Carolyn went to Vacation Bible School every summer, for three weeks; two years of confirmation classes, on Saturday morning, in junior high school; every youth event; every church picnic; every progressive dinner; and every other church social activity. Esther quilted at church every Wednesday, and came home with fingers that looked like pin cushions. She played bridge with her friends from church, every week. However, Esther recognized and was not happy that women were not treated equally in the church, and not allowed to participate in the church administration. Carolyn knew from her experience that she was not treated equally or given fair recognition for her efforts, compared to the boys, in church, Sunday school, or confirmation class.

Esther wanted to go back to work as a nurse, but John refused to allow it. Carolyn was saddened to see Esther's wishes subjugated to her husband. Carolyn saw neighbors become widows, who had not been allowed to have a bank account, and were lost financially and in life, when their husbands died. The widows lacked basic financial skills and basic financial rights in society. Carolyn's rebellion grew as the women's movement grew, and she came to understand the limitations put on the women in society. Carolyn wanted more than what her mother and her mother's generation were allowed.

John and Esther encouraged Carolyn's education and academic success. When Carolyn brought home a report card, John would reward her with money for each "A", money which she was expected to save. Carolyn was the oldest in her class, which gave her an advantage that persisted from kindergarten through high school. She was considered one of the thinkers in her peer group, and always took advanced courses. The advanced classes were more interesting, gave extra credit on GPA averages, and the students in the classes were the thinkers and her friends. She graduated from high school in the top two percent of her class, of over six hundred students.

In fifth grade, Carolyn starred in a school play, which required her to memorize eighty pages of script. In sixth grade she crafted a sun dial, and her parents had to write a note to the teacher confirming it was in fact all Carolyn's work. In junior high school, Carolyn wrote a lengthy paper on Zen Buddhism, which surprised her teachers by its quality and length. After the Zen Buddhism paper, Carolyn continued reading, studying, and applying the teachings of Buddhism and the Dali Lama. Buddhist thought helped her make decisions free of drama, preconceived notions, and false assumptions. It shaped her world view and her internal view; and helped her find happiness in life, through her own internal beliefs.

In high school, Carolyn took typing, like girls at that time, and became a very good typist. She enjoyed typing, which was viscerally similar to playing the piano. Her skill in typing allowed her to get summer jobs as a secretary, and earn money for college. Typing became a significant asset in her education and career. Her ability to type allowed her to type her final exams in law school, which gave her the opportunity to overcome poor hand writing, and keep up with her thoughts, when composing lengthy essay answers. When computers and the Internet became available, her typing skill allowed her to work efficiently on a computer, and function more efficiently in law practice. The ability to type allowed her to compose on a typewriter, and to now write this book.

Carolyn always loved exercise, and being athletic. She excelled in sports, in physical education, and in after school intramurals. She was the girl the boys picked first for sports teams, sometimes ahead of other boys. Being the oldest in her grade, being chosen first for teams by boys, and having a boy as her best friend, shaped her view of herself as an outspoken leader who was allowed to play on teams with boys and was an equal to boys.

John encouraged Carolyn to do whatever she aspired to do, and not be limited in her aspirations because she was a girl. He always expected her to go to college and encouraged her to pursue her desire to major in business, at a time when few women studied business. She went to the University of Missouri, majored in business and economics, and was one of only a few women in the business classes.

John and Esther instilled in Carolyn a strong German work ethic—a German belief that work, work, work, was a path to happiness and value in life. They had expectations of diligence, competence and achievement. Carolyn has long had a framed quotation on the home-office wall:

> *Press On*
> *Nothing in the world can take the place of persistence.*
> *Talent will not. Nothing is more common than unsuccessful men with talent.*
> *Genius will not, an unrewarded genius is almost a proverb.*
> *Education alone will not. The world is full of educated derelicts.*
> *Persistence and determination alone are omnipotent.*

Author unknown

Carolyn grew up in the turbulent 60's and 70's, a period of radical social change. In 1962, when she was in junior high school, John Kennedy was assassinated. The year she graduated from high school, Martin Luther King and Robert Kennedy were assassinated; black leaders were demanding civil rights; police were assassinating black leaders; and riots exploded at the Democratic convention, in Chicago. The Weathermen were bombing buildings, and Patty Hearst was kidnapped. Young men were drafted to fight in a controversial war in Vietnam, and being killed and maimed for an ill-defined cause. The youth were demonstrating against injustice. Women and minorities were demanding equal rights in society.

In college, Carolyn demonstrated for voting rights, women's rights, and against the Vietnam War. Seeing Gloria Steinem speak to a crowd so large it had to be held in a parking lot was life changing. A generation of young people who cared were trying to create change. Hippies were the idealists who had a vision of a better world—a more fair and equal world and a world of peace and love. The turbulent times forged new paths for women, for minorities, and for peace. At a college reunion, a friend described her generation as the ones who went to college in a skirt and left in blue jeans, which summed up the radical transformation during her college years. The desire to fight against wrongdoing and speak out for justice continued, for the rest of Carolyn's life.

Friends and family always said Carolyn should be a lawyer, because she had a talent for persuasion. She had an intuition law would be a good career for her. When her father died in September of her senior year in college, she decided to return to St. Louis to help her newly widowed mother. She thought taking a few years off from school to get work experience, before pursuing law school, was a good idea.

Carolyn first worked for General Electric Credit Corporation, as a management trainee. She was a Credit Manager, then a Collection Manager, then a Credit and Collections Manager. Two years later, she was hired by Searle Laboratories, to become the first woman pharmaceutical representative, in Missouri. Searle trained her in medicine, using a systems approach, system by system, for all the bodily systems that were targets for Searle's drugs. Searle sold so many different drugs the training encompassed all the systems in the body, and taught her to see the body as a whole, with feedback loops, signals, responses and reactions. While working at Searle,

Carolyn talked with hundreds of doctors about medicine; and gained the ability to talk and debate medicine, using their language. She gained real world work experience, a talent for sales, and learned to quickly speak to the point, in the short time available to talk to the doctors. Her skills as a pharmaceutical representative proved valuable as a lawyer, and as Dr. Merchant's wife and co-author.

After two years working for Searle, in Missouri, Carolyn was promoted to work as a pharmaceutical and hospital representative, at the University of New Mexico Hospital. When she was offered the promotion, she was not sure where New Mexico was, and knew nothing about Albuquerque. She read New Mexico had passed an Equal Rights Amendment to the State Constitution; and passed the pending Equal Rights Amendment to the United States constitution, which she saw as a positive. She read Albuquerque had the closest ski area to any metropolitan area; and New Mexico had many great ski areas. She had learned to ski after college, and wanted to move to the mountains, where she could ski more often and more conveniently. Carolyn knew it was time to venture west to find her destiny and find adventure in mountains of the Southwest. At the age of twenty-six, Carolyn moved one-thousand miles away from home and friends, to a place she had never been, and where she knew no one. It took courage and independence to move to New Mexico, just as it took courage for her mother to move from Tulsa to St. Louis.

Carolyn loved New Mexico as soon as she arrived. She learned to spell Albuquerque, bought a house close to the law school, and moved in the house ten days after arriving in New Mexico. She hoped if she lived near the law school it would help her someday become a lawyer. She marveled at the lack of rain and abundance of sunshine, after working in Missouri in the rain, out of the trunk of a car, for weeks on end. She saw the love openly expressed in families, and many multi-generational households, unlike the German culture. She was enchanted by the culture, the food, the big skies, the sunsets, and the mountains; and quickly understood why New Mexico is called "The Land of Enchantment". Her eyes adjusted to the beauty of the flat roof architecture, and the water-sparing Southwestern landscaping.

To Carolyn's surprise, in New Mexico she was again the first woman pharmaceutical representative. She had to make sales calls on professional offices and hospitals, which were not as nice or welcoming as she expected. The spirit of the Equal Rights Amendment had not yet filtered down to medical offices accepting a woman pharmaceutical representative. Carolyn had broken barriers for women in pharmaceutical sales in St. Louis, and became weary at times of being the first at things.

Carolyn met Chris three weeks after moving to New Mexico. Chris came to talk to her at a hospital display, at the Family Practice Center. He had heard a cute girl was in the conference room, with donuts. Carolyn felt an instant attraction when he walked into the room, and felt love at first sight. That night, she told her new neighbor she thought she had met "the one". A week later, she hurt her knee at the ski area closest to Albuquerque; and early Sunday morning naively thought the emergency room at the university hospital would not be busy and could check her knee. Shortly after she arrived and was put in a curtained cubicle, to wait for a doctor, Chris came on duty, in the emergency room. He walked into her cubicle and it seemed like fate. Out of all the residents at the university hospital, Chris was the one who came on duty at the very time she was waiting to see a doctor. A few months later they starting dating, and within weeks they spent all their free time together.

Carolyn and Chris complemented each other's strengths and filled in each other's weaknesses. They were kindred spirits, and even wore the same crystal glasses. Carolyn's sense of humor made Chris laugh, and she loved to see him laugh. Carolyn had met the love of her life, who was also a rebel, protester, independent thinker, and person willing to challenge conventional wisdom. Clelia had prepared Chris to marry someone like Carolyn, an outspoken, opinionated, independent, free-spirit, who sought justice for others.

The Bandito motorcycle gang created a turning point in Carolyn's life. In December 1978, she and Chris went to Taos, for a Christmas vacation. They stayed at the DH Lawrence Ranch, which was owned by the University of New Mexico, and was rented to medical residents at a low cost. After two glorious weeks, she and Chris were sad to go home and wanted to stay just one more night, intending to drive home early Monday morning, and go to work. The dirt road from the main highway to the DH Lawrence Ranch was several miles long and very muddy. They were concerned Carolyn's company car would get stuck on the muddy road, so they left her car parked on the side of the dirt road, near the main highway. They got up early Monday morning to leave, drove Chris's car to the spot where they had parked Carolyn's company car, and the company car was gone! The Bandito motorcycle gang had broken into the car, broken all the windows, and the police had towed the car to an impound lot in Taos. The impound lot did not even open until 9:00 a.m. Carolyn had to call her boss at Searle and say she was not going to be at work, because she was stuck in Taos; and the company car had been vandalized. After retrieving the car, Carolyn and Chris drove the car home to Albuquerque with the windows broken out, in the middle of winter.

The encounter with the Bandito gang motivated Carolyn to finally pursue her dream of going to law school. The few years she had planned to work before law school had already dragged on to seven years. She applied to the University of New Mexico Law School on the last day for submitting applications, and had to take the law school entrance exam, on the last day it was offered. Luckily, she had strong skills in logic, did well on the entrance exam, and was accepted to the University of New Mexico Law School. Chris finished his Family Practice Residency, in July 1979; and Carolyn started law school, in August 1979.

On the first day, Carolyn wondered if she made the right decision, because she was not sure what lawyers actually did. The first presenter said, "Well, you are in the club now"; and she wondered, "What club? What have I done?" The presenter warned everyone to be ready to get C's; and she thought to herself as she looked around the room, "Maybe those guys". She also thought, "Nothing they can say or do to me in law school could be worse than what I experienced as a woman working five years as a pharmaceutical representative". Skills she had learned as a pharmaceutical representative were useful when arguing the law. She was diligent in her studies, and loved to play bridge, with fellow law students and professors.

Living close to the law school allowed her to walk to and from law school, for three years.

Chris and Carolyn got married, in September of 1979, at the county courthouse, which seemed fitting for a law student. Carolyn was overwhelmed as a new law student; so Chris planned the entire wedding, and surprised Carolyn with the wedding plans. She came home from class on Friday at noon, Chris had flowers and wedding plans ready, and they went to the courthouse to get married. They celebrated with friends at their house after the wedding, had a dinner party at a favorite restaurant, and then went on a honeymoon for the weekend. A rebel doctor married a rebel future lawyer, and medicine married law.

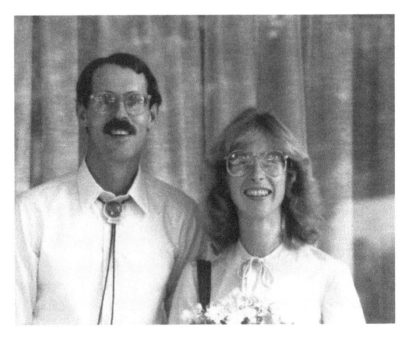

Chris and Carolyn Merchant
Wedding Day, September 1979

Carolyn's intuition was right about law being a good choice for her. She loved her three years in law school, and developed a strong network of friends. She developed her own principles and practices for "How to make A's", which kept the workload in law school manageable. She turned out to be right when she thought, "Maybe them". She graduated *cum laude*, and was awarded an Order of the Coif and the Faculty Award. A professor told her all the professors agreed with her selection for the Faculty Award, and that when they looked at their new class schedules each semester they first checked to see if Carolyn Merchant was on it. The professors liked having her in class, because she was prepared, engaged, sat in the front row, asked insightful questions, was willing to raise her hand to answer the professor's questions, and was fearless debating the professors, when others kept their head down hoping not to be chosen. She even made jokes on her final essay exams, consistent with her tendency toward humor, which must have amused her professors. Carolyn graduated from law school, in 1982, with life-long friends, and a network of friends in law and politics.

Carolyn wanted to be a plaintiff's personal injury lawyer, known as a tort lawyer, which would allow her to use her background in medicine and fight for justice for others. She got a job at a well-known plaintiff's law firm; but as fate would have it, the firm split-up the week before graduation, and she had no job. After passing the bar exam, she took a job working as a defense lawyer for a year, but the job never felt right. She refused to adopt the attitude that plaintiffs were all frauds and malingerers, trying to get money from innocent defendants. She disliked some of the lawyers in the firm, the work culture, and even her hermetically sealed office eight floors up an elevator.

In 1984, Carolyn started her own plaintiffs' personal injury practice. She started working on disability claims, mental health commitments, and car accidents. In 1984, she took on her first medical malpractice case, a man with a brain abscess, who had been diagnosed with brain cancer and left to die from a treatable illness. In 1985, she took on her first eye case, a client injured by contaminated contact lens solution.

In 1987, she took on the case of two men who were blinded in one eye each, by a defective intraocular lens implanted in cataract surgery. The jury found Surgidev knowingly sold a defective, close-loop, anterior chamber intraocular lens, that caused a high rate of sight-threatening complications. When doctors in big cities realized the danger of the lens, and started using posterior chamber intraocular lenses, Surgidev started marketing their anterior chamber lens in small towns, without warnings, to doctors unaware of the danger. When doctors in the small towns realized the danger, Surgidev sold the inventory in bulk to foreign countries. Surgidev manufactured the intraocular lens for thirty cents, and sold it for more than three-hundred dollars, which is a typical percentage profit on many medical devices; and a motive for manufacturers to knowingly conceal dangers and continue to sell defective products.

By the end of the Surgidev case, in 1995, Carolyn had gotten a large jury verdict, including punitive damages, and won three New Mexico Supreme Court writs. A year after the verdict, the court awarded monetary sanctions for discovery abuse, prior to trial. The case generated two appellate opinions, one upholding the verdict and establishing new law; and the other upholding the sanctions awarded for pretrial discovery abuse, while the case was on appeal.[6] The <u>Surgidev</u> case gave Carolyn the knowledge and experience to represent other clients with eye injuries, and other clients injured by defective medical devices. She started to become known as the eye lawyer, and started getting referrals from all over New Mexico and from people she did not know.

In the early 1990's, Carolyn began to represent clients who were injured by RK surgery (refractive keratotomy), in Phoenix, Arizona. Gary Hall, an Arizona ophthalmologist, held marketing seminars, to recruit patients from New Mexico and surrounding states, to fly to Arizona to have RK surgery. Carolyn represented nineteen people against Gary Hall, of the fifty people who brought cases against him. During and after the RK cases, clients came with injuries caused by ALK (automated lamellar keratotomy), then PRK (photorefractive keratotomy), then LASIK (laser in situ keratomelieusis), then variations on LASIK. She represented clients injured by refractive surgery, cataract surgery, glaucoma procedures, glaucoma surgery, retinal injuries, and retinal detachments. She represented clients who were injured by defective medical devices, including injured by equipment used in refractive surgery, intraocular

---

[6] *See* <u>Gonzales v. Surgidev</u>, 120 NM 133, 899 P. 2d 576 (1995); <u>Gonzales v. Surgidev</u>, 120 NM 151, 899 P. 2d 594 (1995).

lenses, contact lens solution, glaucoma devices, implanted defibrillators, lasers used in dermatology, jaw implants, hip implants, and knee implants. She learned from her cases, the FDA does not protect us; and how medical device manufacturers hide adverse events and knowingly sell defective and highly profitable medical products.

Carolyn represented many hundreds of people who were injured by refractive surgery, and ophthalmology or optometry malpractice; and became widely known as the eye lawyer, around the country. She represented many clients from New Mexico; and also represented clients from California, Arizona and Utah. She met ophthalmology experts around the country; and was proud and amused to learn she was the subject of conversation among ophthalmologists, in the hallways of national ophthalmology meetings. She earned an A-5 rating from Martindale Hubbell, the highest available rating for legal ability and ethics, based on evaluations by lawyers and judges. She spoke at a convention of optometrists, opticians and eyeglass manufacturers in Aspen, Colorado; and assured the attendees their business would not end because of refractive surgery, but rather would expand. She spoke at national trial lawyer conventions three times, on issues relating to eyes.

As a lawyer, each case presented a puzzle in need of a coherent legal theory that left no known facts inconsistent with the theory. If any facts did not fit, it was the wrong theory. She observed, collected facts, contemplated what it meant, and thought about how the story fit together. She was able to discern the missing pieces of the puzzle, including identifying medical records that had been deleted or withheld. She used study, investigation, reasoning, common sense, and her desire to make sense of things—to understand the bigger picture, in the case. She believes when she does not know the answer to a question, to take a step back and examine the issue from a bigger or different perspective; and ask bigger or different questions, then the answer can reveal itself and be obvious. She would exhaustively disclose facts and the theory of her case to defendants, and ask defendants to prove where she was wrong.

Carolyn studied the eye almost daily, and developed a deep understanding of eyes. Each case was unique, requiring knowledge of new medical issues, which added to her understanding of the entire body. In every case, multiple medical experts testified and debated what they knew about standards of care, medicine, surgery, eyes, medical devices, economics, biomechanics, vision loss and most any field one can imagine. Each case had to be researched, studied and analyzed, to be able to argue and refute competing medical experts. Carolyn had the opportunity to learn more with every case, by study and by listening to experts testify and debate medical issues. She was a fascination to the experts in ophthalmology and optometry, because of her knowledge of eyes, and of the interaction between eyes and the law. Carolyn's five years as a pharmaceutical representative, and thirty-five years as a lawyer, allowed her to recognize the eye is a microcosm of the body—to understand the eye is to understand the body. The eye is a window into the body, and the window into health.

Carolyn views medicine from the perspective of a lawyer, applying reasoning, healthy skepticism, and common sense. Her experience selling drugs to more than a thousand doctors, marrying a doctor, and suing doctors and makers of medical devices for thirty-five years, allowed her to see doctors as human beings; and seeing the fallibility of the medical profession made her even more willing to question what was said or written by medical professionals. As a pharmaceutical representative and as a lawyer, she looked at the whole person. As a lawyer, she put complex information together in a unified whole. Medicine looks at thousands of separately named body parts, cells, and parts of cells, and identifies thousands of different diseases, findings and syndromes, without considering the person as a whole or the common findings in chronic disease. She came to believe medicine overthought issues, and looked at small details, when what was needed was a broader perspective and structure, to understand the causes of chronic disease.

Carolyn's thinking is not limited by what other people say they know, and she is not intimidated by the authority and education of others, if the other person's explanation does not make sense. Carolyn is willing to question accepted thought, question authority, and seeks understanding of the bigger questions in life, for which the answer is not yet known and thought unknowable. The first level of thinking is concrete thinking, relating to the two-dimensional world. The second level of thinking is abstract thinking, relating to theories, hypothesis, and scientific reasoning. The third level of thinking is computers and technology, which has led to multi-tasking and computer aided intelligence. The fourth level of thinking is pondering the bigger questions in the universe, to understand things not yet known. The fourth level of thinking requires reasoning and deduction to understand things unknown or thought unknowable. Carolyn is fascinated by Einstein, who was engaged in the fourth level of thinking. His theories went beyond what was known, at the time, and his theories were only later proven true. Einstein said, "We cannot solve our problems with the same thinking we used when we created them". He said, "The true sign of intelligence is not knowledge but imagination...Creativity is intelligence having fun."

Carolyn is analytical, intuitive, logical, and creative. She can readily see commonalities and patterns in complex situations; and has the ability to connect ideas, from diverse areas of thought. She used curiosity, reasoning, common sense, and desire to know, to understand chronic disease. She studied intensely and thought deeply about the issues with Chris, for decades. Her "Show Me State" upbringing, her training and experience as a pharmaceutical representative, and her legal perspective on medicine, allowed her to think, learn, and collaborate with Chris. She and Chris sought to find patterns and put diverse information together in medicine, in a simplified structure that explains chronic disease. Her knowledge and skills augmented those of Dr. Merchant. She had the skills to use technology, and to research what others thought about medical issues, to determine whether what was already known confirmed or conflicted with the discussions. Almost daily another example or observation would confirm their belief in a common link, and principle of the whole, in all chronic diseases.

Carolyn is a thinker, who is dedicated to answering the bigger questions in chronic disease. Her knowledge comes from training, experience, interest, research, medical and scientific knowledge, and her ongoing conversations with Dr. Merchant. Enlightened knowledge combined with diligence and interest can lead to breakthroughs in science; and radical new advancements can come when specialized knowledge from different fields are combined. She came to believe no single medical specialty can find the causes and cures for chronic disease; because the answer can only be found by combining knowledge across specialties and across professions.

Carolyn is motivated to help people, and stop the suffering and waste in medicine. She feels an obligation to speak her mind, and to speak on behalf of others when she sees unnecessary suffering and medical mismanagement. Carolyn supported Chris in expressing his opinions and doing what he knew to be right, even if his opinions were not popular. Carolyn realized Dr. Merchant was a visionary, who expressed opinions on the causes of chronic disease before his time, and over and over he was later proven right. She supported him in staying true to his moral values. Chris was the instrument of her inspiration and she of his. Their discussions evolved into new visions in medicine, to solve the mysteries of chronic disease.

As we observed, discussed and studied, over the decades, the desire grew stronger to speak out in a larger forum, and help more people. On their 36th wedding anniversary, in 2015, Carolyn composed the following statement to be read over a megaphone at an outdoor arts festival. The lines were read by a speaker atop a ladder, over a megaphone that echoed for the crowd. The statement expresses Carolyn's thoughts, then and now:

> *To my dear husband Chris*
> *I again pledge my eternal love on our 36th wedding anniversary*
> *It was love at first sight and since that time we have built so much together*
> *I love you now more than ever*
> *I respect you now more than ever*
> *The person you have become*
> *We are ready to move into the next phase of life*
> *And fulfill our dream of helping the greatest number of people*
> *Namaste*
> *I love you*
> *Forever*
> *Carolyn*

CHAPTER 2

THE EVOLUTION OF KNOWLEDGE
FUELED REBELLION

Rather than love, than money, than fame, give me truth.

Henry David Thoreau

Dr. Merchant finished his Family Practice residency, in July 1979. He was offered an academic track at the medical school, but chose to work as a family doctor in an under-privileged area. He went to work for the Family Health Center, a federally funded clinic, where he and two nurse practitioners saw one-hundred fifty patients a day, or more. Dr. Merchant quickly observed endemic gastrointestinal disease in the patients; and believed the patients were sicker, younger, and had a higher than expected rate of cancer, hypertension, arthritis, diabetes, and mental illness.

In the South Valley, residents drank water from shallow water wells, adjacent to poorly constructed septic tanks, in an area with a shallow water table. Dr. Merchant realized patients who drank from the shallow wells, or were exposed to people who did, had an alarming rate of stomach disease and systemic chronic diseases. His medical research confirmed the likely cause of endemic gastrointestinal disease, in his patients, was the parasite giardia lamblia, acquired from drinking contaminated well water. His knowledge and thinking about parasitic disease expanded rapidly, from study, experience, necessity, and interest. He began to apply a simple principle—diagnose what you can, and treat what you can diagnose!

Dr. Merchant began to recognize commonalities in the signs and symptoms of giardia. By history, the patients burped rotten eggs at meals and at night; had intermittent diarrhea; and their stools smelled of sulfur. Many of the patients had big bellies, which resembled a "pregnant man", as Hippocrates described in people who drank bad water, two-thousand five-hundred years ago![7] Some patients had a thin or gaunt appearance, from diarrhea, nausea, malabsorption and a poor appetite. Many described pain in the upper mid-abdomen, above the belly button. Many had recurrent respiratory infections, with mycoplasma or chlamydia pneumonia. Many patients had ulcers and/or had been diagnosed with "irritable bowel syndrome". Many had fatigue, depression and anger. Many were agitated and had increased belligerence. He observed the longer the patient reported a history of the gastrointestinal complaints, and the more constant the symptoms, the more likely the patient had a chronic disease. He observed long-standing parasitic infection caused a cascade of malabsorption, fungal infection, and reduced immunity, leading to new acute infections and recurrent infections, and chronic disease. He observed disturbing patterns of co-morbidities; and the patients developed different chronic diseases and different co-morbid disease from the same longstanding parasitic infection and co-infections.

Giardia selectively blocks absorption of folic acid and B12, nutrients needed for mental stability, and the absence of which can trigger a chronic disease. Dr. Merchant did blood tests on patients with chronic gastrointestinal disease, for folic acid and B12. The patients had low folic acid, low B12, and signs of chronic malabsorption; and patients with low folic acid and B12 developed a decrease in cognitive function, a propensity to violence, and mental illness. As he treated patients for parasitic disease, he saw gastrointestinal symptoms, co-morbid chronic diseases, *and* mental instability improve. He confirmed for himself treatment of parasites and recurrent infections; and supplementing folic acid and B12, could improve chronic disease.

Dr. Merchant spoke out to his employer, peers, and the community, to report the water in the South Valley was causing endemic parasitic disease, and endemic low folic acid and B12, before it was common knowledge low folic acid and B12 were risk factors for mental illness, cancer and other

---

[7] Hippocrates. The Corpus, The Hippocratic Writings. (Kaplan Classics of Medicine). 2008. Kaplan Publishing.

chronic diseases. Dr. Merchant said the well water in the South Valley was making patients sick, and community water and sewer lines needed to be extended to the area. It was apparently heretical to suggest the water was making people sick, and water could cause chronic gastrointestinal and systemic diseases. It was like the story in Ibsen's play, <u>Enemy of the People</u>, in which a doctor was criticized and ostracized for saying the townspeople were getting sick from drinking the town's well water.[8]

Dr. Merchant reached out to the New Mexico State Epidemiologist, Jonathan Mann, MD, MPH, deceased. Dr. Merchant knew Dr. Mann from a residency rotation at the New Mexico State Penitentiary; and knew he was a great physician and teacher. Dr. Mann agreed to conduct a study of gastrointestinal and diarrheal disease in the South Valley. The study documented eighty times the anticipated attack rate of diarrheal disease, in the South Valley. Eventually, as a result of Dr. Merchant's advocacy and the study by Dr. Mann, city water and sewer lines were extended to the South Valley.

Dr. Merchant treated many Vietnam veterans, with PTSD. He treated parasitic infections and recurrent immortal infections, restored lost nutrition, and observed PTSD improve. In 2016, forty-two years after the end of the Vietnam War, the Veterans Administration noticed many Vietnam veterans were dying of unusual cancers, particularly liver cancer. The Veterans Administration conducted a study and discovered the Vietnam veterans were dying a slow death from a liver fluke, a parasite acquired in Vietnam, which was common in the rivers and streams of Vietnam.

Dr. Merchant had worked at the Family Health Center five years, when he was recruited by a large HMO, to work as the doctor-in-charge, at a new clinic being built in the South Valley. At the new HMO clinic, Dr. Merchant saw the same patients, who drank from shallow water wells next to septic tanks; had endemic gastrointestinal disease; had a high rate of mental distress and chronic disease, including in young patients; and a high rate of recurrent respiratory infections. Dr. Merchant decided he

---

[8] Ibsen H. 1882. <u>Enemy of the People.</u>

would do blood tests, for folic acid and B12, on the next one-hundred patients who came through the door. The one-hundred blood tests showed eighty-five percent were below normal, ten percent were borderline low, and five percent of the blood tests were lost by the lab. The high percent of patients with low folic acid and B12, confirmed Dr. Merchant's belief parasitic disease was endemic in the South Valley; and the frequency of mental illness and cancer in his patients was related to low folic acid caused by chronic parasitic disease.

After five years working in the South Valley, and after the one-hundred blood tests for folic acid and B12, of which none were clearly normal, Dr. Merchant felt ethically obligated and required by law to contact the CDC to report endemic giardia in the South Valley. His HMO superiors were angry he had not told the medical director, and gone up the chain of command before contacting the CDC, so the powers above him could make sure the information was blocked before it got to the CDC. The outspoken rebel was supposed to go through channels.

While working for the HMO clinic, Dr. Merchant treated ulcers and irritable bowel syndrome as an infection. The establishment thinking was ulcers and irritable bowel were caused by stress, and Dr. Merchant's desire to treat gastrointestinal disease as an infection created conflict with the HMO. He was called before the Medical Director and told to stop spending money on blood tests and treatment of HMO patients. The HMO did not want him to treat parasitic disease, or to treat ulcers as an infection. Dr. Merchant was told to ignore the patients' gastrointestinal disease, call it all "irritable bowel syndrome", and give the patients "Librax", a cheap symptomatic medication that works like valium for the gut. The HMO thought blood testing for folic acid and B12 was a waste of their money, even though the tests showed widespread depletion of folic acid and B12 in the patients, and patients reported a health benefit from B12 supplementation. They did not want him to give B12 shots, because B12 shots cost the HMO money. The HMO did not want Dr. Merchant to diagnose, treat, or engage in preventive medicine on anyone. The final straw came when the HMO ordered him to stop giving flu shots to HMO Plan patients, because flu shots cost the HMO money. Principles did not matter—prevention of disease did not matter—the correct diagnosis did not matter—it was all about money and the bottom line.

Dr. Merchant and the HMO parted ways, as incompatible. He could not in good conscience ignore the illnesses he diagnosed; and palliate the patient with cheap symptomatic treatment for life. He resolved never again to work in a position in which superiors attempted to block him from doing what was right, in the name of profit. He could not work anywhere administrators and insurance company clerks controlled his medical decisions, and put profit ahead of the best interest of the patient. He started a small private practice in the South Valley, and within a year, a pharmaceutical representative suggested he contact Dr. Fitzpatrick. Dr. Fitzpatrick was an open-minded older family doctor, in solo practice; and a maverick with radical ideas of his own. Dr. Merchant contacted Dr. Fitzpatrick, and in 1984, joined him in private practice.

Dr. Fitzpatrick believed respiratory infections should be treated with erythromycin or tetracycline; and a shot of gamma globulin and B12. Dr. Fitzpatrick did not know specifically why his treatments worked, but many years of observation and loyal patients proved to him the patients did better with erythromycin than with penicillin. The patients reported the gamma globulin and B12 shots made them recover more quickly and feel better. Dr. Merchant continued to diagnose and treat intestinal diseases, and used azithromycin for acute respiratory infections, instead of erythromycin. He continued to prescribe supplemental folic acid; and gave B12 and gamma globulin shots, for acute and chronic infection. He added gamma globulin shots to his treatment regimen for patients with rheumatoid arthritis, multiple sclerosis, and cancer.

Dr. Merchant's experience in diagnosis and treatment of parasitic infections and secondary infections, and observation that his treatment of parasites improved or resolved chronic disease and co-morbid conditions, caused us to write the 1988 article, "Chronic Giardiasis: The Enigmatic Parasite".[9] We proposed chronic infection was a cause of chronic disease; giardia

---

[9] Merchant CC and Merchant CN. 1988. Chronic Giardiasis: The Enigmatic Parasite. *unpublished.*

caused loss of folic acid and B12; and chronic infection caused an infectious cascade of secondary infections and development of chronic disease. We wrote about the interaction between parasites and bacterial infections, including mycoplasma and viral infections. The article was submitted to three journals, and all three journals rejected it. Even worse, someone who read the article while it was being reviewed, stole our ideas, without credit to us; and started to profit from the ideas. A radio show host began broadcasting our ideas, and patients started to tell Dr. Merchant someone on the radio was stealing his ideas. Our experience writing the giardia article was discouraging. We believed what we knew was important and should be shared, but 1988 was not yet the right time.

Our thinking evolved from giardiasis and mycoplasma, to include chlamydia, H-pylori, all forms of intestinal parasites, and toxoplasmosis. Chlamydia pneumonia had been reported by scientists, in 1982 or 1983. Chlamydia pneumonia was not identified as a separate species of intracellular chlamydia, until 1988; and in 1999, the full genome for chlamydia pneumonia was completed.

Dr. Merchant bought and studied textbooks and scientific literature on chlamydia. He realized chronic immortal intracellular infections cause chronic disease; and the greater the infectious burden and longer the immortal infection persisted, the more likely the patient had developed a chronic disease. He observed the immune system response to the infection, and observed patients with longstanding immortal infection developed impaired immunity, recurrent acute infections, and a chronic disease. He saw patients with both giardia and chlamydia, and continued to observe the cause and effect relationship between chronic infections and chronic disease; and between multiple co-infections and chronic disease. He saw the infectious cascade start with parasites or immortal bacteria, followed by new acute infections as immune function declined, fungal invasion, and dispersion of abnormal proteins, which became a chronic disease. He became convinced chlamydia pathogens were the cause of many chronic diseases, alone or in conjunction with other pathogens and parasites.

In 1999 and 2000, we purchased more texts on chlamydia, and books discussing chronic infection and chronic disease. Dr. Merchant studied a textbook on chlamydia, which we refer to as the "Big Red Book" or the "CHLAMYDIA book".[10] The CHLAMYDIA book explained the molecular biology and cellular effect of chlamydia; and gave greater insight into the infectious cascade caused by chlamydia, on a cellular level. The CHLAMYDIA book described many forms of chlamydia, each traced to specific animals; and reported chlamydia pathogens are "associated" with or "connected" to chronic disease. Richard Stephens reported the "association" between chlamydia pneumonia and heart and lung disease is well established, and noted a dizzying array of chronic diseases in patients with chlamydia trachoma. The CHLAMYDIA book explained, at a cellular level, how chlamydia causes chronic disease.

Dr. Merchant's ongoing study and experience caused him to believe asthma was caused by chlamydia pneumonia, damaging the endothelium in the lung and the immune system. He saw asthma and lung function improve when treated with azithromycin and clarithromycin. He saw asthma and lung function worsen when treated with penicillin, amoxicillin and cephalexin. He treated Alzheimer's as a chronic chlamydia pneumonia infection, and saw elderly Alzheimer's patients improve when treated with macrolide antibiotics.

Dr. Merchant's research and experience treating many different chronic diseases as an infection, confirmed to him chronic infections caused chronic disease. He tested patients for infectious immortal pathogens, knew the pathogens he diagnosed in his patients, observed how the infections correlated with the chronic disease, and observed the success of treatment. He observed the type of chronic disease was dependent on the type of infection, combination of chronic infections, the duration of infections, and the overall infectious burden. He observed different chronic diseases could develop from the same pathogens; and the same chronic diseases could develop from different pathogens. As he treated patients for immortal infections, he observed co-morbid diseases improve,

---

[10] Stephens R (*ed*). 1999. CHLAMYDIA Intracellular Biology, Pathogenesis and Immunity. Washington, D.C.: ASM Press.

and patients reported even unreported symptoms improved. He continued his practice of taking good history, doing a physical examination, doing laboratory testing, and making diagnostic decisions and treatment plans, using creative solutions that benefited the patients with chronic disease.

Around 2000, patients who knew Dr. Merchant's interest and belief chronic infection was a cause of chronic disease, started bringing articles to him. One patient brought him a copy of an article entitled "The New Germ Theory", about an evolutionary biologist, Paul Ewald, Ph.D.[11] The patient gave Dr. Merchant the 1999 article in the Atlantic Monthly, *after* he was already treating chronic disease as an infection. The Atlantic Monthly article reported Dr. Ewald's thoughts on the genetic cost of chronic disease. The genetic cost is when patients afflicted with chronic diseases have a reduction in fertility over time; thus, less children, which is the genetic cost of chronic disease. He proposed the genetic cost of a chronic disease would eliminate genetically caused chronic diseases, within a few generations. Dr. Ewald argued genetics was implausible as the sole cause of chronic disease, because if the cause was genetics, each generation should have a lesser occurrence of chronic diseases—not a greater prevalence of chronic diseases. He questioned why chronic diseases are expanding exponentially, rather than diminishing in the population, if genetics are the root cause, because every chronic disease has an established genetic cost.

Dr. Ewald was the author of Evolution of Infectious Disease, which focused on how pathogens acquired increased virulence, when rapidly transmitted between hosts[12]; Plague Time: The New Germ Theory[13]; and Plague Time: How Stealth Infections Cause Cancers, Heart Disease and other Deadly Ailments.[14] He proposed infectious disease would be discovered as the cause of many chronic diseases, based on the timeless logic of evolutionary fitness, and his background in zoology and as an evolutionary

---

[11] Hooper J. Feb. 1999. The New Germ Theory. Atlantic Monthly. Feb. 1999. Doi: www.theatlantic.com.
[12] Ewald PW. 1996. Evolution of Infectious Disease. New York: Oxford University Press.
[13] Ewald PW. 2000. Plague Time: The New Germ Theory, 2nd Ed. Anchor Books.
[14] Ewald PW. 2002. Plague Time: How Stealth Infections Cause Cancers, Heart Disease and other Deadly Ailments. New York: Free Press.

biologist. He argued symptoms are either a defense to a pathogen, or the pathogens' manipulation of the human body to survive; and all diseases and syndromes are no doubt pathogens or multiple pathogens. We did not obtain a copy of any of Dr. Ewald's books, until 2016, while doing additional research for this book.

Dr. Ewald gave schizophrenia and other psychiatric disorders as examples of conditions which have a high genetic cost; and should be decreasing in frequency, not increasing in frequency. He hypothesized heart disease, Alzheimer's, cancer, major psychiatric disorders, multiple sclerosis, thyroid disease, obesity, and eating disorders, are all likely caused by infectious pathogens; and argued cancer had to be caused by infections. He noticed symptoms of schizophrenia were similar to St. Vitus Dance and rheumatic heart disease; and postulated streptococcus as a common cause, because streptococcus was already a known cause of rheumatic heart disease. Toxoplasmosis has also been proven to cause schizophrenia, which does not exclude the fact streptococcus and other pathogens can also cause schizophrenia.

Dr. Ewald noted Robert Koch won a Nobel Prize, in 1905, for his work in identifying tuberculosis as an infectious pathogen. Dr. Koch's presentation of the microscope and the bacterium causing tuberculosis, on March 24, 1882, left the audience in stunned silence. Koch's Postulates, for experimental scientific discovery, are: is the pathogen found in an animal or person with a disease; is the germ isolated and grown in a culture; has the pathogen been injected in a healthy animal and produced disease; and is the pathogen recovered from the diseased animal and shown to be the same pathogen. Dr. Ewald observed in <u>Plague Time: The New Germ Theory of Disease</u> that Koch's Postulates do not work well for the discovery of infectious causes of chronic disease. Observational science, and conclusions based on observation of success in treating patients, does not fit within Koch's postulates. What Koch's postulates did indirectly prove is the same pathogens cause the same diseases, in both animals and humans.

Dr. Ewald's books and articles were published more than a decade after Dr. Merchant had formed his opinions about chronic infection causing chronic disease, and acted on his beliefs by treating patients. Dr. Merchant was already asking why childhood cancers, asthma, diabetes, multiple sclerosis, rheumatoid arthritis, gastrointestinal cancer in young adults, and brain cancer were increasing in frequency. In Plague Time: The New Germ Theory of Disease, Dr. Ewald twice attributes his thinking about infectious causes of chronic disease to Gregory Cochran, Ph.D., and their many discussions.[15] Dr. Cochran is an optical physicist, who moved to Albuquerque, in 1993 or 1994. By 1990, many in the community knew of Dr. Merchant's beliefs, including patients, pharmacists, and other doctors. Dr. Ewald also referred to Jonathan Mann, MD, for his work in HIV,[16] who is the same Dr. Mann who was instrumental in the study of diarrheal disease in the South Valley, with Dr. Merchant.

Whether Dr. Ewald's and Dr. Cochran's ideas originated with Dr. Merchant or not, we do not know. Dr. Merchant was already treating patients in the community for infectious causes of chronic disease and had been for more than ten years, when their discussions began. Dr. Ewald majored in zoology and biology, majors that often precede acceptance to veterinary school. He came to essentially the same conclusions on infectious causes of chronic disease, looking at the issue from a different perspective and different base of knowledge; and using his knowledge of infectious causes of disease in animals. He deduced an answer that made sense, and was consistent with his knowledge of zoology, evolutionary biology, and the theories of Darwin. Dr. Ewald had beliefs that sprang from education, experience, observation, and deep thought. The fact he arrived at the same conclusion using his independent knowledge supports the truth of what we say. Dr. Ewald also added important thoughts on the topic of infectious causes of chronic disease. Perhaps Albuquerque is a new cradle of genius, a city with a high proportion of Ph.D.'s and groundbreaking research, where ideas converge to become new important discoveries. We are now eighteen years past the publication of Plague Time: The New Germ Theory of Disease, and the diagnosis

---

[15] *Id.* @ 57, 271.
[16] *Id.* @ 84.

and treatment of immortal infections as a cause of chronic disease has still not reached mainstream medicine.

In 1998, Brian Balin, D.O., and his team, at the Hahnemann School of Medicine and John's Hopkins, began reporting on chlamydia pneumonia found in Alzheimer's brains, at autopsy. They identified chlamydia pneumonia beneath Alzheimer's lesions, and in cells adjacent to the Alzheimer's lesions and plaque. The plaque was cultured and grew chlamydia pneumonia.[17] Recently, a Harvard professor proposed the idea, as if it is new, and as if it was his idea alone, that chlamydia pneumonia causes Alzheimer's.

In 2003, Louis A. Dvonch and Russell Dvonch published The Heart Attack Germ.[18] The cover of the book displays vials labeled chlamydia pneumoniae, helicobacter pylori (H-pylori), cytomegalovirus, and herpes simplex virus. The book reported the "association" between chlamydia pneumonia and heart attacks, strokes, and Alzheimer's disease. In 2004, Dr. Peter Salgo identified chlamydia pneumonia as the cause of heart disease in The Heart of the Matter: The Three Key Breakthroughs to Preventing Heart Attacks.[19] After publication of The Heart Attack Germ and The Heart of the Matter, patients and friends again started coming to Dr. Merchant saying others were taking his ideas and he needed to hurry and publish his ideas.

---

[17] Balin B, *et al.* 1998. Identification and localization of Chlamydia pneumoniae in the Alzheimer's brain. Med Microbiol Immunol. 1998 Jun;187(1):23-42. PMID: 9749980; *see* Arking EJ, *et al.* 1999. Ultrastructural Analysis of Chlamydia Pneumoniae in the Alzheimer's Brain. Pathogenesis (Amst). 1999; 1(3): 201–211. PMID: 20671799: PMCID: PMC291092. NIHMS157873. PMC 2010 Jul 28; Balin B and Appelt D. 2001. Role of infection in Alzheimer's disease. S2 JAOA. Vol 101. No 12. Supplement to Dec 2001. Part 1. PMID: 11794745; Balin B, *et al.* 2008. Chlamydophila Pneumoniae and the Etiology of Late-Onset Alzheimer's Disease. Journal of Alzheimer's Disease. Apr 2008. Vol 13 (4): 381-391. Doi: 10.3233/JAD-2008-13403.

[18] Dvonch LA, Dvonch R. 2003. The Heart Attack Germ. New York: Writer's Showcase.

[19] Salgo P, Layden J. 2004. The Heart of the Matter: The Three Key Breakthroughs to Preventing Heart Attacks. New York: William Morrow.

In 2005, Dr. Merchant wanted more books, on the subject of chlamydia. Carolyn ordered five books on Amazon, which seemed interesting and related. When the books arrived, we were surprised to find a book entitled Chlamydia and Chlamydia-Induced Diseases, published in 1971, by Johannes Storz, DVM, Ph.D., a veterinarian and microbiologist.[20] Dr. Storz was the head of the Department of Veterinary Microbiology and Parasitology, at LSU; and was awarded the Alexander von Humboldt Prize, for his groundbreaking work on chlamydia. His book reported observations and findings of importance on the topic of chlamydia; and unfortunately, despite his groundbreaking work, the interest in his work was primarily limited to veterinarians.

In 2005, we purchased *Chlamydia pneumoniae* and Chronic Diseases, by Johanna L'age-Stehr (Ed), reporting the proceedings of the State-of-the Art Workshop in Berlin, in March 1999.[21] We also purchased THE INFECTIOUS ETIOLOGY OF CHRONIC DISEASES: Defining the Relationship, Enhancing the Research, and Mitigating the Effects.[22] In the Prologue of THE INFECTIOUS ETIOLOGY OF CHRONIC DISEASES: Defining the Relationship and Enhancing the Research, and Mitigating the Effects, the author states:

> The belief that many long-recognized chronic diseases
> are infectious in origin goes back to the mid-nineteenth
> century, when cancer was studied as a possible infectious
> disease. In the 1950's and 1960's, much biomedical
> research was directed, unsuccessfully, at the identification
> of microorganisms purportedly causing a variety of
> chronic diseases. In recent years, the picture has begun to
> change. One chronic disease after another has been linked,

---

[20] Storz J. 1971. Chlamydia and Chlamydia-Induced Diseases. Springfield, Illinois: Charles C. Thomas.

[21] L'age-Stehr J (*ed*). 2000. *Chlamydia pneumoniae* and Chronic Diseases. Berlin Heidelberg New York: Springer-Verlag.

[22] Knobler S (*ed*), *et al.* 2004. THE INFECTIOUS ETIOLOGY OF CHRONIC DISEASES: Defining the Relationship, Enhancing the Research, and Mitigating the Effects. National Institute of Medicine of the National Academics, Workshop Summary. Washington D.C.: The National Academies Press.

in some cases definitively, to an infectious etiology...
Evidence implicating microorganisms as etiologic agents of
chronic diseases with substantial impact of mortality and
morbidity, including atherosclerosis and cardiovascular
disease, diabetes mellitus, inflammatory bowel disease,
and a variety of neurological and neuropsychiatric
diseases, continues to mount.

Many presenters at the conference reported chlamydia infections, h-pylori, viral infections, and parasitic disease caused a variety of chronic diseases. The conference presenters reported chlamydia pneumonia "caused" heart and lung disease, and chlamydia trachoma "caused arthritic" diseases. The presenters reported diseases "associated" with chlamydia include cardiovascular disease, atherosclerosis, coronary artery disease, abdominal aneurysms, carotid stenosis, adult-onset asthma, chronic obstructive pulmonary disease, lung cancer, Alzheimer's disease, arthritis, reactive arthritis, juvenile diabetes, demyelinating disease, multiple sclerosis, mental illness, and epilepsy. The authors reported toxoplasmosis from cats can cause schizophrenia and epilepsy, particularly when young children are exposed to cats. The presenters suggested future research directions to identify infectious causes of chronic disease.

The authors reported many bacteria, viruses, and parasites had already been linked to chronic disease. The authors concluded an overall infectious burden triggered chronic disease; and the younger the patient when the infections were acquired and the longer the infections persisted, the more likely the patient would develop a chronic disease. The authors reported infections hide inside the white blood cells, and could be transported throughout the body by immune cells; and can hide within cells in the endothelium of the cardiac vessels and lung. The studies reported the patients who had been treated for chlamydia showed improvement or cures, a reduction in heart attacks, and increased survival from heart attacks. The authors also theorized that chronic infection triggered some viral co-infections common in the population, to cause chronic disease.

No one at the conference said "go forth and treat" your patients, or go forth and educate those not present at the conference. The scientists retreated to weaker "association" language, and important knowledge did not change medical thinking or reach the front-line medical practitioners. Fourteen years later, international conferences have still not moved the knowledge from international conferences to the practice of medicine.

The authors at the conference reported science was having difficulty sorting out which infections caused chronic disease, and postulated different infections could cause the same chronic disease. Medicine has difficulty grasping and proving more than one infectious pathogen can cause the same or different chronic diseases. If the patients with a chronic disease do not all show the same infectious pathogen, it can only be called an "association". Relying on the safety of reporting it as an "association" avoids the constraints of the scientific method and fear of criticism from stating a definitive cause, and later having others report a different pathogen causes the same disease. Sir William Osler stated, "In seeking absolute truth, we aim at the unattainable, and must be content with broken portions." So far, we have the broken portions of a whole in medicine, which needs to be put back into a cohesive whole.

In 2005, Barry Marshall, MD, won a Nobel Prize for proving what Dr. Merchant had been saying for decades: Ulcers are a bacterial infection that can be cured with antibiotics. Dr. Marshall proved the spiral curved bacteria H-pylori was the cause of ulcers, by infecting himself with H-pylori, then treating himself with clarithromycin and bismuth salts, to cure his ulcer. Dr. Marshall first published his findings ulcers were caused by an H-pylori infection, in 1983; and again, in 1987. Dr. Marshall said, in 1988, "(e)veryone was against me, but I knew I was right." The National Enquirer reported on Dr. Marshall's discovery, on March 13, 1990, which informed the public ulcers were caused by an infection; and thereafter treatment of ulcers as an infection became the standard.

We recently bought <u>Rheumatoid Diseases: Cured at Last</u>, describing the story of Jack M. Blount, MD, a doctor trained in Mississippi and at George

Washington University.[23] Dr. Blount became afflicted with crippling rheumatoid arthritis, while in medical school. He believed an intestinal parasite, the limax amoeba, caused rheumatoid arthritis; and after curing himself with antibiotics, he began treating rheumatoid arthritis patients with broad spectrum antibiotics and antiparasitic medication, for six to seven weeks. He reported more than three-hundred species of pathogenic amoeba could be treated with available and inexpensive antiparasitic medication. He reported his belief many chronic diseases were caused by the limax amoeba, including some forms of cancer.

Dr. di Fabio cited many older articles, back to the 1950's, in support of infectious causes of chronic disease. He cited Dr. Roger Wyburn-Mason's discovery, in 1920, showing the limax amoeba was found in the human tissue in *all* cases of collagen and autoimmune diseases, and in *all* cases of leukemia and lymphoma. Professor Roger Wyburn-Mason's research was summarized, in 1976-1977, and published in "The Causation of Rheumatoid Disease and Many Human Cancers".[24]

Dr. Blount spoke out about the infectious cause of rheumatoid arthritis, and the potential for a treatment and cure. The medical community responded by calling him before the Medical Board, and threatening revocation of his license. His medical license was suspended; and he only regained his license after agreeing not to discuss his beliefs, not to act on his beliefs, and to practice only within the agreement to ignore infectious causes of rheumatoid arthritis. The Medical Board thereafter sent a fake patient seeking help for rheumatoid arthritis, in an effort to entrap Dr. Blount, and prove he was violating the agreement. Dr. Blount was called back to the Medical Board for violation of the agreement; and ultimately prevailed. Dr. Blount did not hide behind the absence of scientific studies, when he knew he was right; and he was persecuted for his outspoken opinions, and attempts to improve the lives of his patients. Dr. Blount, like

---

[23] Di Fabio A. 1982. <u>Rheumatoid Diseases: Cured at Last</u>. 4th ed. Franklin, TN: The Rheumatoid Disease Foundation.

[24] Wyburn-Mason R. 1983. The Causation of Rheumatoid Disease and Many Human Cancers. Fairview, TN: Arthritis Trust of America/Rheumatoid Disease Foundation.

Dr. Merchant, focused on treating the patient and observing the success of treatment.

Dr. Blount went on to establish the Roger Wyburn-Mason and Jack M. Blount Foundation for Eradication of Rheumatoid Disease. Dr. Blount claimed success in treating more than sixteen thousand patients suffering from rheumatoid arthritis. He and others at the foundation came to the conclusion that over one-hundred differently named collagen tissue diseases, including rheumatoid arthritis, scleroderma, psoriasis and many other diseases, were all caused by infection with the limax amoeba.

In 2017, Dr. di Fabio published a new edition of <u>Rheumatoid Diseases: Cured at Last</u>, which expanded upon Dr. Blount's theory the limax amoeba caused rheumatoid arthritis and other chronic diseases.[25] Dr. di Fabio reported infection is the root cause of many chronic diseases, as Dr. Merchant has said for decades. The 2017 edition of <u>Rheumatoid Diseases: Cured at Last</u> acknowledged many different infectious pathogens can cause a variety of chronic disease. Dr. di Fabio reported various infections with bacteria, viroid's, parasites, fungus and even prions (stripped down viruses now known by various names, all describing an abnormal protein) were the cause of rheumatoid arthritis and other chronic diseases. He reported symptoms classifications are not descriptions of primary causes! He said, "Symptomatic treatment of arthritis never cured a patient" and the front-line practice of medicine was disconnected from research. He argued medicine today was out of touch with the needs of patients. Dr. Blount initially focused on one specific amoeba, to the exclusion of other pathogens. However, antiparasitic medications treat many types of parasites and intestinal pathogens, chlamydia trachoma, and chlamydia psittacosis. Treatment of rheumatoid arthritis as a parasitic infection, with antiparasitic medications, would treat parasites and a variety of chlamydia pathogens capable of causing arthritis.

Dr. Merchant said arthritis was a chronic infection long before reading about Dr. Blount's experience. He had successfully treated a teenager

---

[25] Di Fabio A. 2017. <u>Rheumatoid Diseases Cured at Last</u>. Franklin, TN: The Arthritis Trust of America.

with juvenile rheumatoid arthritis, by treating immortal infections with macrolides and gamma globulin. Dr. Merchant had discussed his belief arthritis was caused by infection, with a rheumatologist in Albuquerque. The rheumatologist had independently come to the same conclusion, and had compiled his own research and evidence of infectious causes of arthritis. The rheumatologist had remained silent about treating arthritis as an infection; because his beliefs were not welcome and not appreciated by the medical community or his employer.

In 2005, the UNMH Department of Community Health obtained a grant to study chronic diseases on the Navajo Reservation. We collected our references and resources, and made a sincere and honest presentation to the head of the Department of Community Health about infections causing chronic diseases, suggesting how the grant could be used to find the infectious causes of chronic disease on the Navajo Reservation. The chairman rolled his eyes and ignored everything we said. He refused to consider the scientific literature or evidence. He wasted the grant money on issues of no long-term benefit to the Navajo people, and which gave no insight into the infectious causes of chronic disease on the Navajo Reservation. It was a discouraging experience, and again made clear we had to write a book to explain what we believe to be true about infectious causes of chronic disease.

In 2007, Dr. Merchant gave a talk on chlamydia as the cause of chronic disease, to a group of naturopathic doctors. Naturopaths focus on alternative medicine and nutrition. In his talk, Dr. Merchant said chlamydia species caused asthma, heart disease, coronary artery disease, arthrosclerosis, arthritis, and fibromyalgia. The naturopaths listened, were open-minded, began to apply the knowledge, and began to use Dr. Merchant as a resource for consultation and referrals.

In 2017, I Contain Multitudes, the Microbes Within Us and a Grander View of Life described the bacteria within us that make us who we are.[26] The microbiome is a delicate balance, in which good bacteria

---

[26] Jong E. 2016. I Contain Multitudes, The Microbes Within Us and a Grander View of Life. 1st ed. Harper Collins.

perform valuable functions, in cooperation with other good bacteria and good fungus. Good fungus creates a scaffolding for good bacteria to accomplish digestive functions, and good bacteria and good fungus live in peaceful co-existence. Bacteria, viruses, and fungi, work in cooperating communities, to accomplish necessary body functions. Some bacteria and groups of bacteria cooperate in the fight against pathogens. Science has not identified all the good bacteria; and is just beginning to know how good bacteria and fungus, and bad bacteria and fungus, work in cooperating cultures. Only a fraction of the good bacteria has been identified and described, and some of the most important good bacteria have not yet been replicated in a laboratory; thus, cannot be provided in any supplement. In the United States, the diversity of the microbiome has been steadily decreasing. I Contain Multitudes supports Dr. Merchant's longstanding practice of recommending probiotics, for promotion of health.

Our thoughts on chronic disease began long before the Internet, but after Internet we were able to more easily research and confirm our beliefs, and buy new books on the topic. We were able to rapidly check medical literature across every specialty; and verify and validate our belief as observational science drew our attention to new issues. Every insight was researched to compare with what was known. Today, scientists have reported a study on almost everything, but few conclusions as to the causes of anything. The studies report associations and provide discussions of the study, but rarely conclude by giving a cause or suggesting new treatments.

Books and conferences have discussed infection and chronic disease for a century, with a significant acceleration in publications, since 2000. World conferences have been held on infectious causes of chronic disease, and the findings and conclusions do not reach beyond the conference to medical practice. Anecdotal evidence has been growing that treating a variety of chronic diseases with specific antibiotics improves chronic diseases. Yet, the knowledge of infectious causes of chronic disease does not seem to move beyond the academic and esoteric, from research to practice, or from talk into action, to benefit patients.

Dr. Merchant is a medical visionary, with a desire to think beyond what is known. He was right in saying the water-borne parasites were causing an epidemic of chronic disease. He was right saying ulcers were an infection, and treating ulcers with antibiotics. He was right to say irritable bowel syndrome was not a diagnosis; and irritable bowel syndrome is an infection that responds to treatment with antibiotics and antiparasitics, and probiotics and prebiotics. He was right to say parasites and low folic acid were causing higher rates of cancer, in younger patients. He was right to say Alzheimer's is a chronic immortal infection, before others discovered chlamydia pneumonia under and adjacent to Alzheimer's lesions and plaque. He treated multiple sclerosis as an infection and saw the disease improve, before others reported chlamydia infection was found in the spinal fluid of patients with multiple sclerosis. He treated rheumatoid arthritis as an infection, before others proved it was caused by chlamydia pneumonia and byproducts of chronic infection. He was right in saying not to give penicillin to acute chlamydia pneumonia, because penicillin can cause conversion of the infection into asthma, and worsen lung function.

Dr. Merchant had the courage to put his visionary ideas into practice, in the face of criticism; and was willing to implement what science already knew into practice. With each new patient, the theory was challenged; and over and over again, the theory proved true. He tested his beliefs thousands of times as he questioned himself. He observed, listened, examined, and performed blood and urine tests to document immortal infections. He had the courage to think, find new ways to treat patients with chronic diseases based on science and reasoning, and the courage to do what was right to help his patients. He was never able to disprove his beliefs; and to the contrary, decades of medical practice and observation confirmed his beliefs that chronic infection causes chronic disease. He watched chronic diseases and co-morbid conditions improve, by treating immortal infections and parasites. He has been a voice crying out in the wilderness, for decades.

> *The very first step towards success in any occupation is to become interested in it…The best preparation for tomorrow is to do today's work superbly well…There is no more difficult*

art to acquire than the art of observation…For some men, it is quite as difficult to record an observation in any brief and plain language…Observe, record, tabulate, and communicate…Use your five senses. Learn to see. Learn to hear. Learn to feel. Learn to smell…Know by practice alone you can become an expert.

Sir William Osler, English physician, 1849-1919.

CHAPTER 3

OBSERVATIONAL SCIENCE FUELED REBELLION

Aristotle is recognized as the inventor of the scientific method. The scientific method is an empirical method of knowledge acquisition, used for forming hypothesis and coming to scientific conclusions. The scientific method includes careful observation, rigorous skepticism about what is observed, and avoiding cognitive assumptions about how the world works that can influence how one interprets a percept. The scientific method involves formulation of hypothesis by induction, based on observations; experimental testing and measurement of deductions drawn from the hypothesis; and refinement or elimination of hypotheses based on experimental findings. When a particular hypothesis becomes very well supported, a general theory may be developed.[27]

Observational science goes back to Galileo, and is the subject of renewed interest and advocacy in medicine. Dr. Elazer R. Edelman, a cardiologist and Director of the Harvard-MIT Biomedical Engineering Center, spoke to the World Congress on Animal Models in Drug Discovery and Development, on September 27, 2017, on the topic of the roots of "Reverse Translational Medicine". Dr. Edelman defined "Reverse Translational Medicine" as scientific discovery by observing what works in practice, in other words, scientific understanding arising from experience and observation in medical practice. He reported the rise of research on the basis of observed clinical issues; and emphasized the importance of scientific advocacy. He viewed clinical challenges as an opportunity to harness science and technology. He urged scientists to be better at admitting what

---

[27] Wikipedia. Scientific Method. Doi: en.wikipedia.org/wiki/Scientific_method.

they know and what they don't, referring to his own personal motto, "Priam sciere", or "Above all, seek to understand."

Medicine no longer closely adheres to the scientific method; and the importance of observation, experience, rigid skepticism, and avoidance of assumption has faded. Careful observation has given way to looking at computer screens and a fascination with data, technology, and testing. Rigorous skepticism has been abandoned in favor of compliance with what they were taught; and obtaining information from drug companies who have manipulated studies and have secondary gain. Formulating hypothesis by inductive reasoning, has been replaced with narrow hypothesis, and deductions influenced by cognitive assumptions about medicine and the world. Refinement or elimination of hypothesis has been impaired by the limitations of the studies, failure to observe objectively, and reliance on those conducting biased studies and with secondary gain. Research searches infinite small details, hoping an answer will be revealed.

Scientific law is a body of knowledge, which describes what phenomenon occur. Scientific theory explains why phenomenon occur. The scientific law and scientific theory are circles of knowledge that overlap, and in the center of the overlap of theory and law is repeated successful predictions. Hypotheses lead to predictions which can be tested, to develop a general theory. [28]

We propose a general theory, based on known science, known constructs, scientific law, observation, experience; and based on repeated predictions confirmed by successful outcomes, in chronic disease. We propose a scientific theory that explains the cause of chronic disease in a unified whole, and provides is a new construct for medical practice and diagnosis, to benefit patients.

---

[28] Wikipedia. Scientific Method. Doi: en.wikipedia.org/wiki/Scientific_method.

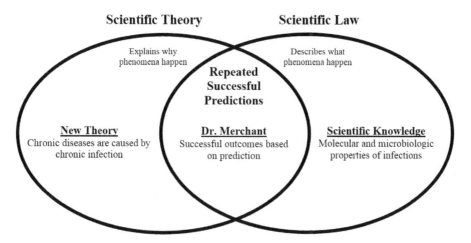

Scientific Theory   **Scientific Law**

Explains why
phenomena happen

**Repeated
Successful
Predictions**

Describes what
phenomena happen

New Theory
Chronic diseases are caused by
chronic infection

Dr. Merchant
Successful outcomes based
on prediction

Scientific Knowledge
Molecular and microbiologic
properties of infections

SCIENTIFIC THEORY DIAGRAM

We engaged in Reverse Translational Medicine and observational science, for four decades. We approached medical knowledge with rigid skepticism. We abandoned bias and sought to understand. We tried to prove ourselves wrong, testing the theory of chronic disease over and over, and could not. We observed unnecessary suffering due to a lack of understanding, in friends, family, acquaintances, and the public domain. At the same, we observed Dr. Merchant's experience and successes, in treating chronic diseases with the understanding chronic disease is caused by chronic infections. The observation of unnecessary suffering fueled our desire to engage in scientific advocacy, and set forth a new vision in chronic disease.

A Dateline television show was devoted to a family with five children, all five of whom had cardiomyopathy. The oldest child was sixteen, had been subjected to medical procedures, heart surgeries, and a heart transplant; and was being considered for a second heart transplant. The second oldest child was waiting for her first heart transplant. The three younger children had also been diagnosed with the same heart condition. Neither parent had heart disease; yet, the heart surgeons and family assumed the heart condition, in all five children, was genetic. The children were subjected to life-altering surgeries and the terror of doing what the doctor said or die, most of their life; and each sibling saw their future, in the suffering of the older siblings. No one considered infection and re-infection within the family had caused the children's heart disease, and failure of the oldest child's first heart transplant. The medical system spent millions on each of these children, and no one investigated pathogens known to cause heart disease and/or cardiomyopathy.

The more likely explanation for the children's heart disease was disclosed when Dateline cut to commercials. Each time, the father was galloping on his horse on their farm, in rural America. In less than five minutes, research on cardiomyopathy revealed a type of chlamydia common in horses, chlamydia psittacosis, can cause heart disease and cardiomyopathy— the same chronic disease in these five children. Chlamydia pneumonia, a community acquired infection, can also cause cardiomyopathy. Mice are common on farms, and carry and transmit forms of chlamydia known to cause cardiomyopathy, endocarditis, myocarditis, and dilated cardiomyopathy. The children may have had a genetic predisposition, but more likely the infections from animals, in the family, and in the community triggered their heart disease.

The parents of the five children reported they had "the best doctors in the country". The surgeons assumed nothing could be done to save the children but more heart surgeries—because they were surgeons. The best cardiac surgeons in the country are not well-versed in infectious causes of heart disease, or knowledgeable or interested in the medical management of heart disease. The cardiac surgeons were not knowledgeable about pathogens in horses, mice or other farm animals, known to cause the same heart disease these children had; or the children's past exposure to these pathogens. The surgeons had not considered transmission of animal pathogens known to cause cardiomyopathy, passed from person-to-person or child-to-child within the family, or animal-to-child. The surgeon did not consider re-infection may have caused failure of the oldest child's heart transplant. No one attempted to diagnose and treat pathogens known to cause cardiomyopathy, to which the children were likely exposed.

Television is inundated with commercials advertising cancer treatment. The actors in the commercials, who allegedly have cancer, are kissing a dog, or petting the dog while sitting on furniture with the dog. Dogs transmit immortal infections and parasites, back and forth between dog and owner, which over time can cause cancer. Animal pathogens causing chronic disease in humans are not always symptomatic in animals. Cancer is not contagious, but the infections that cause cancer are contagious. Caregivers and spouses of cancer patients have an increased risk of cancer, because caretakers can become infected with the same pathogens that infected the cancer patient.

Years ago, we saw a television commercial for an expensive new TNF-inhibitor to treat disabling arthritis, showing the female actress kissing a bird! Kissing a bird can transmit immortal infections, particularly chlamydia psittacosis. It was ludicrous for the actress in the commercial to be kissing a bird, because kissing a bird exposes a person to the pathogen that causes arthritis. A patient with disabling rheumatoid arthritis, came to Dr. Merchant too weak to walk, on 120 mg. of prednisone a day. She had been told nothing else could be done, and she was dying. After careful tapering and discontinuation of the steroids, and treatment of infections, the patient stabilized, on intermittent azithromycin. Dr. Merchant saw many other patients with reactive arthritis who improved with treatment of immortal infections.

A caretaker, spouse or family member can have the same pathogens and develop a different manifestation of chronic disease. Maria Menounos revealed she had a golf ball size meningioma (cancer) in her brain, after she had cared for her mother with stage four brain cancer; and now her seventeen-year old dog has the same type of brain cancer. Phil Mickelson disclosed he has psoriatic arthritis, which he developed at approximately the same time or shortly after his wife was diagnosed with breast cancer. Both arthritis and cancer can be caused by immortal pathogens, which can be acquired through close contact with family members, in the community, traveling, or on a golf course. The infections caused or triggered the same or a different manifestation of chronic disease, in the caretaker, family member, and pet.

Two teenage boys were friends and lived next door to each other, in the South Valley; and both drank contaminated well water. Both boys developed bone cancer, at the same time. The chance of two teenage boys who are friends, on the same street, getting the same bone cancer, at the same time, was extremely remote. One boy took a water sample when he went to a cancer center on the West Coast, and was told the water was so bad he should not even bathe in the water. The teenage boys had chronic parasitic disease from drinking contaminated water, which depleted folic acid and triggered cancer; and chronic infection. These two boys with bone cancer were one of the early motivators for Dr. Merchant to become more aggressive in speaking out about the danger of contaminated well water, in the South Valley. The two boys contributed to his belief patients in the South Valley were getting more cancers, at a younger age; and low folic acid and B12 from chronic parasitic infection was a trigger for cancer.

A Northern New Mexico town seemed to have a high concentration of gastrointestinal disease. Northern New Mexico had issues related to contaminated water for generations, and at one time giardia was found in a community water system. (The water system was later upgraded.) Mountain communities often have water contamination issues, because animals have open access to mountain streams and lakes; and the people drink well water and use septic tanks. The area had a constellation of risk factors for gastrointestinal disease, which is represented by the 'WOAs'— contaminated water, outdoor activities, and animals. The doctors in the community failed to diagnose infectious pathogens and parasites, and treated the gastrointestinal complaints symptomatically, causing a proliferation of gastrointestinal disease; worsening morbidity; bowel surgeries to remove infected portions of the bowel; and even death.

A young woman was the subject of a newspaper article, disclosing she suffered from disabling Crohn's disease. After being subjected to expensive and harmful TNF-inhibitors, at a cost of $14,000 per treatment, she planned to go out-of-state to have part of her intestine surgically removed. Surgery can temporarily reduce symptoms of Crohn's and surgeons may need to remove parts of the bowel damaged beyond repair; but ordinarily the symptoms of Crohn's return after surgery. The infections are not treated, and the infection returns but now with a part of the bowel removed. None of her doctors tried to diagnose and treat intracellular infections or parasites. Dr. Merchant treated a thirty-eight-year-old patient with Crohn's disease, who had previously seen a gastroenterologist in New York, and presented with significant weight loss and diarrhea. After aggressive treatment over the course of two and a half years, with macrolides, antiparasitics, and antifungal medications, his disease went into remission.

The death of Beau Biden from brain cancer was tragic; and painful to watch. He was a healthy and vibrant young man, until he was deployed to Iraq for a year. When he returned, he developed an unexplained seizure disorder. Within two years, he was diagnosed with glioblastoma, a type of brain cancer. Shortly after his death, an article in the New York Times reported an abnormal protein was at the center of *all* gliomas, causing brain tissue to stick together.[29] Chronic infections alter normal proteins, and generate abnormal proteins that are sticky and malformed. The abnormal proteins spread to the brain, through the blood and lymphatics; and in time cause cancer where the abnormal proteins cause the glial cells to stick together. Parasitic infections are also capable of migrating or metastasizing to the brain, causing sticky tissue and creating a focus for epilepsy and/or cancer. By history, Beau Biden likely acquired an immortal pathogen or parasite while deployed in the Middle East, which caused a chronic infection. Beau Biden's seizures prior to the diagnosis of brain cancer were an early manifestation of the cancer, caused by brain cells sticking together; and the immune battle against pathogens and abnormal sticky proteins, which became the focus for brain cancer.

An acquaintance developed leukemia, after a severe respiratory infection and travelling over the holidays. During the travel, he may have been exposed to a second infection, such as whooping cough, mycoplasma, influenza, or another form of chlamydia. The pathogens likely infected his immune cells; and the combination of co-infections overwhelmed the immune system's ability to fight the infections, causing a rapid proliferation of white blood cells. He had a history of benzene exposure, a known environmental hazard with a risk for cancer. He was diagnosed

---

[29] Kolata G. 2015. Brain Cancers Reveal Novel Genetic Disruption in DNA. New York Times (Health). Dec. 23, 2015. Doi: https://www.nytimes.com/2015/12/24/health/brain-cancers-reveal-novel-genetic-disruption-in-dna.html.

with acute leukemia. He chose treatment with chemotherapy and a bone-marrow transplant, and survived; but suffered ill effects from the disease and treatment.

Around the same time another acquaintance, who was about the same age and worked in the automotive field, developed leukemia. His ex-wife told him to take Tequin before chemotherapy and before his bone marrow transplant. At that time, Tequin was the only antibiotic on the market, which could penetrate bone and attack infection inside the bone marrow. The patient did so well his cancer doctors could not understand why he did so well, better than expected, and better than other leukemia patients. He is still alive, doing well, without any significant ill effects, and required little additional treatment.

Ellen DeGeneres had a teenager on her show, who was completely blind. He was sighted at birth, and at age six or seven he started losing his sight. When he began losing his sight, the doctors gave no hope to save his vision. The teenager did not know why he lost his sight, and the doctors were never able to provide an answer. Research showed he had the classic picture of a child who acquired cytomegaly virus (CMV) *in utero*. CMV can destroy eyesight or hearing when acquired *in utero*, and the signs of vision loss or hearing loss begin to develop six or seven years after birth. Toxoplasmosis acquired *in utero* could also explain his blindness, because toxoplasmosis acquired *in utero* can also manifest as sight loss, years after the birth.

A software developer publicly reported his two-year old daughter lost her hearing, and was progressing to blindness. He developed a software program to introduce Braille to his daughter, while she could still see. The doctors thought the child had a form of progressive retinitis pigmentosa. CMV and toxoplasmosis can infect a fetus and cause blindness, years after a child is born; and H-pylori can attack the retina and cause loss of vision, similar to the presentation of retinitis pigmentosa. No diagnosis of pathogens or treatment was offered, and the father was never told why his child lost her hearing or was going blind.

An acquaintance had glaucoma and retinal degeneration. Many years before she had taken in a stray cat. She had co-morbid conditions, including rosacea, thyroid disease, and gastrointestinal disease. No one attempted to diagnose and treat immortal pathogens or parasites, which could potentially cause glaucoma or retinal degeneration. An astute ophthalmologist treated her with doxycycline, for her "ocular rosacea", which delayed the progression of her glaucoma and her vision loss. Her glaucoma specialist was astonished at how much the doxycycline helped her glaucoma, and praised the ophthalmologist who prescribed the doxycycline as brilliant.

Two small communities seemed to have clusters of trachoma. Trachoma has a predilection to attack reproductive tissue and ocular tissue. In one community the pathogen attacked reproductive tissue and in the other attacked ocular tissue. Trachoma can be sexually transmitted, transmitted by the Musca Sorbens fly, or transmitted to the eyes by self-inoculation. Trachoma in the reproductive tract can infect the urinary tract, and cause "interstitial cystitis", another description of a symptom meaning the urinary tract is inflamed. One surgeon in the community removed a patient's bladder, for "interstitial cystitis", without considering trachoma, even though the patient had been diagnosed with trachoma a decade earlier and had never properly been treated. When doctors fail to diagnose and adequately treat immortal infection, the pathogen can spread in the patient and in the community, and morbidity and mortality increases.

A second small community seemed to have a higher than expected rate of ocular trachoma. The small community was near another isolated community, which had open sewer pits and farm animals that attracted flies. The small community was infested with flies in the summer. The Musca Sorbens fly migrates across the Southwest each summer, and feeds on ocular trachoma, then transmits ocular trachoma to the next person. A picture of the child in Africa with a face covered with flies is pathognomonic of ocular trachoma. Flies know no city or state boundary, and when ocular trachoma is in the geographic area, flies can spread ocular trachoma in the community and to nearby communities. When doctors fail to diagnose ocular trachoma, it becomes more widespread in the community; with greater opportunity for transmission and morbidity.

A third small community appeared to have a higher than expected rate of retinal detachments. The rate of retinal surgeons nationally is about one per one hundred thousand people. In one county, with a population of one-hundred-twenty thousand, four to five retinal surgeons serve the county, in two locations providing eye surgery. Pathogens that attack the retina may be spread within the community, and cause retinal disease and retinal detachments; or the community may be engaging in activities, such as swimming in a river, that exposes them to pathogens that attack the retina. Ophthalmologists identify retinal detachments and perform surgery to repair retinas. Ophthalmologists do not look for infections in the community causing a high rate of retinal detachments; or consider why the community has an unusually high need for retinal surgeons.

Many celebrities publicly discuss fertility problems; and their fertility treatments. Chlamydia trachoma, chlamydia abortus, and chlamydia *suis*, can all cause infertility and miscarriages. Toxoplasmosis from cats can cause miscarriages and congenital toxoplasmosis in the fetus. Fertility specialists do not investigate immortal pathogens in the mother; take a history of contact with animals; or consider chronic infection as the cause of infertility. A daughter of an acquaintance tried for ten years to get pregnant. She was deployed overseas in the military, and while overseas got an acute respiratory infection. The doctors gave her an antibiotic for her respiratory illness that incidentally also treated the immortal infection causing infertility. Shortly thereafter, she had an unexpected surprise, she got pregnant and had a normal, full-term baby.

Looking back at Elvis Presley, Michael Jackson, and Prince, they all likely had immortal infections from their lifestyle and frequent travel; and tragically suffered and died from undiagnosed infections and doctors who prescribed pain and sleeping medications instead of investigating to find a medical diagnosis. Elvis Presley died of heart disease, aggravated by chronic use of pain medication and sedatives. Michael Jackson developed vitiligo after a tour in Africa as a child, most likely from a fungus or unusual pathogen acquired in Africa. Michael Jackson also had a menagerie of animals and had a monkey for a pet, which added to his risk for multiple chronic infections and unusual infections. He suffered chronic pain and inability to sleep, common in chronic infection and chronic disease; and he took pain medication and required sedation to sleep that caused his death. Prince died of an accidental overdose of pain medication, after he was prescribed pain medications for joint degeneration and intractable pain. All of the celebrities had personal physicians willing to give pain medications as a palliative measure, *in lieu* of diagnosis and treatment of the root causes of their pain.

We observed absurd medical costs, because doctors fail to understand that infectious pathogens cause chronic disease. Dr. Merchant saw patients who had spent countless thousands of dollars on medical care, without ever getting a diagnosis or treatment of infections. He saw one patient who had spent more than $1,000,000 on medical care, and had seen specialists around the country, including infectious disease specialists; and no one could explain the symptoms. On the first visit, Dr. Merchant diagnosed two immortal infections and a chronic urine infection, which had not been diagnosed or treated by her infectious disease specialists or primary care doctors.

While helplessly observing tragic story after tragic story of unnecessary suffering, among family, friends, acquaintances, and in the public domain, including many more stories than described, we observed Dr. Merchant's successes in treating chronic disease. He had the courage to diagnose and treat the patients; and has decades of experience observing the success of treatment, by diagnosing and treating infectious pathogens causing the chronic disease. The successes of treatment confirmed to him infectious pathogens were causing chronic disease.

Dr. Merchant treated a patient with cardiomegaly who had completely clogged arteries, with clarithromycin, and saw the disease improve. The patient lived four more years, with quality of life. He treated a patient with transient ischemic episodes and antiphospholipid syndrome, with clarithromycin, and the transient ischemic episodes completely resolved.

The heart conditions improved, contrary to reported studies of the hopelessness of cardiomegaly, ischemic heart disease, and transient ischemic attacks.

He treated a leukemia patient with a potent fluoroquinolone, antifungal therapy, intravenous vitamin C, and diet, and her leukemia resolved. He treated a seventy-year-old smoker with end stage lung disease, who was told he had less than a year to live, by treating multiple forms of chlamydia, and the patient is still alive four years later. He treated a female with asthma, with intermittent macrolides; and she improved to the point of no lung or heart limitations during exercise.

Dr. Merchant treated patients with Alzheimer's with macrolides, and saw the symptoms stabilize and improve. One Alzheimer's patient lived an additional five years, after being put on hospice, with high cognitive function until the end of life. He treated a patient with Parkinson's disease and neuromuscular changes with a macrolide, for six years, and many of the Parkinson's disease symptoms improved.

Dr. Merchant treated a patient with adult onset diabetes, high blood pressure, elevated cholesterol, reactive arthritis, and congestive heart failure, by treating infections, and the patient claimed he felt better than he had in thirteen years. His adult onset diabetes improved, his blood pressure was lower, and he was able to exercise.

He treated a patient with multiple sclerosis for immortal infections, and stopped the progression of multiple sclerosis. He treated a sixty-year old woman diagnosed with systemic lupus and multiple sclerosis, solely with antibiotics and thyroid medications, and she had no significant medical consequences from lupus or multiple sclerosis. He treated a patient with muscular dystrophy and a seizure disorder for chlamydia pneumonia, and the patient's condition resolved, to the point the patient needed only a cane for ambulation and became seizure free. An ALS patient, diagnosed at the Mayo Clinic, was given less than three months to live, and when treated for chlamydia pneumonia, lived four additional years before dying of leukemia in another state.

A young woman was waking-up blind in one eye, then the other eye. Each time, she was hospitalized and given steroids, because the doctors did not know what else to do. She was given a diagnosis of "optic neuritis". Anything referred to as "itis" is not a diagnosis, but rather a description of inflammation—her optic nerve was inflamed. She had two major work-ups at the university hospital, by a neurologist and rheumatologist. Her MRI showed white spots in the brain, and she was rapidly progressing to a diagnosis of multiple sclerosis. She went to Dr. Merchant for a second opinion, and was diagnosed and treated for two chronic infections, over the course of fifteen months. The optic neuritis disappeared, *and* the white spots on her MRI disappeared! Her ophthalmologist and neurologist were shocked to see her recovery, and did not understand how the optic neuritis and white spots on MRI could have disappeared. Yet, neither her ophthalmologist nor her neurologist contacted Dr. Merchant to ask what he had done to cure the patient of an incurable disease; or how he made white spots, which are typical of multiple sclerosis, disappear on an MRI.

A thirty-five-year-old acquaintance was told she had retinitis pigmentosa and would be blind within five years. When she first saw Dr. Merchant, she had difficulty seeing in a dimly lit room, was limited in her ability to drive, and could not drive at night. Dr. Merchant tested her for immortal pathogens, and she was diagnosed with H-pylori and psittacosis. When asked about contact with birds or pigeons, she said her family ate pigeons when she was young, when the family was poor and hungry. Psittacosis is well known to attack the eye, and is associated with eye cancer in people and birds. H-pylori can attack the retinal epithelium; and H-pylori has been "associated" with "idiopathic central serous chorioretinopathy" (ICSR), a disease very similar to retinitis pigmentosa. "Idiopathic" means the doctor does not know, and it must be something inherently wrong with the patient. Treatment of H-pylori, in ICSR, has been shown to improve the disease and preserve vision. The patient was treated for psittacosis and H-pylori, and her vision improved to the point she can drive without limitation, and was able to return to driving at night. Her contrast sensitivity vision significantly improved. Her friends and family were astonished.

We want to fulfill the obligation of scientific advocacy that is integral to Reverse Translational Medicine and observational science, and return to the bedside to bench approach, with use of older and effective medications. We seek to improve medical care. We hope to benefit patients suffering from chronic disease, or who may develop chronic disease in the future. We hope to generate discussion and encourage a new understanding of chronic disease. We hope to help mankind manage chronic disease, have improved outcomes, prevent chronic disease, and conquer chronic disease.

We feel a strong desire to speak the truth that others deserve to know. We must speak out about the origins of chronic disease, the false cognitive assumptions, and lack of rigid skepticism in the medical system, just as Vincenzo Crespi, IV spoke out against hypocrisy in the Catholic Church; and just as Brittie spoke out against the corrupt military dictatorships, in Panama. We must speak out, as so many of our ancestors have done, for the benefit of others, even if unpopular. We are the next generation who has an obligation to speak out for the good of all. Our time has come.

> *If there is a book that you want to read that has not been written yet, you must be the one to write it.*
>
> Toni Morrison

CHAPTER 4

THE PRINCIPLE OF THE WHOLE—THE ORIGIN OF DISEASE: *The War Within*

But the years of anxious searching in the dark for truth that one feels but cannot express, the intense desire and the alterations of confidence and misgiving until one achieves clarity and understanding, can only be understood by those who have experienced them.

Albert Einstein

Since Hippocrates, physicians have sought a unifying principle in medicine. Hippocrates was the first to report disease was not a curse sent by God—disease had a cause. Hippocrates based his medical practice on observation, documentation, and study of the human body. He documented detailed observations of the symptoms, and different diseases occurring in different seasons. He documented the time course of diseases, the duration of illness, whether the patient relapsed, and the patients' recovery or demise. Many diseases described by Hippocrates can be identified as acute and chronic immortal infections that persist today, by his description of the organ attacked, the duration of illness, whether the patient relapsed, and the outcome of recovery or demise.

Doctors motivated to ease suffering, reduce the burden of disease, and improve the quality of life of patients, have been criticized, ridiculed, and ostracized for expressing new ideas. Hippocrates was criticized for saying diseases had a cause. In 1847, Dr. Ignaz Samelweiss, a Hungarian physician, proposed deaths of infants delivered in the hospital were caused by transmission of germs on the doctors' hands and from dirty sheets. He separated the mothers into a group cared for exclusively by nuns, with antiseptic technique and washed sheets; and a group of mothers who were cared for exclusively by the doctors, who arrogantly dismissed the need for antiseptic technique. Dr. Samelweiss proved sterile technique reduced the death rate of infants in the hospital from thirty percent to slightly over one percent. He was rewarded, by first being denied assistance in caring for his patients, then being fired from the hospital staff and ostracized by the profession. Dr. Koch delivered his discovery of the bacteria causing tuberculosis to an audience who sat in stunned silence. Dr. Rous was ridiculed for his discovery of an infectious cause of cancer in chickens, and his discovery was finally acknowledged fifty years later. Dr. Blount said arthritis was a parasitic infection, and the medical board tried to take his medical license. The fact many doctors have been ridiculed and persecuted, for expressing new ideas has created a chilling effect, preventing doctors from expressing new and unpopular ideas, and interfering with innovation and discovery.

Some argue it is a fool's errand to try to find a unifying principle for chronic disease, which belief arises from cognitive assumptions and biases, and the complexity of thought medicine has imposed on itself. It is a fool's errand to attempt to make sense of chronic disease by dividing medicine into diverse specialties; and divide immortal infection into thousands of symptoms, findings, syndromes, and diseases. It is a fool's errand to continue searching small details, without a purpose and direction, hoping for an answer; treating patients symptomatically without knowing the cause; and ignoring the bigger picture and commonalities in chronic disease across medical specialties. The small details support what we say, but alone cannot provide an answer.

Many scientists and thinkers, over the course of centuries and millennia, from veterinary medicine, to medicine, to Ph.D. scientists, have postulated infectious causes of disease; or reported an "association" between infectious disease and chronic diseases. During the Civil War, tight chest (cardiovascular disease) was thought to be from infection. In 1880, the germ theory of disease was accepted. In 1903, Sir William Osler proposed infection was the cause of atherosclerosis. Inclusion bodies, were first described, in 1907, and cause lumps, bumps and clots common in many chronic diseases. In 1926, T. Howard Plank, MD, suggested numerous chronic diseases were caused by infection, including heart disease, myocarditis, asthma, bursitis, rheumatism, arthritis, chronic sinusitis, rhinitis, diabetes, nephritis, ulcers, colitis, enterocolitis, prostatitis, boils, pimples, and more.[30] Other scientists said heart disease, Alzheimer's, Hashimoto's, cerebral palsy, obesity, chronic fatigue, lupus, and eating disorders have an infectious cause. Even without the ability to identify specific pathogens, scientists have long believed chronic infection could spread throughout the body and cause many different symptoms, and many different chronic diseases, in different patients.

Stanford professor of immunology and microbiology, David A. Relman, said diabetes, sarcoidosis, inflammatory bowel, lupus, Wegner's, cirrhosis, and Kawasaki are all caused by infection. He also said less than half of one percent of bacteria have been identified. Ninety-nine percent of the bacteria in this world may be unknown, and no one knows of nano-particles and nano-bacteria in microfilm layers.

The answer is more likely true, when independent thinkers over centuries have reached the same conclusion. The answer to a complex question is more likely true, when the answer provides a unified principle of the whole, which incorporates known facts, reason and common sense; and leaves no facts outside the principle of the whole. Dr. Merchant's experiences and success diagnosing pathogens and treating patients with chronic disease for immortal pathogens supports the truth of a unified principle of the whole.

Scientific knowledge, reasoning, experience, observations, and common sense support a principle of the whole for chronic disease. Human experience functions on the principle of the whole. We observe the world around us and hear symphonies using a principle of the whole. We learn early in life to make broad generalizations based on limited information, consistent with a principle of the whole. We learn language based on a principle of the whole. An infant told the word dog intuitively knows that means a type of animal, not the name of the breed or the name of the dog.

---

[30] Plank TH. 1926. <u>Actinotherapy and Allied Physical Therapy</u>. Chicago: Manz Corporation.

A unifying principle for chronic disease must exist, because the universe and our body functions on a unified principle of the whole. How could chronic disease be an outlier in the universe, existing without a principle of the whole?

The human body does not act—it reacts and responds to signals, in specific ways. Our body functions as a whole, with feedback loops sending signals to other parts of the body, to react and make necessary adjustments to keep the body in balance, or fight a pathogen. The balance of salt and potassium is maintained by a feedback loop between the endocrine system and kidneys. The professional immune system gets a signal from tissue to go to the location of the infection to fight the pathogens, with a programmed immune response. The endocrine system functions as a unit to allow reproduction. We are one person, the sum of the parts—not just separate parts. Our organs and systems act and react passively together, to sustain life.

Medicine has divided the body, diseases, and specialties; and parsed each body part and disease from one into many, down to the cellular level. Constellations of symptoms and findings were named after the first doctor to describe the symptoms, findings and syndromes, before the medical community had the knowledge and tools to diagnose infectious pathogens. Specialists have given different names to diseases that are symptoms, findings, and syndromes, as various pathogens attack in different ways and symptoms are noticed by specialists, at different points in the infectious cascade.

We need to move beyond studying biochemistry and naming diseases, toward diagnosing the pathogens causing chronic disease. We need to revisit the cause of symptoms, findings, and syndromes, and use cross specialty collaboration to discover causes and cures for chronic disease. The answer to chronic disease cannot be found in one specialty alone, or one pathogen alone—it is found in all specialties together. Medicine must first understand the cause of chronic disease is infectious pathogens, and then understand more than one pathogen can cause the same disease and the same pathogen can cause different diseases.

Research is a sub-specialty of each specialty, and a specialty unto itself. Each research specialty searches for part of the answer, rather than a principle of the whole. Research has become esoteric, consumed by small details, and infected with bias, which prevents important discoveries or important discoveries are overlooked. Research is limited by the desire to find one infectious cause per disease, when more than one pathogen or combinations of pathogens can cause the same disease. If the research results do not prove all patients had the same chronic infection, it becomes an "association" and never a cause. Medical practitioners will not act to diagnose and treat a patient based only on a reported "association". Science looks at small details of cell microbiology and Cluster Differentiations, hoping an answer will reveal itself; and no one is looking at common patterns and current knowledge across specialties and across chronic disease, to find and recognize larger patterns.

In every decade, research into infectious causes of chronic diseases has lagged far behind genetic research. Funding in cancer research has been divided between the genetic cause camp and the infectious cause camp, with significantly less funding dedicated to the infectious causes of cancer. The genetic camp has produced significantly less advancement in identifying the cause of cancer, while the infectious causes of cancer camp had tangible success in identifying causes of cancer. The percent of cancer thought to be from infectious causes steadily rose, from less than one percent, then three percent, then ten percent, then twenty percent. Today, some propose only five to twenty percent of cancer is *not* from an infectious cause. <u>Plague Time: The Germ Theory of Disease</u>. Fearing or ignoring the truth that infectious pathogens cause chronic disease does not change the truth. Fear and bias against infectious causes only diverts attention away from meaningful solutions.

Medicine lives in prison of complicated thought, which interferes with understanding and discovery of answers to broader questions. The medical community has been unable to recognize and accept intracellular animal pathogens cause chronic disease in humans. Medicine must re-unite its fragmented parts, now separated by specialty, body part, and disease. The medical community is not organized in a way that allows seeing the big picture; or refuses, or rejects the knowledge—chlamydia, in its many forms, and parasites, cause chronic disease in humans. Patterns in chronic disease supporting a principle of the whole cannot be seen by one medical specialty alone—it is found looking at all specialties together.

Medicine must diagnose and treat the root infectious causes of chronic disease, and not just give a meaningless name to a disease, symptom or syndrome, then treat the patient symptomatically. Medicine must gain a new appreciation for co-morbid conditions, which may be caused by the same immortal pathogens as the presenting chronic disease.

It is time to abandon cognitive bias, assumptions, associations, symptoms and syndromes. The same pathogens are reported to be "associated" with chronic diseases over and over, in various specialties and sub-specialties; yet, no one seems to be willing to say chronic infection with an immortal pathogen is the "cause" of anything. "Associations" are empirical observations, not scientific fact. It is time to deduce the answer to causes of chronic disease from experience, observation, known science, reasoned logic, diagnosis of immortal pathogens, outcomes from treatment, and repeated scientific studies finding the same association. It is time to move medicine beyond research, academic conferences, and publications; to implementation of what we know. It is time to replace "associations" with a finding of actual causes. It is time to take an accepted body of knowledge and develop a general theory of causation for chronic disease.

Chronic disease is caused by chronic infection with immortal intracellular pathogens and parasites that crossed over from animals, and the ongoing war between the immune system and the immortal pathogens. The more immortal infections a person has, and the longer the infections persisted, the more likely the person will have chronic disease. We acquire good and bad bacteria, from gestation to death—through the placenta, in the birth canal, and throughout life. We are conceived, we get infected, we wage an internal war between the immune system and the pathogens, we get chronic disease, and we die.

Chlamydia species are the only pathogens capable of becoming intracellular, consuming ATP, causing fermentation, causing angiogenesis, generating inflammation, generating TNF-alpha, infecting immune cells, causing reduced immunity by invading the professional immune cells, causing loss of normal apoptosis, and becoming immortal. The cellular effects of chlamydia reflect the molecular cellular findings in many chronic diseases. We focus our discussion on chlamydia pathogens, as the most important and under-recognized pathogens causing chronic disease; the most common co-infections in chronic disease; and the most common cause of diseases of unknown origin, to explain a principle of the whole in chronic disease.

Other known and unknown pathogens can cause chronic disease by the same processes that occur with chlamydia. Knowledge chronic infection with immortal pathogens causes chronic disease, and understanding the infectious cascade starts with acute infection and becomes a chronic disease, can transform the chaotic quest to name a symptom, finding, or syndrome, into a search for the pathogens causing the chronic disease. When doctors approach the diagnosis of chronic disease as a search for immortal pathogens; and begin to routinely diagnose infectious pathogens, medicine will begin to understand the infectious causes of chronic diseases and move toward solutions. Science can begin to repurpose drugs we already have; to find new solutions to prevent, interrupt and reverse the process of chronic disease.

Chlamydia species are immortal, intracellular, parasitic bacteria that crossed over from animals-to-humans. Chlamydia species are microscopic organisms that live inside a host cell, and replicate inside the cell. Chlamydia species exist in two forms, the elementary body and the reticulate body. The elementary body is the infectious form, which has a rigid outer membrane that binds to host cells. When chlamydia invades a host cell and becomes intracellular, it becomes a reticulate body, and it is protected from the immune system by the host cell wall. The reticulate body is the non-infectious form of chlamydia, which is metabolically active and replicates by division. When the reticulate body replicates, it creates new elementary bodies, which are released from the host cell into the body, to infect new host cells. When the host cell dies, the infectious form is released to spread within the body. The chlamydia bacteria can proliferate and infect new host cells within hours. When penicillin is used to treat chlamydia, penicillin destroys the cell wall but not the pathogen. Penicillin causes the reticulate body to change shape and become larger, make more elementary bodies, and extends the life cycle of chlamydia from thirty hours to seventy-two hours.

Chlamydia species can cause the same disease in different people, or different diseases in different people, depending on the predilection of each pathogen, the patient's predisposition, time, co-infections and triggering events. Different combinations of immortal pathogens can cause the same diseases in different people, or different diseases in different people. The attack on particular tissue and organs and the chronic disease caused by the pathogens may depend on the person's unique genetic make-up, weak links, time the pathogen persisted, loss of key nutrition, co-infection, environmental triggers, and prior medical treatment.

A huge diversity and wide distribution of chlamydia species are found in nature. Chlamydia has been recovered from one-thousand years old sludge. Chlamydia strains have been activated from the sludge of acanthamoeba species, supporting chlamydia can be a parasite of acanthamoeba. Ancient chlamydia may have been part of a host, and spread to soil through fecal contamination from birds and animals. Chlamydia pneumonia grew in a culture, after being recovered from a human brain at autopsy. Some species of chlamydia, such as trachoma and psittacosis, have been known for many decades. Research emerged, in the 1970's, identifying more species of chlamydia; and chlamydia pneumonia was identified as a separate species, in 1988.

Animals have been domesticated for 10,000 years. Close contact between humans and animals allowed new animal pathogens to enter the human microbiome. Our microbiome contains ancient viral DNA embedded in our DNA, which is not understood. The fragments of DNA may be evidence of immortal chlamydia pathogens, from ancient times, similar to debris generated by chronic chlamydia infections. In ancient Egypt, the aristocracy owned pets; and scientists found significant atherosclerosis in mummies, suggesting chronic chlamydia pneumonia infection.

Chlamydia pathogens are a family of intracellular pathogens, and each chlamydia species is associated with a particular species of animals. Chlamydia was originally transmitted from animals-to-humans, then evolved into forms capable of person-to-person transmission. Today, chlamydia pneumonia can be acquired during community-wide outbreaks. All forms of chlamydia can be acquired by close contact within the family; from pets, domesticated animals or birds; and some species are acquired from flies or through sexual activity. Chlamydia can be transmitted from animal-to-human, from human-to-animal, and from animal-to-animal. All animals can transmit parasites to humans, and shed parasites on the ground and in water sources. Cats are the vector for the toxoplasmosis parasite. Chlamydia species and parasites can migrate and spread from the lung, intestine, or reproductive tract, to distant sites in the body, to cause chronic disease.

Transmission of chlamydia from pets and domesticated animals to humans is well established. Chlamydia pneumonia is easily transmitted to experimental animals, including mice, monkeys and rabbits. Chlamydia infections have crossed over to humans from cattle, horses, pigs, sheep, goats, guinea pigs, birds, dogs, cats, snakes, and monkeys. When chlamydia is transmitted from one animal to another type of animal, cross-species transmission can create the evolution of new forms of chlamydia.

All pets and domesticated animals create a risk of acquiring and transmitting intracellular animal pathogens, and parasites and worms transmitted by animal feces, at some time over the life of the animal. Animals go outside or live outside, have contact with other animals that can transmit immortal infections from animal-to-animal, animals are not concerned with hygiene, and the animal's lifespan is much shorter than the lifespan of the owner. Any animal infected with immortal pathogens and/ or parasites can be a vector for human infection and re-infection, over the animal's lifetime, and ultimately transmit pathogens to the owner.

Scientists identified community acquired pneumonia caused by animal pathogens, in an area with a high density of animal farms. The community acquired pneumonia was from a gram-negative intracellular bacteria, harbored in sheep, goats and cattle.[31] Farmers have greater close contact with domesticated animals, livestock, horses, cats, dogs, mice, and dirt contaminated with animal feces; and are known to be at higher risk for many chronic diseases.

Veterinarians recognize immortal infection and parasites cause chronic disease in animals, infections and parasites can be transmitted from pet-to-owner, and the same chronic diseases occur in animals and humans. Pets acquire many of the same diseases as people, and people acquire the same diseases as pets. Animal diseases may have the same name as human diseases, or be given a different name when the same disease occurs in an animal. It is time for the medical doctors to recognize it!

Different animal species carry different species of chlamydia. As many as three-hundred fifty species of chlamydia are thought to exist. Science is aware of at least fifteen species of chlamydia, and additional serovars (sub-types) within each species. Medical diagnostic laboratories routinely test for only three chlamydia species that are recognized as pathogenic in humans—chlamydia pneumonia, chlamydia trachoma and chlamydia psittacosis. Laboratories do not ordinarily test people for all known chlamydia species. New chlamydia pathogens and new serovars of existing forms of chlamydia are still being discovered and identified as pathogenic in humans. Undiscovered and new species of chlamydia, such as para-chlamydia, chlamydia waddelia, and chlamydia simcania, may interfere with traditional diagnostic tests for chlamydia pneumonia. Emerging species of chlamydia such as *suis*, abortus, pecorum, gallinacean, and muridarum; and new serovars of known chlamydia species, are not part of blood testing, and are not well studied or understood.

---

[31] Hiujskens E, *et al.* 2015. Evaluation of Patients with Community-Acquired Pneumonia Caused by Zoonotic Pathogens in an Area with a High Density of Animal Farms. Zoonoses and Public Health. Doi: 10.1111/zph.12218.

Scientists speculate other known and unknown species of chlamydia are not prevalent in humans, or are prevalent in animals but do not infect humans; yet, have not supported their assumption. More than three primary species of chlamydia likely infect humans and cause chronic disease, because people and animals have the same chronic diseases; and chlamydia species that are known to infect people cause the same chronic diseases in people as the pathogens cause in animals. Chlamydia species are known to attack any cell with a nucleus and to cause chronic diseases in animals; thus, transmission of new species of chlamydia, from animals, poses a threat to humans, and investigation into the new species of chlamydia provide the opportunity to identify new causes of chronic disease. Common chronic diseases in humans are caused by species of chlamydia alleged to be rare; thus the pathogen must be more common than recognized.

Any opening in the body is a portal for immortal infection with animal pathogens. Pathogens can enter the body through the mouth, nose, and eyes; and through sexual activity. Chlamydia can be acquired by inhaling pathogens from an infected person or infected animal; by hand-to-face contact; or through sexual contact with an infected person. Each form of chlamydia has a predilection to attack specific types of tissue or organs, and are acquired by a preferred route. Chlamydia pneumonia is acquired as a respiratory infection, and attacks the heart, lung, smooth muscle, vascular system, and brain. Chlamydia trachoma is most often sexually transmitted or transmitted by a fly; and can occasionally become airborne and cause a severe respiratory infection. Chlamydia trachoma attacks the reproductive system, urinary system, and eyes. Psittacosis is acquired primarily from birds, through direct contact and self-inoculation with bird feces, or by inhaling particles of bird feces, and can cause an acute life-threatening respiratory infection. Psittacosis can cause chronic disease in the lymphatic system, and causes many forms of lymphoma. Chlamydia pneumonia, chlamydia trachoma and chlamydia psittacosis can attack the joints, and leave debris in joints, causing reactive arthritis and rheumatoid arthritis; and attack the central nervous system, causing central nervous system disease.

Tissue throughout the body consists of five layers, whether it be skin, vascular tissue, corneas, or organs. The outer layer is the epithelium, the inner layer is the endothelium, and the central layer is stroma. The stroma is separated from the epithelium and endothelium by thin membranes. A collagen matrix in the stroma makes spaces to hold fluid to keep tissue hydrated, with fluid pumped in and out of the tissue, by the endothelium. Immortal chlamydia pathogens attack the epithelium or the endothelium, or both, depending on the species. The H-pylori bacterium attacks epithelium, and then burrows down to attach to collagen. Pathogens starting at the endothelial or epithelial layers migrate toward the center, and cause disintegration of the membrane separating layers, leaving the inner and outer layers less able to function properly, and the collagen and stroma vulnerable to attack, inflammation, and atrophy (thinning). When pathogens reach the stroma, the immune battle causes inflammation and atrophy, and it may be diagnosed as collagen vascular disease. Co-infections can work synergistically to enhance the damage to tissue, and trigger chronic disease.

Chlamydia pneumonia attacks endothelial cells; and can attack throughout the body, causing impaired endothelial function. When chlamydia pneumonia damages the endothelium, the endothelium cannot pump fluid into and out of the tissue and interstitial spaces, to keep the tissue hydrated. As endothelial function fails, tissue may swell, or atrophy, from dehydration or excessive fluid. Blood vessels have endothelium on the inside of the vessel, and the cardiovascular system is a major site for attack by chlamydia pneumonia. Chlamydia pneumonia causes plaque in the cardiovascular system and brain, and soft plaque inside the lining of the vessels. In the brain, chlamydia pathogens and abnormal proteins create plaque, and cause tissue to stick together, to cause Alzheimer's lesions and brain cancer.

Chlamydia trachoma and chlamydia psittacosis attack epithelial and endothelial cells. The intestinal tract has epithelium on the inside of the intestinal tract, making the stomach lining susceptible to pathogens that attack epithelium. Nerves have epithelium forming the protective sheath around nerves. The corneas have epithelium on the surface, and endothelium on the underside of the cornea; and the retina has epithelium on the inside surface. Attack on the epithelium damages the surface of the cells or structure, causes loss of adhesion in the layers of tissue, and damages protective nerve sheaths. H-pylori attacks epithelium and attaches to collagen, and can work synergistically with immortal pathogens and fungus to cause chronic disease, particularly in and along the gastrointestinal tract and in the eyes. The damaged epithelium allows other pathogens and fungus to invade the deeper layers of tissue, and cause a chronic disease.

Acute chlamydia pneumonia causes widespread community outbreaks of respiratory infections, causing an extended respiratory illness, lasting six to twelve weeks, followed by a persistent cough lasting four months or longer. Chlamydia pneumonia may be referred to, in the vernacular, as "walking pneumonia". Mycoplasma and whooping cough also cause community outbreaks of an extended respiratory illness and pneumonia, lasting six to twelve weeks, followed by a persistent cough for four months or longer; and if combined with chlamydia as an acute co-infection, may trigger more immediate chronic disease. Treatment can shorten the acute illness, prevent the development of a prolonged cough, limit wheezing, limit the infectious burden, limit the spread in the community, and delay development of chronic disease. People do not acquire long-term immunity to immortal animal pathogens; and re-infection can occur. Repeated re-infections increase the infectious burden, and can trigger secondary adverse events such as stroke or heart attack.

Acute chlamydia can become a chronic sub-clinical infection, which spreads in the body invading any hospitable tissue; and causes chronic disease, over years and decades. The chlamydia pathogens live as long as the host lives, and as long as the pathogen has a host cell. Chlamydia infection starts an infectious cascade of reduced immunity, new immortal infections and parasites, fungal invasion, and the proliferation of abnormal proteins and debris generated by the immune battle with the pathogen. Chlamydia infections create a perpetual and never-ending war within, between the immune system and the animal pathogens. The evolution of chronic disease is determined by the immortal infections and parasites we acquire, the infectious burden, the combination of co-infections, how long the infections have persisted, and how the infections have been treated. Chronic disease can emerge years or decades after the acute infection.

Intracellular animal pathogens may infect the body by one route; and migrate to adjacent tissue, or metastasize to new hospitable host cells through the immune system and lymphatics. Chlamydia can spread by self-inoculation when touching one's eyes, nose or mouth; and when touching the face with cell phones. Chlamydia pneumonia can live and spread through vessels, the immune system, the smooth muscles, and the vagus nerve; and can live in endothelium, spongy or porous organs, and in cholesterol. Pathogens can migrate from the stomach to other vital organs along the intestinal tract; and via the vagus nerve, a large nerve connecting the brain and vital organs, to the eyes and brain. The pathogens can migrate from the gastrointestinal tract to the urinary tract, by direct migration or self-inoculation; and from the urinary tract to the prostate or kidney by ascending up the urinary tract. Sexual activity can spread pathogens from the gastrointestinal tract or reproductive tract, to the urinary tract and kidney. Chlamydia trachoma in the vagina can migrate upwards into the uterus and fallopian tubes, causing reproductive diseases; or in the male, migrate up the penis to cause inflammation and scarring of the lumen and prostate.

Chlamydia pathogens cannot create their own energy. The pathogens survive by consuming the ATP energy created by the host cell, creating fatigue. Normal cells synthesize ATP to create energy, through a positive charge. The chlamydia pathogen takes control of cell functioning, consumes ATP created by the cell, and reverses the energy charge of the cell. Infected cells have substantially less ATP, which impairs the ability of the cell to bring oxygen across the cell wall, into the cell. When ATP in the cell is depleted, the pathogen consumes sugar to make energy. The sugar is converted to alcohol, through fermentation, fostering the development of fungus. Fungus feeds the infection and protects the pathogens from immune system. The loss of ATP in the cell, and the pathogen's consumption of sugar for energy causes weaker and weaker replicas of cells, less able to make ATP. Chlamydia impairs normal apoptosis (cell death); and new cells are no longer identical copies of the host cell, and are infected with the intracellular pathogen. Loss of ATP causes impaired cellular and organ function, and fatigue. Low ATP and fermentation impair the ability of the host cell to metabolize glucose, and to maintain the glucose balance in the cells and body. Chlamydia and the response of the immune battle against the pathogen generates inflammatory signals, TNF-alpha, and angiogenesis (new blood vessel formation).

Chlamydia depletes folic acid and B12, through direct competition for nutrients, and malabsorption of nutrients caused by damage to the intestinal villi and mechanical blockage. Some chlamydia strains directly consume B12 and folic acid. Some strains synthesize folic acid from material obtained inside the cells, use folic acid precursors, and significantly inhibit the cell's ability to produce and utilize folic acid. Trachoma and psittacosis pirate folic acid produced in the Krebs cycle (basic human cell biochemistry). The absence of folic acid intracellularly leads to broken chromosomes and mutant cancer cells. Co-infection with parasites causes additional competition for nutrients and blocks absorption of nutrients in the gastrointestinal tract.

Chlamydia pathogens are destructive, erosive, and sticky. Chlamydia generates abnormal proteins, and changes normal proteins to abnormal proteins. The pathogens and the sticky byproducts cause inflammation, mis-folding of proteins inside the cells, dispersion of abnormal proteins attached to the pathogen, and clogging of passive body functions. Abnormally shaped and folded proteins can get stuck in aberrant locations, and attach to and alter genes, creating genetic abnormalities and abnormal gene expression. Bodily functions have to passively accommodate the effects of the pathogens, just as falling water passively moves around a rock, and the universe passively arcs around a black hole. Interruptions to passive function, with clogging, sticky tissue, or inclusion cysts, become a focus for development of chronic diseases.

Medicine discovered 42,000,000 proteins inside each cell. Intracellular pathogens and the immune battle generate sticky molecules, which can cause proteins to fold into abnormal shapes. The intracellular pathogens can alter how proteins are formed and folded, creating abnormal shapes.

Science is now trying to define a proteinbiome, which would reflect the infections each person carries inside the cell. The variations in the shape and design of proteins has led to naming new Cluster Differentiations, based on the abnormal proteins attached to the outside of cells and generated by the cells infected with immortal pathogens.

The species of chlamydia may determine the type and shape of abnormal proteins. Abnormal proteins attached to the outside of the pathogen compound the infectious burden, and confuse the immune system. When host cells die, fragments of nucleus and abnormal proteins are released into the blood and lymphatic system, which are not compatible with passive function. Plasmids (pieces of the cell) and abnormal proteins are not alive; therefore, cannot be killed. The pathogens, abnormal proteins, and plasmids circulate in the body and clog and dam passive functions, interfere with passive function, and provide an inclusion cyst and/or focus for development of cancer and other chronic disease. The immune system attacks abnormal proteins, in a futile attempt to kill abnormal proteins that cannot be killed, then attempts to sequester the pathogen or abnormal protein.

Biofilm is created over the pathogens, and can contribute to the composition of pus and plaque. The white blood cells generate sticky pus; and attempt to kill the pathogen and dispose of waste products of infection. The pus created by the immune system starts as biofilm, then soft pus, then soft plaque inside the vessel walls; and may be covered by a harder cap, created by the vessel wall at the site of attack. Soft pus becomes soft plaque, and soft plaque becomes hard plaque. Biofilm, pus, and plaque covering the pathogens is a passive immune system defense, to wall off the infection and pus. The type and consistency of pus and plaque may differ, based on location of the pathogen, the composition, and time, but the principle is the same: Infection causes the immune system to attack, leading to inflammation, biofilm, and pus; then the pus becomes soft and hard plaque, in response to the immune system failure to fully eradicate the pathogens and harmful debris.

Chlamydia infects and replicates within the immune cells, impairing and confusing immune function, reducing immunity, and leading to new acute infections. Chlamydia species invade host cells, and when the immune system attempts to fight the pathogen, the immune cells become infected. The chlamydia pathogen becomes the Trojan horse of the immune system, hiding inside and spreading via the immune cells. New infectious forms of the pathogen and waste products are dispersed into the blood and lymphatics, and invade new cells in the body.

Each type of immortal pathogen attracts specific types of immune cells. The immune cells which attack the pathogen become infected with the intracellular pathogen, and spread the pathogen through the blood stream and lymphatics, to new host cells. When the immune system is unable to eradicate the intracellular pathogen, the immune cells generate TNF-alpha, which is a more aggressive immune response. C-reactive proteins formed in the liver are also generated and cause inflammation. TNF-alpha is considered a super family of proteins, in the naming of Cluster Differentiations, with subcategories within the Cluster Differentiations for the TNF family. C-reactive protein is correlated with the CD-4 in the list of Cluster Differentiations, and is considered a marker of systemic inflammation in the body. The C-reactive proteins are intended to clear apoptotic cells, debris, and bacteria. Both C-reactive proteins and findings of CD-4 in research are common in many chronic diseases.

The immune system does not attack healthy tissue—it reacts to a chemical signal in a feedback loop directing a futile attack against intracellular pathogens. New blood vessels form to provide oxygen, to oxygen-deprived cells. The immune cells generate TNF-alpha, as a stronger inflammatory attack against the intracellular pathogen the immune cells could not destroy. The stronger inflammatory attack by the immune system, with TNF-alpha, can damage adjacent healthy tissue and cause atrophy of the tissue.

Compelling evidence supports chlamydia can affect genes, by creating abnormal proteins that attach to genes and alter gene expression. The abnormal genes and gene expression can be passed down in the family to the next generation. Research to develop ways to rid the body of abnormal proteins may be an important method to improve health, after acute and chronic infection, and to fight the development of chronic disease.

Chlamydia species cause inclusion bodies, also referred to as inclusion cysts, which can become granulomas or mini-tumors, sheltering chlamydia from the immune system. The immune system engulfs the chlamydia pathogen and/or abnormal proteins in inclusion cysts, to sequester the pathogens and abnormal proteins, which the immune system cannot eradicate. The chlamydia inclusion body is separated from the eukaryotic endocytic pathways, and chlamydia may modify the inclusion membrane through insertion of chlamydia derived components, including abnormal proteins generated by chlamydia.[32] The ongoing immune system attack creates an inclusion cyst, with particles of the pathogens and host cells, abnormal proteins, fungus, and indigestible particles. The immune battle continues to enlarge the inclusion cyst and can transform the inclusion cyst into a tumor. Bodily functions have to passively arc and change to accommodate the presence of the inclusion body created by the immune battle against the pathogen.

More than one immortal infection at the same time confuses and complicates the immune defense. Co-infection puts added stress on an already weakened immune system and creates unusual patterns of abnormal proteins attached to the pathogens that confuse the immune system. Multiple chronic infections with more than one type of immortal bacteria; more than one type of chlamydia; and/or infection with any combination of bacteria, parasites, fungus, viruses and environmental triggers, accelerate development of chronic disease. The greater the infectious burden, the longer the infections have persisted, the weaker the immune system, the greater the likelihood a person will develop a chronic disease.

The more immortal pathogens the patient harbors, the more likely pathogens will attack multiple organs and organ systems. Multiple chronic infections are analogous to repeated assaults in the war being waged by

---

[32] Pannekoek Y, *et al*. March 2006. Inclusion Proteins of Chlamydiacea. Drugs Today. 2006. 42 Suppl A: 65-73. PMID: 16683046.

the immune system. Pathogens will attack tissue from both the inside out (endothelium), and from the outside in (epithelium). Different types of immune cells are called to fight different types of pathogens, and a greater diversity of immune cells become infected. As the pathogen damages a greater number of host cells, infects a greater number and different types of immune cells, and dangerous byproducts are dispersed in the immune system war against the pathogen, a chronic disease develops. A high infectious burden with multiple forms of chlamydia; or a combination of chlamydia and other immortal pathogens or parasites, can accelerate the infectious cascade, reduce immunity, and trigger secondary adverse events. The immortal pathogens synergistically damage the cells in the body, and further impair the function of the cells and the immune cells.

Endo- and ecto-symbionts are pathogens that live inside the cell (endo-symbiont) or attach to the outside of the cell (ecto-symbiont). Pathogens can become endo- and ecto- symbionts of other pathogens and parasites, and independently or synergistically cause disease. Whether the pathogen becomes an endo- or an ecto-symbiont is determined by size, and the ability of the pathogen to invade the cell or pathogen. Smaller pathogens can invade larger pathogens and become an endo-symbiont, and larger pathogens attach to the outside of other pathogens as an ecto-symbiont. Chlamydia can host other bacteria and viruses; and other bacteria, parasites, and viruses can host chlamydia, as endo- or ecto- symbionts. Chlamydia can spread by becoming a parasite of another pathogen and traveling with the pathogenic host, or spread pathogens that are parasites attached to the chlamydia bacteria.

Parasitic infection can be acquired secondary to reduced immunity. Parasites are microscopic organisms, originating from animals, which are larger than chlamydia and can serve a host cell for chlamydia. Parasites can host bacteria and viruses as endo- and ecto-symbionts; and generate fungus, in the gastrointestinal tract, which aggravates the overall infectious burden, and can accelerate malabsorption of key nutrients and development of chronic disease. Parasites include amoebas, giardia, cryptosporidiosis, toxoplasmosis, schistosomes, and other parasites. Worms are bigger than other parasitic infections, and may be visible to the naked eye. Parasitic disease is generally acquired by ingestion, from animal-to-person, person-to-person, or accidental ingestion of parasites shed in animal feces. Parasites set in motion a cycle of eggs and cysts, as the infection persists, spreads, and becomes a chronic infection.

Parasites have preferred locations in the intestine, in the stomach, small intestine, or large intestine. Parasites can migrate from the intestine to adjacent organs, including the liver, gallbladder and pancreas, to become a focus for disease; and other parts of the body along the vagus nerve or through the lymph system. Parasites have been found in abdominal organs, inside tumors in abdominal organs, and in the brain. Worms usually establish themselves in the intestine, most often in the lower intestine and rectum, but can migrate to other parts of the body. The toxoplasmosis parasite, acquired from contact with infected cat feces, by ingestion or inhaling the toxoplasmosis parasite, can start in the intestinal tract and migrate to attack the brain and cause a variety of mental illnesses.

Parasitic infection in the intestinal tract damages intestinal villi and clogs the intestine, impairs digestion, impairs absorption of nutrients, and causes leaky gut syndrome. Parasitic infections cause malabsorption of folic acid and B12, which have been "associated" with a variety of chronic diseases. Depletion of folic acid has been "associated" with cognitive decline; and low folic acid and low vitamin D are thought to be triggers for cancer.

Some immortal infections and parasites causing chronic disease are more common outside the United States. The schistosome parasite, liver flukes, and leishmaniosis are common in the Middle East and Africa. Chlamydia psittacosis, in humans, is common in the Middle East, where bird handling is part of the culture. Psittacosis is endemic in pigeons worldwide; and infects virtually all of the pigeons in Italy, where people are in closer contact with pigeons. Brazil has the highest rate of pet ownership in heavily populated areas, and one of the highest rates of toxoplasmosis. In Turkey and Greece, an unusual streptococcus serovar is common and is known to attack the heart and kidneys; and to cause a systemic blistering skin disease. The pathogens can be acquired in foreign countries and brought back to the United States, and may not be recognized by United States doctors, due to lack of training, lack of awareness, and lack of interest in infectious diseases around the world.

The Principle of the Whole is a unifying principle of chronic disease: Chronic infection with immortal pathogens cause chronic disease, and the more immortal pathogens and parasites a person has, and the longer the infections persisted, the more likely the person will develop a chronic disease. The Principle of the Whole offers a new paradigm for how we can improve the diagnosis and treatment of all chronic diseases. The Principle of the Whole provides structure and meaning to the vast segmented knowledge and varied specialties, in medicine. The Principle of the Whole puts the person back together and the specialties back together, united in the diagnosis of the root infectious causes of chronic disease. Patients can have renewed hope, because the Principle of the Whole offers new pathways for treatment, and new pathways for research, with the potential for important discoveries in the diagnosis and treatment of chronic disease.

> *If something is important enough, even if the odds are against you, you should still do it.*

Elon Musk

CHAPTER 5

INTRACELLULAR CHLAMYDIA PATHOGENS

Much has been written about chlamydia since 1988, when Dr. Merchant attempted to publish an article reporting chronic giardia was causing low folic acid and B12, recurrent respiratory infections, reduced immunity, and chronic disease.

The medical literature now reports chlamydia is "associated" with many chronic diseases, across all medical specialties. Medical providers retreat from diagnosis and treatment of immortal pathogens, because scientific literature retreats to "associations" rather than causes. Different medical specialties are not aware of similar reports of chlamydia causing chronic disease in other specialties, to be aware of the patterns or commonalities between chronic disease and chronic chlamydia infection. Few recognize a pattern of chlamydia causing chronic diseases; or that treatment of chlamydia can prevent, improve or reverse chronic diseases.

Just searching Google for references on chlamydia generates references in the millions. Searching "chlamydia pneumonia" or just "chlamydia" combined with a search term for any chronic disease, gives references to articles supporting chlamydia as a cause of chronic disease. A Google search for "chlamydia" gave 10,200,000 references, spanning every medical specialty; "chlamydia and cancer" gave 9,980,000 results; "chlamydia pneumonia" gave 1,480,000 results; "chlamydia and trachoma" gave 2,484,000 results; "chlamydia and chronic disease" gave 587,000; "chlamydia and heart disease" gave 484,000 results; "chlamydia and psittacosis" gave 352,000 results; "chlamydia and atherosclerosis" gave 381,000 results, and "chlamydia and cardiomyopathy" gave 163,000 results. "Chlamydia and multiple sclerosis" gave 963,000 results;

"chlamydia and Alzheimer's gave 796,000 results; and "chlamydia and chronic fatigue" gave 246,000 results. "Chlamydia and eye disease" gave 2,510,000 results. "Chlamydia animal to humans" gave 7,450,000 results; and "chlamydia in animals" gave 572,000 results. No doubt many of these references overlap or are duplicates; however, the sheer number of references demonstrates extensive reports in the public domain suggest chlamydia is a cause of chronic disease. It is time to convert the vast reports of "associations" between chlamydia and chronic disease, and other immortal pathogens and chronic disease, into a coherent theory that states a cause, and provides new direction to doctors and researchers for diagnosis and treatment of chronic diseases.

Chlamydia previously had two names, chlamydia and chlamydophila; and has various spellings in the European literature, such as chlamydiae and chlamydiacea. In 1999, the term chlamydophila was replaced with more specific naming of the species of chlamydia. A formerly single genius, chlamydia, was expanded to include at least nine species recognized in animals (abortus, caviae, felis, muridarum, pecorum, pneumoniae, psittaci, *suis*, trachoma); and two additional species were recently discovered (avium and gallinacean).[33] Veterinarians may still refer to chlamydia infection as chlamydophila or chlamydiosis, when present in animals.

The MERCK MANUAL: VETERINARY MANUAL describes chlamydia bacteria as ubiquitous obligate intracellular gram-negative bacteria that replicates within a host cell, via a unique developmental cycle, and competes with the host for intracellular nutrient pools.[34] It states virtually any chlamydia organism can infect any eukaryotic host cell, which is any cell with a nucleus. If true, all chlamydia species have the potential to infect humans, not just the three or four species currently diagnosed by chlamydia PCR blood testing or the nine species currently recognized.

---

[33] *Id.*
[34] Sykes J, *et al.* 2016. MERCK MANUAL: VETERINARY MANUAL. 2016. 11th ed. Overview of Chlamydial Conjunctivitis, Etiology and Epidemiology. (Sykes J, *et al.*). Doi: merckvetmanual.com/eye-and-ear/chlamydial-conjunctivitis/overview-of-chlamydial-conjunctivitis.

The MERCK MANUAL: VETERINARY MANUAL states, "Chlamydiaceae have been associated with conjunctivitis in the host species they infect, including Chlamydia caviae (guinea pigs), C *suis* (pigs), C psittaci (birds), and C pecorum (cattle and sheep)...Chlamydia conjunctivitis in cats, caused by C felis (formerly Chlamydophila felis)...C pneumoniae has been detected in cats with conjunctivitis... Transmission to people occurs as a result of direct, close contact between cats...C psittaci has been isolated from dogs with keratoconjunctivitis and respiratory signs, in a dog breeding facility.[35]

Veterinarians have studied chlamydia extensively, documented chlamydia in a wide variety of animals, and documented transmission of chlamydia from animals-to-humans. Chlamydia was identified in parrots (1930), and parakeets (1930); in geese, ducks, and in chicken, pheasants, black-headed gulls, turkeys, willets, pigeons (1940), doves (1941). It was found in conjunctivitis in dogs (1942); in cattle encephalomyelitis (1942); in opossum encephalitis (1949); in pneumonia in sheep (1952); in pneumonia in goats (1953); in pneumonia in dogs (1954); in pneumonia in cattle (1955); in polyarthritis in sheep (1959); in the ferret, mouse, hamster, guinea pig, snowshoe hare, domestic rabbit, and muskrat (1966); in pneumonia in cats (1960, 1966); in conjunctivitis in cats (1969); in pigs with intestinal infections, pneumonia, conjunctivitis, and abortion (1963, 1965); in poly-arthritis in cattle (1964); in opossum pneumonia (1965); and in horse pneumonia (1968). In 1967, chlamydia was recognized as endemic in one-hundred thirty different species of birds. Resistance of the chlamydia organisms to penicillin was recognized, in 1960 and 1961.

In 1954, Enright and Sadler detected a rising antibody titer to chlamydia, in veterinarians working in stockyards. In 1956, in the Congo, Giroud and Associates isolated several strains of infectious agents with chlamydia properties from the lung of an aborted human fetus; and from the placentas of aborting women who had contact with sheep, goats, or cattle, suffering from pneumonia or abortions. In 1956, Meyer and Eddie recovered a chlamydia agent causing sporadic bovine encephalomyelitis, from the blood of a patient after an accidental laboratory infection. In 1957, Giroud

---

[35] *Id.*

and Associates isolated a chlamydia agent from the cerebral spinal fluid of a febrile child, who was in contact with a flock of sheep experiencing abortions. In 1967, Roberts and coworkers studied a woman who aborted in the sixth month of pregnancy and who had been exposed to sheep, and found a high chlamydia titer. Prat (1955), Fiocre (1959), Sarateanu, and coworkers (1961), suspected that human chlamydia infections were contracted from cattle infected with chlamydia bronchopneumonia; and suggested man contracts chlamydia infections from domestic animals.

Chlamydia pneumonia was found in birds, cats, cattle, mice, rhesus monkeys, sheep, goats and humans, prior to 1971. Chlamydia has been reported in rodents, sheep, goats, cattle, horses and koalas. Chlamydia pneumoniae respiratory pathogens have been detected in cats, dogs, horses, koalas, iguanas, boas, chameleons, turtles, and frogs. Chlamydia trachoma was found in sheep and piglets with subclinical keratoconjunctivitis; and chlamydia trachoma urogenital infection and lymphogranuloma venereum was found in pigs. Chlamydia *suis* is found in swine, formerly known as porcine serovar of chlamydia trachoma, and affects multiple sites in the swine. Chlamydia muridarum was found in a mouse colony with pneumonia.

Veterinarians recognize pigeons and sparrows are major reservoirs for chlamydia psittaci, and chlamydia psittaci causes sheep and goat abortions. Chlamydia psittaci can be transmitted to humans by parrots, pigeons, cats, and dogs. Chlamydia pneumonia, chlamydia trachoma, chlamydia psittaci, chlamydia pecorum; and chlamydia enteritis, encephalomyelitis, and polyarthritis, have been identified in many animals, including amphibians such as frogs. When a seal pulled a young girl into the water, she required treatment with tetracycline, to avoid "seal-finger" disease, caused by an animal pathogen, like mycoplasma or a mycobacterium, which can cause significant adverse consequences to health, if not promptly treated. Reports of seal-finger disease note amphibians, as opposed to terrestrial animals, carry a host of bacteria uncommon to land mammals, which require humans be treated promptly.

Wild animal species identified as harboring chlamydia included lions, zebras, spotted hyenas, the African buffalo, cheetahs, gazelles, elephants, jackals, bat eared foxes, dogs, mongooses, giraffes, and impala wildebeests. Virtually all mainland koalas had chlamydia pneumonia and chlamydia pecorum; and chlamydia infections in koalas were associated with ocular infections and genital tract infections, linked to infertility.[36] The South African buffalo had mixed chlamydia abortus and chlamydia pneumonia. Chlamydia abortus was found in fifty-four animals and fourteen mammalian species; and in all animal samples tested at the Serengeti Animal Preserve.[37]

Chlamydia abortus (formerly classified as a chlamydia psittaci serotype 1), causes abortion in small ruminants (sheep, cattle, antelope, deer, giraffe), mainly sheep and goats. In sheep, it is called ovine enzootic abortion, also now known as ovine chlamydiosis. Chlamydia abortus has been found in cattle, swine, wild suidae (pigs, hogs, and boars), horses and birds. Chlamydia abortus has been suggested as a cause of abortion and fetal demise, when transmitted to humans from sheep or goats. Chlamydia caviae is found in guinea pigs, and causes ocular and urogenital infections. Chlamydia felis is associated with acute and chronic conjunctivitis, rhinitis, and bronchopneumonia, in stray and domestic cats. Chlamydia felis is transmitted by close contact with infected cats, their aerosol, and fomites (materials around them, clothes, utensils, furniture, any non-living object that carries bacteria and transfers to another). Chlamydia gallinacea has been found in chickens and other domestic birds in China; and chlamydia gallinacea is found in poultry and can affect developing chicken embryos. Chlamydia avium has been identified in pigeons and in psittacines (parrot family). Chlamydia pecorum is ubiquitous in cattle herds with multiple organ manifestations. Tasmanian devils carry a form of chlamydia that causes cancer, when one animal bites another animal.

---

[36] Polkinghorne A, *et al.* 2013. Recent Advances in Understanding the Biology, Epidemiology and Control of Chlamydia Infections in Koalas. Vet Microiol. 2013. 165(3-4): 214-223. PMID: 23523170. Doi:10.1016/j.vetmic.2013.02.026.

[37] Pospischil A, *et al.* 2012. Evidence of Chlamydia in Wild Mammals of the Serengeti. Journal of Wildlife Diseases. October 2012. Vol. 48(4): 1074-1078. Doi: doi.org/10.7589/2011-10-298.

In 1971, in <u>CHLAMYDIA AND CHLAMYDIA INDUCED DISEASES,</u> Dr. Johannes Storz, described chlamydia induced diseases in animals. Chlamydia induced diseases included abortions in cows, chronic diseases in fetuses, ovine pig abortions, and placental reactions to chlamydia infection. He reported chlamydia was found in birds, including chickens, ducks, egrets, parrots, partridges, pheasants, sea gulls, and turkeys; and because of their migratory routes, birds were reported as a vector for the spread of chlamydia infections. He also noted a relationship between ticks and chlamydia.

Dr. Storz reported chlamydia had the same cellular effects in animals, as are known to occur in humans. Chlamydia had amino acid requirements that affected energy metabolism in the infected cells. Chlamydia arrested the cell cycle of apoptosis; and folic acid was synthesized by some chlamydia strains. Chlamydia induced a lethal toxin in chicken embryos. He reported chlamydia conjunctivitis in cats, dogs, cattle, sheep, pigs, parakeets, mice, pigeons, and guinea pigs. Guinea pigs were particularly susceptible to inclusion conjunctivitis from chlamydia. Chlamydia can be fatal to pathogen free pigs, when the pigs are exposed to conventionally raised pigs. Chlamydia in dogs caused gastrointestinal disorders, granulomatous hepatitis, encephalitis, and pneumoencephalitis. Chlamydia infection caused polyarthritis in cows, dogs, and pigs. Dr. Storz recognized genital chlamydia infections in endometritis, epididymitis, LGV non-specific urethritis, proctitis, seminal vesiculitis syndrome; and the venereal nature of inclusion conjunctivitis. Dr. Storz stated, "Human chlamydia infections are traceable to mammals" and either occurred infrequently or remained unrecognized and unreported in humans.

Chlamydia can be transmitted from one animal species to another, such as birds-to-cattle, birds-to-horses, and sheep to cattle; and animals may be co-infected with more than one type of chlamydia. Each animal has its own form of chlamydia, and each animal form of chlamydia can cross over to other animals and humans. Chlamydia pneumonia is thought to have originated in birds and ducks; and can now be found in many animals, and is frequently found in cattle. Chlamydia pneumonia in sheep and cattle is closely connected to widespread clinically unapparent intestinal chlamydia infection in sheep and cattle. Each species of bird has specific psittaci serovars; and psittaci is capable of recombination in co-infected animals to become a new species of chlamydia psittaci. Chlamydia psittacosis has been isolated from fecal samples in two dogs that were exposed to avian/ bird chlamydia; and has been found in cats, dogs, and horses. Chlamydia pecorum has been found in cattle, sheep, goats, pigs, koalas, guinea pigs, and Tasmanian devils. Chlamydia abortus has been found in sheep, cattle and goats.

The classification of chlamydia species based on host and/or association with disease has not had a high degree of consistency. Chronic chlamydia creates plasmids, or pieces of DNA separated from the cell, making it more difficult to relate a particular type of chlamydia to a particular animal species. Cross species transmission confuses the diagnosis. Failure to identify the chlamydia species, and generalizing chlamydia into only three types of chlamydia (pneumonia, trachoma, psittacosis), has hampered recognition of the pathogenesis of all chlamydia species, in humans.

Chlamydia pneumonia in koala bears was studied, using the sequence of the genome (the organism's hereditary information). The DNA sequence of chlamydia pneumonia in koalas, in Australia, matched the chlamydia pneumonia in humans, suggesting humans were originally infected with chlamydia pneumonia from animals. In Brazil, the genome sequence of pathogens in animals, including cats and dogs, has been studied extensively; and more research has been dedicated to understanding pathogens in animals, than to understanding pathogens in humans.

"Diseases We Catch from Our Pets, Zoonotic Illnesses of Dogs Cats and Other Pets", listed and described numerous pathogens transmitted from companion animals to humans.[38] The pathogens included bacteria (salmonellosis, shigella, pasteurellosis, campylobacter, streptococcus, staphylococcus, tuberculosis, plague, parrot fever (psittacosis or orinthosis), anthrax, leptospirosis, brucellosis, helicobacter pylori, bartonellosis, Q-fever,

---

[38] Hines R. 2nd Chance. Ron Hines, DVM, Ph.D. Hines R. Diseases We Catch from Our Pets, Zoonotic Illnesses of Dogs Cats and Other Pets. Doi: 2ndchance. info/zoonoses.

and tularemia. It includes parasites (hookworm, roundworm, tapeworm, dog heartworm, giardia, cryptosporidium, toxoplasmosis); skin parasites (sarcastic mange, scabies); viruses (viral encephalitis, West Nile virus, hantavirus in rodents, the ORF virus, rabies, B-virus herpes in monkeys); tick borne diseases (Lyme disease, Rocky Mountain Spotted Fever); fungi (ringworm); and even prion diseases (spongiform encephalopathy).

Cats and dogs share common diseases with humans, including heart disease, lung disease, asthma, allergies, cancer (including lymphoma), epilepsy, endocrine disease, Addison's disease (adrenal disease), diabetes, arthritis, gastrointestinal disease, liver disease, obesity, reproductive diseases, kidney disease, urinary tract disease, lupus, multiple sclerosis, conjunctivitis, cataracts, blood disorders, immune diseases, HIV (feline immunodeficiency virus), tuberculosis, Lyme disease, influenza, acne, and more. Cats infected with toxoplasmosis have the same types of mental illness as occurs in humans infected with toxoplasmosis.[39]

Published articles, by veterinarians, written as far back as the 1940's, discussed the pathology of chlamydia, and its relationship to disease in animals. The veterinary literature refers to intracellular animal chlamydia pathogens as a cause of chronic disease; and veterinarians know chronic chlamydia infections in animals cause chronic disease. Veterinarians know household pets and other companion animals get all the same chronic diseases as people. In COMMON DISEASES IN COMPANION ANIMALS, Alliece Summers, MS, DVM, describes diseases in animals which have remarkable similarity to chronic diseases in humans.[40] The chronic diseases are the same, because the pathogens causing the chronic diseases are the same. All forms of chlamydia are intracellular, cause similar cell damage, damage ATP production, impair apoptosis, generate abnormal proteins, alter genes, and start an infectious cascade. Animals

---

[39] Gartner M, *et al*. 2014. Personality Structure in the Domestic Cat (Felis silvestris), Scottish Wildcat (Felis silvestris grampia), Clouded Leopard (Neofelis nebulosi), Snow Leopard (Panthera uncia), and African Lion (Panthera leo). Journal of Comparative Psychology. 2014. Vol 128(4): 414-426. Doi: 10.1037/a0037104.

[40] *See* Summers A. 2014. COMMON DISEASES IN COMPANION ANIMALS, 3rd Ed. China: Mosby.

have the same chronic diseases as humans, caused by the same intracellular pathogens. Veterinary literature reports, "Infections acquired from wildlife, known as zoonotic infections, are one of the most significant growing threats to global human health".[41]

The pathogens in dog and cat mouths are different than in humans. The microbiome in cats and dogs are fifty-percent similar to each other, but neither cats nor dogs have a microbiome similar to humans. Humans do not have immunity to pathogens in the mouths of animals. When pathogens from the animal's mouth get into a wound or through broken skin, the pathogens can cause necrotizing fasciitis, septicemia, amputations, and death; or the infection can become chronic and evolve into a chronic disease. Cats have millions of pathogens on their fur from licking themselves, which can be transmitted from the fur to owners. Just petting a cat or dog will transfer at least one-hundred fifty new animal pathogens onto the skin, which live on the skin for hours, and can be self-inoculated to the eyes, nose or mouth. Pets allowed to sleep on the bed can transmit the pathogens to the bed and to the humans who use the bed.

Animal pathogens cannot ever peacefully merge into the human microbiome. Animal pathogens in the human microbiome create a never-ending war within. Animal pathogens live by consuming the energy generated by the host cells; and generate debris that is harmful, interferes with passive function, and can alter genes. The immune system cannot eradicate intracellular pathogens; and the pathogens fight for dominance and survival, creating a destructive infectious cascade and downward spiral to development of chronic disease. When animal pathogens infect a human, it can cause chronic disease years or decades later.

Veterinarians know pets and domesticated animals transmit chlamydia pathogens to humans. Veterinarians know people transfer chlamydia pathogens to their pets, and infections can be passed back and forth between pets and people. Veterinarians know pets have parasites and

---

[41] 2010. Animals Linked to Chlamydia Pneumoniae". Science Daily. Queensland University of Technology. Feb 22, 2010. Doi: sciencedaily.com/releases/2010/02/100222094805.htm.

worms, and can transmit parasites and worms to humans. Veterinarians know animals can make their owners sick, and the owners can make their animals sick! Veterinarians have the courage to say a disease is "caused" by an infectious pathogen. Naturopaths know pathogens and parasites from animals cause malabsorption and chronic disease! Why don't the medical doctors understand the relationship between animal pathogens and chronic disease? Medical doctors should know as much about chlamydia and intestinal parasites as veterinarians and naturopaths. Testing for immortal intracellular infections and parasites should be routine and widespread in humans, with any chronic disease or severe acute disease.

Prior to the 1890's, veterinarians and medical doctors were one profession. When the professions split, medical doctors established their own system of training; and veterinarians appear to have taken important knowledge about infectious causes of chronic disease with them. The medical establishment today does not interact with veterinarians, or consider their knowledge, on infectious causes of disease. The infectious cause of chronic disease, and the diagnosis and treatment of immortal pathogens and parasites, get little or no attention in medical training. Minimal teaching is done on infectious causes of chronic disease and training in parasitic disease is waning. The medical establishment should know what veterinarians know, about infectious causes of chronic disease, because the knowledge is critical to understanding the origin of chronic disease in humans.

In <u>CHLAMYDIA Intracellular Biology, Pathogenesis and Immunity</u>, the authors described the history of discovery of various types of chlamydia in humans, back to the mid-nineteenth century, when an infection was thought to cause heart disease, and was referred to as "tight chest" or clogged arteries. Chlamydia infections were first identified in man, in 1895; and again in 1930 (four people). Chlamydia trachoma was identified in man, in 1907, including conjunctivitis, cervicitis and non-specific urethritis, by three groups of authors, who reported their findings in 1909. Chlamydia psittacosis was identified in man, and named parrot fever, in 1917, after an outbreak of severe respiratory infection in Brazil. Airborne transmission of chlamydia agents was reported, in 1943 and 1944. Chlamydia was identified in Reiter's Syndrome, in 1966. Some abortions in woman were identified as related to chlamydia, in 1966, when subclinical chlamydia infections were recognized, without knowing the specific species of chlamydia. Chlamydia conjunctivitis was identified, in 1968. Chlamydia pneumonia was identified, in 1988.

Einstein said every reaction has an equal and opposite reaction; and for all matter, anti-matter must exist. Einstein believed his rules of physics were universal, and it was not possible for the laws of physics in the universe to differ from quantum physics in the body. Intracellular animal pathogens and parasites trigger responses and reactions arising from the war within, between the immune system and the animal pathogens. The war against the immortal intracellular pathogens generates redness, heat, swelling, pain, scarring, biofilm, pus, plaque, sticky, clogging, erosion, and atrophy, which causes a change in quantum physics. The immortal pathogens feed off the energy of the cell, alter the functioning of the cell, interfere with apoptosis, cause angiogenesis, increase TNF-alpha, and cause fatigue in the cells. Chronic fatigue and high TNF-alpha are present in virtually all chronic diseases. Quantum physics may only differ from the universal laws of physics when passive functions in the body change in response to chronic infection with animal pathogens. Intracellular animal pathogens may be the equivalent of anti-matter to healthy human cells.

Chlamydia Pneumonia

Chlamydia pneumonia was once thought to be rare. It is now recognized as a major cause of community-acquired pneumonia worldwide. Chlamydia pneumonia may be more prevalent in warm climates. Chlamydia pneumonia becomes an airborne epidemic every two to three years, and quickly spreads from person-to-person. Those acquiring repeated infection may have a less severe course, but are at greater risk of secondary adverse events and chronic disease. Chlamydia pneumonia can be acquired at any age, and the prevalence increases with age. Fifty percent of young adults and seventy-five percent of elderly patients have serologic evidence of previously having had chlamydia pneumonia.

Chlamydia pneumonia was first recognized to cause disease in humans, in 1963. Chlamydia pneumonia caused a community outbreak, in Taiwan, in 1965, which caused severe pneumonia and wheezing; however, the pathogen was thought to be an influenza virus, and was identified as the TWAR strain. Chlamydia pneumonia was isolated, in 1971, while researching eye disease; and was thought to be a new strain of trachoma, because trachoma was already known to cause conjunctivitis and other eye diseases. In 1978, an outbreak of chlamydia pneumonia occurred in Seattle, at the University of Washington. In 1985, advances in cell cultures and the electron microscope allowed researchers to distinguish chlamydia pneumonia, as a separate species from chlamydia trachoma. In 1988, chlamydia pneumonia was identified as a separate species of chlamydia; and in 1999, the full genome sequence of chlamydia pneumonia was published.

In "Chlamydophila" (multiple forms of chlamydia), the authors reported chlamydia pneumonia was first isolated in the 1960's; however, its role as a human pathogen was not fully defined until 1983, when it was recognized as an important cause of community acquired respiratory infections, pneumonia, and acute bronchitis. In 1991, chlamydia pneumonia was "associated" with asthmatic bronchitis, adult onset asthma, and wheezing. Chlamydia pneumonia can trigger wheezing; and generates abnormal proteins in chronic respiratory illness, which have been "associated" with asthma severity. Chlamydia pneumonia was hypothesized to be involved in maintaining or worsening diverse chronic conditions, such as COPD, asthma, atherosclerotic disease, Alzheimer's, and multiple sclerosis. Chlamydia pneumonia has also been "associated" with acute respiratory exacerbation in acute chest "syndrome", cystic fibrosis, chronic obstructive pulmonary disease, adult onset asthma, and sickle cell disease,

Chlamydia pneumonia begins as an acute respiratory infection. Chlamydia attacks a healthy cell using projections on the outside of the pathogen to penetrate the cell wall. Within a half hour of exposure, the elementary body has breached the cell wall and become intracellular. In twelve to twenty-four hours the elementary bodies have formed new reticulate bodies; and the reticulate bodies are multiplying by division, inside the cell. In twenty-four to forty hours the cell is full of reticulate bodies and forming new elementary bodies. Within forty-eight to seventy-two hours, new elementary bodies are released from the cell back into the body to invade new host cells. The process repeats itself in each new infected cell. Antibiotics are only active against the infectious/elementary body form. The developmental cycle of all species of chlamydia are similar, as depicted in the diagram for chlamydia trachoma.

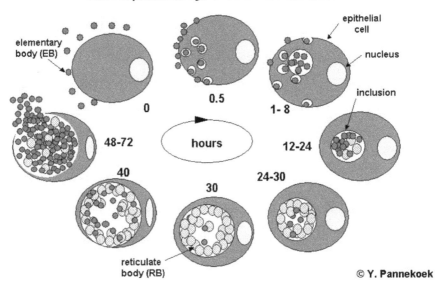

Life Cycle Trachoma by Pannekoek

Chlamydia pneumonia thrives and replicates in airway and vascular endothelium, smooth muscle cells, and macrophages. Researchers have found macrophages (white blood cells) adherent to endothelial cells. The professional immune cells come to the site of infection to attack the pathogen, and the chlamydia pneumonia then infects the immune cells, allowing the chlamydia pneumonia pathogen to spread via the immune system to new host cells. Chlamydia spreads through the bloodstream, smooth muscles, immune cells, and lymphatics, to preferred tissue and weak links. The pathogen may opportunistically attack any hospitable tissue to live and thrive. Chlamydia pneumonia may invade the heart and other hollow and spongy organ systems; attack endothelium in the vascular system; and can hide in cholesterol, plaque, and inclusion bodies.

Chlamydia pneumonia attacks endothelial tissue throughout the body; and has a predilection for attacking endothelium in the heart, lungs, brain and eyes. The endothelium is the inner layer of tissue in the vessels, which controls the movement of fluid in and out of the cells, tissue, and organs. Chlamydia pneumonia impairs the ability of the endothelial cells to function, deprives the cells of energy, and impairs the fluid balance and oxygen transport, in tissue and organs. Chlamydia pneumonia generates an immune reaction that causes biofilm, pus and plaque formation.

Many chronic diseases originate from endothelial dysfunction and plaque formation. Many existing syndromes and diseases are defined by endothelial dysfunction and/or plaque, including heart disease, coronary artery disease, and corneal disease. Some diseases and syndromes have even been named "endothelial dysfunction". Chlamydia attacks the endothelium of the cornea, causing "endothelial dysfunction", leading to corneal thinning; attacks the anterior chamber angle, causing loss of intraocular pressure control; and attacks the back of the eye, and the blood vessels in the eye, causing endothelial damage and plaque inside the vessels of the eye, reduced blood flow to the back of the eye, macular degeneration, clots, and other chronic eye diseases.

Chlamydia pneumonia hides and is sheltered from the immune system, by living inside the cells, inside inclusion cysts, in biofilm, and under plaque. The immune system is signaled to bring white blood cells to the site of the pathogen, and white blood cells generate inflammatory molecules and pus to fight the infection. The immune battle against chlamydia pneumonia in the heart and lungs causes pus, which becomes plaque, and which clogs the cardiovascular system. Pus develops in the lumen and the walls of vessels, and over time hardens to become plaque. The vessels create a harder cap over the pathogen and pus, to wall-off the infection. Plaque in the cardiovascular system is evidence of an immune system response to chlamydia pneumonia.

The immune system attacks the cells infected with chlamydia pneumonia, and the chlamydia pathogen infects the immune cells. Chlamydia replicates inside immune cells, and inside immune cells is capable of long-term survival. Chlamydia can hide and reproduce in mast cells, monocytes, macrophages, neutrophils, lymphocytes (T-cells), and plasma cells, which allows the pathogen to spread from the respiratory tract to new host cells, via the bloodstream. Infection of immune cells aids efficient propagation and immune protection of the chlamydia pneumonia organism, within the host.[42] Chlamydia pneumonia infected immune cells can breach the blood-tissue barriers and blood-brain barrier, and spread chronic infection to any tissue. In the brain, chlamydia pneumonia and its byproducts can cause Alzheimer's disease and brain cancers; and in the central nervous system can cause neurodegenerative diseases such as ALS and multiple sclerosis.

Chlamydia pneumonia gains control over apoptotic regulation in the cell, and impairs programmed cell death, by inhibiting apoptotic signaling cascades within monocytes, epithelial cells, and microglial cells. Loss of apoptosis causes a proliferation of weak copies of immortal cells, and each new cell is formed by division and infected with chlamydia. Infected cells continue to make weaker and weaker copies, rather than die and be replaced by new normal cells. Chlamydia pneumonia impairs T-cell apoptosis, which leads to the persistence of the chlamydia organism.

Loss of normal apoptosis is one of the hallmarks of cancer.[43] The hallmarks of cancer included self-sufficiency in growth signals, insensitivity to anti-growth signals, evading apoptosis, limitless replicative potential, sustained angiogenesis, and tissue invasion and metastasis, which are all consistent with chronic chlamydia infection. In 2011, the researchers updated the hallmarks of cancer to add the reprogramming of the energy of the cell,

---

[42] Rupp J, *et al*. 2009. Chlamydia Pneumonia Hides Inside Apoptotic Neutrophils to Silently Infect and Propagate in Macrophages. PloS Onei. Jun 23, 2009. 4(6). Doi: https://journals.plos.org/plosone/article?id=10.1371/journal.pone.0006020.

[43] Hanahan D and Weinberg RA. 2000. The Hallmarks of Cancer. Cell. 100(1): 57-70. (Jan 2000). Doi: https://doi.org/10.1016/S0092-8674(00)81683-9.

to support the continuous growth and proliferation of a cancer cell; and the ability of the cancer cells to evade immune detection.[44]

The hallmarks of many chronic diseases mimic the cellular properties of chlamydia infections. Chlamydia interferes with apoptosis—the loss of normal programmed cell death. Chlamydia takes control of cell function, and alters the basic cellular mechanism of producing energy. Chlamydia consumes the ATP energy made by the cell, and damages the ability of the cell to create ATP. Chlamydia damages the mitochondria, the molecules in the cell generating energy; and inhibits the development of macromolecules, which are large molecules formed intracellularly, critical for building cells and cell function. Chlamydia reprograms the energy metabolism to support continued growth and proliferation. Chlamydia causes sustained angiogenesis. When chlamydia causes destruction of the cell, debris is released into the system, in the form of fragments of the cell and abnormal proteins, to create new focus for an immune battle and chronic disease.

Proteins are the building blocks of all cells and the immune system. Chlamydia pneumonia generates abnormal proteins; and is capable of altering genes, when abnormal proteins and byproducts of the chronic infection attach to genes. Chlamydia pneumonia creates gene products (primarily heat shock protein-60), which lead to a cascade of cytokine release and up-regulations of adhesion molecules. Cells infected with chlamydia pneumonia are characterized by increased quantities of heat shock protein-60 (hsp 60), which is a highly immunogenic abnormal protein that has been "associated" with the pathogenesis of chronic inflammatory diseases. The chlamydia bacterium causes angiogenesis, homocystinemia, elevated TNF-alpha, and elevated levels of C-reactive protein, markers of inflammation. An emerging body of evidence, including the known host immune response to chlamydia hsp-60, links chlamydia pneumonia

---

[44] Hanahan D and Weinberg RA. 2011. Hallmarks of Cancer: The Next Generation. Cell. 144(5): 646-74. Doi:10.1016/j.cell.2011.02.013. PMID 21376230.

infection to a spectrum of chronic inflammatory diseases, asthma, chronic bronchitis, and COPD, long thought to be diseases of unknown etiology.[45]

Chlamydia pneumonia is difficult to culture, which has delayed recognition by doctors of the significance of chlamydia pneumonia and its relationship to chronic disease. Chlamydia can be detected through identification of chlamydia DNA, in a blood test known as a polymerase chain reaction test (PCR). Prior treatment with penicillin can cause a false-negative PCR test, and numerous heart studies have proven chlamydia pneumonia can be infecting and damaging the heart tissue, even when a patient has a negative PCR test. TNF-inhibitors can impair the ability of the immune system to fight the infection, by inhibiting the aggressive immune response of TNF-alpha against the pathogen.

Specific antibodies to chlamydia do not develop in most young children. PCR antibodies to chlamydia pneumonia have been found in 28% of children with pneumonia. A Swedish study assessed the prevalence of chlamydia pneumonia, in healthy children, compared to those with respiratory infection. The study found the PCR for chlamydia pneumonia was positive in forty-five percent of eighty-five sick children, and only five percent of ninety-three healthy children.[46]

Meta-analysis showed an "association" with atherosclerosis and coronary artery disease, and supports prior infection with chlamydia pneumonia creates an increased risk of lung cancer. Chlamydia pneumonia has been identified in atherosclerosis, by direct analysis of plaque. A meta-analysis of children admitted to the hospital for pneumonia showed an increased risk for developing leukemia, lymphoma and brain cancer, in the short and long term. Chlamydia pneumonia has also been found in the cerebral spinal fluid of patients with multiple sclerosis.

---

[45] Biosci F. 2002. Chlamydia Pneumonia as a Respiratory Pathogen. Front Biosci. Mar. 1, 2002. 7:e66-76. PMID: 11861211.

[46] Falck G, *et al.* Prevalence of Chlamydia pneumoniae in Healthy Children and in Children with Respiratory Tract Infections. Pediatric Infectious Disease Journal. Oct 1997. 16:549-554. Doi: https://europepmc.org/abstract/med/9194103.

In animal studies, rabbits exposed to chlamydia pneumonia developed respiratory symptoms, including bronchitis, pneumonia and a generalized vasculitis. Pigs exposed to chlamydia pneumonia developed acute respiratory infections, and in two weeks developed endothelial dysfunction in the lungs. Genetically altered mice, resistant to atherosclerosis, when infected with chlamydia pneumonia and fed a high fat diet, developed lesions of atherosclerosis in fourteen days. A high fat diet was thought to accelerate the effect of the chlamydia pneumonia infection.

Chlamydia Trachoma

Records discovered in China suggest chlamydia trachoma existed as far back as the 27th Century BC. Drawings from ancient Egypt depict treatment of eye disease that was likely trachoma. The Napoleonic Wars, from 1803 to 1815, spread sexually acquired trachoma throughout Europe, raising awareness of the infection. Historically, rape is part of war, and war fosters the spread of trachoma. In 1836, trachoma was isolated and described. In 1907, trachoma was described, but assumed to be a virus. A century after trachoma was isolated, the trachoma pathogen was recognized to cause vaginitis.

Wars, the sexual revolution, and birth control, have contributed to the worldwide spread of sexually transmitted disease; an increase in the global burden disease; and an increase in reproductive disease. Infection and re-infection with chlamydia trachoma causes destruction of tissue, thinning of tissue, a proliferation of fibroblasts, scarring, and chronic diseases. Temporary immunity may occur after a trachoma infection, but re-infection is inevitable in endemic areas.

Each year, ninety-two million new cases of trachoma are diagnosed. Trachoma is more common in dry and dusty climates, and is widespread in North Africa, the Middle East, and certain regions of Southeast Asia; with pockets of trachoma worldwide. The incidence of chlamydia trachoma infections in graduating high school seniors, in the United States, is alarming. In endemic areas in North Africa and the Middle East, most children are infected by age two, by *in utero* transmission or transmission by flies. Flies have been recognized to transmit infections for four-hundred years. The

Musca sorbens fly transmits ocular trachoma, by landing on the face of an infected person, and transmitting ocular trachoma to the next person. Musca Vetustissima flies are thought to transmit trachoma in the eyes, nose or mouth, from one person to another.

Chlamydia trachoma has many subtypes, known as serovars. Many strains of chlamydia trachoma have extra-chromosomal plasmids, meaning small DNA molecules of chlamydia trachoma, which are physically separated from the chromosomal DNA and can replicate independently outside the cell. Trachoma types Ab, B, Ba, and C attack the eyes, and can lead to blindness; and are not the same serovars as sexually acquired trachoma. Chlamydia trachoma in the eye can be transmitted by flies or hand-to-eye contact. Serovars D-K cause urethritis, pelvic inflammatory disease, ectopic pregnancy, neonatal pneumonia, and neonatal conjunctivitis. Chlamydia trachoma can ascend up the reproductive and genitourinary tracts to cause chronic disease in adjacent tissue, in the urinary tract and kidney. Serovars L1, L2, and L3 cause lymphogranuloma venereum, an infection in the lymphatic system which can also cause lymphogranuloma venereum conjunctivitis. The same serovars of chlamydia trachoma are transmitted within the family by close contact within the family, through direct contact, towels, and bedding.

Chlamydia trachoma has a strong predilection for attacking the reproductive system, the eyes, the central nervous system, and the joints. Chlamydia trachoma is one of the more dangerous forms of chlamydia, because it can attack both endothelium and epithelium. When infections attack the endothelium and epithelium, and infect the immune cells, the infection and the infectious cascade can progress rapidly to a chronic disease, as tissue is being damaged from both the inside out and the outside in, and the infection is spread by the immune system.

Chlamydia trachoma has long been known to be a sexually transmitted disease. Sexual activity is a risk for acquiring chlamydia trachoma, through a vulnerable portal. Observation of poor health and early demise in patients infected with sexually transmitted diseases, including trachoma, syphilis, and gonorrhea, may be the reason modern cultures developed a goal of one sexual partner. Observation of the relationship between sexually transmitted disease and cancer may be the reason cancer was at one time considered embarrassing. Cancer was thought to reveal sexual promiscuity.

An estimate of five to twenty-two percent of pregnant women have trachoma infection in their cervix. Sexually transmitted chlamydia trachoma, in women, can cause pelvic inflammatory disease and cervicitis, endometriosis, infertility, and cancer. Trachoma infection doubles the risk of ovarian cancer. Powder has long been "associated" with ovarian cancer, caused by indigestible particulate in the reproductive tract, which becomes a focus of cancer. Some powder is alleged to have contained asbestos, a known focus for cancer. Women who have trachoma and use powder in their private areas are at significantly increased risk for ovarian cancer.

In Sweden, a new variant of sexually acquired trachoma was discovered, in 2006.[47] The study reported an all-time high for chlamydia trachoma in Sweden, and estimated eight-thousand cases had never been reported. Forty-six of forty-eight specimens showed the identical new variant of chlamydia trachoma. Positive tests for the new variant, in different areas of Sweden, ranged from sixty-four percent to seventy-eight percent. The emergent mutant strain of chlamydia trachoma created a public health concern, when health officials noticed the trachoma infections caused reproductive disease, ectopic pregnancies, and infertility. The new variant of trachoma was rarely observed outside Sweden. The study reported concern the new variant of trachoma may escape detection, by routine tests; and did not address the consequences to men who acquired the new variant of chlamydia trachoma.

Chlamydia trachoma can be transmitted to a fetus, *in utero*. In a fetus who acquires the pathogen *in utero*, the chlamydia trachoma will proliferate in their body, for their whole life. Trachoma in the lungs induces thick mucus and low oxygen, which may cause chronic lung disease. Infection with chlamydia trachoma, chlamydia pneumonia, or chlamydia psittacosis, *in*

---

[47] Herrmann B, *et al*. 2008. Emergency and Spread of Chlamydia Trachomatis Variant, Sweden. Emerging Infectious Disease Journal. Sep 2008. Vol. 14(9). Doi:10.3201/eid1409.080153.

utero, causes chronic disease in the fetus, particularly diseases affecting the heart and lung. Chlamydia trachoma acquired in the birth canal causes neonatal conjunctivitis, nasopharyngitis, otitis media, and pneumonitis, which is why the standard is to treat newborns for trachoma eye infections. Cystic fibrosis is consistent with the presentation of chronic chlamydia trachoma, in the lung of a newborn or infant.

Men harbor trachoma in their prostate, and can pass trachoma infection to their sexual partners. Trachoma can cause chronic disease in men, including Peyronne's disease, chronic prostate disease, and prostate cancer. The highest incidence of testicular cancer occurs at ages seventeen to thirty, when males become sexually active and are exposed to chlamydia trachoma.

Chlamydia trachoma is the leading cause of blindness in the third world; and is on the World Health Organization (WHO) list of the most neglected diseases, requiring diagnosis and treatment. Chlamydia trachoma causes a variety of eye ocular surface diseases, ranging from inflammation in the follicles, inclusion cysts, inversion of the eyelashes, blood vessel formation, and corneal scarring. Chlamydia trachoma can invade the internal structures of the eye, and cause glaucoma, retinal damage, and blindness.

Chlamydia Psittaci

Chlamydia psittacosis (ornithosis) was first described in humans, in 1879, in Europe, after seven people were exposed to tropical birds and developed pneumonia. Outbreaks of psittacosis occurred in Germany, in 1879, and in other European countries. An outbreak occurred Paris, in 1890, which caused mortality in one-third of the victims. The European outbreaks were caused by contact with sick exotic birds. In 1917, in Brazil, an outbreak of chlamydia psittacosis pneumonia, led to the discovery of psittacosis in parrots, and the disease was named parrot fever. An outbreak of psittacosis also occurred in the United States, in Pennsylvania, in 1917, caused by birds stored in the basement of a Pennsylvania department store.[48]

---

[48] Ramsay, EC. 2003. The Psittacosis Outbreak of 1929-1930. Historical Perspective. Journal of Avian Medicine and Surgery. 17(4):235-237. 2003.

Chlamydia psittacosis has been referred to as avian chlamydia, because chlamydia psittacosis originated in birds. In animals, it has been called avian chlamydiosis and/or orinthosis. Chlamydia psittacosis was a cause of abortions in herds of dairy cattle; and was known as mammalian chlamydia psittaci abortion, until the feline and guinea pig strains were named as new species—chlamydia felis, and chlamydia caviae.

Chlamydia psittacosis is found in birds and cats. Birds are the primary reservoir for psittacosis. Psittacosis has spread worldwide, in pigeons, and other types of birds and mammals. Psittacosis has been found in parrots and pigeons worldwide; and has been found in doves, parakeets, canaries, cockatoos, cockatiels, sparrows, macaws, chickens, ducks, turkeys, and tortoises. Birds spread psittacosis to cats and mice, and mice can also spread psittacosis to cats.

Psittacosis and trachoma were originally thought to be part of the same genus of chlamydia. After electron microscopy, in the 1960's, psittacosis was recognized as a unique bacterium. Limitations on the ability to diagnose pathogens in prior decades, the merging and later divisions of chlamydia species, and reports in the scientific literature chlamydia was a virus or a different species of chlamydia, has led to confusion and delayed recognition of the importance of chlamydia infections in causing chronic disease. Some still refer to chlamydia psittacosis as a virus. The use of many different names for the pathogen; laboratories being unable to definitively identify the type of chlamydia; and laboratories limiting testing to only three main types of chlamydia, makes it difficult in retrospect to clarify or confirm the exact species described in some scientific reports.

In 1986, Thomas Grayston, M.D., thought he had found trachoma in the eye of a child with conjunctivitis, in Thailand. Psittacosis was previously known to occur in people with pet birds and poultry farmers; but was thought to only be acquired by animal-to-person transmission. Dr. Grayston identified the pathogen as a new species, psittacosis in the eye, which was a new variant of bird psittacosis. Dr. Grayston found fifty-percent of middle aged adults who had contact with poultry had been infected with psittacosis; and proved psittacosis is not just as a pathogen transmitted from bird-to-person, but also a pathogen transmitted from person-to-person.

Psittacosis has nine serovars, each highly correlated with the host bird species, and capable of being transmitted to humans and other animal species.[49] Psittacosis serovars are identified by the alphabet, and letters are added as new serovars are discovered. Chlamydia psittaci serovar A is endemic among psittacine birds (two toed birds), and causes sporadic disease in humans. Serovar C and D are recognized as occupational hazards for slaughterhouse workers and people in contact with birds. Serovar E, arises from avian hosts worldwide. Serovar M56 and WC were isolated during outbreaks in mammals. Psittacosis can change hosts frequently, and is capable of cross-species transmission. Psittacosis can undergo rapid recombination in a host and mix phenotypes, to generate new or more virulent strains.

Psittacosis has been found in humans and animals worldwide; and all strains of psittacosis are considered readily transmissible to humans. Psittacosis can be transmitted from animal-to-person; from animal-to-animal, such as birds-to-cats, birds-to-horses, birds-to-dogs, and birds-to-cows; from person-to-person; and by inhaling or ingesting particles of bird droppings. Chlamydia psittacosis can be transmitted to people from domestic and wild birds, and from other animals. Birds transmit psittacosis to other animals, and the animals then infect humans. Rodents acquire chlamydia psittacosis, which can then be transmitted from rodents to cats. Birds and rodents transmit psittacosis to cats, and cats transmit psittacosis to humans. Ownership of pet birds is considered a public health concern, due to the risk of transmission of psittacosis.[50] Seventy percent of human cases of psittacosis pneumonia had a known source of contact with birds or bird droppings.

---

[49] Pannekoek Y, *et al*. 2010. Multi Locus Sequence Typing of Chlamydia Reveals an Association between Chlamydia Psittaci Genotypes and Host Species. PLoS ONE. 2010. 5(12). Doi:10.1371/journal.pone.0014179.

[50] Lindmayer V. 2015. Psittacosis Associated with Pet Bird Ownership: A Concern For Public Health. JMM Case Reports 2. Doi: 10.1099/jmmcr.0.000085.

Psittacosis was previously considered an occupational disease of zookeepers and pet store owners; and outbreaks have occurred in veterinary centers. In Belgium, among people who had contact with birds, one-hundred-forty-four out of five-hundred-forty patients had evidence of psittaci infection; and parrots, canaries and pigeons created the highest risk. Feral pigeons present a substantial zoonotic risk, because feral pigeons are highly infected with psittacosis.[51] Zoonotic risk is not limited to direct contact with birds, and is also associated with a rural environment and outdoor activities, such as gardening and mowing lawns.[52] Psittacosis transmission to humans has been "associated" with cats, dogs, horses, livestock, and rodents; and outbreaks of psittacosis in dogs have been reported. Prior infection with psittacosis does not provide immunity to re-infection.

Periodically, psittacosis can become an airborne respiratory infection, transmitted in the community from person-to-person. Psittaci can also be transmitted by airborne particles from the droppings of infected birds and animals, including pigeons nesting on the rooftops.[53] Psittacosis in the respiratory tract requires aggressive treatment, or the psittacosis infection can be fatal or become a chronic disease. Untreated, acute psittacosis can cause acute respiratory failure and death, in up to one-third of adult cases

---

[51] Dovc A, *et al.* 2005. Long-term Study of Chlamydophilosis in Slovenia. Vet Res Commun. 2005. 29 (Suppl 1): 23–36; Heddema, *et al.* 2006. An outbreak of psittacosis Due to Chlamydophila Psittaci Genotype A in a Veterinary Teaching Hospital. J Med Microbiol. Nov 2006. 55 (Pt 11):1571-5. Doi: 10.1099/jmm.0.46692.0; Tanaka C, *et al.* 2005. Bacteriological Survey of Feces from Feral Pigeons in Japan. J Vet Med Sci. 2005. 67: 951–953. Doi: 10.1292/jvms.67.951; Harkinezhad T, *et al.* 2009. Prevalence of Chlamydophila Psittaci Infections in a Human Population in Contact with Domestic and Companion Birds. Journal of Medical Microbiology. 2009. 58:1207–1212. Doi: 10.1099/jmm.0.011379-0.

[52] Fenga C, *et al.*, 2007, Serologic Investigation of the Prevalence of Chlamydophila Psittaci in Occupationally-Exposed Subjects in Eastern Sicily. Ann Agric Environ Med. 2007. 14; 93-96. PMID 17655184; Tefler B, *et al.* 2005. Probable Psittacosis Outbreak Linked to Wild Birds. Emerg Infect Dis. Mar 2005. 11(3): 391-397. Doi:10.3201/eid1103.040601.

[53] *See* Mair-Jenkins J, *et al.* 2015. A Psittacosis Outbreak Among English Office Workers With Little or No Contact with Birds, August 2015. Doi: 10:ecurrents. outbreaks.b646c3bb24f0e3397183/81823bbca6. Online version published April 27, 2018. Doi: https://www.ncbi.nlm.nih.gov/pmc/articles/PMC5951689/.

with psittacosis pneumonia; and some hospitalized patients who receive treatment require ventilation support. Acute psittacosis causes a severe and prolonged respiratory infection and pneumonia, particularly in infants and children, immunocompromised adults, and laboratory workers. Chlamydia psittacosis respiratory infection will cause low oxygen concentration during the acute infection, and has the potential to cause asthma and exercise induced asthma.

Chronic psittacosis can attack both the epithelium and endothelium; and attack the lung, vessels, eye, lymphatics, and joints. Chronic chlamydia psittacosis, in the lymphatic system, spreads to other parts of the body via the lymphatics. Complications of psittacosis include endocarditis, pericarditis, myocarditis, arterial embolism, glomerulonephritis/tubule-interstitial nephritis, hemolytic anemia, disseminated intravascular coagulation, pancreatitis, reactive arthritis, transverse myelitis, meningoencephalitis, Guillain-Barre syndrome, and transmission of the psittacosis pathogen to a fetus.

Psittacosis has been "associated" with acute transverse myelitis, since 1996. Mycoplasma pneumonia, a small bacterium that attacks cell membranes, has also been associated with acute transverse myelitis. Acute transverse myelitis begins early in the course of the acute infection; and can resolve, improve, or be avoided, with prompt treatment of psittacosis or mycoplasma. However, without treatment with antibiotics, psittacosis or mycoplasma manifesting as transverse myelitis, can cause longstanding neurologic deficits and paralysis.

Chronic chlamydia psittacosis can invade the lymphatic system, and has been "associated" with lymphoma. Psittacosis has been found inside primary lymphoma tumors. Hodgkin's lymphoma, non-Hodgkin's lymphoma, MALT lymphoma, and lymphoma attached to breast implants, have all been "associated" with psittacosis. Lymphoma was reported in breast implant patients who have implants with rough surfaces, which allowed psittacosis in the lymphatic system to attach to the breast implant and caused lymphoma. Psittacosis can cause MALT lymphoma in the eye; and psittacosis has been found in patients with Waldenstrom "syndrome". Psittacosis has been "associated" with many different types of eye cancer, cancer in tissue around the eye, and with melanoma. Scientists have reported psittacosis is a common pathogen "associated" with cancer.

Psittacosis is endemic in pigeons in Italy, and psittacosis infects virtually one-hundred percent of the pigeons. Italy has one of the highest rates of lymphoma in the world, and the rate of lymphoma has been steadily increasing, since 1996, contrary to the trend of reducing rates of lymphoma in developed countries.[54] Italy has a higher rate of lymphoma, rare cancers, and eye cancers; and is experiencing an increased rate of melanoma, despite the darker skin of Italians. The Italian patients with Sjögren's syndrome, parotid gland marginal zone B-cell lymphoma, and MALT lymphoma, were found to have a high rate of chlamydia psittacosis infection.[55] Pigeons are flying rodents, and should never be encouraged to interact with people. People should avoid contact with pigeons and pigeon droppings, which can cause a variety of chronic diseases, including blinding eye diseases and cancer.

In the Middle East, including the United Arab Emirates (UAE), bird handling is part of the culture. In the UAE, primary extra-nodal non-Hodgkin's lymphoma and sarcoidosis occur at a higher rate. The UAE also has an abundance of eye diseases, including glaucoma and loss of vision; likely caused by psittacosis and/or psittacosis combined with chlamydia trachoma, which is also known to be widespread in the Middle East. In non-Hodgkin's lymphoma, the risk of infection, morbidity and mortality was increased in the presence of co-infections, such as Epstein Barr Virus.[56] Co-infections with other virulent pathogens, including trachoma and

---

[54] Massimilliano S, *et al.* 2014. Epidemiological Overview of Hodgkin Lymphoma Across the Mediterranean Basin. Mediterr J of Hematol Infect Disease. 2014. 6 (1). Doi: 10.4084/MJHID.2014.048.

[55] Fabris M, *et al.* 2014. High Prevalence of Chlamyophila Psittaci Subclinical Infection in Italian Patients with Sjogren's syndrome, Parotid Gland Marginal Zone B-Cell Lymphoma, and MALT Lymphoma. Clin Exp Rheumatol. Jan-Feb 2014. 32 (1) 61-65. PMID: 24447326.

[56] Castella A, *et al.* 2001. Pattern of Malignant Lymphoma in the United Arab Emirates - A Histopathologic and Immunologic Study in 208 Native Patients. Acta Oncologica. 2001. 40(5): 660-664. (2001) Doi: 10.1080/028418601750444231.

immortal viruses, can accelerate the development of chronic disease in patients with psittacosis.

In 2002, an outbreak of psittacosis, in the Blue Mountain region of Australia, was linked to wild birds. In 2004, a psittacosis outbreak occurred at a veterinary teaching hospital, when psittacosis was transmitted from infected birds-to-people; causing the death of thirty percent of the victims, before the laboratory identified the psittacosis pathogen. The remaining victims were given antibiotic treatment for psittacosis and survived.[57] Dr. Heddema also documented the prevalence of chlamydia psittacosis in birds, in the Netherlands, and in hospitalized patients.

Horses acquire psittacosis from birds, by cross-species transmission; and then transmit psittacosis infection to people. In 1982, chlamydia psittaci was isolated from the lungs of a horse with a fatal respiratory infection. When the psittaci pathogen was introduced into a Shetland pony intrathecally, the pony developed local and metastatic lesions in the lung and liver. Post-mortem the pony showed microscopic evidence of generalized chlamydia psittacosis infection. Lesions of interstitial pneumonia and focal hepatic necrosis were observed, and chlamydia psittaci was isolated from lung tissues. The conclusion was chlamydia psittaci can become invasive and produce generalized infection.[58] In 1992, nasal and conjunctival swabs of three hundred horses showed fifteen (five percent), were positive for chlamydia psittacosis, without evidence of disease.[59]

In 2014, a cluster of respiratory infections occurred at a veterinary school in New South Wales, in Wagga Wagga, Australia. Five of the nine people exposed to the aborted fetal membranes of a horse became ill with respiratory and flu like symptoms, and two were hospitalized. The foal

---

[57] Heddema, *et al.* 2006. An Outbreak of Psittacosis Due to Chlamydophila Psittaci Genotype A in a Veterinary Teaching Hospital. J Med Microbiol. Nov 2006. 55 (Pt 11):1571-5. Doi: 10.1099/jmm.0.46692.0.

[58] McChesney S, *et al.* 1982. Chlamydia Psittaci Induced Pneumonia in a Horse. Cornell Vet. 1982. 72:92-97.

[59] Mair T and Wills J. 1992. Chlamydia Psittaci Infection in Horses: Results of a Prevalence Survey and Experimental Challenge. Vet. Res. May 9, 1992. 130(19):417-9. Doi: https://dx.doi.org/10./1136/vr.130.19.417.

died a week later, and the mare tested positive for chlamydia psittacosis. Psittacosis in horses has been "associated" with abortions in mares. The human cases of psittacosis all had arisen from exposure to the infected equine fetal membranes, and contact with birds was not associated with the illnesses. The exposure was believed to be via airborne transmission or direct inoculation from the fetal membranes of the infected horse.[60] In 2015, a cluster of psittacosis was identified in office workers, who had no contact with birds. Investigation found the source of the psittacosis was pigeons nesting on the roof.[61]

Chlamydia psittacosis infects mucosal cells and macrophages, in the respiratory tract. The pathogen can become localized in epithelial cells and macrophages of most organs, the conjunctiva, and the gastrointestinal tract. Psittacosis pathogens can become a host cell for other bacteria and viruses, which can replicate inside the psittaci pathogen. When psittaci serves as a host to other bacteria and viruses, it allows the parasitic pathogens to move throughout the body with the psittaci pathogen, in the blood or lymphatic system.

The Spanish Flu pandemic started in January 1918, and ended in December 1920. World War I lasted from July 1914, to November 1918. The Spanish Flu pandemic was attributed to soldiers returning from World War I, bringing home the H1N1 form of influenza. The H1N1 influenza virus is an influenza-A virus, which is an avian influenza originating in birds. The Spanish Flu pandemic killed many millions of people worldwide, and up to one-third of the population.

The Spanish Flu pandemic came in three waves, with each wave becoming deadlier. The Spanish Flu caused a W-pattern of death, with a greater rate

---

[60] Chan J, *et al*. 2017. An Outbreak of Psittacosis at a Veterinary School Demonstrating a Novel Source of Infection. One Health. June 2017. Vol. 3: 29-33. Doi: https://doi.org/10.1016/j.onehelt.2017.02.003; Weese S. 2017. Psittacosis From A Horse. Worms & Germs Blog. Aug 3, 2017. Doi: wormsandgermsblog.com.

[61] Mair-Jenkins J, *et al*. 2015. A Psittacosis Outbreak Among English Office Workers With Little or No Contact with Birds, August 2015. Doi: 10:ecurrents.outbreaks. b646c3bb24f0e3397183/81823bbca6. Online version published April 27, 2018. Doi: https://www.ncbi.nlm.nih.gov/pmc/articles/PMC5951689/.

of death in young adults and pregnant women, than in children and the elderly. Influenza viruses normally cause higher rates of mortality in the very young and very old, in a "U" pattern of mortality and age. High rates of spontaneous abortion and preterm birth were reported; and one study showed greater than fifty-percent of pregnancies, in which the pregnant woman had influenza and pneumonia, were not carried successfully to term.[62] Scientists hypothesized the high mortality in young adults, during the Spanish Flu pandemic, was because of a high level of heat shock proteins, causing a stronger immune response to the infection in young adults.

A psittacosis outbreak occurred in Pennsylvania, in 1917, related to birds stored in the basement of a department store. Psittacosis was identified in Brazil, in 1917, and exotic birds shipped around the world spread the disease. Psittacosis was identified in the United States, during the 1929-1930 psittacosis outbreak. The psittacosis outbreak of 1929-1930 started with pet parrots, in Annapolis, Maryland, and spread to twelve countries; however, the specific serovar was never identified.

Psittacosis respiratory infection causes a high rate of mortality in middle aged adults, and a greater mortality rate in young adults than in children, in a W-shaped pattern of mortality. Psittacosis can cause mortality in one-third of infected adults; and cause death in up to eighty percent, in pregnant women. In the 1929-1930 psittacosis outbreak, no one under the age of thirty died. The same pattern and rate of mortality occurred in numerous epidemics of psittacosis. The mortality rates of untreated psittacosis in middle aged adults and pregnant women is consistent with the death rates and pattern of deaths, during the Spanish Flu pandemic.

The Spanish Flu, of 1918, also spread to become an epidemic, in swine. Humans or birds transmitted the H1N1 virus to swine, who had no immunity; thus the H1N1 virus spread rapidly and became an epidemic among pigs. Swine are common vectors for influenza, and are capable of harboring infections and creating new mixed infections and new serovars,

---

[62] Rasmussen S. 2008. Pandemic Influenza and Pregnant Women. Emerging Infectious Diseases. 2008. Vol. 14(1). www.cdc.gov/eid.

which can then be transmitted to other animals and people. Pigs are susceptible to avian, human and swine influenza viruses, and may be infected with influenza viruses from different species (e.g., ducks and humans) at the same time. Pigs can be infected with both human and avian influenza viruses, in addition to swine influenza viruses, and may exhibit signs of acute illness similar to humans, such as a cough, fever and runny nose. Pigs could have developed or harbored psittacosis at the same time the pigs became infected with H1N1; and/or an epidemic of psittacosis could have spread from birds to pigs, which was mis-identified as a virus or influenza. The H1N1 virus may have infected pigs and mixed with psittacosis, and rapidly spread with increasing virulence. It is possible the genes of the H1N1, and the psittacosis pathogens mixed and created a new more virulent pathogen in pigs, during the pandemic.[63]

The H1N1 avian strain of influenza re-emerged, in the summer of 2009, and was traced to swine in Mexico. The Swine Flu epidemic, of 2009, was caused by an *avian* influenza virus in a pig, not an influenza virus originating in pigs. The Swine Flu pandemic, of 2009, was caused by the H1N1 bird flu virus, which had been transmitted to pigs, during the Spanish Flu pandemic; and was transmitted to humans from pigs, in 2009. The Swine Flu epidemic, in 2009, was estimated to have caused between 151,700 and 575,400 deaths, and caused a higher rate of death among pregnant women. The Swine Flu epidemic did not cause the same high rate of mortality overall, a higher rate of death in young adults, or a W-shaped pattern of mortality in the population, as occurred during the Spanish Flu pandemic. The different pattern of deaths and total deaths during the Spanish Flu pandemic, and the Swine Flu epidemic caused by the same bird influenza virus, suggests other pathogens may have contributed to the high rate and pattern of deaths during the Spanish Flu pandemic.

The high mortality in the Spanish Flu pandemic of 1918-1920; high rate of mortality in young adults and pregnant women; the corresponding epidemic of Spanish Flu in swine; the corresponding outbreak of psittacosis

---

[63] *See* Center for Disease Control and Prevention. National Center for Immunization and Respiratory Diseases. April 12, 2017. Doi: www.cdc.gov/flu/about/viruses/transmission.htm.

in Brazil and Pennsylvania, in 1917; and the lower mortality from the H1N1 virus in 2009, suggest a co-morbid outbreak of psittacosis pneumonia may have played a role in the high rate of deaths and pattern of deaths, during the Spanish Flu pandemic. Birds shipped around the world continued to spread psittacosis; and the outbreak, in Pennsylvania, could have persisted in the population when the Spanish Flu struck Philadelphia, in July of 1918, causing significant mortality.

The H1N1 bird influenza virus and chlamydia psittacosis could have been co-infections, or co-epidemics, spreading in the population through humans and birds. Co-infection and co-existing epidemics, of H1N1 *and* chlamydia psittacosis, would explain the high rate of mortality in the Spanish Flu pandemic, a high level of heat shock proteins, the high rate of fetal demise and death among pregnant women, the increasing virulence during three waves of the pandemic; and the "W" pattern of deaths among middle aged adults, from 1918-1920, that did not occur in 2009. The H1N1 virus may have become a bacteriophage of psittacosis, and became a pandemic of dual pathogens during the Spanish Flu pandemic, creating a high rate of mortality and premature demise. Those who survived the Spanish Flu were later found to have a ten-year reduction in life expectancy, which is consistent with a shortened life expectancy from an immortal pathogen such as psittacosis.

Scientists were not able to distinguish influenza and psittacosis, during the Spanish Flu pandemic. Microbiology identification and specificity was not developed, and even in the 1929-1930 outbreak of psittacosis, in the United States, scientists still referred to psittacosis as a virus. Psittacosis may have been overlooked or misidentified during the Spanish Flu pandemic, in patients and swine, because psittacosis (parrot fever) was a newly discovered pathogen, scientists had limited ability to identify specific pathogens, and scientists were not aware, in 1918 or 1929, that chlamydia psittacosis could be spread from person-to-person or from animals-to-person, other than from parrots.

The incidence of psittacosis in the adult population has been estimated to be as low as one percent, which seems a vast under-estimation. Dr.

Grayston found fifty percent of adults who had contact with poultry had evidence of a prior psittacosis infection. Researchers found psittacosis in a high percent of Italian patients with numerous types of cancers. Multiple types of lymphoma are caused by psittacosis; and retinitis pigmentosa, eye cancer and transverse myelitis can be caused by psittacosis. Scientists have postulated psittacosis may be responsible for one-fifth of pneumonia cases. Psittacosis must be more prevalent than recognized, because of the prevalence of birds and other animals that harbor psittacosis and transmit psittacosis to humans, the high number of cats and a high rate of cat ownership, and prevalence of chronic diseases in humans that are caused by psittacosis.

Psittacosis is not often recognized in humans, or recognized to cause chronic disease. The true prevalence of human psittacosis infection is unknown, because psittacosis is not being diagnosed in respiratory infections, lymphoma, melanoma, autoimmune diseases, sarcoidosis, diseases of the eye, or other chronic diseases known to be caused by psittacosis. Physicians do not take a history to know the patient's risk for chlamydia psittacosis, do not test patients for chlamydia psittacosis, and seldom diagnose chlamydia psittacosis, even in patients with pneumonia, lymphoma, melanoma, sarcoidosis, eye disease, eye cancer, recurrent miscarriages, fetal demise, or transverse myelitis. Implementation of a model to diagnose and treat chlamydia psittacosis in medical practice is slow, as it has been for other forms of chlamydia.

Chlamydia Abortus, Chlamydia Suis, Chlamydia Pecorum, Chlamydia Muridarum

A former single genius of chlamydia has now been divided into at least nine species (abortus, caviae, felis, muridarum, pecorum, pneumoniae, psittaci, *suis*, trachoma); and two additional species have been discovered (avium and gallinacean), and are widespread in some species of birds. New species continue to be defined, and new serovars of each species continue to be discovered and reported. Some species are almost identical, and require close observation to distinguish the correct species, such as chlamydia trachoma and chlamydia muridarum, which appear more than ninety-five percent identical.[64] Transmission to humans and the pathogenic potential of new species is not well understood; however, knowledge of transmission and the pathogenic potential of other chlamydia species, to any cell with a nucleus; and knowledge other chlamydia species cause the same diseases in animals and humans, suggest new species can similarly infect humans and cause chronic disease.

Chlamydia abortus is a sexually transmitted disease in animals, including sheep, goats, and cows. In sheep, goats, and cows, chlamydia abortus causes late-term abortions, miscarriages, stillbirths, prematurity, birth defects, and weak offspring. The male animal can acquire the infection and transmit the infection to the female animal. Chlamydia abortus can be transmitted from animal-to-animal, causing abortions throughout a herd. Ewes seldom abort more than once, but remain persistently infected and shed chlamydia abortus from their reproductive tract, for two to three days before and after ovulation. In non-pregnant animals, chlamydia abortus becomes a latent infection, possibly harbored in lymphoid tissue; and in sheep, the primary infection may become established in the tonsil, and disseminated by blood or the lymphatics to other organs.

Elementary bodies for chlamydia abortus have been found in the placenta and in the vaginal discharge of infected animals. The placenta may be necrotic, reddish brown; and thickened, and in some areas covered by exudates. Chlamydia abortus is transmitted to the fetus; and the offspring may develop ascites, lymphadenopathy, liver congestion or lung disease. Chlamydia abortus is thought to be a cause of EAE (experimental autoimmune encephalomyelitis), which describes inflammation of the brain in an infected animal.

Contamination of the environment by an infected animal can act as a source for transmission of chlamydia abortus to humans. A human case of chlamydia abortus was reported after isolation of chlamydia abortus from the patient's sputum, which confirmed chlamydia abortus can attack the lung of humans and cause atypical pneumonia. The patient developed respiratory

---

[64] Greenwood D. *et al (eds)*. 2012. <u>Medical Microbiology</u>. 18th Ed. 2012. Elsevier Ltd. Chlamydia. D. Mabey and Peeling RW.

symptoms, breathing problems, and a high fever. Chlamydia abortus attacked the patient's villi, in the inner lining of the lung, causing thickening of the lung tissue, typical of some "syndromes" involving the lung.

Most recognized human cases of chlamydia abortus occurred in pregnant women, who developed a life-threatening illness. Transmission occurred after contact with livestock who had recently given birth, or in a research setting. The United Kingdom recognizes the problem of chlamydia abortus in sheep and goats; and has reported one or two cases per year of chlamydia abortus in pregnant women. The fetus survived in only a few cases, after being delivered by cesarean section. Pregnant women are advised not to work with pregnant sheep, particularly if abortions are occurring in the animals.

Chlamydia abortus can be passed from mother-to-fetus in an animal, and can likely also be passed from mother-to-fetus in a human. Doctors fail to consider chlamydia abortus in women with infertility, recurrent miscarriages, late term fetal demise, an infant with a weak constitution, or birth defects; or in an infant with abnormalities consistent with chlamydia abortus, including abnormalities in the brain, persistent lung infections, liver abnormalities or lymphadenopathy. Too often doctors dismiss miscarriages as a genetic problem in the fetus; and fail to check the mother or the infant for chlamydia pathogens.

The prevalence of chlamydia abortus in humans is unknown. No commercially available testing is available for chlamydia abortus, and chlamydia abortus appears similar to chlamydia trachoma on serological testing. Doctors fail to consider the risk of patient contact with sheep, goats, and cows, in settings such as farming, fairs, or petting zoos; and do not inquire into a history of contact with pets or livestock. Any woman who suffers infertility, miscarriages, late-term abortions, stillbirths, prematurity, birth defects, weak offspring miscarriages, or fetal death, should be asked for any history of animal contact; and tested for chlamydia abortus and all other forms of chlamydia that attack the reproductive tract or fetus, or which are known to cause the abnormalities that developed in the fetus.

Chlamydia pecorum strains are serologically and pathogenically diverse. The word "pecorum" comes from the Latin word for flocks of sheep or herds of cattle. Chlamydia pecorum has been found in herds of sheep and cattle. Prior to 1993, chlamydia pecorum strains were thought to be part of the chlamydia psittaci species, sharing many similar phenotypic characteristics, including formation of inclusion bodies, the absence of glycogen in inclusions, and resistance to sulfadiazine. The first isolation of chlamydia pecorum was reported by McNutt and Waller, in cattle with sporadic encephalomyelitis.

Chlamydophila pecorum has only been isolated from mammals. Chlamydia pecorum has been found in cows, sheep, koalas (marsupials), and pigs. Chlamydia pecorum is commonly found in the intestine and vaginal mucus of infected cows and sheep, and the animal can appear healthy. In cattle, chlamydia pecorum colonization begins at three months of age, when young animals start to graze. The persistence of chlamydia pecorum strains in the intestine and vaginal mucus of ruminants may cause a long-lasting sub-clinical infection. Chlamydia pecorum can be transmitted from animals to humans, but is thought to be rare, in part due to lack of consideration of the pathogen and lack of blood tests to diagnose chlamydia pecorum, in humans.

In animal species, chlamydia pecorum has been associated with conjunctivitis, encephalomyelitis, enteritis, polyarthritis, pneumonia and abortion. Chlamydia pecorum, in cattle, has been "associated" with conjunctivitis, arthritis, and orchitis (inflammation of the testes). Chlamydia pecorum in cattle causes sporadic bovine encephalomyelitis, polyarthritis, enteritis, vaginitis, endometritis, and pneumonia; and can reduce fertility. Chlamydia pecorum was found in symptomatic flocks of Australian sheep with conjunctivitis and polyarthritis.[65] Chlamydia pecorum was recovered from the joint fluid of a sheep with polyarthritis. In pigs, chlamydia pecorum has been associated with pneumonia,

---

[65] Jelocnik M, *et al.* 2014. Evaluation of the Relationship Between Chlamydia Pecorum Sequence Types and Disease Using a Species-Specific Multi-Locus Sequence Typing Scheme (MLST). Vet Microbiol. 2014. 7:174 (1-2): 214-22. Doi: 10.1016/j.vetmic.2014.08.018.

polyarthritis, pleuritis, pericarditis and abortion. In sea lions, chlamydia pecorum causes premature birth and abortions. (Sea lions can also harbor chlamydia trachoma and chlamydia psittacosis.)

Chlamydia pecorum is common in koalas. In koalas, chlamydia pecorum is considered the most important infectious disease, and the most pathogenic.[66] In the koala, chlamydia pecorum causes conjunctivitis, urinary tract disease, reproductive tract disease, infertility, and death. Young koalas have a high level of chlamydia pecorum, and fifty-eight percent of the infections involve both ocular and urogenital infections, suggesting mother-offspring transmission is a major transmission route among koalas. In male koalas, chlamydia pecorum causes prostatitis. Chlamydia pecorum may reduce the number of offspring in endangered animals.

The study of the genome of chlamydia pecorum in koalas found unique serovars of chlamydia pecorum, most similar to chlamydia pneumonia.[67] Koalas are also heavily infected with chlamydia pneumonia; and thus, may have co-infections with different forms of chlamydia, and harbor chlamydia pneumonia and chlamydia pecorum. The study suggests the adaptation and evolution of chlamydia pneumonia in koalas, co-infections with other types of chlamydia, misidentification of chlamydia pecorum, or giving a known type of chlamydia a different name when found in an animal. Co-infections with chlamydia pneumonia and chlamydia pecorum, and potentially other immortal co-infections, is decreasing the well-being and health of koalas, creating a genetic cost, and creating the danger of extinction of koalas.

Chlamydia *suis* is endemic in domestic pigs, in Europe, and is the predominant chlamydia species found in fecal samples of pigs. Chlamydia *suis* causes inclusion cysts; and conjunctivitis, enteritis, pneumonia and reproductive failure in pigs. The pathogen is similar to various chlamydia

---

[66] Wikipedia. Chlamydia Pecorum. Doi: en.wikipedia.org/wiki /Chlamydophila pecorum - cite_note-6.

[67] *See* Bachmann N, *et al*. 2014. Comparative Genomics of Koala, Cattle and Sheep Strains of Chlamydia Pecorum. BMC Genomics. 2014. 15(1): 667. Doi: 10.1186/1471-2164-15-66.

trachoma serogroups, and has been documented in pig farmers, based on pharyngeal and rectal samples. Chlamydia *suis* DNA was found in pigs on all farms tested, and eight of nine farmers were positive in at least one anatomical site. Nine porcine (pig) chlamydia *suis* isolates were retrieved, originating on three farms. Drug resistant strains of chlamydia *suis* were also isolated.[68] Chlamydia *suis* is not recognized and diagnosed in humans, and no blood testing is available for chlamydia *suis* in humans; however, the evidence of chlamydia *suis* found in farmers suggests it is a pathogen capable of infecting humans and causing chronic disease similar to the chronic diseases caused in animals.

Chlamydia muridarum was found in a colony of mice with pneumonia. Scientists deny chlamydia muridarum can be transmitted to humans. Hantavirus from mice is transmitted to humans, and virtually all other forms of chlamydia can be transmitted from animals-to-humans; thus, chlamydia muridarum is likely transmissible to humans. The reason scientists believe chlamydia muridarum is not transmitted to humans may be because doctors do not test for chlamydia muridarum, or study the effects of chlamydia muridarum, in humans.

A recent study of pathogens in the mice in New York City showed the mice were crawling with pathogens; and carried new pathogens and drug resistant pathogens, which were formerly unknown. The scientists did not know if the pathogens posted a risk to humans; or consider whether the mice contracted these pathogens from the inhabitants, or the mice independently carried new forms of pathogens and drug-resistant pathogens.[69] The fact the drug-resistant pathogens in mice matched the drug-resistant pathogens in New York hospitals suggests the mice may have contracted pathogens from the people.

---

[68] De Puysseleyr L, *et al.* 2017. Assessment of Chlamydia *Suis* Infection in Pig Farmers. Transbound Emerg Dis. June 2017. 64(3): 826-833. Doi: 10.1111/tbed.12446. Epub Nov 18, 2015.

[69] Weintraub K. 2018. Trolobites. New York Mice Are Crawling With Dangerous Bacteria and Viruses. New York Times. (Health) April 17, 2018. Doi: nyti.ms/2H6gXat.

CHAPTER 6

THE INFECTIOUS CASCADE
OF PARASITIC DISEASE

The infectious cascade is the adverse processes between acute infection and chronic infection, and between chronic infection and chronic disease. The infectious cascade is a process which begins with acute infection with immortal pathogens and/or parasites, and the pathogens then cause a cascade of adverse responses and reactions in the body and by the immune system, which cause the development of chronic disease. The infectious cascade starts with acute infection, the immune cells become infected and develop impaired immune function, the immune cells spread the pathogen to new tissue, fungus develops, and we acquire new acute infections, in the march toward chronic disease.

Immortal pathogens invade the body, attack the host cell, and become intracellular. The pathogens replicate inside the cell, and release new infectious forms of the pathogen into the body. The pathogens spread through the blood, lymphatics, smooth muscles, and immune cells; and by direct migration to adjacent tissue. How acute immortal infections are treated and with what antibiotics can alter the course of the infectious cascade. Penicillin changes the shape of the chlamydia reticulate bodies, extends the life cycle of the pathogen, increases the number of elementary bodies produced, and causes a false-negative chlamydia blood test.

The chlamydia pathogen lives off the energy produced by the cell; and changes the ability of the cell to create energy, creating cellular, organ and body fatigue. Immortal pathogens damage oxygen transport into the cell, damage sugar transport into the cells, cause inflammation, generate inflammatory markers, and generate and release abnormal proteins and cell fragments. Intracellular pathogens produce HSP 60 and LPS, inducing cell wall adhesion. The pathogen impairs normal apoptosis, and generates infinite weak replicas of infected cells. When the energy of the cell is depleted, the pathogen consumes sugar and causes fermentation. Depletion of ATP, use of sugar for energy, and fermentation lead to development of fungus, and makes a more hospitable environment for parasites to attack and thrive. Fungus hides pathogens and parasites, clogs the digestive system, exacerbates malabsorption, and blocks the functioning of good bacteria. Parasitic infection aggravates fungal development and loss of key nutrients, when parasites clog and compete for nutrients in the intestine.

TNF-alpha is generated by the immune cells, when the immune system is unable to eradicate the pathogens. Monocytes are large white blood cells in the bloodstream, and macrophages are in extracellular fluid that bathes tissue. Monocytes generate macrophages, and TNF-alpha is primarily generated by macrophages; however, any immune cell can generate TNF-alpha. Macrophages are scavengers, consuming dangerous cells, bacteria, and abnormal proteins that may present a threat to health. TNF-alpha is intended to fight cancer cells, and destroy cells which could become cancer. Macrophages infected with chlamydia produce interleukin 6, and infected T-lymphocytes produce interleukin-6 and a higher level of TNF-alpha. TNF-alpha is a more aggressive immune response, with a higher level of inflammation. Generation of TNF-alpha against chlamydia pathogens suggests the immune system attacks chlamydia as if it was cancer.

The pathogens are covered in abnormal proteins, which confuse the immune system. The intracellular pathogen creates abnormal proteins inside the host cell, as sticky substances cause the proteins inside the cell to fold in abnormal patterns. Abnormal proteins are dispersed and can lodge in locations which clog or cause tissue to stick together, and become a new focus for immune system attack. Abnormal proteins created by the pathogen can attach to genes, and cause a genetic abnormality.

The pathogen triggers the immune cells to mount an attack, with immune cells specific to the pathogen; and the immune cells fighting the pathogen become infected and spread the pathogen in the body. The pathogens can replicate in the immune cells, and infected immune cells cause reduced immunity to new infections, parasitic infection, and fungus, which leads to an increase in the total infectious burden. Co-infections work synergistically to accelerate and cause chronic disease.

Parasitic disease can be the primary infection, or an opportunistic infection after a patient develops reduced immunity from chronic chlamydia. Parasites can initiate the infectious cascade, and decline in the immune system; or be the opportunistic result of reduced immunity from immortal infections and fungal development. Parasites make a person more vulnerable to chlamydia, and chlamydia makes a person vulnerable to parasites. A person can be infected and re-infected from pets and other animals, and have more than one type of parasite.

The longstanding war between the immune system and immortal pathogens causes an infectious cascade, which leads to new infections with immortal pathogens and parasites. The end result is chronic infection, an impaired immune response, and chronic disease.

Intestinal Parasites (Giardia, Cryptosporidiosis, Amoebas)

Dr. Merchant's belief chronic infection causes chronic disease began with giardia lamblia, an intestinal parasite. He observed people who drank contaminated water had bloated bellies, and the appearance of bloated bellies was related to chronic disease. Dr. Merchant wrote about the health consequences of chronic giardia, in 1988, including the infectious cascade of malabsorption, dysbiosis (imbalance in the microbiome), lowered immunity, damage to mental health, and chronic disease. Dr. Merchant's thinking about chronic infection causing chronic disease expanded, to include chlamydia, other types of parasites, toxoplasmosis, and h-pylori, but the principle chronic infection causes chronic disease has not changed.

In the South Valley, Dr. Merchant advocated for clean water, to reduce the burden of water borne parasitic disease. Dr. Merchant believed the human cost of endemic chronic intestinal disease was far greater than the cost of extending city water lines. The greatest impact on extending life and reducing disease has been to supply clean water, with indoor plumbing;

and adequate housing to avoid mosquito borne diseases. It was astonishing the resistance and ostracism Dr. Merchant endured because he advocated for clean water, and the denial by the medical community that water could cause acute or chronic disease; particularly considering Hippocrates, the Father of Medicine, knew drinking contaminated water caused disease 2,500 years ago.

When Dr. Merchant began to study parasitic disease, and the role of chronic infection in chronic disease, he wondered to himself, "Why was this not taught in medical school?" Parasitic diseases are largely ignored in medical training. Parasitology training is limited and waning, and inconsistently taught in medical schools and residency programs. Parasitology may be part of an undergraduate or graduate course; however, medical schools typically include less than thirty hours of didactic training in parasites, and in some medical schools less than ten hours. Medical schools do not offer clinical training in parasitology. Limited parasitology training is provided in residency and fellowship training, in gastroenterology, internal medicine, pediatrics and infectious disease. Obstetrical residency training in parasitology is limited to toxoplasmosis. In practice, doctors seldom have the time to devote to a patient, or the awareness of chronic parasitic disease, necessary to make a diagnosis of parasites. If intestinal complaints require more than five minutes of the doctor's time, the patient is referred to a gastroenterologist, who also seldom diagnoses parasitic infections.

All living organisms get parasites. Parasites are part of nature, and part of living and dying. Parasites are common in all mammalian species, and are some of the most neglected diseases in the United States. Many types of parasites exist throughout the world, and different types of parasites are endemic in different parts of the world. The CDC and WHO recognize parasitic diseases are common, and neglected diagnoses; and list antiparasitic medications as essential drugs. The failure to diagnose parasitic infections has limited the understanding of the importance of parasitic infection in chronic disease. The failure to diagnose and treat parasitic infection has caused the public to lose important antiparasitic drugs, which were removed from the market because the drugs were not used frequently enough. Antiparasitic drugs are still available; however, have become extremely expensive.

The principle that chronic infection causes chronic disease remains the same, regardless of the type of immortal infection; and regardless of whether the chronic infection is an immortal intracellular infection, a parasitic infection, or both. Chronic parasitic infection can cause different manifestations of disease in different patients; and symptoms can vary or change in the same patient over time. Parasites can migrate to organs adjacent to the intestine and to distant sites, causing different chronic diseases. The damage caused by chronic parasitic infections depends on the duration of infection, the extent of malabsorption, co-existing infections, the overall infectious burden, the extent of reduced immunity, the burden of infectious byproducts, and manner in which the parasite spread.

Parasites originating in animals are transmitted from animal-to-person; and person-to-person, through close familial contact, contaminated surfaces, and food handling. People with pets or in contact with domesticated animals are vulnerable to parasitic infection transmitted from the animals or from animal feces. Parasites capable of infecting humans are shed in animal feces; and are found in lakes, rivers, streams and public swimming pools. Public swimming pools have been linked to outbreaks of giardia and cryptosporidiosis. People engaged in outdoor activities such as camping, fishing, boating, contact with lake water, or drinking from lakes or streams, are vulnerable to parasitic infection. Swimming in lakes or rivers can expose a person to parasites. Parasites have been found in community water systems served by unprotected surface water; and in water systems, households, and buildings, in which sewer lines contaminate water lines.

A recent study found the highest amount of feces contamination in surface water comes from birds. The next most common types of feces found in surface water were from dogs, people, rodents, cows, and other domesticated and wild animals.[70] Pets and domesticated animals are more likely to drink

---

[70] Westphal D. 2017. Does a Bear…in the River? No, But Plenty of Others Do. Albuquerque Journal. Sep 18, 2017. Doi: ejournal.abqjournal.com/popovers/ dynamic_article_popover.aspx?artguid=2d87718e-ec))-4b92-855d-5744b64728f9.

contaminated water from a stream or lake, which can cause parasitic infection in the animal. When a pet becomes infected, the pet can bring parasites into the household which can be transmitted from pet-to-person and person-to-person. Pets contaminate surfaces with parasites, including furniture and floors; and an owner can acquire parasites by contact, ingestion, and self-inoculation. Veterinarians know pets transmit parasites to humans and treat the animals for parasites, but medical doctors seldom take a pet history or diagnose and treat the parasites in animal owners.

At least fifty percent of households have at least one pet. Dr. Rabinowitz, a professor at Yale University School of Medicine, reported humans contract millions of infections per year from cats, dogs and other pets, ranging from skin infections to life-threatening illnesses; and said "(M)ost human infectious diseases are zoonotic in origin, consequently, many infections can pass between pets and people". Toxoplasmosis, toxocara, and hookworm are common parasitic infections transmitted to humans from pets.

In 1987, four million pet-related infections were estimated to occur annually, and the direct cost of pet-related infections was estimated to be three hundred million dollars per year. Yet, surveys suggest doctors are uncomfortable advising patients of the risks of animal contact. A history of pets and animal contact should be a routine part of every medical history, and parasitic disease should be considered in any pet owner and any patient who had contact with pets or domestic animals.[71] Dr. Rabinowitz suggested the extent of the problem of zoonotic diseases is not understood, because the conditions are not diagnosed or reportable; and suggested medical doctors and veterinarians need to collaborate, to improve prevention and treatment of conditions caused by animal pathogens.

Parasites infect us primarily through the mouth, and establish infection in the gastrointestinal tract; however, parasites can also infect by other routes, such as the respiratory tract or bite of an insect. Common gastrointestinal parasites include giardia, cryptosporidiosis, amoebas, and worms. Giardia is a parasite found in drinking water; and cryptosporidiosis closely

---

[71] *See* Rabinowitz P, *et al.* 2007. Pet Related Infections. American Family Physician. Nov 2007. 76(9): 1314-1322. www.aafp.org/afp/2007/1101/p1314.html.

resembles giardia, and has been isolated from public swimming pools. Amoebas are a more virulent type of water borne parasite, which cause gastrointestinal disease, blinding eye infections, and can even lead to enucleation of the eyeball. Schizophrenyrendidae Acanthodea (named similarly to schizophrenia), is an amoeba for which the name alone suggests it can migrate from the intestine to the brain and cause mental illness. Naegleria-fowelri is a brain eating amoeba found in warm lakes, which until recently has been uniformly fatal when ingested through the nose or mouth. Worms come in many sizes and shapes, and in many species. Worms are ordinarily transmitted by the feces of an infected animal.

Gastrointestinal parasites start with an acute infection. Parasites have an egg and cyst cycle; and start as cyclical intestinal symptoms. Over time, the symptoms become more constant, and a chronic disease. The duration of the life cycle of parasites is different, depending on the parasite. Re-infection can occur from the same vectors, accelerating the volume of parasitic infection, and the spread and constancy of symptoms.

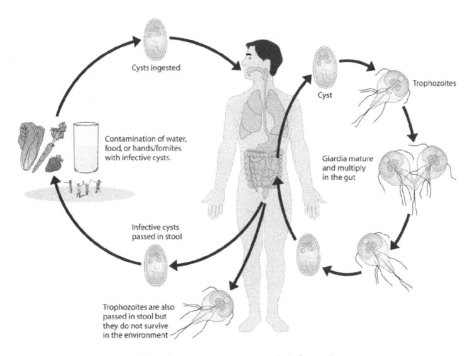

Cysts ingested

Trophozoites

Cyst

Contamination of water, food, or hands/fomites with infective cysts.

Giardia mature and multiply in the gut

Infective cysts passed in stool

Trophozoites are also passed in stool but they do not survive in the environment

Giardia ingestion, spread, life cycle

Parasitic disease can cause a variety of symptoms, and the person may appear thin, gaunt, and wasting, from periodic or constant diarrhea; and/ or have a big belly, and wide girth, with constipation. Parasitic disease can cause excessive burping and gas. Gastrointestinal parasites damage the villi, clog the intestine, block absorption, compete for nutrients, create fungus, and cause malabsorption and dysbiosis. Giardia depletes folic acid and B12, nutrients necessary for mental health and cognitive functioning. Loss of folic acid and B12 impact mental stability and cause cognitive decline; and low folic acid and B12, and low vitamin D, can trigger the development of cancer. A parasitic infection causes inflammation and reduced immunity, and the patient becomes more susceptible to new acute and chronic infections.

Patients with parasites acquire co-infections with immortal bacteria, and the parasites can host other viruses and bacteria, which compounds the infectious burden. A bacteriophage is a virus that can replicate within a bacteria or parasite. Parasites host intracellular chlamydia bacteria and viruses, as endo- and ecto-symbionts—parasites have parasites! When parasites host other chlamydia or viral pathogens, the co-infections can act synergistically to cause greater harm, and treatment is more difficult. The parasites and co-infections can create and host abnormal proteins that are dispersed throughout the blood and lymphatic system and block passive function, fostering an environment for cancer to develop and new focus for a futile attack by the immune system.

Parasites generate fungus, which protects the parasites from the immune system and feeds the parasites. The more co-infections, the more deterioration of the balance in the microbiome and normal pH, the greater the dysbiosis, the greater the fungal burden, the greater the impairment to the immune system, the more the infectious cascade is accelerated.

Parasites can migrate to organs adjacent to the intestinal tract, such as the liver, gallbladder, bile ducts, and pancreas, to cause chronic disease; and to remote sites in the eye, sinus and brain. Giardia has been found inside pancreatic masses, and the authors speculated the giardia may have caused the patient's lymphoma.[72] During different stages of the parasitic cycle, the parasite may migrate and live in different parts of the intestine, starting in the stomach, moving to the small intestine, and then the large intestine. Chlamydia pneumonia in the intestine is thought to alter other intestinal pathogens such as e-coli, causing e-coli to move to a different part of the intestine where e-coli can cause disease. Parasites can migrate to the brain and the eye, by moving along the vagus nerve; or invade the brain and eye through the blood stream and lymphatics.

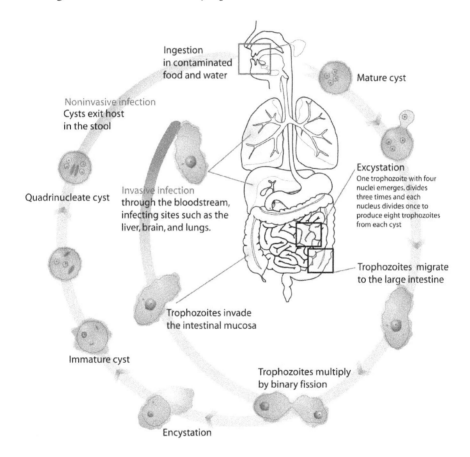

Giardia invasion and spread in the human body

[72] *See* Shah R, *et al.* 2017. Giardia-filled Pancreatic Mass in a Patient with Recently Treated T-cell Rich B-cell Lymphoma. Cureus. Feb 9, 2017. 9(2): e1019. Doi: 10.7759/cureus.1019.

Dr. Merchant tested many patients for ova and parasites, and it became clear inspection of the stool under a microscope was inadequate to diagnose parasitic infections. The ability to diagnose parasites by examining stool is highly dependent on whether the patient was shedding cysts at the time of the test, and the diligence of the examiner. The diagnosis of parasites was made based on a thorough history and physical examination, and blood testing suggestive of a parasite, including high monocytes, abnormal liver function tests, and low folic acid and B12. Patients with positive and negative stool tests had the same symptoms, and all of the patients benefited by treatment. Dr. Merchant's experience was chronic parasitic infection caused chronic disease, including systemic chronic disease beyond the gastrointestinal tract; and treatment of parasites caused symptoms of chronic disease to improve, even when the chronic disease was not the target of treatment.

In the 1982 edition of <u>Rheumatoid Diseases Cured at Last</u>, Dr. Rodger Wyburn-Mason and Dr. Jack M Blount hypothesized a limax amoeba caused rheumatoid arthritis. The authors reported finding amoebas in "all" body tissues, in all cases of human leukemia (disease of blood forming organs) and lymphoma (disease of lymphoid tissue); and in all cases of collagen and autoimmune disorders, including at remote sites, such as salivary glands, the spleen, muscles, thyroid, lymph nodes and the central nervous system. They reported amoebas were found in a large number of human and animal malignant tumors, but found less in malignant tumors than in other tissues. Dr. Blount believed pathogens were responsible for many scourges of chronic disease. Dr. Blount was criticized, for his beliefs and for treating patients for amoebas, despite his success in treatment of rheumatoid diseases by treating parasitic disease.

In the 2017 edition of <u>Rheumatoid Diseases Cured at Last</u>, the authors noted diagnostic tools were limited, in 1982; and broadened the range of infections which caused chronic rheumatologic diseases. The 2017 edition acknowledged additional pathogens could cause rheumatoid disease, and rheumatoid disease could develop in response to abnormal protein products or waste products of the microorganism. Dr. Blount may have inadvertently treated numerous pathogens with the potential to cause rheumatoid arthritis, by treating the patients with antiparasitic drugs. He was correct in saying rheumatoid arthritis was caused by an infection, and what was important was the patients were cured; even though the limax amoeba is not the only pathogen that causes rheumatoid arthritis, nor the only pathogen treated by antiparasitic drugs.

Scabies is a common skin parasite. Less common skin parasites are Leishmaniasis (sand fleas) and Morgellons's Disease. Leishmaniasis is common in the Middle East. Skin parasites cause itching, and the most intense itching often occurs at sunrise and sundown. Scabies leaves a linear track pattern of itchy skin and scabs. Sand fleas leave a linear tunnel track and cause intense itching. Scabies in the hair, and hair lice, cause a pattern of scabs and moles along a hairline, hat or helmet.

Doctors should become aware of the symptoms and consequence of parasites, and treat patients when intestinal symptoms and/or patient history and blood testing are suggestive of parasitic infection. Pediatricians should recognize parasitic infection in infants and children with gastrointestinal symptoms, who have pets in the household or contact with domesticated animals. We need more effective serologic tools to diagnose parasites and the type of parasite; and for doctors to recognize the cascade of parasitic infection, and depletion of critical nutrients that damage mental health and cause chronic disease. Recognizing and accepting the fact that parasitic infection exists in humans, diagnosing parasitic disease, and treating patients for parasites, is part of effective medical management, and can improve the health of patients and prevent chronic disease.

Worms

The CDC and WHO put worms (Helminths) on the list of the most neglected diseases. Doctors in the United States denied helminths existed in the United States, and are just starting to recognize worms and parasitic diseases are endemic in the United States, particularly among patients with pets and world travelers. Recently, American doctors "re-discovered" hookworm, a type of helminth. Helminths cannot be eliminated in the United States, because the United States has a high population of household pets, who harbor parasites. Hookworm, pinworms, roundworms, flatworms, threadworms, tapeworms, and other pathogenic worms have always been with us, and in the animals around us.

Worms are most often transmitted by ingestion of the worms or the larvae. Worms begin by invading the gastrointestinal tract; although some types of worms, like hookworm and the Thelazia Gulosa worm, invade through the skin. A pet can spread worms or larvae by direct pet-to-person transmission, and fecal contamination inside the home. Worm larvae can remain on the ground where infected animals defecated. Hookworm hides in soil and attaches to grass, and can be transmitted through the skin, to a person walking barefoot in the grass. Some pathogenic worms can be transmitted by flies, or by the bite of a fly.

Helminths are a family of worms, including hookworm, whipworm, pinworm, liver fluke, pork tapeworm, and bovine tapeworm. Each type of intestinal worm has a favored location in the intestinal tract; and any intestinal worm can migrate into new locations in the intestinal tract, or spread to organs connected to the intestinal tract. Helminths infecting the intestinal tract block absorption of nutrients. Worms can migrate to the eye and brain along the vagus nerve. When worms invade the brain, the patient may have seizures. Reflux and vomiting may transfer parasitic infection from the intestine to the sinus, providing another route for infection in the eye and brain, via the sinus. Helminth Unlimited reports new water borne diseases are more prevalent in foreign countries, and anyone traveling to certain underdeveloped parts of the world, for travel, work, or military deployment, particularly where hygiene is limited, are at risk for new diseases not recognized by American doctors.

Hookworm is a blood-sucking parasite that lives in the small intestine. The hookworm enters through the skin, most often by walking barefoot in grass where the parasite was shed by a pet or animal. Hookworms from feces attach to grass, to wait for the next host. Hookworms rob the body of necessary nutrients, clog and impair passive function in the intestine, and cause anemia. Hookworm can enter the bloodstream and migrate to the lung, causing a chronic cough; and to the brain and cause neurologic diseases. Ignorance of parasitic disease, and bias against parasitic diseases, prevents doctors from recognizing hookworm in patients with anemia or other gastrointestinal conditions caused by hookworms.

HOOKWORM

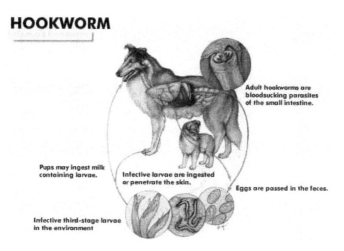

Hookworm in Dog

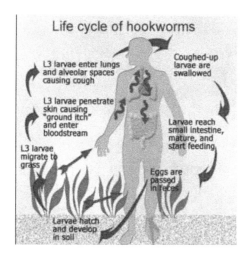

Life Cycle of Hookworm[73]

The toxocara parasite is a roundworm, which lives in the intestines of cats and dogs, particularly in stray animals. The microscopic eggs are shed in the animals' feces, contaminating yards, playgrounds and

---

[73] Courtesy of Metapathogen.com

sandboxes. The infectious particles cling to the hands of children playing where feces were shed, and are ingested. Toxocara parasites can infect the liver and lungs, and cause a damaging inflammatory reaction. The eggs hatch, releasing larvae that wriggle through the body and can migrate to the brain; or to the eye. Scattered scientific articles have reported finding toxocara worms in the central nervous system. Toxocariasis has been called visceral larva migrans (VT or VLM), or ocular larva migrans (OT or OLM), depending on the site of attack and degree of eosinophilla. Toxocaria in the eye can lead to blindness. The various names for toxocariasis include Weingarten's disease, Frimodt-Moller's syndrome, and eosinophillic pseudoleukemia.

Toxocara has been linked to lower intelligence and epilepsy, can cause developmental delays, and may damage learning and cognition. Children who tested positive for toxocara had lower mean test scores. The greater the magnitude of the toxocara infection the greater the impairment.[74] The implication of roundworm infections acquired on public playgrounds and in public parks causing lower intelligence, epilepsy, and developmental delays; and decreased learning, cognitive function, and lower mean test scores, is significant, particularly in places where pet ownership is common and no one cleans feces from the sidewalks and parks.

Dr. Peter Hotez, Dean of the National School of Tropical Medicine at Baylor College of Medicine, called toxocara one of the most common and the most neglected parasites in the United States. A CDC survey found eighty-five percent of pediatricians had only passing familiarity with toxocara, and even given the symptoms could rarely correctly diagnose the infection as roundworms. It has been estimated approximately sixteen million people carry antibodies to toxocara, indicating current and chronic parasitic disease. Few scientists study the infection, most doctors are unaware of it, and no funding has been provided to study the parasite. Lance Erickson, sociology professor at Brigham Young University, said, "What we don't

---

[74] Beil L. 2018. The Parasite on the Playground. New York Times. (D1). Jan 16, 2018. Doi: https://www.nytimes.com/2018/01/16/health/toxocara-children-new-york-playgrounds.html.

see is easy to ignore".[75] Hulda Regehr Clark, Ph.D., N.D., attributes many chronic diseases to various types of helminth worms and worm larvae.[76]

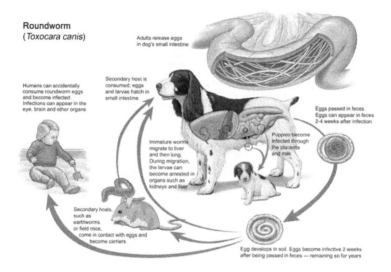

Roundworm
(*Toxocara canis*)

ROUNDWORMS IN DOG

Pinworms are common in dogs, and in dog owners. Pinworms can be transferred animal-to-person, and reproduce in the small intestine. Adult pinworms worms adhere to the lining of the intestine. Pinworms can move to the lower intestine and rectum, lay eggs in the anal area, and exit the rectum at night, causing itching around the rectum. Pinworms lead to chronic disease in the middle and lower intestine, and rectum. Pinworms are likely an overlooked cause of hyperactivity in children. A blood morphologist, who examines whole blood for the purpose of diagnosis and treatment, verbally reported to Carolyn that sixty percent of all blood samples she examined had evidence of pinworm. Hulda Regehr Clark, a naturopath, suggested pinworms were a cause of many chronic diseases, in 1995.[77]

---

[75] Beil L. 2018. The Parasite on the Playground. New York Times. (D1). Jan 16, 2018. Doi: https://www.nytimes.com/2018/01/16/health/toxocara-children-new-york-playgrounds.html.

[76] Clark HR. 1995. THE Cure for All Diseases, With Many Case Histories. New Century Press: California.

[77] *Id.*

The schistosome parasite is a parasitic flatworm known as a blood-fluke, which afflicts more than two-hundred million people worldwide, killing thousands. Schistosomes are a snail parasite, transmitted through the skin by a snail that lives in fresh water; and is endemic in the Middle East, South America, and sub-Saharan Africa. In some locations, WHO has advocated widespread treatment of communities to fight schistomiasis. Shistomiasis has been named "snail fever"; and can cause blood clumping, an overactive bladder, and bladder cancer. The schistosome parasite is thought not to exist in the United States; but cannot be ignored in patients with symptoms of a schistosome parasite, particularly if the patient has a travel history to the Middle East, South America, or sub-Saharan Africa. A global economy, worldwide travel, and soldiers stationed in the Middle East, make it reasonable to believe shistomiasis exists in patients exposed to the schistosome parasite, in other parts of the world.

A relative of Dr. Merchant, from Panama, was diagnosed with bladder cancer, and scheduled for radical bladder surgery. Dr. Merchant treated him with antibiotics and antiparasitic drugs, before he returned to his doctor for surgery to remove his bladder. After Dr. Merchant's treatment, upon re-examination, the doctor was astounded he could no longer find cancer, and cancelled the impending bladder surgery. The doctor never asked how Dr. Merchant had cured bladder cancer.

Failure to diagnose worms in the gastrointestinal tract causes lifelong suffering, and the patient is vulnerable to worms migrating outside the gastrointestinal tract to cause additional chronic diseases. Hookworms can cause anemia, and liver flukes can cause liver cancer. Veterinarians know pets get worms, and pets transmit worms to their owners. Antiparasitic drugs are widely available and widely used in animals, but people who own the pets are seldom diagnosed and treated for worms by medical doctors. Medical doctors ignore or are not knowledgeable about parasites acquired from pets, and do not attempt to diagnose or treat worms, which can cause chronic disease. Medical doctors are reluctant to warn patients about the danger of animal pathogens, and unwilling or unable to collaborate with veterinarians to assure continued health of the owner and pet.

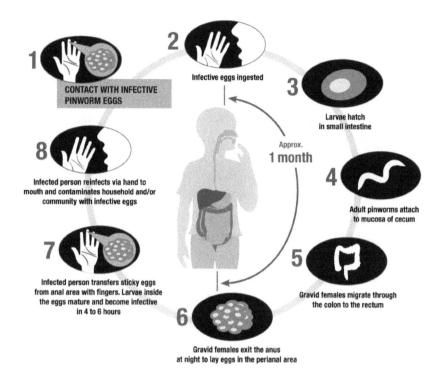

1 CONTACT WITH INFECTIVE PINWORM EGGS

2 Infective eggs ingested

3 Larvae hatch in small intestine

Approx. **1 month**

4 Adult pinworms attach to mucosa of cecum

5 Gravid females migrate through the colon to the rectum

6 Gravid females exit the anus at night to lay eggs in the perianal area

7 Infected person transfers sticky eggs from anal area with fingers. Larvae inside the eggs mature and become infective in 4 to 6 hours

8 Infected person reinfects via hand to mouth and contaminates household and/or community with infective eggs

Pinworm Ingestion and Spread

Taenia Solium is a tapeworm acquired from eating undercooked pork from an infected pig. The Taenia Solium worm lodges in the small vessels and muscles of pork. In the larvae form, the Taenia Solium tapeworm can be acquired through contact with the feces of an infected pig or human; and after infecting the intestine, the tapeworm can spread to other tissues. When the larvae form of the tapeworm enters the nervous system or the brain, it causes neurocysticercosis, which can cause epilepsy. Almost one-third of epilepsy cases in countries where the Taenia Solium worm is prevalent have evidence of having had neurocysticercosis. In Peru, scientists found thirty-seven percent of the population tested positive for the Taenia Solium worm.

In humans, the Taenia Solium worm burrows into the person's bloodstream, gets swept through the body by the bloodstream, and can form cysts in the brain. As the cyst grows, it can clog and block pathways in the brain, interfere with function, and dam the flow of the cerebral spinal fluid. Any cyst in a susceptible area of the brain can cause seizures, and those lodged near regions that signal commands to muscles can trigger violent convulsions.[78] The immune system attacks the cyst and can cause the surrounding brain tissue to swell, bringing more immune cells; and the brain tissue becomes inflamed.

No one knows how many people in the United States harbor the Taenia Solium tapeworm. Brain parasites are not often diagnosed in the United States, limiting knowledge of the rate of tapeworm infection, and the relationship between tapeworms and chronic disease.[79] Many domesticated and wild animals infected with tapeworms have tapeworms in the animal's brain[80], making it likely humans who are infected with tapeworms also have tapeworms in the brain.

Spirometra tapeworm (Loa Loa worm) lives in the intestines of cats and dogs; and the larvae is shed in feces. The Loa Loa worm is a nematode worm that causes filariasis, a skin and eye disease. The larvae can live in water, invading certain small crustaceans, or end up in frogs and snakes. The larvae can be transmitted to humans through ingestion or direct contact with infected animals or feces of infected animals.

Humans acquire loa filariasis through the bite of a deer fly or mango fly. After infecting the human, an adult Loa worm migrates throughout the subcutaneous tissues of humans, and occasionally crosses into subconjunctival tissues of the eye. The Spirometra tapeworm can migrate to the eye and the brain, causing tissue damage, blindness, paralysis and even death.

The Dirofilaria Repens is another nematode which causes filariasis. The worm is most often found in the Mediterranean region, sub-Sahara Africa and Eastern Europe. The Dirofilaria Repens infects dogs, cats,

---

[78] *Id.*

[79] Zimmer C. 2012. Hidden Epidemic: Tapeworms Living Inside People's Brains. Discover. Doi: discovermagazine.com/2012/jun/03-hidden-epidemic-tapeworms-in-the-brain.

[80] *Id.*

wolves, coyotes, foxes, muskrats, and sea lions. The worm is transmitted by mosquitoes, and can infect humans. Italy has the highest burden of dirofilaria in Europe, followed by France, Greece and Spain. Infection in humans often manifests as a subcutaneous nodule, which is trapped by the immune system. The worm can migrate in the body and has rarely been reported in organs, including the lung, male genitals, female breast and the eye. The worm most often occurs in adults, but for in Sri Lanka, where children as young as four months have been infected.[81]

The Thelazia Gulosa is a worm spread by "face flies" that feed on tears. The Thelazia Gulosa worm lives in the intestines of dogs, cats, sheep, cattle, foxes and wolves. Doctors previously believed the Thelazia Gulosa worm could not be transmitted from cattle to humans. Recently, the Thelazia Gulosa worm was diagnosed in the eye of an Oregon woman; and a surgeon removed fourteen worms from her eye. She acquired the worm while living at an old cattle ranch, with only one cow, and riding horses. She was the first recognized case of transmission of the Thelazia Gulosa worm to a human. A parasitic worm acquired from flies that can migrate to the eye confirms worms are not confined to the intestine, and can be acquired by routes other than ingestion, to cause significant acute and chronic disease.

Capillaria Aerophila and Aelurostrongylus Abstrusus, known as lungworms, are two of the most common worms found in cats, and may also infect dogs and horses. Cats become infected by drinking contaminated water; or by eating an infected snail, slug, mouse, rat, frog, lizard or bird. Sixteen percent of stray cats are infected; however, any cat can become infected. The lungworm can be transmitted to people, and causes symptoms such as coughing and shortness of breath (dyspnea). The coughing is caused by worm larvae laid in the airway, which in turn cause difficulty breathing and mucus accumulation.[82]

---

[81] Wikipedia. Dirofilaria repens. *Accessed* 6/22/18. Doi: en.wikipedia.org/wiki/Dirofilaria_repens; *See also* Kartashev V and Simon F. 2018. Migrating *Dirofilaria repens*. N Eng J Med. 378:e35. Doi: 10.0154/NEJMicm1716138 (worm nodule moving, removed from face of woman).

[82] Pet MD. Lungworms in Cats. Doi: petmd.com/cat/conditions/respiratory/cctlungworms.

Tropical parasites are also moving north into the United States, due to global warming. The rat lungworm was recently discovered throughout Florida. Rat lungworms are a particularly dangerous parasite, which attacks the lung and can get into the brain. Rat lungworm has been found in eosinophilic meningitis, and the incidence of rat lungworm in humans is rising.

Onchocerca volvulus is the worm that lives in water, in sub-Saharan Africa, and causes river blindness. The Onchocerca worm is the target of widespread eradication efforts, to prevent suffering and blindness in Africa.

Medical doctors rarely diagnose worms, particularly worms in the brain and eye. In past days, children were routinely treated for worms, a practice derived from wisdom that has been forgotten.

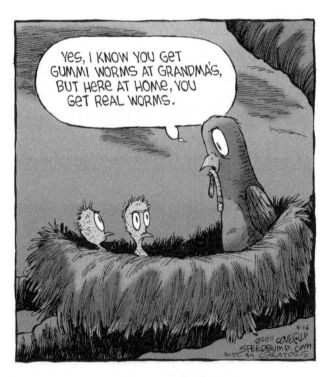

Grandma's Worms

Toxoplasmosis

Cats are the only known animal reservoir in which the toxoplasmosis parasite can replicate, and the only animal known to transmit toxoplasmosis to humans. Cats transmit toxoplasmosis to humans, rodents and other animals. Toxoplasmosis is thought not thought to be transmitted from person-to-person, or from rodents or other infected animals to humans. Toxoplasmosis has been called the love parasite, because cats with toxoplasmosis are able to attract prey to them, by the smell of toxoplasmosis in the urine. Toxoplasmosis in rodents causes epigenetic remodeling, which alters behavior and causes a reduced aversion to the smell of cats.

Toxoplasmosis is an intracellular parasite, which is immortal and lives in the host as long as the host lives. Toxoplasmosis is transmitted to humans through ingestion or inhalation of the toxoplasmosis cysts; and can be transmitted by touching and ingesting anything that has been in contact with infected cat feces. Toxoplasmosis feeds off the nutrients provided by the cell, consumes folic acid, and destroys normal apoptosis. Toxoplasmosis generates abnormal proteins, which attach to and change genes. Toxoplasmosis causes a variety of serious chronic diseases, causes mental illness, and can cause catastrophic neurologic damage to a fetus.

Many domesticated and wild animals can be infected with toxoplasmosis. Toxoplasmosis can infect livestock, including pigs, sheep, goats, cattle, and horses. Toxoplasmosis can infect primates, giant pandas, macaques, marsupials, wild boars, rodents, and marine animals. In the United States and across the world, pigs have the highest rate of toxoplasmosis. Animals kept outdoors and in free-range environments, are at higher risk of acquiring toxoplasmosis than animals raised indoors. Some animals die within weeks of acquiring toxoplasmosis, and others harbor toxoplasmosis as a chronic infection.

The toxoplasmosis parasite presents a significant danger to human health. In 1908, Charles Nicolle and Luis Manceaux first described the toxoplasmosis organism in a rodent, in Tunisia. The organism was differentiated from leishmaniosis, in 1909, and given the name toxoplasma gondii, to describe its curved shape during the infectious stage. In 1909, the organism was independently identified, in a rabbit, in Brazil. In 1923, the first case of congenital toxoplasmosis was reported in an infant with hydrocephalus and chorioretinitis (disease of the retina), but not identified as toxoplasmosis. In 1937, Sabin and Olitsky analyzed toxoplasmosis in monkeys and mice. In 1939, toxoplasmosis was shown to be transmissible from animals-to-humans and identified as a human pathogen, when Wolf, Cowen, and Paige, identified toxoplasmosis in an infant delivered at full term, who developed seizures and chorioretinitis in both eyes, three days after birth. The infant developed encephalomyelitis and died at one month, at which time toxoplasmosis was identified in brain tissue.

In 1940, Pinkerton and Weinman reported the first adult case of toxoplasmosis, in a twenty-two-year-old man from Peru, who died from a bacterial infection and fever. In 1941, toxoplasmosis transmission during pregnancy, from mother to child, was confirmed. In 1948, Sabin and Feldman developed the first test to diagnose toxoplasmosis in the blood, which became the standard. In 1965, Desmonts and others, demonstrated toxoplasmosis could be acquired from eating raw or undercooked meat. In 1974, Desmonts and Couvreur demonstrated transmission of acute toxoplasmosis to a fetus caused the greatest harm when the mother was infected in the first two trimesters. In the 1970's and 1980's, patients with lowered immunity from HIV were found more susceptible to toxoplasmosis.[83]

The risk of transmission of toxoplasmosis from a cat to the owner is greatest when litter boxes are used indoors, by kittens; and when litter boxes are not cleaned daily. Any cat infected with toxoplasmosis can shed the pathogen in feces. Kittens and cats shed large quantities of toxoplasmosis, in the first three weeks after acute infection. Toxoplasmosis in cat feces, in a litter box, can become airborne after twenty-four hours, contaminate the environment, and be inhaled by the cat owner.

Cats are a fertile reservoir for mixed infections. Cats acquire psittacosis from birds; and acquire additional forms of chlamydia from rodents. Toxoplasmosis can host chlamydia pathogens and viruses as bacteriophages.

---

[83] Wikipedia. Toxoplasmosis. Doi: en.wikipedia.org/wiki/Toxoplasmosis.

Toxoplasmosis can host HIV, the Borna virus, and the Zika virus, as bacteriophages. Transmission of toxoplasmosis, along with bacteriophages, increase the infectious burden, and introduces co-infections with more than one type of dangerous pathogen. Toxoplasmosis and the Borna virus have been found in schizophrenic brains; and both toxoplasmosis and Borna virus can be acquired from cats.

Toxoplasmosis is assumed to be asymptomatic, in cats and in humans. Cats that are symptomatic with acute toxoplasmosis may have compromised immune systems with fever, lethargy and lack of appetite; and some get pneumonia, and their eyesight and nervous system is affected. Cats also develop mental health symptoms, when infected with toxoplasmosis. It is reasonable to believe toxoplasmosis could attack humans in similar ways.

Toxoplasmosis may begin in the intestinal tract, as a symptomatic or asymptomatic infection. Doctors dismiss the importance of toxoplasmosis because the infection can be asymptomatic or cause mild flu-like systems, which are assumed to resolve without treatment. Acute toxoplasmosis can become chronic toxoplasmosis, and can insidiously persist and proliferate, to cause mental illness and systemic disease, months or years after infection. Moreover, diarrhea has been reported as a presenting symptom of disseminated toxoplasmosis in an immunocompromised host, who had thickening of the ascending colon and cecum; and treatment of the patient with pyrimethamine (Daraprim), sulfadiazine and leucovorin caused complete resolution of the symptoms.[84] The report of disseminated toxoplasmosis which resolved with treatment negates the claim toxoplasmosis is always a self-limiting disease. Toxoplasmosis may cause symptoms that go unnoticed or dismissed in a pet or by a patient, as the parasite causes slow and insidious changes, not noticed from day to day; in part because doctors and patients fail to understand the connection between the toxoplasmosis infection and the symptoms.

---

[84] Glover M, *et al.* 2017. Case Report: Diarrhea as a Presenting Symptom of Disseminated Toxoplasmosis. Hindawi. Case Reports in Gastrointestinal Medicine. Volume 2017. Article ID 3491087. Doi: https://doi.org/10.1155/2017/3491087.

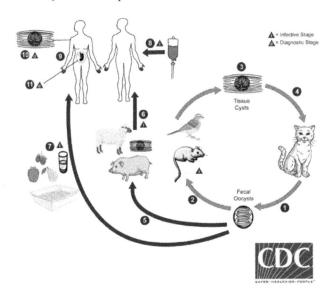

Transmission of Toxoplasmosis[85]

Toxoplasmosis causes a variety of chronic illnesses, brain disease, central nervous system disease, lung disease, and skin disease, years after acute infection. The NIH has reported toxoplasmosis can migrate from the stomach to the eye and the brain along the vagus nerve, or can be transferred via gastrointestinal reflux into the sinus and then from the sinus to the eyes and brain. Toxoplasmosis has been "associated" with epilepsy, movement disorders, Alzheimer's disease, demyelinating diseases, and cancer, including brain cancer. Toxoplasmosis proteins (protein 15) were shown to induce apoptosis in choriocarcinoma.[86] Toxoplasmosis has been "associated" with the development of seizures, particularly in infants; and causes regressive developmental disorders in a fetus. The severity of seizures is dependent on the number of cysts in the brain, the location of the cysts, the duration of infection, and the scar tissue in the brain left by

[85] Center for Disease Control and Prevention. Toxoplasmosis. https://www.cdc.gov/dpdx/toxoplasmosis/index.html.

[86] Wei W, *et al.* 2018. Toxoplasma Gondii Dense Granule Protein 15 Induces Apoptosis in Choriocarcinoma JEG-3 Cells Through Endoplasmic Reticulum. Parasites & Vectors. 2018. 11:251. Doi: https://doi.org/10.1186/s13071-018-2835-3. PMID: 2553092. PMCID: PMC4270089.

the infection. Toxoplasmosis can migrate to abdominal organs, and cause disease in the liver and pancreas; and has been "associated" with obesity.[87]

Toxoplasmosis causes a variety of mental illness, including schizophrenia, depression, anxiety, obsessive compulsive disorder, bipolar disorder, hostility, anger, emotional outbursts disproportionate to the circumstance, and reckless behavior. Toxoplasmosis increases testosterone in male brains, and has been linked to outbursts of anger and aggression. Patrick House, a Stanford neuroscientist, reports males with toxoplasmosis are more aggressive and less inhibited. Toxoplasmosis has been "associated" with reckless and dangerous behavior, including an increased risk of car accidents, self-harm, and self-mutilation. University of Chicago researchers found toxoplasmosis played a role in impulsive aggression; and found a link between toxoplasmosis and intermittent explosive disorder (IED), a psychiatric disorder characterized by recurrent, impulsive, problematic outbursts of verbal or physical aggression that are disproportionate to the situations that trigger the outbursts.

A study of the mental status of cats showed cats with toxoplasmosis had the same mental illnesses as humans, when infected with toxoplasmosis, including depression, anger, outbursts of violence, intermittent explosive disorder, and cats are killers.[88] Both animals and humans infected with toxoplasmosis undergo similar, subtle, long-term hormonal and mental health changes, causing the same mental illnesses. The term "crazy cat lady" arose because mental illness was noticed in women who acquired toxoplasmosis, from close contact with cats. Male owners of cats likely also have mental health effects from toxoplasmosis, including an increase in testosterone and reckless behavior, which are not recognized as different from male stereotypes.

---

[87] Oz HS. 2014. Toxoplasmosis, Pancreatitis, Obesity and Drug Discovery. Pancreat Disord Ther. Sep 2014. 4(2): 138. PMID: 2553092. PMCID: PMC4270089.

[88] Gartner M, *et al*. 2014. Personality Structure in the Domestic Cat (Felis silvestris catus), Scottish Wildcat (Felis silvestris grampia), Clouded Leopard (Neofelis nebulosi), Snow Leopard (Panthera uncia) and African Lion (Panthera leo). Journal of Comparative Psychology. 2014. Vol 128(4): 414-426. Doi: 10.1037/a0037104.

Transmission of toxoplasmosis from cats may present a significant risk to owners and members of the household. Toxoplasmosis presents a risk of chronic medical illness and a risk of mental illness. Lady Gaga reported she has fibromyalgia, chronic fatigue, and is in chronic pain, which developed shortly after giving her boyfriend a feral cat, the most dangerous pet in terms of transmission of toxoplasmosis and psittacosis. She also owns a sphynx cat, and sphynx cats are also infected with toxoplasmosis. Toxoplasmosis has been "associated" with both fibromyalgia and chronic fatigue. Mariah Carey, reports she has bipolar disorder, which is strongly "associated" with toxoplasmosis; and she is a well-known cat-lover who owns and has close contact with many cats. Toxoplasmosis has been "associated" with bipolar disorder and depression; and can insidiously progress after acute infection to chronic mental illness. A third celebrity, Selena Gomez, reports she has lupus, and co-morbid depression and anxiety. She also had cats, and had contact with cats owned by others. Toxoplasmosis is "associated" with lupus and with depression.

Cat owners are at risk for central nervous system disorders, and demyelinating disease. Toxoplasmosis has been identified as a leading cause of focal nervous system disease, and is commonly acquired by patients with HIV.[89] Toxoplasmosis is the most common central nervous system infection in patients with acquired immunodeficiency syndrome (AIDS), who are not receiving treatment for HIV.[90] Viral pathogens, including HIV, hide inside the toxoplasmosis parasite, and are sheltered from the immune system. HIV causes reduced immunity, and increased vulnerability to toxoplasmosis infection; and the HIV can then become a bacteriophage of toxoplasmosis, and/or a bacteriophage of a co-existing chlamydia infection.

Toxoplasmosis can cause blinding infections in the eye, by direct contact of the parasite to the eye, and by migration and metastasis into the eye. If a cat with toxoplasmosis scratches the cornea, it can cause a blinding

---

[89] Uppal G, *et al*. 2017. CNS Toxoplasmosis in HIV. Medscape. July 11, 2017. Doi: emedicine.medscape.com/article/1167298-overview.

[90] Gandhi R, *et al*. 2016. Toxoplasmosis in HIV-Infected Patients. UptoDate. Doi: uptodate.com/contents/toxoplasmosis-in-hiv-infected-patients.

infection. When toxoplasmosis invades the layers of the retina and causes inflammation, it is named "choroiditis", a medical term for inflammation in the choroid (middle) layers of the retina. The inflammation in the retina may also be called chorioretinitis, the same condition described in fetuses born with congenital toxoplasmosis, in 1923 and 1939. Pictures of a retina damaged by chronic toxoplasmosis may show de-pigmented areas, where retinal tissue has been destroyed by the parasite and inflammation.

Toxoplasmosis can cross the placenta, and be transmitted to a fetus. The earlier in the pregnancy the toxoplasmosis is acquired, the more severe the impact on the fetus. Pregnant women are advised to avoid cats and litter boxes, because toxoplasmosis is known to cause miscarriages; and fetal nasal malformations, brain damage, and damage to the eyes. Toxoplasmosis in a fetus can cause severe developmental disorders. Congenital toxoplasmosis damages the brain and/or central nervous system of the fetus. Babies born in the winter and early spring are more likely to develop mental illness during their life, which coincides to the time pregnant women have greater contact with litter boxes, when cats and kittens are kept inside.

Toxoplasmosis in a fetus is insidious, and symptoms may not appear until months or years after birth. Months or years after birth the fetus can develop a central nervous system disease, such as epilepsy. A fetus infected with congenital toxoplasmosis may appear normal at birth, and at six to eighteen months show signs of developmental regression. Congenital toxoplasmosis causes developmental regression and physical symptoms, which are very similar to numerous named syndromes identifying developmental regression syndromes in infants. Any infant with a regressive disability syndrome, vision impairment, or central nervous system disease, who develops regression of milestones, months or years after birth, may have congenital toxoplasmosis.

Toxoplasmosis is diagnosed through PCR blood testing, including serology, histology and molecular testing. Toxoplasmosis may be difficult to diagnose, during an inactive phase; and can be difficult to distinguish from primary central nervous system lymphoma. We need better and faster serologic tests to identify toxoplasmosis, anywhere in the body.

Daraprim treats blood borne parasitic infection, including toxoplasmosis. Toxoplasmosis can be treated with Daraprim, plus sulfadiazine (a sulfa antibiotic). Daraprim is a folic acid antagonist, meaning it prevents the body from making folic acid. Daraprim was developed by a Nobel Prize winning American scientist, Gertrude Elion (1918-1999), who was a biochemist and pharmacologist. WHO reports Daraprim is one of the most effective and safest medicines, needed in a health system. In clinical trials, Daraprim has been shown effective treating HIV, retinochoroiditis (retinal inflammation), and ALS (Lou Gehrig's disease). Daraprim may slow the progression of Tay-Sachs disease, a syndrome in which nerve cells in the brain and spinal cord are destroyed. Use of Daraprim has increased by 7,000 percent, because of the success of treating a variety of chronic diseases with Daraprim, in clinical trials.

In the United States, Daraprim has become prohibitively expensive, and unavailable to those in need. Martin Shkreli bought Turing Pharmaceuticals, owner of the patent on Daraprim. Turing Pharmaceuticals owns and controls the distribution of Daraprim. Martin Shkreli raised the price of Daraprim from $13.50 per pill to $750 per pill, which amounts to $75,000 for one month of treatment. Treatment for toxoplasmosis, with Daraprim, sulfa, and folic acid, may be six weeks or longer. In other countries, Daraprim is sold for ten cents to ten dollars per pill. Turing Pharmaceuticals has also blocked generic competition, by preventing potential generic competitors from gaining access to patented Daraprim. The FDA requires generic competitors to submit studies comparing the safety and effectiveness of the generic drug to the patented drug; and without the patented Daraprim, no generic competitor can perform the required studies to gain access to the market. Martin Shkreli is in jail for fraud, because he raised the price on Daraprim and other important drugs, to cover his fraud in a prior business; but he and Turing Pharmaceuticals still control the price and distribution of Daraprim and the price remains prohibitively expensive.

Daraprim should not be a "rare" drug, and should not be prohibitively expensive, because it is a valuable and needed treatment for many chronic diseases. The FDA needs to loosen restrictions on generic Daraprim, under an important drug exception; and allow generic competitors to submit alternate evidence of safety and efficacy, or force Turing Pharmaceuticals to provide patented drugs needed for testing, to break the stranglehold of Turing Pharmaceuticals over a drug needed for toxoplasmosis. Congress needs to control drug companies who abuse their position of trust as healthcare providers, exploit profit to the detriment of public health, block generic competition, and keep needed and reasonably priced important drugs from patients who need them.

CHAPTER 7

THE INFECTIOUS CASCADE
OF CO-INFECTIONS

Helicobacter Pylori

H-pylori is an ubiquitous gram-negative spiral bacterium that has been found in fifty percent of the population. H-pylori is transmitted from person-to-person, by saliva, food handling, contaminated water, feces, and poor hygiene. Swimming in contaminated water sources or drinking contaminated water in developing countries can be a source for acquiring H-pylori; and likely in developed countries as well. Once acquired, any spiral bacterium can be difficult to eradicate because it weaves into tissue. H-pylori can migrate deeper into collagen beneath the epithelium, and hide in organs adjacent to the gastrointestinal tract. High concentrations of antibiotics are necessary to treat H-pylori.[91]

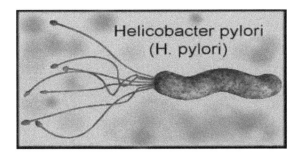

H-Pylori Bacteria[92]

---

[91] Dubois A, *et al.* 2007. Helicobacter Pylori Is Invasive and It May Be a Facultative Intracellular Organism. Cellular microbiology. 2007. 9(5): 1108-1116. Doi:10.1111/j.1462-5822.2007.00921.x.

[92] Helicobacter Pylori. H Pylori Assignment Point. Doi: https://www.assignmentpoint.com/science/medical/helicobacter-pylori.html.

In 1874, Arthur Boettcher, a pathologist and anatomist, discovered a small curved bacterium, in ulcers. In the 1940's, residents trained at Mt. Sinai in New York were taught to treat ulcers with antibiotics, because doctors observed antibiotics cured the ulcers, without knowing the pathogen. In the 1950's, knowledge ulcers were caused by a spiral bacterium and that ulcers were an infection was deleted from medical texts and medical training; and forgotten by mainstream medicine and gastroenterologists. Dr. Merchant said ulcers were an infection when he worked in the South Valley, based on observational science and the success of treatment, when conventional medicine still attributed ulcers to stress.

In 1982, Dr. Marshall proved H-pylori caused ulcers, by infecting himself, and curing himself. When Dr. Marshall reported the cause and cure for ulcers, the scientific community did not respond and apply the knowledge, and treat ulcers with antibiotics effective against H-pylori. It took until 1990, eight years later, when an article about Dr. Marshall's discovery appeared in the National Enquirer, for the medical establishment to notice and act on his discovery. In 2005, twenty-three years later, Dr. Marshall was awarded the Nobel Prize, for proving ulcers are caused by an H-pylori infection.

H-pylori is the bacterium now recognized to be the cause of stomach ulcers and stomach cancer. H-pylori lives in the intestinal tract, and attaches to epithelium. Penetration of a large number of H-pylori pathogens into gastric epithelial cells is "associated" with cell damage and cell disintegration. H-pylori can cause loss of normal apoptosis; invade and destroy immune cells, particularly neutrophils; and generate sticky proteins. Gastrointestinal symptoms of H-pylori include a variety of complaints, such as excessive burping or bloating, nausea, vomiting, loss of appetite, anorexia, weight loss, and bad breath.[93] H-pylori can independently cause chronic disease, or work synergistically with chlamydia and other co-infections, to increase the infectious burden and risk of developing chronic disease.

---

[93] Helicobacter. Assignment Point. Doi: assignmentpoint.com/science/medical/helicobacter-pylori.html.

The human mouth and human feces are the only confirmed reservoir for H-pylori. The human mouth plays a crucial role in both H-pylori transmission and gastric infection; and the oral cavity is considered the main reservoir for H-pylori. In "Helicobacter Pylori and Its Reservoirs: A Correlation With The Gastric Infection" [94], the authors report finding H-pylori in the oral cavity (dental plaque, saliva, tongue, tonsil tissue, root canals, oral mucosa) in humans and animals; and in the human stomach. Scientists have found "correlations" between H-pylori infection in the oral cavity and periodontal disease, oral tissue inflammation, and gastric re-infection.

Discovery of H-pylori as the cause of ulcers and stomach cancer has been called the tip of the iceberg. H-pylori has many strains, and not all strains and not all modes of transmission have been identified. Scientists identified possible animal reservoirs for H-pylori, and theorized a parallel development of H-pylori in animals and humans, which may have an unknown common ancestor. Animal reservoirs implicated as a reservoir for H-pylori include cats, pigs, sheep, monkeys, and house flies. Later studies suggested H-pylori may have transferred from humans to pigs.[95]

H-heilmannii is in the H-pylori family, and has been found in gastric biopsies. H-heilmannii has been strongly "associated" with contact with cats, dogs, cattle, pigs, and primates. Logistic regression analysis showed contact with cats, dogs, and pigs, leads to a significant risk of H-heilmannii infection. The conclusion was that cats, dogs, pigs, and primates, are reservoirs for the transmission of H-heilmannii. The fact animal reservoirs for H-pylori and H-heilmannii exist, and H-heilmannii is "associated" with animals and has been found in humans in gastric biopsies, supports transmission of H-pylori and H-heilmannii from animals-to-people, and animals as a vector for infection and re-infection with variants of H-pylori and H-heilmannii.

---

[94] Payão SL and Rasmussen LT. 2016. Helicobacter Pylori and Its Reservoirs: A Correlation With the Gastric Infection. World J Gastrointest Pharmacol Ther. Feb 6, 2016. 7(1):126-32. Doi: 10.4292/wjgpt.v7.i1.126.

[95] Megraud F and Broutet N. 2000. Review Article, Have We Found the Source of H-pylori?. Aliment Pharmacol Ther. 2000. 14 (supp 3):7-12; Doi: https://doi.org/10.1046/j.1365-2036.2000.00095.x; *see also* Payai SL and Rasmussen LT. 2016. Helicobacter Pylori and Its Reservoirs: A Correlation With the Gastric Infection. Doi: 10.4292/2jgpt.v7.i1.126.

Current high-throughput technology may help in determining the origin and vectors for H-pylori and H-heilmannii.

H-pylori can attack epithelium anywhere in the body. H-pylori invades mucosal cells, then burrows deeper to inner layers of collagen; and attaches itself to the collagen matrix below the epithelium. As H-pylori migrates through the layers of tissue, it damages membranes separating layers of tissue and causes loss of adherence between tissue layers, damages collagen structures, and eventually causes thinning and atrophy of tissue. H-pylori can migrate from the stomach to the lower intestine, and to other parts of the body, particularly adjacent abdominal organs, and along the vagus nerve or sinus, into the eye and brain. H-pylori can also spread to the eye through self-inoculation.

H-pylori cannot replicate intracellularly; however, H-pylori may be able to hide intracellularly in a host cell. Some suggest H-pylori can hide temporarily intracellularly, to avoid the immune system and stomach acid.

H-pylori can become more pathogenic when combined with other pathogens, because other pathogens may allow H-pylori pathogens to reach areas in the body where the H-pylori pathogen alone could not reach. When H-pylori damages the epithelium, the damage allows other pathogens and fungus to invade deeper into tissue, through the damaged epithelium, to cause disease. H-pylori can cause atrophy in the intestine, by damaging the inner layers of the intestinal tissue.

H-pylori has been "associated" with Parkinson's disease, and treatment of H-pylori can reduce motor fluctuations.[96] H-pylori and chlamydia psittacosis have been "associated" with lymphoma, including Hodgkin's lymphoma, non-Hodgkin's lymphoma, MALT lymphoma of the stomach, MALT lymphoma of the small intestine, MALT lymphoma of the eye, and MALT lymphoma of the skin. Chlamydia psittacosis has been "associated" with MALT lymphoma of the eye, and with

---

[96] Camci G and Ogfuz S. 2016. Association Between Parkinson's Disease and Helicobacter. J Clin Neurol. 2016; 12(2):147-150. Doi: https://dx.doi.org/10.3988/jcn.2016.12.2.147.

melanoma. Research suggests patients with co-morbid chlamydia psittacosis are at higher risk of developing MALT lymphoma, Sjögren's syndrome, Hashimoto's thyroiditis, Borrelia Burgdorferi infection (Lyme disease), Campylobacter Jejuni, and rheumatoid arthritis.

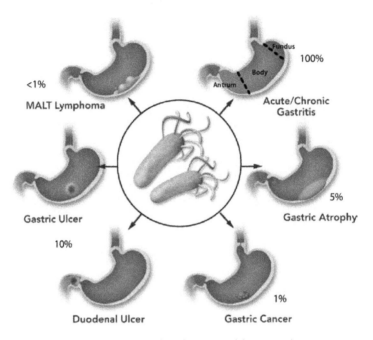

Diseases recognized to be caused by H-pylori[97]

H-pylori can become an originating cell or trigger for cancer; and is an accepted cause of stomach cancer. H-pylori can infect neutrophils and cause hyper-segmentation in the neutrophils that appears similar to cancer. H-pylori can cause MALT lymphoma, supporting H-pylori can migrate via the lymphatic system, and cause cancer at remote sites in the body. Patients with H-pylori are six times more likely to develop a MALT lymphoma tumor, and some MALT lymphoma patients have been cured by treatment of H-pylori.[98] The first-line treatment for lymphoma is treatment of H-pylori, which may eradicate the disease.

---

[97] Sachs G and Scott D. 2012. Helicobacter Pylori: Destruction or Preservation. F1000Reports MEDICINE. Figure 1. April 2, 2012. P. 1-5. Doi: https://f1000.com/reports/m/4/7.

[98] National Cancer Institute. Helicobacter Pylori and Cancer. Doi: www.cancer.gov.

H-pylori causes a variety of eye diseases, including corneal disease, glaucoma, and retinal disease. In the eye, the cornea has epithelium on the front surface of the eye, and inside the eye the retina has epithelium on the front surface. On the cornea, H-pylori attacks the epithelium, then burrows through membranes separating the layers of tissue, attaches to collagen, causing loss of adherence of the corneal layers of tissue, atrophy, and weak spots on the cornea. When H-pylori reaches the collagen structure, it can damage and thin the cornea, causing abnormally shaped corneas that bulge forward. Ophthalmologists have many names for corneal thinning, bulging, and abnormally shaped corneas; and all of the named diseases and syndromes should be investigated as an infection, including H-pylori and all chlamydia species.

H-pylori can migrate into the eye and along internal structures of the eye, to the anterior chamber angle and the back of the eye. Inside the eye, H-pylori can attach to the epithelium in the anterior chamber angle and many articles have reported H-pylori is "associated" with primary open angle glaucoma. H-pylori diagnosis and treatment has not been incorporated into ophthalmology training, or routine ophthalmology or glaucoma practice.

H-pylori can attack and infect retinal tissue. Retinal specialists have many names to describe weak, loose, or damaged retinal epithelium. Retinal specialists may name loose retinal epithelium RPE (retinal pigment epithelium), to describe retinal epithelium that is poorly adherent, loose, or has a change in pigment. H-pylori can cause separation of layers, loose surface tissue, chorioretinopathy, and serious retinopathy. Chronic H-pylori attacking the retina can cause a tear, hole, or detachment. Patients with a loose retinal epithelium and a retinal detachment are recognized by ophthalmologists and retinal specialists to have "co-morbid" stomach disease, but retinal specialists generally ignore the connection between the stomach and eye, and the fact stomach pathogens in the eye cause retinal disease.

H-pylori causes ICSR (idiopathic central serous chorioretinopathy), a "rare" disease formerly attributed to an unknown cause. Idiopathic means the doctor does not know the cause; thus, attributes the disease to something unique about the patient or their defective genes. The patient is told nothing can be done to halt the progression of the blinding disease. In ICSR, serous fluid bubbles form in the middle layers of the retina, which bubble to the surface and leave holes in the retina, causing micro-detachments in the retina. In 2001, treatment of H-pylori was reported beneficial for ICSR, and provoked faster reabsorption of sub-retinal fluid.[99] Several subsequent scientific reports confirmed H-pylori caused ICSR, and treatment of H-pylori was effective in treating ICSR.

Mycoplasma pneumonia

When Dr. Merchant first recognized chronic infections caused chronic disease, chlamydia pneumonia had not yet been discovered and identified as a separate species of chlamydia. His focus was on giardia and mycoplasma. The mycoplasma bacterium is a single cell life form that mimics mushrooms and ferns; hence the name, "myco" or "like a mushroom". Mycoplasma spreads by airborne spores. Mycoplasma causes acute respiratory infection and pneumonia, lasting four to six weeks or more, which has been referred to as "walking pneumonia". Mycoplasma has been "associated" with many chronic diseases, similar to chlamydia; and the chronic diseases are not limited to the respiratory tract. Mycoplasma can generate an infectious cascade, to cause chronic disease in a manner similar to chlamydia.

Mycoplasma was initially thought to be an extracellular bacterium; however, further study of the genome proved mycoplasma is more like an intracellular bacterium. It is a cell-wall deficient bacteria.[100] Mycoplasma is an atypical bacterium, which has more than twenty species. Mycoplasma has been found in animals, including cats, sheep, pigs, goats, and calves. Mycoplasma is common in cats, and an infected cat can transmit mycoplasma to the

---

[99] Rahbani-Nobar M. 2011. The Effect of Helicobacter Pylori Treatment on Remission of Idiopathic Central Serous Chorioretinopathy. Mol. Vis. Jan 2011. 11(17): 99-103. Doi: https://www.ncbi.nlm.nih.gov/pubmed/21245962. PMID: 21245962. PMCID: PMC3021578.

[100] Meseguer M, *et al.* 2003. Mycoplasma Pneumoniae: A Reduced-Genome Intracellular Bacterial Pathogen. Infe. Genet Evol. May 2003. 3(1): 47-55. Doi: https://doi.org/10.1016/S1567-1348(02)00151-X.

owner. Once infected, the mycoplasma bacteria can become immortal in cats and humans. (Cats also carry chlamydia pneumonia).

Mycoplasma is a stealth pathogen, which can become a chronic intracellular pathogen, and cause damage in the body. Mycoplasma has been found in joints in rheumatoid arthritis, and in lupus.[101] Mycoplasma can cause central nervous system disease, neuropathy, brain abscess, super antigens, and abnormal stimulation of cytokines such as IL-2. Mycoplasma causes induction of multi-state oncogenic cancer processes leading to chromosomal alterations, toxic oxygen radials creating oxidative stress, lesions in the heart, liver, kidneys, and central nervous system; and induces loss of normal apoptosis. Some argue a wide-spread plague of auto immune diseases in humans, is caused by contact with cats.[102]

Feline mycoplasma transmitted to a human has been "associated" with lupus, scleroderma, and rheumatoid arthritis. The link between cats and rheumatoid arthritis has been known, since at least 1939, when Dr. Thomas McPherson Brown isolated mycoplasma bacterium in rheumatoid joints.[103] Sudden onset joint pain and arthritis was reported after acute human exposure to feline mycoplasma.[104] Some suggest feline mycoplasma causes chronic fatigue; and some suggest a super strains of mycoplasma infected troops in Iraq.[105]

Streptococcus

Streptococcal disease was first described by Hippocrates, and has been studied by scientists through the centuries. The first vector for

---

[101] Hernandez A. The Danger of Human Contagion of Mycoplasma from Animals and Its Role in Arthritis and Chronic Pneumonia. https://www.masterjules.net/catlung.htm.

[102] *See Id.*

[103] Brown TM, Swift HF. 1939. Pathogenic Pleuropneumonia-Like Microorganisms From Acute Rheumatic Exudates and Tissues. Nature Journal. Mar 1939. 24(89). (2308): 271–272. DOI: 10.1126/science.89.2308.271.

[104] *See* Hernandez S. Warning: CAT DISEASES THAT CAN INFECT HUMANS. Hernandez S. Warning: Cat Diseases That Can Infect Humans. Doi: https://www.luckinlove.com/mycat.htm. *Accessed* 6/13/18.

[105] *Id.*

streptococcus is believed to be soil, and streptococcus has been found in sewage. Streptococcus pathogens are gram positive bacteria, and the many species of streptococcus have varying levels of virulence. Streptococcus can deplete folic acid, and can attach to other host cells and pathogens. Streptococcus can attack many different cells and organs, and cause different chronic diseases.

Streptococcus starts as an extracellular pathogen, and covers itself in abnormal proteins, to protect its surface from attack by the immune system. As the immune system fights the pathogen, the abnormal protein byproducts can become intracellular. Abnormal protein molecules covering the streptococcus pathogen range from coiled to globular, and the virulence of streptococcus is determined by the type of abnormal proteins on the surface of the pathogen. Streptococcus has a variant known as streptococcus *suis,* which is common in pigs and can be transmitted to humans. Streptococcus *suis* in humans has the potential to cause meningitis.

Doctors know streptococcal infections require treatment with antibiotics, because untreated streptococcal infections can cause significant morbidity. Post streptococcus infection has been "associated" with reactive arthritis in children and adults, heard damage and kidney damage.

One particularly virulent species of streptococcus is streptococcus type-M, named for the M-proteins on the surface of the pathogen. Streptococcus type-M is a virulent strain that causes rheumatic fever (heart valve damage) and glomerulonephritis (inflammation of the tubules in the kidney). Some forms of streptococcus adhere to the wall of the intestine. Streptococcus and the abnormal proteins attached to it can invade the brain, and cause strep-induced seizure disorders. The abnormal proteins can invade the kidney and cause impaired kidney function. A streptococcal endophthalmitis almost always leads to blindness.

Streptococcus and mycoplasma are the only two pathogens known to have M-proteins attached to the surface of the pathogen. M-proteins have been "associated" with rheumatic fever and glomerulonephritis. Multiple myeloma is cancer in the plasma cells; and is diagnosed by the presence of M-proteins in the blood and urine. Streptococcus or mycoplasma can become an intracellular infection in the plasma cells; and plasma cells carry the infection to the bone marrow. The diagnostic significance of M-proteins in multiple myeloma make it reasonable to consider whether streptococcus and/or mycoplasma cause multiple myeloma by infecting the plasma cells with the pathogen and/or with M-proteins, during or after the streptococcus infection. Are M-proteins found on the surface of the streptococcus and mycoplasma bacteria, and M-proteins used as the diagnostic criteria for multiple myeloma, one and the same? Are the M-proteins diagnostic of multiple myeloma the fragments of what started as an M-protein attached to mycoplasma or streptococcus, and was engulfed by the macrophages and plasma cells? Streptococcus and mycoplasma can be treated with antibiotics; however, M-proteins are not alive, and science will have to find new ways to remove M-proteins from the body, and the immune cells, with medications or plasmapheresis.[106] If the M-proteins attached to forms of streptococcus are completely unrelated to multiple myeloma, then science should stop naming different things by the same name, and stop naming the same thing by different names.

Peptostreptococcus is a form of streptococcus that resides in the intestine and can only grow in an anaerobic environment. Peptostreptococcus can live in all areas in the body, including the mouth, head, neck, chest, central nervous system, abdomen, pelvis, bone, joints, gastrointestinal tract, reproductive tract, skin, and soft tissue. Peptostreptococcus also has many sub-species. The pathogenesis of peptostreptococcus alone or in combination with other pathogens has been debated. It is not known whether peptostreptococcus is pathogenic, or only becomes pathogenic when dysbiosis causes the microbiome to be out of balance. Peptostreptococcus is often overlooked in the diagnosis of gastrointestinal disease, because the pathogen is difficult to isolate and identify as pathogenic versus normal intestinal bacteria.

---

[106] *See* Ricci J, *et al.* 2016. Novel ABCG2 Antagonists Reverse Topotecan-Mediated Chemotherapeutic Resistance in Ovarian Carcinoma Xenografts. Molecular Cancer Therapeutics. Doi: 10.1158/1535-7163.MCT-15-0789.

Peptostreptococcus is thought to be slow growing and synergistic with other pathogenic organisms. Peptostreptococcus has been found in patients with leukemia and multiple myeloma; and found at higher levels in patients with Crohn's disease. Crohn's disease may be caused by pathogenic bacteria, or normal intestinal bacteria that has become pathogenic, alone or in combination with other pathogens. The confusion between normal and pathogenic bacteria in the intestine complicates a diagnosis in Crohn's disease; and the fact a "normal" intestinal pathogen could become pathogenic makes the diagnosis of pathogenic causes of intestinal disease more difficult. Gastroenterologists do not attempt to diagnose pathogens in Crohn's disease. Crohn's disease is ulcers in the lower intestine, similar to ulcers in the stomach caused by H- pylori. H-pylori may combine with peptostreptococcus or e-coli in the intestine, to cause Crohn's disease.

Diagnosis of pathogens in Crohn's disease has been complicated by a bias against infectious causes, deletion of infectious causes of gastrointestinal disease from textbooks, and lack of interest in diagnosing infectious causes. Gastroenterologists do purges before scopes and remove evidence of pathogens, and the gastroenterologist does not examine or culture the fluid expelled by the purge, to find infectious pathogens or other clues to the infectious causes of Crohn's disease. The gastroenterologists do not test the blood or tissue in the colon for pathogens, virulence, or antibiotic resistance, to better understand an infectious etiology of Crohn's disease.

Laboratories often fail to distinguish the many different strains of streptococcus. The laboratory may call all streptococcus "strep-A", and not distinguish or report on the many sub-types of streptococcus. It is important to know the type of streptococcus causing disease, particularly streptococcus type-M, because streptococcus type-M proteins are a significant finding in a number of chronic diseases, and are a virulent pathogen that cause chronic disease. It is difficult to recognize strep type-M is the cause of chronic diseases, when laboratories do not differentiate streptococcus-A from streptococcus-A type-M on laboratory reports.

Viruses

In 1898, Friedrich Loeffler and Paul Frosh found evidence the cause of foot-and-mouth disease in livestock was an infectious particle, smaller than a bacterium, which provided the first clue to the nature of viruses. Viruses are smaller than bacteria, can invade normal host cells, and can become bacteriophages of other pathogens. Viruses need a host cell to replicate; and can live and replicate inside a host cell, including immune cells, living off the energy of the host cell.[107] Viruses can exist outside a host for a limited time, which allows viruses to be transmitted from person-to-person.

Viruses are acellular organisms, meaning the virus lacks a cell wall. Some viruses have a protein coat or "capsid", some viruses have a membrane on the surface, and some are enclosed in an envelope of fat and protein molecules. The capsid or membrane protects the virus from the immune system. Viruses can transfer genetic material between species, which is why viruses are used in genetic engineering. Viruses cause many diseases, ranging from what is referred to in the vernacular as the common cold, to smallpox, chickenpox, influenza, shingles, herpes viruses, polio, parvovirus, rabies, Ebola, Hantavirus, hepatitis, hand-foot-and-mouth, HIV and AIDS, and hemorrhagic fevers. Some viruses resolve after an acute infection and the remnants of the viral infection provide immunity or partial immunity. Other viruses become a chronic disease or a bacteriophage to other pathogens.

Ancient viruses have been identified in the human microbiome and genes.[108] An ancient mummy of a child was found to have evidence of hepatitis-B infection. Egyptian royalty had monkeys as pets, which created a risk of transmission of viruses from monkeys-to-humans; and HIV and Ebola viruses are believed to have originated in monkeys and were transmitted to humans from monkeys. Monkeys are a sexually promiscuous species, leading to increased virulence of the viruses in the monkeys, and an increased overall infectious burden.

---

[107] Emiliani C. 1993. Extinction and Viruses: Introduction to Viruses. BioSystems. 31: 155-159. Doi: ucmp.berkeley.edu.
[108] Jong E. 2016. I Contain Multitudes, The Microbes Within Us and a Grander View of Life. 1st ed. Harper Collins.

Chronic viral infections live in the host for the life of the host, and wreak havoc when combined with other immortal infections. Some of the most dangerous viral infections are already recognized to cause cancer, including CMV, EBV, HPV-1, HPV-2, HIV-1 and HIV-2, and hepatitis B and C. Hepatitis-A is believed to have originated in small mammals and bats. Hepatitis-B is believed to have originated in birds. Hepatitis C is believed to have originated in horses. Diseases like hepatitis, herpes, human papilloma virus, Epstein Barr (EBV), HIV, and CMV are cumulative in causing chronic disease, because each pathogen can destroy different parts of the body and different layers of tissue.

Immortal viruses combine with chronic chlamydia and parasites, as bacteriophages, to cause, trigger, or worsen chronic disease. In <u>THE INFECTIOUS ETIOLOGY OF CHRONIC DISEASES, Defining the Relationship and Enhancing the Research, and Mitigating the Effects</u>, the authors postulated when a patient is previously infected with these viruses, immortal infections such as chlamydia may trigger chronic disease. Parvovirus is recognized as dangerous and potentially fatal in dogs; and the human form of parvovirus is "associated" with leukemia and arthritis. Cats carry feline HIV, known as FIV, which is a form of animal HIV; and feline mycoplasma, which can be transmitted to humans.

A number of epidemiology studies have linked an increased risk of acquiring HIV infection to chlamydia pneumonia and chlamydia trachoma. Co-infection, with chlamydia pneumonia and HIV, accelerates the development of AIDS; which may be determined by the overall burden of infectious disease and co-existing chlamydia infection. The molecular biology of chlamydia pneumonia and trachoma, as a persistent infection in immune cells, are more immunosuppressive than HIV, HPV-1, HPV-2, EBV, and H-pylori. HIV replicates in immune cells, and chlamydia also infects and replicates in immune cells. When a person has an intracellular virus and intracellular chlamydia, as co-infections in the immune cells, these co-infections accelerate the loss of immune function and cause HIV to progress to AIDS. The patients who progress to AIDS have an increased risk of co-morbid heart disease, from co-existing chlamydia pathogens.

Science has shown it takes ten to twelve years for HIV to progress to AIDS, which is the time it takes for HIV to invade a sufficient number of immune cells to destroy immune function. Dr. Merchant's experience treating an HIV patient with azithromycin, and changing no other parameters of care, was the patient had a marked decrease in the viral load and increased numbers of functioning lymphocytes. Treating parasites can also help fight the HIV infection. Treatment of chlamydia and parasites will delay progression of the HIV to AIDS, and improve the quality of life for HIV patients.

Smallpox has been hypothesized to have originated in ancient African rodents, and transmitted to humans, ten millennia ago. Smallpox was documented to exist in the 3rd century BC, in Egyptian mummies. Smallpox killed three to five hundred million people before the virus was eradicated, through widespread vaccination. Hantavirus is a potentially fatal respiratory virus, acquired from exposure to feces of a deer mouse. Different types of Hantavirus live in different types of rodents, and all forms may be transmitted to people. Hantavirus seems to attack people born after 1972, when smallpox vaccinations were discontinued. Hantavirus may be similar enough to the smallpox virus that prior immunization against smallpox provides partial protection against Hantavirus.

Arboviruses include all viruses transmitted by arthropods. Arthropods are mosquitoes, ticks, insects, fleas, midges, spiders and crustacean. Tiboviruses are any virus transmitted by ticks; and are a subcategory of arboviruses, which are considered a super-virus of the arbovirus type. Plasmids and fragments of other pathogens attach to arboviruses and tiboviruses, and arboviruses and tiboviruses attach to intestinal parasites and chlamydia as ecto- and endo-symbionts. Arboviruses and Tiboviruses combine with other pathogens and cause chronic disease; and when attached to parasites and chlamydia can metastasize to other targets in the body with the host pathogen, which the virus cannot reach alone.

Mosquitoes transmit hemorrhagic viruses, which can be fatal. Ticks transmit spirochetes, the spiral bacterium that causes Lyme disease; and tiboviruses, from the Flaviviridae, Reoviridae, and Bunyaviridae family of viruses. Spirochetes are difficult to eradicate because the spiral shape becomes tangled in tissue. Spirochetes live and hide inside red blood cells, and travel with the red blood cells. Spirochetes may be a co-infection with other immortal infections, inside the immune cells, and as a co-infection may trigger blood cancers.

The Black Death, a pandemic of plague in the Fourteenth Century, killed up to sixty percent of the population, and has long been blamed on rodents. Scientists in Norway now suggest it was more likely a rodent-flea transmission of the plague. The fleas were infected, the fleas bit the rodents, fleas bit humans, and fleas transmitted the plague to humans. Human body lice or fleas may have been the main transmission routes in medieval pandemics.[109] Boris Schmid, a computational biologist at the University of Oslo, referred to the pandemic as an example of a disease coming from wildlife and spreading like wildfire.

In 2015, Brazil suffered an outbreak of microcephaly, believed to be caused by the Zika virus. Brazil was not the only country to have the Zika virus, nor the only place to have microcephaly in newborn infants; but microcephaly occurred at a higher rate in Brazil than in other countries. The Zika virus was thought to be a relatively large pathogen, which was unable to penetrate the blood-brain barrier; thus, how the Zika virus could cause microcephaly was not understood. Scientists converged on Brazil looking for Zika infected patients, trying to understand why microcephaly was worse in Brazil than in other countries, and how Zika got into the brains of a fetus. The scientists failed to investigate co-infections in the mothers of babies born with microcephaly, to find pathogens that could act as a host for the Zika virus, allowing the Zika virus to get into the brain of a fetus.

Brazil has a high concentration of people living in cities; one of the highest rates of pet ownership of cats and dogs, in densely populated cities; and animal waste is not cleaned up in the streets or parks. Brazil has a high

---

[109] Guarino B. 2018. The Classic Explanation for the Black Death Plaque Is Wrong, Scientists Say. The Washington Post. (Speaking of Science). Jan 16, 2018. Doi: https://www.washingtonpost.com/news/speaking-of-science/wp/2018/01/16/the-classic-explanation-for-the-black-death-plague-is-wrong-scientists-say/?noredirect=on&utm_term=.23e6cbb35686.

rate of toxoplasmosis in cats; thus, the population in Brazil, particularly owners of the cats, are likely to have a high rate of toxoplasmosis. Pets in Brazil are riddled with endo- and ecto-parasites; thus, also necessarily transmit endo- and ecto-parasites to pet owners. Women of child bearing age in Brazil are estimated to be infected with toxoplasmosis at a rate of fifty to eighty percent.[110] Brazil also has one of the highest rates of sexually transmitted chlamydia trachoma and one of the highest rates of H-pylori infection, in the world.

The high rates of toxoplasmosis, chlamydia trachoma, and H-pylori, in Brazil, suggest chronic co-infections with immortal pathogens are the explanation for a greater number of cases of microcephaly in Brazil. The Zika virus likely became a bacteriophage of toxoplasmosis, chlamydia trachoma, or H-pylori, to get into the brain of a fetus. Toxoplasmosis can cross the placenta and cause microcephaly in a fetus, even without the Zika virus; and when acquired during pregnancy can cause regressive developmental disorders, mental retardation, and other mental disorders in the child. If Zika was able to attach to toxoplasmosis as a bacteriophage, the Zika virus could cross the placenta and the blood brain barrier, along with the toxoplasmosis parasite. Toxoplasmosis with Zika as a bacteriophage would enhance the effect of both pathogens on the brain of a fetus, and increase the risk of microcephaly.

Chlamydia trachoma and H-pylori can also serve as a host to the Zika virus; and trachoma and H-pylori can enter the central nervous system and brain. Chronic infection with immortal pathogens can also reduce the effectiveness of the blood brain barrier, making it easier for pathogens to enter the brain. The high rates of toxoplasmosis, chlamydia trachoma, and H-pylori, in humans and pets, explains why microcephaly is more common in Brazil than in other countries.

Chlamydia psittacosis was identified in Brazil, in parrots, in 1917. An outbreak of psittacosis killed one third of victims in Paris, in 1890; and

---

[110] Oz HS, *et al.* *Toxoplasma gondii* (Toxoplasmosis), 2nd Ed. Authors 2nd ed. (Jose G. Montoya, M.D., Jacques Couvreur, M.D., Caterine Leport, MD). Doi: antimicrobe. org/new/b130.asp.

an outbreak of psittacosis occurred in Pennsylvania in 1917. Infected birds from South America were shipped worldwide, spreading psittacosis. A psittacosis epidemic spread to twelve countries, by the winters of 1929-1930. Psittacosis now infects birds and cats, worldwide. Psittacosis is likely still common, in birds and cats in Brazil, and is another pathogen to which Zika could become an endo- or ecto-symbiont, to cross the placenta and cross the blood-brain barrier of a fetus.

The influenza virus is categorized as influenza A, B and C. Influenza-A has been responsible for the major flu pandemics, in modern history, including the Spanish Flu pandemic, of 1918-1920; the Asian Flu pandemic, of 1957; the Hong Kong Flu pandemic, of 1968; and the Swine Flu pandemic, of 2009. Influenza-A comes from birds and bats; and includes twenty-nine different sub-types of influenza, defined by the proteins attached to the surface of the virus. Influenza-A is divided into low pathogenicity and high pathogenicity, based on the molecular characteristics of the virus, and the ability of the virus to cause disease and mortality in chickens.

Birds are the reservoirs for twenty-seven sub-types of influenza-A, and bats are the reservoir for the remaining two sub-types of influenza-A. Aquatic birds, including gulls, terns, waterfowl, and shorebirds, are reservoirs for influenza-A. Influenza-A is found in cats, ducks, chickens, pigs, whales, horses, and seals. Influenza-A may be asymptomatic or cause mild illness; however, in birds, two types of influenza-A can cause widespread illness and death. In animals, influenza-A can combine with other pathogens, to create new strains of influenza. Eight new variations of the influenza virus have been found in Asian domestic ducks, wild birds, and domestic poultry. In 2013, in China, an influenza virus was created by the combination of pathogens in domestic ducks, wild birds, and domestic poultry. Reports allege transmission influenza-A from animals to humans is rare; however, human infection and human outbreaks of influenza-A transmitted by animals have been reported.[111] Influenza can occur in both humans and

---

[111] Center for Disease Control and Prevention. Control and Prevention Report. Transmission of Influenza Viruses from Animals to People. Doi: www.cdc.gov/flu/about/viruses/transmission.

animals, and many believe influenza can be transmitted from human-to-animal or animal-to-human.

Pigs can be infected with avian influenza, and are known reservoirs for swine influenza. Pigs can be infected with avian influenza from ducks, and other forms of influenza at the same time. In pigs, the genes of the influenza virus mix and create new strains of influenza. When pigs are co-infected with more than one strain of flu at the same time, new viruses are created and known as "variant viruses". The re-assortment of the genes in the viruses changes the type of flu and virulence of the influenza virus, in humans and animals.

Transmission from animals-to-humans, and the risk of acquiring the influenza as a co-infection with chlamydia and/or parasites cannot be excluded. The Swine Flu pandemic, of 2009, was caused by a bird flu, which was traced to pigs in Mexico—the same stain of bird flu that was transmitted from humans to pigs during the Spanish Flu pandemic. Humans transmitted the H1N1 avian influenza virus to pigs, in 1918; and pigs transmitted the H1N1 bird influenza virus to humans, in 2009.

Outbreaks of dog influenza have occurred in clusters, and two types of influenza are known to infect dogs. However, no dog-to-human transmission has been reported. Influenza-A in dogs is referred to as "canine influenza virus". Cats can be infected with influenza viruses, including avian influenza strains. Cats can transmit the influenza virus to other cats, in the same manner as human influenza spreads, by direct contact, sleeping together, nasal discharge, and contaminated surfaces. Some suggest influenza can be transmitted from humans-to-cats, but the risk of cat-to-person transmission is unknown. Cats can transmit feline mycoplasma, toxoplasmosis, and other pathogens and parasites to humans; thus, cats can also likely transmit influenza to humans.

Viruses are difficult to culture; but can be diagnosed by a blood test. Blood tests to confirm a viral pathogen are seldom done. Viral pneumonia can be life-threatening, and a vaccination is available. Some forms of chlamydia infections can also cause life threatening pneumonia. The misdiagnosis of chlamydia infections as viruses has caused confusion in understanding the role of chlamydia pathogens in chronic disease. All forms of chlamydia have previously been mis-identified as a virus, before modern technology allowed scientists to differentiate pathogens. Thus, prior epidemics and pandemics could have been mis-identified as a virus, and other types of pathogens could have caused morbidity and mortality, alone or as a co-infection.

Antibiotics do not treat a virus, but can treat secondary bacterial infection. Influenza often causes a secondary bacterial infection, within twenty-four to forty-eight hours, which requires treatment. The only treatment for an acute viral infection is an anti-viral medication, anti-flu medication, or doing nothing until the acute viral infection resolves. The best treatment for acute influenza is Tamiflu, early in the course of acute infection, which is now available in a generic form. Anti-viral medication or anti-flu medication for influenza shortens the duration of the illness, and mitigates the severity of the illness. Aspirin should be avoided in all cases of influenza, because the combination of aspirin and influenza can cause Reye's syndrome and death from liver failure.

CHAPTER 8

THE INFECTIOUS CASCADE OF ABNORMAL PROTEINS, INFLAMMATION, ALTERED GENES, AND FUNGUS

Our forty-year discussion of infectious causes of chronic disease began with a discussion of the categories of infectious pathogens—bacteria, parasites, fungus, and viruses. Medicine has since added the categories of abnormal proteins and inflammation as being "associated" with chronic diseases. The quantity of scientific knowledge concerning abnormal proteins and inflammation has expanded, but has not necessarily advanced knowledge on the cause of chronic disease. Abnormal proteins and inflammation are caused by immortal pathogens. Genetic abnormalities can be caused by immortal pathogens. Fungus develops in all chronic diseases, during the downward spiral of an infectious cascade, caused by immortal pathogens.

Abnormal Proteins

Scientists are attempting to map the proteinbiome, and are rapidly identifying variations in normal and abnormal proteins. Scientists have identified three-hundred-sixty-three Cluster Differentiations, which are the small details and shapes of small molecules and proteins in the body. Many of the Cluster Differentiations are abnormal proteins. A super category of Cluster Differentiations is devoted to TNF-alpha, which is a substance generated by the immune system in response to immortal pathogens, that causes enhanced inflammation. Scientists are struggling to understand the significance of what they observed, documented, and named; and the relationship of their findings to chronic disease. They do not know why the abnormal proteins are created, where the abnormal proteins come from, the effect of abnormal proteins in causing chronic disease, or how to remove abnormal proteins from the body.

Proteins are an essential part of the human body, and are the building blocks of our body. We have forty-two million protein molecules inside each cell. The immune system uses proteins to make antibodies to fight infection. Abnormal proteins are not an independent disease, but rather are caused by chronic infection with immortal pathogens, and the immune response to the pathogens. The abnormal proteins are attached to the outside of the pathogens, and released in the body; and the sticky intracellular environment created by the immortal pathogens and the immune battle cause protein molecules to stick together and fold into abnormal shapes.

Abnormal proteins have many different names, and each specialty and field of research may describe abnormal proteins by different names. Abnormal proteins have been called prions, heat shock proteins, tau proteins, bent proteins, twisted proteins, M-proteins, Lewy body proteins, and many other variations describing the sticky and abnormally shaped proteins. All of the terms refer to an abnormally shaped chain of molecules that are attached to the outside of the cell and released into the system when the cell dies; or are abnormally shaped. The abnormal proteins do not passively move through the body, can become stuck in tissue, and can become a focus for immune system attack. Different intracellular and extracellular pathogens have distinct types of abnormal proteins attached to the surface, or cause unique or similar variants in abnormal proteins. The more chronic infections a person has, and the longer the infections have persisted, the more abnormal proteins and different types of abnormal proteins are created by the immortal pathogens and immune battles against multiple pathogens and abnormal proteins.

Abnormal proteins on the surface of pathogens protect the pathogen from the body's defense system. The immune system works on pattern recognition, to form antibodies to attack pathogens; and abnormal shapes of proteins confuse the immune system. When the host cell dies, broken parts of the cell and the abnormal proteins are released into the blood and lymphatics. Abnormal proteins are sticky, damming, bulky, and block passive flow. Abnormal proteins can become stuck in organs, as the abnormal proteins move through the blood vessels, lymphatics and organs;

and destroy passive functions. The abnormal proteins become a focus for immune system attack. Abnormal proteins cannot be killed; thus the immune system can only attempt to digest or engulf the abnormal proteins. As the infectious burden increases, or the patient acquires multiple chronic infections, the number and types of abnormal proteins also increase.

Scientists have now described three-hundred-sixty-three "Cluster Differentiations", which are also known as "Cluster Designation" or "Classification Determinant", and all are abbreviated as CD followed by a number, or by numbers and letters. The Cluster Differentiations describe the variations in shapes of the normal and abnormal proteins, and normal and pathogenic molecules. The Cluster Differentiations describe proteins in the body or generated by the immune system, such as TNF-alpha and C-reactive proteins; and the abnormal protein molecules on the surface of pathogens, created by the immune battle with pathogens, the abnormal folding of proteins, and which have attached to genes. The number of abnormal proteins to be categorized into Cluster Differentiations are as vast as the infections that create the abnormal proteins; the randomness of proteins folding and molecules sticking to each other; of sticky proteins attaching to pathogens and to each other; and of abnormal proteins attaching to genes.

Diseases thought to be caused solely by abnormal proteins are acquired by eating undercooked pork and fish, and by engaging in cannibalism. Jacob-Crutzfield disease and mad cow disease are examples of diseases believed to be caused by abnormal proteins that destroy the brain and end in death. Jacob-Crutzfield disease is thought to have originated in sheep, which were fed to cows, and the cows became a vector for mad cow disease in humans. The abnormal proteins found in fatal brain diseases leave holes in the brain; and the protein disease spreads throughout the brain causing death. How abnormal proteins spread in the brain is unclear, because the abnormal proteins are not alive; however, damage to the brain could occur from an aggressive immune response attacking the abnormal proteins, causing inflammation that damages brain tissue. If abnormal protein brain diseases are caused by immortal pathogens, additional abnormal proteins could continue to be released, spread, and deposited in the brain.

Lewy bodies are abnormal aggregates of proteins that develop inside nerve cells in Parkinson's disease, Lewy Body dementia, and other brain diseases. An aggregate of abnormal proteins can occur when the normal or abnormal proteins stick together. Lewy Body proteins may be from a specific type of abnormal protein, generated by immortal infection. H-pylori is one of the immortal infections "associated" with Parkinson's and Lewy Body dementia; and H-pylori can generate abnormal proteins, infect neutrophils, and cause profound changes in neutrophils. H-pylori is one of the likely causes of Parkinson's disease and Lewy Body dementia; and the most likely cause of abnormal protein aggregates identified as Lewy bodies. Low dose doxycycline has been shown effective in mice, in treating Parkinson's disease, supporting an infectious cause.[112]

The New York Times recently reported abnormal sticky proteins were found at the bottom of *all* glioma brain cancers. The sticky abnormal proteins caused glial cells in the brain to stick together and become a focus for a failed immune system attack, and development of brain cancer. The article reported Dr. Bradley E Bernstein, a pathologist at Massachusetts General Hospital, said he already found a similar phenomenon in about a dozen other tumors.[113]

Some scientists suggested ALS and frontal-temporal dementia are related to abnormal proteins. Dr. Merchant treated ALS patients for immortal infections, and saw improvement in the ALS. One elderly ALS patient lived four additional years before dying of leukemia, not ALS. Another patient was treated for six months with azithromycin, the condition stabilized during treatment, and the patient lived much longer than expected.

Identification of the type and virulence of cancer, and targeted cancer treatment, rely on the identification of abnormal proteins attached to the tumor. In breast cancer, the difference between HER-2 positive and

---

[112] De-Bel E and Barbosa A. 2017. Antibiotic Doxycycline May Offer Hope for Treatment of Parkinson's Disease. Scientific Reports. May 2017. Doi: https://www.sciencedaily.com/releases/2017/05/170503134119.

[113] Kolata G, 2015. Brain Cancers Reveal Novel Genetic Disruption in DNA. New York Times (Health). Dec. 23, 2015. Doi: https://wwwnytimes.com/2015/12/24/health/brain-cancers-reveal-novel-genetic-disruption-in-dna.html.

HER-2 negative cancer is whether abnormal proteins are attached to the outside of the tumor. If a patient has abnormal proteins on the surface of the tumor, they have immortal infection creating the abnormal proteins, which may have caused the cancer and could be treated to improve the cancer prognosis.

Scientific research is needed to discover which infections generate which types of abnormal proteins, and how to clear abnormal proteins from the body. New methods to clear the abnormal proteins from the body after acute or chronic infection could potentially provide protection against the development of chronic diseases. Chemotherapy fails in ovarian cancer when abnormal proteins block the effectiveness of the chemotherapy drugs. A new drug, developed at the University of New Mexico Hospital, clears abnormal proteins after failed chemotherapy for ovarian cancer, and improves the effectiveness of the next round of chemotherapy.[114] Potentially, use of a drug that clears abnormal proteins could be expanded to new indications, to clear abnormal proteins generated by infection before the cancer develops and to improve the prognosis in other types of cancer and other chronic diseases.

Inflammation

Science is now studying "inflammasomes", a new medical term, describing clumps of abnormal proteins shaped in different patterns, causing inflammation. Scientists studying inflammasomes believe inflammasomes initiate an inflammatory cascade. Scientists study and describe every stage of inflammation, during the inflammatory cascade. Scientists do not understand why tissue becomes inflamed, the relationship between inflammation and immortal pathogens, and the relationship of immortal pathogens and chronic disease. The immune system is responding to intracellular pathogens, and the immune battle is causing the inflammation.

Inflammasomes are hypothesized to create an inflammatory cascade. Apoptosomes are hypothesized to activate the apoptotic cascade. The

---

[114] Ricci J, *et al.* 2016. Novel ABCG2 Antagonists Reverse Topotecan-Mediated Chemotherapeutic Resistance in Ovarian Carcinoma Xenografts. Molecular Cancer Therapeutics. Doi: 10.1158/1535-7163.MCT-15-0789.

categorization of inflammasomes is describing the patterns of abnormal proteins stuck together, on the inside and outside of cells, and in tissue. The abnormal proteins get stuck in tissue, and the immune system reacts, causing inflammation. The intracellular pathogen is causing the abnormal proteins, and the inflammatory reaction is to the pathogen and the abnormal proteins. The pathogen causes the loss of normal apoptosis, not the inflammation as a stand-alone cause of the loss of apoptosis.

Inflammation is not a diagnosis—inflammation is a description of a symptom and a finding in many chronic diseases. What is causing the inflammation, now thought to be "associated" with so many different chronic diseases? An overactive immune system against what? Tissue becomes inflamed in reaction to something—infection! The hallmarks of infection are redness, heat, swelling and pain. Inflammation is the redness and heat components, which are hallmarks of infection. Inflammation is the result of the immune response to chronic intracellular infection. Heat is generated by the war between the immune system and the pathogen, and from energy released from dying cells. Inflammation can have a protective role, or can damage tissue and cause atrophy, as the inflammation persists or recedes. Treating inflammation alone will not treat the cause of inflammation, can make the diagnosis more difficult, and can worsen the disease and the prognosis.

Many chronic diseases now thought to be inflammatory diseases are caused by underlying immortal infections. Inflammation is evidence the body is responding to the infection. Inflammation is the immune system reaction to an intracellular pathogen that hides inside cells, inclusion cysts, cholesterol and fungus. Chlamydia infected cells produce interleukins, cytokines, and TNF-alpha, all of which are part of an immune response, and cause inflammation. TNF-alpha is a higher level of inflammation, generated by the immune cells and particularly macrophages, when the immune system is unable to eradicate the pathogens or proteins and mounts a more aggressive inflammatory response to the chronic infection. Chlamydia increases C-reactive proteins, a common marker in the blood for inflammation; and generates heat shock proteins. Immortal infection becomes chronic and widespread, causes widespread inflammation, and causes chronic disease. The inflammation and the chronic disease are caused by the same pathogen, and the immune battle against the pathogen.

Scientists are finding and describing the small details in cell microbiology, and describing the proteinbiome, Cluster Differentiations, inflammasomes, and apoptosome, hoping a scientific discovery will emerge from the study of minute details and categorization of every variation in abnormal proteins. Categorization and research into inflammasomes are diverting research away from infectious causes of the inflammation. The scientists studying Cluster Differentiation, the proteinbiome, inflammasomes, apoptosomes, and gene research, should combine knowledge, to find new understanding in the minute details of cell microbiology and abnormal proteins.

Inflammation is the immune response to pathogens. Chronic chlamydia infections cause inflammation, immune dysfunction, abnormal apoptosis, endothelial dysfunction, angiogenesis, TNF-alpha, C-reactive protein, heat shock proteins, and more. Research should be directed to which pathogens are causing which "inflammasomes", apoptosomes, abnormalities described in the proteinbiome, and Cluster Differentiations, to discover the root cause of chronic disease and further enlighten diagnosis and treatment of chronic disease and inflammation, based on findings of specific abnormal proteins.

Genes and Genetic Causes of Disease

Hippocrates was a revolutionary when he suggested diseases had a cause, and were not sent from God. Doctors still do not know what causes most chronic diseases, and often attribute chronic disease to something unknown about the patient, or a genetic abnormality. Genetic defects are the modern version of the chronic disease was sent from God.

Dr. Merchant has suggested immortal infections can alter genes and gene expression. Dr. Glidden argued doctors talk about genetic causes when the doctor cannot offer an explanation for the disease.[115] Talking about genetic causes leads the patient to bow to the superior knowledge of the

---

[115] Glidden B. 2010. <u>The MD Emperor Has No Clothes-Everybody is Sick and I Know Why</u>, 3rd Ed. San Bernardino, CA.

doctor, stop asking questions, accept their fate as abnormal genes, and accept symptomatic treatment for their disease. Dr. Ewald argued if genes were the cause of chronic disease, chronic diseases would be eliminated or reduced in every generation, because of the genetic cost of chronic disease. Dr. Ewald suggested pathogens cause alteration of genes; and reported it is already known that genes are driven and changed by infection with bacteria and viruses.[116]

Science has observed, mapped and identified our DNA, mapped genes, studied gene expression, and identified abnormal genes and gene variations, in chronic disease. Science makes diagnoses based on genetic abnormalities, but have not considered nor confirmed if the genetic defect caused the disease or the disease caused the genetic defect. Science cannot understand why gene abnormalities and gene variations are not consistent, between people with the same chronic disease or among people living in different geographic areas. Science has not explained why genetic abnormalities occur, why the chronic disease persists in the population, or offered any treatment or cures based on knowledge and findings of genetic abnormalities. A doctor makes a diagnosis of a genetic defect when the doctor observes a gene abnormality, and does not know any other cause to explain the chronic disease.

Identifying abnormal genes is an observation, rather than a diagnosis of the cause. Chronic infection can alter genes and gene expression. Research to identify and correlate which pathogens cause which abnormal proteins, and which pathogens and abnormal proteins change which genes, would be helpful in finding the root infectious causes of chronic diseases now thought to be genetic. Understanding that chronic infection can change genes offers hope to those with a chronic disease diagnosed as a genetic defect.

Human DNA is most similar to chimpanzees. A person has about three billion nucleotide bases that form our genes, with four fundamental types

---

[116] *See* Hooper J. The New Germ Theory. Atlantic Monthly. Feb. 1999. Doi: www.theatlantic.com; Ewald PW. 2002. Plague Time: The New Germ Theory, 2nd Ed. Anchor Books.; Ewald PW. 2000. Plague Time: How Stealth Infections Cause Cancers, Heart Disease and other Deadly Ailments. New York: Free Press.

of bases comprising our DNA, commonly abbreviated as A, C, G, and T. Within the three billion nucleotide bases, we only have about 20,000+ genes that make us unique as human beings. The 20,000 genes unique humans are studied in the field of epigenetics.

Genes are specific sequences of bases that provide instructions on how to make important proteins that trigger biological actions to carry out life functions. Genes and epigenetics give instructions that direct the activities of cells. Genes and epigenetic signaling evolve with the microbiome and exposure to infectious pathogens. Proteins direct genes, and sticky abnormal proteins generated by immortal intracellular pathogens attach to genes. The abnormal proteins impair or damage epigenetic signaling to the cells, and reduce the ability of the genes to properly function.

Epigenetics studies the changes in genetic signaling, caused by modification of gene expression, rather than alteration of the genetic code.[117] Gene expression represents the directions from the gene being turned on or off, which impacts the directions from the genes to the cells. Epigenetics determine how genes are read by cells, and how proteins are created. Some circumstances can cause genes to be silenced or expressed over time; and, at any given time, genes can be turned off (become dormant) or turned on (become active). Gene expression may also change with the seasons.[118] The study of epigenetics has revealed fragments of DNA from ancient pathogens, fragments of viral genes, inside the cells, and some viral genes have been integrated into human genes.

Epigenetic signaling can be changed by infections acquired in a person's lifetime, the combinations of infections, and the abnormal proteins created by the immortal infections. One study reported *only* animal pathogens and the abnormal proteins from the animal pathogens were

---

[117] 2013. A Super Brief and Basic Explanation of Epigenetics for Total Beginners. Jul 30, 2013. Doi: whatisepigenetics.com/what-is-epigenetics/.

[118] Dopico X, *et al.* 2015. Widespread Seasonal Gene Expression Reveals Annual Differences in Human Immunity and Physiology. Nature Communications. May 2015. Article 6:7000. Doi: 10.1038/ncomms8000.

capable of altering genes and gene expression[119], which includes all chlamydia pathogens originating in animals. The alterations in genes caused by immortal pathogens can be passed on to the next generation, and be identified as a genetic defect. The genes children inherit from their parents includes alterations in epigenetic signaling caused by abnormal proteins attached to the parents' genes. The abnormal genes may then be identified as a genetic abnormality or weakness in the child.

Intracellular chlamydia creates junk DNA, a non-coding DNA fragment, which can create pseudo genes; and alters the genes and epigenetic signaling with sticky abnormal proteins. Junk DNA, plasmids and abnormal proteins, play a role in developing cancer cells and create a focus for chronic diseases.

Identical twin studies, on twins separated at birth, repeatedly confirm genes change during our life. Twenty years after separation, the genes of identical twins no longer matched! The epi-genes had changed, based on the variety of immortal infections and environmental triggers the person experienced in their life. Pathogenic bacteria, particularly chlamydia species, cause genetic changes; and one must ask whether the genetic defect is causing the chronic disease, or the immortal infections in the family are causing the gene defect and the chronic disease. The twin studies suggest genetic defects are caused by an immortal pathogens acquired in life, and pathogens can cause both chronic disease and a genetic defect.

Experts searched for common variations in genes in common chronic diseases, and found it was not as simple as expected. Researchers studied groups of people who had chronic diseases in common, and expected to find common variations in genes. They did not! Epigenetic studies showed different genetic variants can cause the same disease, and rare variants can cause the same disease. Researchers were unable to find common gene variations in various chronic diseases. Researchers found different genetic mutations caused the same disease on different continents; and that different gene variations on different continents can cause the same disease. Researchers found different rare gene variations in common diseases, in different people

---

[119] Bierne H, *et al.* 2012. Epigenetics and Bacterial Infections. Cold Spring Harb Perspect Med. 2(12). a010272. Dec 2012. Doi: 10.1101/cshperspect.a010272.

The finding patients with the same chronic disease had different genetic mutations, on different continents; and rare genetic mutations, and different combinations of genetic mutations, were found in the same chronic disease, is consistent with infectious pathogens altering genes, altering epigenetic signaling, and causing chronic disease. Chlamydia pathogens and abnormal proteins generated by infectious pathogens can attack different genes in different people. Different immortal infections and combinations of infections can alter genes in the same or different ways in different people; and the same immortal infections and combinations of infections can cause the same or different diseases in different people, which is consistent with variations in genetic mutations between people who have the same chronic disease.

Chlamydia and parasitic infections are transmitted between family members, and can cause the same chronic infections in family members and the same genetic changes. Abnormal genes and abnormal gene expression can arise from common familial infections and unique abnormal proteins from the infections. The same combinations of infections can be present in all of the family members, causing the same alterations in genes, and the same or different chronic diseases. Genes may play a role in predisposition or vulnerability, to a chronic disease, once a gene variant develops from chronic infection or is inherited, and may change the manifestation of chronic disease—but immortal infections common to members of the household and pets in the household generate abnormal proteins that alter the genes and epigenetic signaling. Whether chronic disease is inherited in the form of abnormal genes, or chronic infections alter genes *and* cause chronic disease or a predisposition to chronic disease, is not clear.

Infections, genes, and genetic signaling have a constantly evolving relationship, in a battle between the immune system and the pathogen. Each type of immortal pathogen causes its own unique abnormal proteins and genetic mutations, and its own unique chronic disease. The greater the infectious burden, and the more abnormal proteins spawned from immortal infection, the greater the potential for genetic defects and chronic disease.

Gene theory alone cannot account for chronic disease, because, if true, the genetic cost of chronic disease would eliminate many chronic diseases from the population within a few generations. The higher the genetic cost, the sooner the disease would be eliminated. It is infections, not genes, underlying chronic disease *and* genetic abnormalities. Abnormal genes and abnormal signaling can impact the development and manifestation of chronic disease, but abnormal genes are the result of the immune battle against chronic infection.

When the rate of a chronic disease is increasing rather than decreasing, the chronic disease cannot be explained by abnormal genes. Why are diseases, like childhood cancer, hypertension, diabetes and obesity occurring in even greater numbers, if the cause is genetics? Chronic diseases caused by animal pathogens cannot be genetic, because human genes are not the same as animal genes? If chronic diseases are genetic, how could humans develop the same chronic diseases as animals, from the same animal pathogens; and how could pathogens and chronic diseases be passed from animals-to-humans?

Medical bias favors diagnosis of genetic causes over diagnosis of infectious causes, which limits the ability of doctors and researchers to identify infectious causes of chronic disease. Doctors fail to inquire as to the health of all family members, including family members who are not blood relatives, pets, and contact with domesticated animals. Chronic and persistent infection is harder to recognize than acute infection, and requires work and time, particularly when infectious causes of chronic disease were never taught in medical school. Immortal infections, among family members and animals, and in the household, are as important, or more important, than genetics, in causing genetic abnormalities and chronic disease.

Billions of dollars have been spent on genetic research, which has yielded minimal answers as to the cause of chronic disease. The billions spent on genetic research overlooks the fact genes can change over time in response to chronic infection; and immortal infections create abnormal proteins that alter the genes, cause random variations in genes, and alter epigenetic signaling. Research into small details of cell microbiology should be directed to the cause and cure of immortal infections, and determining which genes are targeted by which immortal infections and which abnormal proteins.

Fungus

Fungus is similar to a plant or mushroom. Fungus is a part of life, and every living thing has some fungus. The fungus types within our body comprise the mycobiome, which includes 5.1 million species of fungus, three-hundred species of which can cause disease. More than one-thousand bacterial species are found in the gut. Scientists do not understand all the types of fungus, and which are good and bad. Fungus may be referred to as yeast, candida, and other names in medicine. The predominant species of fungus affecting the health of humans are saccharomyces, mallassezia, and candida.

I Contain Multitudes describes fungus as part of the culture within us. Good bacteria work alone or in combination with good fungus, and good fungus aids digestion by creating scaffolding for good bacteria. Good bacteria and good fungi work together to fight pathogens. Bad fungus, or an overgrowth of fungus, can occur when the microbiome and mycobiome are out of balance. Bad fungus damages the intestinal scaffolding, impairs absorption of nutrients, hides pathogens from the immune cells; and feeds and potentiates pathogens and parasites.

Fungus can be harmless, or pathogenic; and can become pathogenic when immune function declines, the microbiome is out of balance, or the epithelium is damaged. A person with fungal overgrowth likely has co-infections with intracellular pathogens, causing reduced immunity, increasing dysbiosis, and increasing the fungal burden. Co-infection with H-pylori can damage the epithelium, which then allows fungus to invade the lining of the intestine and cause leaky gut and dysbiosis.[120] Fungus is part of the infectious cascade, and eventually develops in every chronic

---

[120] *See* 2017. Q&A on Candida with the Scientist Who Named the Microbiome (Mahmoud Ghannoum, Ph.D.). SCIENCE. Doi: biohmhealth.com/blogs/science/a-q-a-on-candida-with-the-scientist-who-named-the-mycobiome.

disease. Science has not yet recognized fungus is a common finding, in every chronic disease.

Fungus can invade or develop in any organ or body systems. It can develop in the digestive tract; or outside the digestive tract, including in the sinus and brain, to cause secondary disease. Fungus can invade deeper into tissue whenever the epithelium has been damaged by other pathogens. Fungus and an increase in pH allows intestinal bacteria to infect and thrive in the urinary tract, and create an environment for frequent urinary tract infections. Fungal infection or frequent urinary tract infections, and recurrent vaginal yeast, should trigger medical investigation into chronic infection.

Patients with advanced heart disease had "vegetation" on their heart valves. The vegetation was a mass of bacteria, cells, and fungus, developing on and around the immortal infection that caused the chronic heart disease. Vegetation is a sign of long-standing infection with chlamydia pneumonia, causing fermentation and fungal development. Those who developed vegetation, on the heart valves, required heart surgery to replace valves.[121]

Histoplasmosis is a type of fungus associated with bird and bat droppings. Within the U.S., histoplasmosis is particularly common in the Ohio and Mississippi River valleys. In demolition projects, in areas that contain bat or bird droppings, the spores may become airborne and can travel hundreds of feet. The fact histoplasmosis is associated with bird droppings suggests it may also associated with psittacosis; and in patients with lowered immunity, histoplasmosis can invade the lung and cause pneumonia. If the histoplasmosis infection spreads throughout the body, it can cause disseminated disease. If the disease progresses without treatment, the patient may develop weight loss, shortness of breath, and fatigue. Ocular involvement in disseminated histoplasmosis can cause loss of vision. If the infection spreads to the central

---

[121] Friedman H, *et al* (*eds*). 2004. *Chlamydia Pneumonia Infection and Disease*. New York: Kluwer Academic/Plenum Publishers. Chlamydia Pneumonia and Myocarditis. (Gnarpe JG and Gnarpe JA). Ch. 13

nervous system, severe symptoms may develop, including seizures, headaches, and confusion.[122]

Coccidiodomycosis is a common type of fungus that is in dust in the Southwest. It is known as Valley Fever or California fever. The incidence of coccidiomycosis increases after dust storms. Coccidiomycosis can cause a respiratory infection and pneumonia.

Ringworm, although called a "worm", is actually a fungal infection on the skin. Ringworm is called ringworm because the skin lesion resembles a worm. Ringworm starts as a scaly, circular brown spot, and over time the ringworm spreads spread out wider, leaving a ring of abnormal raised skin that looks like a worm around the edge of the lesion. Ringworm is highly contagious, and spreads from person-to-person and from animal-to-person, including to and from cats and dogs, by direct contact with the skin.

---

[122] Stoppler M and Davis C (*eds*). Histoplasmosis. MedicineNet.com. *Accessed* Jun 21, 2018. Doi: www.medicinenet.com/histoplasmosis facts/article.htm#histoplasmosis facts.

CHAPTER 9

CHRONIC INFECTION IN
GASTROINTESTINAL DISEASES

Hippocrates said, "Man is not nourished by what he swallows, but by what he digests and uses." In ancient times, people had less access to clean water and hygiene. Animals transmitted pathogens and parasites to man; and man had a limited ability to treat the pathogens and parasites. In the 1930's, widespread availability of indoor plumbing extended life expectancy, by providing clean water and better hygiene, which reduced the infectious burden of bacteria and parasites. Clean water, hygiene, and barriers to mosquitoes extended the life expectancy more than any medicine.

Dr. Merchant's thinking began with diseases of the gastrointestinal tract. In the South Valley, he observed a characteristic big belly, in men who drank contaminated well water. He observed patients with big bellies, wasting, and recurrent respiratory infections. Giardia patients often developed hives, and increasing sensitivity to food and drugs. He observed the patients had low folic acid and B12, causing mental instability and belligerence, and a high rate cancer. He observed patients with parasitic infection had high eosinophils and high monocytes. Eosinophils attack parasites and worms, by surrounding the parasites; and release cytoplasmic granules to disable or kill the parasite. Monocytes then engulf and digest the parasites if possible. In endemic areas, many patients have high monocytes, and doctors need to recognize high eosinophils and high monocytes can be related to endemic parasitic infection in the community; and the findings should not be dismissed as unimportant, merely because doctors frequently see the same symptoms, and the same high eosinophils and high monocytes.

More and more scientists and thinkers are starting to agree with Dr. Merchant that chronic diseases can start in the gastrointestinal tract. More and more scientists and thinkers are describing and investigating the "gut-brain connection". Some have now reported the gastrointestinal tract is a key to health, and reporting numerous conditions are linked to gastrointestinal health, including pain, mood disorders, schizophrenia, depression, autism and Parkinson's disease.[123] A balance in the microbiome and mycobiome is necessary to maintain gastrointestinal health, and prevent an overgrowth of pathogenic bacteria and fungus.

The mouth is the major route by which pathogens and parasites enter the intestines. Pathogenic bacteria and parasites live off the energy in the cells, and the nutrients provided in the gastrointestinal tract; cause fungal invasion; generate abnormal proteins and plasmids; and combine with other pathogens to cause dysbiosis. Immortal pathogens and parasites compete for nutrients; and the immortal pathogens and the byproducts of the pathogens clog the gastrointestinal system, causing malabsorption. Immortal pathogens and parasites cause chronic disease in the gastrointestinal tract, and migrate or metastasize outside the gastrointestinal tract to cause chronic disease throughout the body.

The gastrointestinal tract is a complex anaerobic culture of micro-organisms and fungus. The gastrointestinal tract lacks sufficient oxygen to support most aerobic pathogens. Some intestinal bacteria are good, and aid body functions; and other bacteria are pathogenic. Some bacteria are beneficial in one part of the gastrointestinal tract, but can become pathogenic when in a different part of the gastrointestinal tract or in other organ and systems. Scientists understand less than one percent of the microorganisms in the gastrointestinal tract.

Diagnosis of intestinal pathogens has been limited by the inability of gastroenterologists to distinguish normal intestinal bacteria from pathogenic bacteria; and limited understanding of the microbiome.

---

[123] Cenit MC, *et al.* 2017. Influence of gut microbiota on neuropsychiatric disorders. World J Gastroenterol. Aug 14, 2017. 23(30): 5486-5498. Doi: 10.3748/wjg.v23.i30.5486.

Carolyn Merchant, JD & Christopher Merchant, MD

Even when bacteria in the intestine are identified in a chronic disease, the tendency is to dismiss the results of testing as not important, or the pathogen is alleged to be normal intestinal flora. Even normal intestinal bacteria can cause disease when in an aberrant location in the intestine or body, or when it combines with other pathogens.

Gastrointestinal disease can be divided into upper, middle, and lower gastrointestinal tract disease. The location of the complaints, in the upper, middle, or lower digestive tract, can be a clue to the pathogens and parasites causing the symptoms. Upper gastrointestinal disease in the esophagus and stomach is most likely H-pylori. Upper and middle intestinal tract disease in the stomach and small bowel is more likely parasites, such as giardia and cryptosporidiosis; and can be from H-pylori. Some types of worms live in the small intestine and liver, such as hookworms and liver flukes. The pathogens and parasites in the upper and middle gastrointestinal tract migrate to organs adjacent and attached to the gastrointestinal tract, including the liver, gallbladder, biliary tract, and the pancreas, causing chronic disease.[124] Lower intestinal disease, in the colon and rectum, may be caused by chlamydia; worms; or streptococcus, combined with other immortal infections and parasites. Toxoplasmosis can invade the small intestine and cause inflammation in the lining of the intestine.

Chlamydia, giardia and cryptosporidiosis, worms, amoebas, H-pylori, and toxoplasmosis, are the most common intestinal tract infections. Chlamydia causes a weak gastrointestinal environment, vulnerable to attack by intestinal pathogens and parasites; and fosters development of biofilm, mucous, pus, plaque and fungus. Chlamydia consumes folic acid and B12, depletes folic acid and B12, clogs the digestive tract, and damages the villi in the intestine, which promotes dysbiosis. Chlamydia infection in the gastrointestinal tract causes a generalized immunodeficiency and dysbiosis, allowing new infections with pathogens and parasites. Parasites also compete for folic acid and B12; and generate pathogenic fungus, accelerating the infectious cascade. Fungus develops from fermentation

---

[124] *See* Onsioen C, *et al.* 2008. Chlamydia is a Risk Factor for Pediatric Biliary Tract Disease. European Journal of Gastroenterology & Hepatology. Apr 2008. Vol. 20(4): 365-366. Doi: 10.1097/MEG.0b013e3282f340f1.

and an alteration of pH, and further damages the villi and worsens the clogging of the digestive tract. Fungus hides the pathogens from the immune system and worsens the malabsorption of nutrients.

Immortal pathogens and fungus create weak immunity and make an environment hospitable for parasites. The parasites infect and reproduce in the host, in a cycle of eggs and cysts, and the eggs and cysts spread the parasite. As the eggs hatch, develop, mature, spread, and die, the symptoms may become dormant, during parts of the life cycle of the parasite. As the burden of parasitic infection increases, all phases of the life cycle of the parasite are present and constant, and the symptoms can change and become constant. Parasites can start in a preferred part of the intestine, depending on the type of parasite, and can migrate to new locations over time, to avoid stomach acid or find other hospitable environments.

Chronic diseases in abdominal organs have been "associated" with infectious pathogens and parasites in the gastrointestinal tract. Gastrointestinal pathogens can migrate or metastasize to the liver, gallbladder, pancreas, urinary tract, kidneys, and reproductive tract. The liver, gallbladder, pancreas and biliary tract connect to the intestine in the middle intestinal tract; and pathogens and parasites in the intestine, near where the organs connect to the intestine, can migrate into the adjacent organs to cause chronic disease. The giardia parasite has been found inside pancreatic tumors. Chlamydia, H-pylori, and the infectious byproducts of gastrointestinal pathogens have been found in the fluid around arthritic joints.

People in contact with animals are vulnerable to any pathogen or parasite in the animal. Gastroenterologists do not often recognize or acknowledge chlamydia, giardia, cryptosporidiosis, or worms, even in community outbreaks or endemic areas. Gastroenterologists and many primary care providers have a false assumption the United States has advanced beyond parasitic disease, which interferes with the accurate diagnosis of acute and chronic parasitic disease. Gastroenterologists and primary care doctors only consider the diagnosis of parasitic disease when the patient has a history of foreign travel. Parasitic disease exists worldwide, in all mammals. Parasites have always existed in the United States. World travel and foreign wars, in parts of the world with endemic parasitic disease, have further spread parasitic disease and unusual parasites to the United States.

Veterans acquire parasitic infections during foreign deployments. The Veterans Administration recently noticed a high rate of liver cancer and other unusual cancers in veterans of the Vietnam War. A study confirmed persistent parasitic infection with liver flukes, a worm common in the rivers and streams of Vietnam, which invades the liver and causes cancer over a long period of time. The Veterans Administration delayed forty-two years before noticing Vietnam veterans had unusual parasitic diseases common in Vietnam! Veterans who were not diagnosed and treated for parasites and immortal infections suffered a reduced quality of life and developed chronic disease and cancer years later. Instead of diagnosing and treating parasitic infection and other pathogens, the Veterans Administration channeled the veterans into psychiatric care and psychiatric drugs, ultimately causing a higher rate of suicide among veterans. The veterans had untreated parasitic disease and were given psychiatric drugs which increase the risk of suicide.

Giardia is a common intestinal parasite, and may be indistinguishable from or diagnosed as the less common parasite cryptosporidiosis. Giardia resides in the upper digestive tract, although not the only parasites to inhabit the upper digestive tract. The patients with giardia complain of episodic or persistent abdominal pain, in the upper abdomen above the belly button; and often describe a "comma" pattern of pain, by putting their hand in the upper right and central portion of the abdomen in a comma pattern. Giardia clogs the intestine, competes for folic acid and B12, causes malabsorption of nutrients, causes dysbiosis, and fosters fungus to aid survival and hide from the immune system. Chlamydia and giardia as co-infections potentiate the damage to the intestinal tract and depletion of nutrients, especially folic acid and B12. Giardia and other parasitic infections can hide chlamydia and viruses as endo-symbionts; and pathogens, like H-pylori, can attach to the outside of chlamydia infected cells and parasites as an ecto-symbiont.

Patients may initially dismiss transient symptoms of acute parasitic infection; and only seek medical attention when longstanding parasitic infection has caused malabsorption and chronic disease. The patient may have been infected months or years before seeking medical attention, from drinking water, a public swimming pool, lakes, streams, camping, pets, domesticated animals, soil, or any number of sources long forgotten, and not recognized as the source of the symptoms when the patient seeks medical attention.

Worms are a common cause of gastrointestinal symptoms, particularly in pet owners and people in contact with livestock or wild animals. Virtually all animals acquire worms in their lifetime. Pet owners and household members are at risk of acquiring worms through close contact with pets. Gastroenterologists fail to inquire into a history of pets or contact with domesticated animals, when animals are a vector for many types of immortal infections, parasites, and worms causing diseases in the gastrointestinal tract. A gastroenterologist has to observe and think to diagnose pathogens and parasites; and be knowledgeable as to the locations where parasites reside in the intestine, the effect of different pathogens and parasites, and blood testing abnormalities in patients with parasitic diseases, as a means of diagnosis.

Worms establish themselves in the upper, middle, or lower intestinal tract, depending on the type of worm and duration of infection. Worms deprive the body of nutrients, by competing for nutrients and mechanically clogging the intestine, blocking absorption of nutrients. Hookworms are blood sucking worms that inhabit the small bowel (middle intestine), and can cause anemia. Worms in the lower gastrointestinal tract can be misdiagnosed as irritable bowel. Pinworms inhabit the lower intestine and rectum; and cause rectal itching, particularly at sundown. Worms in the intestine can invade other abdominal organs, and have been found in the liver, gallbladder, pancreas, and brain. Worms in vital organs can cause blockage, and immune system attack, and chronic disease.

Parasites have typically been diagnosed by microscopic inspection of the stool, which is notoriously unreliable; and dependent on the diligence of the examiner. ELISA blood tests are now available to test for giardia and cryptosporidiosis in the stool. The lack of readily available and accurate testing for parasites, has impaired diagnostic acumen with regard to parasites. Blood tests showing high monocytes, high eosinophils, low folic acid, and low B12, give clues to parasitic disease. Most parasitic infections, other enteric infections, and some forms of chlamydia, like trachoma and psittacosis, respond to metronidazole. Pathogens not amenable to treatment with metronidazole can be treated with macrolides and cyclines or other anti-parasitic medications. H-pylori requires a different treatment regimen than chlamydia pathogens or parasites, and often requires combined antibiotic treatment. Gastroenterologists are seldom willing to diagnose infectious causes of intestinal disease or consider using safe antibiotics or antiparasitic drugs.

Veterinarians are well aware of diseases caused by worms, and worms can be spread from pets and domesticated animals to people. Naturopaths reported parasites, worms and other bacteria cause chronic disease, in 1995 and 2010.[125] Why don't gastroenterologists, and all primary care doctors know the animal-to-person transmission of pathogens, parasites, and worms? We treat the pets for parasites—but no one treats the people!

In the 1940's a teaching hospital knew ulcers were an infection, and treated ulcers successfully with antibiotics, even though unable to identify the bacterium. In the 1950's, knowledge of the infectious cause of ulcers was deleted from medical texts and medical training. The 1982, Cecil Textbook of Medicine fails to mention infectious cause of ulcers, and returns to the discussion of risk factors, co-morbid conditions, and attributing ulcers to genes or the psychological make-up of the individual.[126] Dr. Marshall began reporting ulcers were an infection, in the early 1980's, and it took until 1990, after an article in the National Inquirer, for gastroenterologists to begin treating ulcers as an infection. Few gastroenterologists today were taught H-pylori, chlamydia, and parasites are the major causes of chronic gastrointestinal diseases. Some doctors and patients persist in attributing

---

[125] Glidden B. 2010. The MD Emperor Has No Clothes-Everybody is Sick and I Know Why, 3rd Ed. San Bernardino, CA; Clark HR. 1995. THE Cure for All Diseases, With Many Case Histories. California: New Century Press.
[126] Wyngaarden JB and Smith LH (ed). 1982. Cecil Textbook of Medicine. 16th Ed. Part VII. Gastrointestinal Diseases. Philadelphia: WB Saunders Company.

ulcers to stress, or to a bowel that is "irritable", or to something the patient ate last night; and end the diagnostic process with a diagnosis of a symptom, description of a finding, or syndrome named as a disease, such as an "ulcer" or "irritable bowel syndrome".

Up to twenty percent of American adults have gastrointestinal symptoms labeled as "irritable bowel syndrome" (IBS). Medicine persists in alleging irritable bowel is related to psychiatric disorders.[127] IBS is not a diagnosis—it is a description of symptoms. IBS should be more appropriately re-named, "It's Bull Shit". A diagnosis of IBS or inflammatory bowel disease usually shows the doctor does not know why the patient has symptoms, and is clueless about diagnosis and treatment of pathogens and parasites. IBS is related to psychiatric disorders, only to the extent gut pathogens and dysbiosis also cause what doctors are diagnosing as a psychiatric disorders. IBS is only related to psychiatric disorders to the extent immortal pathogens in the gastrointestinal tract cause mood disorders—the gut-brain connection!

IBS is caused by immortal pathogens, parasites, the immune system reaction to pathogens, and the consequences of dysbiosis. Gastroenterologists seldom recognize or acknowledge gastrointestinal pathogens and parasites can cause IBS, and other systemic diseases. Intestinal pathogens and parasites are seldom considered in the differential diagnosis of IBS, or other intestinal disease. No patient over fifty, with blood in the stool, weight loss, or significant diarrhea, should be labeled with IBS unless all infectious causes have been excluded.

A recent debate between gastroenterologists diagnosing IBS versus CIC (chronic idiopathic constipation) demonstrates the gastroenterologists' desire to seem knowledgeable and make-up an answer when they do not know. IBS and CIC are considered diseases of unknown origin. Idiopathic means "the doctor does not know; therefore, it must be you". Neither IBS

---

[127] Fadgyas-Stanculete M, *et al.* 2014. The Relationship Between Irritable Bowel Syndrome and Psychiatric Disorders: From Molecular Changes to Clinical Manifestations. Journal of Molecular Psychiatry. 2014. 2:4. Doi: 10.1186/2049-9256-2-4.

or CIC is a diagnosis. IBS and CIC are descriptions of symptoms; and the debate about which symptoms define IBS versus CIC, should be a debate about which infectious pathogens and parasites cause irritable bowel, diarrhea and constipation. Instead of diagnosing an infectious cause of the intestinal symptoms, doctors are subdividing IBS, into new syndromes of IBS constipation and IBS diarrhea. Both IBS and CIC are caused by immortal pathogens and/or parasites, and both are part of the infectious cascade. Both occur during the evolution of parasitic disease from episodic to constant, at different points in the life cycle of the pathogens and parasites.

Rather than diagnosing the infectious pathogens and parasites causing the bowel to be "irritable", gastroenterologists prescribe symptomatic treatment for diarrhea, constipation, bloating, and pain. They give drugs to stop diarrhea, when diarrhea is the body's clue to an infection and a defense against pathogens! The passive reaction of the body to rid itself of pathogens in the gastrointestinal tract is diarrhea, and preventing the elimination of pathogens with medications to stop diarrhea is itself dangerous. Stopping diarrhea keeps the pathogens in the intestine, where pathogens can become established and cause greater harm. They prescribe drugs to move the bowels when the patient has constipation. They give drugs to treat constipation caused by other drugs. Drugs to treat symptoms can be harmful, and drugs to treat diarrhea or constipation are associated with serious side effects, including bowel perforation, heart attacks, and strokes. Symptomatic treatment of intestinal disease, rather than treatment of the infectious cause, leads to a life-long dependency on the gastroenterologist for symptomatic medications and scopes.

Chlamydia pneumonia has been "associated" with elevated body mass index, in young men. Finnish military recruits who were IgG seropositive for chlamydia pneumonia were studied for six to twelve months. The study showed the "association" between chronic chlamydia pneumonia and obesity, in young men. Persistent chlamydia pneumonia antibodies and/or elevated CRP were found to be significant risk factors for being overweight.[128] Increasing girth is a known risk factor for heart disease and diabetes, which diseases are also caused by chlamydia pneumonia; often with co-infections. Toxoplasmosis has also been "associated" with obesity and anorexia, and pancreatitis.[129]

Today, young adults are developing obesity and getting gastrointestinal cancers at higher rates, and doctors do not seem to be studying the pathogens that cause both obesity and cancer. Patients with obesity are treated by endocrinologists, when the patients should be evaluated, diagnosed, and treated for infectious disease by gastroenterologists. Gastroenterologists should recognize the relationship between obesity and gastrointestinal pathogens, and evaluate the patient for bio-diversity and gastrointestinal pathogens and parasites; and supplement nutrition, particularly folic acid, to avoid triggering cancer.

H-pylori is a spiral bacterium, which causes stomach ulcers and stomach cancer. H-pylori attacks epithelium, and invades deeper into the collagen matrix, below the epithelium, damaging the collagen matrix. Neutrophils are the most common type of white blood cell and a type of immune cell which attacks H-pylori. When neutrophils attack H-pylori, the neutrophils become infected intracellularly with H-pylori. The infected neutrophils changed phenotype, making the neutrophils less able to recognize and kill the H-pylori. The infected neutrophils change from three or four interconnected lobes to six or more segmented lobes, secrete pro-inflammatory cytokines, and cause toxicity in surrounding tissue. The hyper-segmentation of the neutrophils into lobules resembles characteristics

---

[128] Rantala A, *et al*. 2010. Chlamydia Pneumonia Infection Is Associated with Elevated Body Mass Index in Young Men. Epidemiol Infec. Sep 2010. 138(9): 1267-73. Doi: 10. 1017/S0950268809991452. Epub. Dec 17, 2009.

[129] Oz HS. 2014. Toxoplasmosis, Pancreatitis, Obesity and Drug Discovery. Pancreat Disord Ther. Sep 2014. 4(2): 138. PMID: 2553092. PMCID: PMC4270089.

found in tumor-associated neutrophils in mice.[130] The neutrophils do not die as quickly, because normal apoptosis in the neutrophils is destroyed. The toxic secretions from the infected neutrophils damage surrounding tissue and help the H-pylori survive and spread.

One study showed that treatment of H-pylori lowers the risk of stomach cancer, particularly in the elderly.[131] Another study found patients with early stomach cancer who were treated for H-pylori had lower rates of metachronous stomach cancer and more improvement in the grade of gastric corpus atrophy, than patients who received a placebo.[132] Long-term follow-up in China, in an area where rates of gastric cancer are high, showed treatment with antibiotics reduced the incidence of gastric cancer by almost forty percent, during a fifteen year period after treatment.[133] Many patients with MALT lymphoma were cured with antibiotic treatment for H-pylori.[134] It is apparent from these studies, the treatment of H-pylori in patients at risk of stomach cancer, or who already have stomach cancer or lymphoma, can prevent cancer and improve the prognosis of cancer. Studies also found an "association" between H-pylori and pancreatic cancer,[135] proving H-pylori can migrate from the stomach to the pancreas and cause cancer.

---

[130] Whitmore L, *et al.* 2017. Cutting Edge: Helicobacter pylori Induces Nuclear Hypersegmentation and Subtype Differentiation of Human Neutrophils In Vitro. J Immunol. Mar 1, 2017. 198 (5): 1793-1797. Doi: doi.org/10.4049/jimmunol.1601292; Horrom T. 2017. Study Shows How H. Pylori Causes White Blood Cells to Morph. VA Research Communications. March 9, 2017. Doi: https://www.research.va.gov/currents/0317-1.cfm.

[131] Leung W. 2018. Effects of Helicobacter Pylori Treatment on Incidence of Gastric Cancer in Older Individuals, Gastroenterology. Mar 14, 2008. Doi: https://doi.org/10.1053/j.gastro.2018.03.028.

[132] Choid IJ, *et al.* 2018. Helicobacter Pylori Therapy for the Prevention of Metachronous Gastric Cancer. N Engl J Med. 2018. 378: 1085-1095. Doi: 10.1056/NEJMoa1708423.

[133] National Cancer Institute. Helicobacter Pylori and Cancer. Doi: https://www.cancer.gov.

[134] Leukemia & Lymphoma Society. Treatment for Indolent NHL Subtypes. Doi: https://www.lls.org.

[135] National Cancer Institute. Helicobacter Pylori and Cancer. Doi: https://www.cancer.gov.

Crohn's disease and ulcerative colitis are a description of a finding of ulcers in the colon. Chlamydia pneumonia has been "associated" with lower gastrointestinal disease, including Crohn's disease. The description of damage to the intestine in Crohn's disease is similar to damage known to be caused by H-pylori in the stomach. The symptoms of Crohn's disease are also the same as ulcerative colitis, and both Crohn's and ulcerative colitis are considered inflammatory bowel diseases. Co-morbid conditions in Crohn's disease include mood disorders, anemia, skin rashes, arthritis, inflammation in the eye, and fatigue—all of which are caused by the same pathogens causing the Crohn's disease. Chlamydia may directly attack the gastrointestinal tract, in Crohn's disease; or be a co-infection with pathogens like H-pylori, peptostreptococcus, e-coli, parasites or other unknown pathogens that enhance adherence of the pathogens to the wall of the intestine and burrow through epithelium. Crohn's disease and other lower intestinal diseases may be caused by more than one pathogen, or particular combinations of pathogens, parasites and fungus.

Crohn's disease is another disease named after a doctor, who described symptoms and findings he could not explain. Gastroenterologists do not know the cause of Crohn's disease, because they do not look for an infectious cause, and their procedures make it more difficult to identify an infectious cause. Gastroenterologists rely on scoping to view the colon, and prescribe symptomatic treatment and surgery; but fail to inspect stool flushed prior to scoping the colon, utilize blood tests for immortal pathogens, or diagnose and treat parasites and other enteric infection. Some Crohn's disease patients have surgery to remove the damaged part of the bowel, which may give temporary relief; but, the condition often returns, because the pathogens were not diagnosed and treated. Every person with Crohn's disease, or any other lower intestinal tract disease, should be tested for chlamydia, parasites and other immortal pathogens.

H-pylori in the gastrointestinal tract can migrate along the vagus nerve to the eye, sinus and brain; can be transmitted to the sinus by reflux from the intestine, and then migrate to the eye and brain; or be transmitted to the eye by self-inoculation. H-pylori has been "associated" with brain fog, allergies, thyroid disease, and Parkinson's disease. In Parkinson's disease, the infectious byproducts of H-pylori may clump together to form the Lewy bodies characteristic of Parkinson's disease. H-pylori or its infectious byproducts of abnormal proteins may cause brain cancer.

In the eye, H-pylori can cause serious and sight-threatening disease. H-pylori attacks the surface of the eye and invades deeper into the collagen matrix, causing a loose corneal surface, and corneal thinning diseases. H-pylori can migrate from the cornea to the inner structures of the eye, down the iris and into the anterior chamber, where it can cause glaucoma. H-pylori attacks epithelium, and some ophthalmologists have described glaucoma as impaired or damaged epithelium. Chlamydia pneumonia attacks endothelium, and some ophthalmologists have described glaucoma as impaired endothelium. H-pylori can migrate to the back of the eye, where it can cause inflammation in the vitreous, and attack the epithelium of the retina. When H-pylori attacks the retina, it invades the epithelium and the deeper layers, causing loose epithelium, inflammation and bubbles, and retinal damage and retinal detachments.

Neither gastroenterologists nor ophthalmologists recognize the connection between H-pylori or chlamydia, and chronic eye disease; or refer patients for diagnosis and treatment of chlamydia and H-pylori. Failure to diagnose and treat H-pylori infection not only leaves the patient vulnerable to stomach cancer, it also leaves the patient vulnerable to H-pylori spreading to new locations to cause disease, including chronic disease and cancer in adjacent organs, corneal thinning diseases, glaucoma, blinding eye diseases, and Parkinson's disease.

The common method used by gastroenterologists for diagnosis is scoping, which rarely diagnoses intestinal pathogens and parasites. Gastroenterologists spend their life scoping patients to find stomach cancer, bowel cancer, polyps, inflammation, Crohn's disease, ulcerative colitis, etc.; and ignore the immortal pathogens and parasites that are the root cause the gastrointestinal disease. Gastroenterologists can bill as much as ten thousand dollars, in a half day, scoping patient after patient. Gastroenterologists too often rely on scopes, because scoping is quick, easy, and profitable; and scoping addresses the doctors' fear of missing a diagnosis of cancer.

Scoping is no doubt justified in some cases, and important in diagnosing cancer and pre-cancerous polyps. A scope will reveal chronic disease affecting the anatomy, like cancer and polyps; and may show redness, from inflammation in the intestine, caused by intestinal pathogens and parasites. Scopes do not tell the doctor why a patient developed polyps or cancer, or diagnose pathogens and parasites causing the intestinal disease. Scoping is not useful in finding the root cause of the intestinal symptoms, when caused by common enteric pathogens and parasites.

The gastroenterologist purges the patient before the scope, temporarily flushing out pathogens, making it impossible to diagnose the intracellular infections or parasites. The gastroenterologist purges the gastrointestinal tract of visible evidence of infectious pathogens before the scope, then observes the stomach or colon through a scope and says "it looks okay to me". The doctor flushed out the evidence of pathogens with the purge! The scope has a low-power microscope, and even biopsies from the scope may or may not identify microscopic pathogenic organisms. When a gastroenterologist finds no cancer and no ulcers, the effort at diagnosis ends. The patient is told it is in their head, or it is stress, or it is genes; given the diagnosis of a syndrome; and prescribed symptomatic treatment.

The way in which scoping is done is contrary to the basic rules of diagnosis, established by Hippocrates—which is to examine bodily fluids. The gastroenterologist never examines the stool flushed out before the scope, looks at the stool under a microscope, or cultures the material flushed out, where the evidence of the infectious causes could be found. The flush of the intestine before the scope is a lost opportunity to examine body fluids most likely to reveal a diagnosis of the pathogens and parasites. The purge itself can reduce the overall burden of intestinal pathogens, without doing the scope; and may temporarily improve gastrointestinal symptoms. When the effect of the purge wears off, the intestinal complaints return, the doctor gives the patient a syndrome as a diagnosis and prescribes symptomatic treatment.

TNF-inhibitors, and the profit from using TNF-inhibitors, has infected gastroenterology. Gastroenterologists are treating patients with

TNF-inhibitors, to treat inflammation in the bowel, without knowing why the bowel is inflamed. TNF-inhibitors interfere with the natural immune defense to the pathogens, and have significant and dangerous complications. Gastroenterologists are willing to use dangerous and expensive TNF-inhibitors, without knowing the cause of the disease; yet, are unwilling to use effective and safe antibiotics and antiparasitics for gastrointestinal disease, which is consistent with immortal pathogens and parasites.

Nexium (emperazole, omeprazole, "the purple pill"), is frequently prescribed for reflux [esophagitis]. In patients with reflux, the gastrointestinal system is allegedly backing-up, and acid from the stomach is damaging or could damage the esophagus. Nexium is marketed for acid suppression; and treats a symptom of a symptom, caused by the pathogens or parasites. Nexium was tested as an antibiotic to treat H-pylori, and found to be a low-level suppressor of H-pylori infection in the gastrointestinal tract. The fact Nexium has a low-level antibiotic effect and can treat reflux is a clue to the infectious cause of a "syndrome" named gastrointestinal "reflux".

Treatment of gastrointestinal pathogens and parasites should be the mainstay of gastroenterology, not just treatment of symptoms. Gastroenterologists need to diagnose intestinal pathogens and parasites, know when patients need aggressive treatment for infectious pathogens and parasites, and know to avoid potentially harmful medications. Some of the most underutilized medications today are albendazole, mebendazole, metronidazole, tinidazole, and fluconazole, to treat intestinal disease. Vermox (brand name mebendazole), an effective and safe antiparasitic that treats pinworms and other intestinal parasites and pathogens; was taken off the market because it was not being used enough—an inexpensive, safe and effective medication for parasites was not being used! Pharmaceutical companies continue to develop new drugs for gastrointestinal symptoms, rather than methods to diagnose and treat the underlying infectious causes of intestinal disease. What we need are drugs to treat pathogens in the gut, dysbiosis, and imbalances in the microbiome and mycobiome; and to use the drugs we already have for these conditions. New and expensive drugs for IBS are an indication the pharmaceutical companies are in charge—in gastroenterology, the culture of a "pill for every ill" is alive and well.

The specialty of gastroenterology has lost its way and its purpose. Gastroenterology has lost the art of inspection of the countenance, the stool, and the blood. Gastroenterology denied ulcers were an infection for fifty years, and edited knowledge ulcers were an infection from their textbooks. Infectious causes should be in the differential diagnosis for all intestinal diseases. Patients with intestinal complaints should give a thorough history that includes all animal contact, a complete physical examination, a blood test to measure neutrophils and monocytes, PCR tests for chlamydia and H-pylori, tests for streptococcal infection and e-coli, and tests for ova and parasites. Diligence in finding infectious pathogens will help the disease, forestall spread of the chronic infections to new locations, and prevent other chronic diseases from developing over time. The diagnosis and treatment of infections with appropriate medications is more effective, and safer for the patient.

Closed minds, and pressure from the medical establishment, employers, and insurers to do the easiest and cheapest thing—do nothing, scope patients, and prescribe indefinite symptomatic treatment, has left patients to suffer physically and with self-blame. Millions of people suffer with ulcers, Crohn's disease, inflammatory bowel disease, IBS, CIC, and other gastrointestinal diseases. Einstein suffered with an ulcer, and ultimately died of an abdominal aneurysm, most certainly caused by infectious immortal pathogens. Dr. Merchant observed and came to believe ulcers and many forms of gastrointestinal disease are an infection with immortal bacteria and parasites, based on his experience in a patient population suffering widespread gastrointestinal disease from contaminated well water. If gastroenterologists would recognize immortal infections and parasites are causing chronic intestinal disease and systemic disease, many gastrointestinal diseases, systemic diseases, significant morbidity, and the cost to society from infections with animal pathogens could be avoided or minimized.

Those who cannot remember the past are condemned to repeat it.

George Santayana

CHAPTER 10

CHRONIC INFECTION IN CARDIOVASCULAR AND LUNG DISEASES

Heart Disease

Remains of the aristocracy in Ancient Egypt show atherosclerosis. Leonardo de Vinci described atherosclerosis, which he found when performing autopsies; and called it hardening of the arteries. As early as 1853, doctors recognized an infection caused "stiff heart"; and in 1859, Dr. Virchow proposed an infectious cause of heart disease. During the civil war doctors recognized heart disease was caused by infection, and called it "tight chest". In 1908, Sir William Osler proposed an infectious cause of heart disease. In 1911, Dr. Frothingham proposed infection as a cause of heart disease. In 1920, Dr. Ophuls proposed infection as a cause of heart disease.

Between 1989 and 2000, more than twenty pathogens were "associated" with atherosclerosis, including chlamydia pneumonia, mycoplasma, H-pylori, streptococcus, and cytomegaly virus; however, chlamydia pneumonia has the strongest connection and greatest acceptance as a cause of heart disease.[136] Primary care doctors and cardiologists still do not understand chronic infection causes chronic cardiovascular disease, that more than one pathogen can cause the same chronic disease, or that treatment of the immortal infection can benefit the patient. Doctors are not trained to diagnose chronic infection, to treat or mitigate heart disease, to prevent future heart attacks, and prevent other forms of morbidity from chronic disease. Doctors only do what they were taught to do; and

---

[136] Friedman H (Ed), *et al.* 2004. *Chlamydia Pneumonia* Infection and Disease. New York: Kluwer Academic/Plenum Publishers. Chlamydia pneumonia and Atherosclerosis—an Overview of the Association. (Neha J and Gupta S). Ch 9. P. 113-114.

observe, document and treat. The medical system needs to incorporate new thinking into what they are doing, and how they approach the diagnosis and treatment of chronic diseases and heart disease.

The population in Finland has a high rate of heart attacks. In 1986, Finnish researchers found seventy percent of heart attack victims had evidence of current or prior chlamydia pneumonia. The researchers concluded heart attacks and atherosclerosis were caused by chlamydia pneumonia. Their conclusion was received with fascination, suspicion, and ridicule.

In 1990, an Australian pathologist identified chlamydia pneumonia in seventy-nine percent of tissue specimens removed from coronary arteries; and in another study chlamydia pneumonia was found in seventy-one percent of carotid artery specimens. In 1992, an African pathologist, Alan Shor, identified chlamydia pneumonia inside atherosclerotic plaque, which had been removed during bypass surgery. In 1997, chlamydia pneumonia was isolated from a sixty nine percent of sixteen coronary artery specimens, and viable chlamydia pneumonia bacteria was found within atherosclerotic plaque.[137]

In 1998, the Helsinki Heart Study of one-thousand male patients under age fifty, who had a recent heart attack, showed significantly elevated levels of IgA and IgG for chlamydia pneumonia. In March 1999, scientists in the College of Cardiology Scientific Session suggested infective agents, including chlamydia pneumonia, H-pylori, and cytomegaly virus, are increased risk factors for the development of coronary artery disease. In 2001, a study of one-thousand patients infected with chlamydia pneumonia, who had implanted stents for heart disease, showed significant re-stenosis of the implanted stents. Chronic chlamydia pneumonia raises fibrinogen, C-reactive proteins, and clotting factors, and causes endothelial dysfunction, which clogged the stents.

---

[137] Jackson L, *et al.* 1997. Isolation of Chlamydia Pneumonia from a Carotid Endarterectomy Specimen. The Journal of Infectious Diseases. 1997; 176:292-5. Doi: https://www.ncbi.nlm.nih.gov/pubmed/9207386.

Dr. Stratton noted most people get chlamydia pneumonia in their lifetime. He proposed chlamydia pneumonia could be acquired *in utero*, and some get it as early as age four. By age twenty, he said fifty percent of the population has had chlamydia pneumonia; and by age eighty, approximately eighty percent had evidence of a prior chlamydia pneumonia. Dr. Stratton noted other studies had discovered remarkably high antibody levels to chlamydia pneumonia in two-thousand heart attack victims.

Chlamydia pneumonia has a predilection for attacking the heart and lung, and specifically for attacking the endothelium in the heart vessels and lung. The endothelium is the inner most of the five layers in tissue; and is the fluid pump, which balances fluid in and out of the blood vessels, tissue, organs, and interstitial spaces. Chronic chlamydia pneumonia causes endothelial dysfunction in the vessels and smooth muscle. Chlamydia pneumonia can infect and reproduce in endothelial cells, in the coronary arteries and smooth muscle cells; and in macrophages. Chlamydia pneumonia generates sticky plaque and abnormal proteins; and the immune battle against the pathogen creates biofilm, mucous, pus and plaque. The pathogen and immune battle deposits abnormal proteins, debris and cell parts, into the blood and lymphatics. Chlamydia pneumonia can also cause an abdominal aortic aneurysm and a brain aneurysm.

Chronic chlamydia pneumonia infection proliferates in the endothelium and smooth muscle. Chlamydia pneumonia can infect the smooth muscles throughout the body, and smooth muscles are also a vehicle for the spread of chlamydia in the body.[138] The immune cells that respond to fight the chlamydia pathogen become infected, the pathogen replicates in the immune cells, and the immune cells facilitate the spread of the pathogen, throughout the body. Chlamydia pneumonia has been shown to hide in apoptic neutrophils, and propagate in macrophages.[139]

---

[138] Deniset J, *et al.* 2010. Chlamydophila Pneumoniae Infection Leads to Smooth Muscle Cell Proliferation and Thickening in the Coronary Artery Without Contributions from a Host Immune Response. Am J Pathol. 2010. 176(2): 1028-1037. Doi: 10.2353/ajpath.2010.090645.

[139] Rupp J. *et al.* 2009. Chlamydia Pneumoniae Hides in Apoptotic Neutrophils to Silently Infect and Propagate in Macrophages. PLoS ONE. June 2009. Vol. 4. No. 6. Doi: https://journals.plos.org/plosone/article?id=10.1371/journal.pone.0006020.

Chlamydia pneumonia has unique biologic and biochemical properties that allow invasion of cardiovascular tissue and smooth muscle. Chlamydia pneumonia produces heat shock protein 60 and LPS. Heat shock protein 60 activates mononuclear inflammatory cells in cardiovascular disease; induces the macrophage matrix and vascular cell wall adhesive molecules; and is the direct signal that triggers atherosclerosis. Macrophages infected with chlamydia pneumonia produce interleukin 6; and infected T-lymphocytes produce interleukin-6 and TNF-Alpha. Circulating mast cells and macrophages infected with intracellular chlamydia pneumonia can initiate new or re-infection of coronary endothelial cells, promoting atherosclerosis by the release of pro-inflammatory mediators. Elevated TNF-alpha has been shown to accelerate atherosclerosis in mice.[140]

Chlamydia pneumonia causes endothelial dysfunction throughout the body, including in the heart, vessels, lung, and eye. The endothelial cells are deprived of energy, lose normal apoptosis, and the ability of the endothelium to pump fluid into cells and organs and interstitial spaces is impaired. Chlamydia pneumonia induces pathological signaling in the vasculature, causing the vessel to create a cap over the pathogen to wall off the infection. The immune response leads to over expression of cytokines and changes in coronary vessels, which is the biochemical basis of coronary artery disease. Chlamydia pneumonia induces angiogenesis (development of new blood vessels) and inflammation, two events that define atherosclerosis.[141] The development of new blood vessels at the site of ischemia, after myocardial infarction, are a good form of angiogenesis, intended to nourish tissue deprived of blood and oxygen, and reduce tissue death; and reduces future cardiovascular events and improves survival.

Chlamydia pneumonia in endothelial cells lining the coronary arteries cause development of coronary plaque, increased cholesterol, increased

---

[140] Campbell L, *et al.* 2005 Tumor Necrosis Factor Alpha Plays a Role in Acceleration of Atherosclerosis by Chlamydia Pneumonia in Mice. Infection and Immunity. May 2005. Vol. 73. No. 5. P. 3164-3165. Doi: 10.1128/IAI.73.5.3164-3165.2005.
[141] Kern JM, *et al.* 2009. Chlamydia Pneumoniae-Induced Pathological Signaling in the Vasculature. FEMS Immunol Med Microbiol. Mar 2009. 55(2): 131-9. Doi: 10.1111/j.1574-695X.2008.00514.x.

triglycerides, glucose intolerance, hyper-coagulopathy (increase fibrinogen, factors that cause clots), and increased cytokines (interleukin 6, 8, TNF-alpha). Cardiac inflammation, caused by chlamydia pneumonia, is characterized by perivascular and pericardial infiltrates of mononuclear cells, fibrotic changes, and fibrinous occlusion (blockage), originating from blood vessel endothelium. Elevated homocysteine levels caused by chlamydia pneumonia raise the risk of heart disease, stroke and dementia.

The immune system does not attack normal tissue—the immune system attempts to attack an intracellular pathogen, is confused by molecular mimicry, and/or is generating inflammation in the attack that damages normal adjacent tissue. Molecular mimicry occurs when the immune system is confused in knowing what cells to attack. The immune system is confused by inflammatory signals and abnormal proteins on the outside of chlamydia pneumonia pathogens, and fragments of cells and abnormally shaped proteins dispersed by the pathogen and immune battle. Chlamydia pneumonia has abnormal protein surface molecules identical to trachoma, which mimic myosin (heart muscle protein). The resemblance between abnormal proteins attached to chlamydia and cardiac antigens is close enough for the host immune system to mount an exaggerated attack on the pathogens and heart, in the course of mounting an immune system attack against the chlamydia pathogen and abnormal proteins. Chlamydia antigens induce myocarditis, by virtue of molecular mimicry, causing the immune system to attack the infected tissue and heart. Molecular mimicry causing an exaggerated immune response to deposits of abnormal proteins are the likely cause of heart valve damage, after an acute streptococcal type-M infection.

In <u>*Chlamydia Pneumoniae* Infection and Disease</u>, the authors reported studies identifying chlamydia pneumonia in myocarditis, endocarditis, and dilated cardiomyopathy, including patients who survived and patients with a fatal outcome.[142] The authors reported finding chlamydia pneumonia in

---

[142] Friedman H (Ed), *et al.* 2004. <u>*Chlamydia Pneumonia* Infection and Disease</u>. New York: Kluwer Academic/Plenum Publishers. Chlamydia Pneumonia and Myocarditis. (Gnarpe JG and Gnarpe JA). Ch. 13. p. 187-193.

atherosclerosis and cardiovascular disease and describe numerous studies identifying chlamydia pneumonia in myocarditis.[143]

One study discussed six cases of fatal myocarditis, including a twenty-six-year-old man who had sudden death while skiing. The man had a history of pneumonia a couple of months prior to his death, with a cough that lasted two months. On autopsy, his heart showed degenerative changes with monocytes and focal fibrosis in the left ventricle, and antibodies to chlamydia pneumonia.

The second patient was a thirty-seven-year-old male with a sore throat, malaise, and fever, followed by erythema nodosum, in the lower extremities; and reactive arthritis in both ankles and his right wrist. He was admitted to the hospital with pneumonia and myocarditis; and had a high titer for chlamydia pneumonia. He was given penicillin and netilmicin; and after one month he showed improvement in his condition, but complained of chronic fatigue with physical activity.

The third patient was an eighteen-year old male patient who was admitted with a diagnosis of chlamydia pneumonia and flu; and a rising titer to chlamydia pneumonia. He was given erythromycin and cefotaxime, and a course of doxycycline to prevent relapse. His cardiac and renal functions returned to normal.

The fourth patient was a fifty-one-year-old male teacher, who collapsed and was taken to the hospital. He had bilateral pneumonia and an enlarged heart, compared to tests done one month prior. He was given IV penicillin and fluids, and collapsed and died the next morning. The autopsy showed fibro-purulent pericarditis with mild myocardial hypertrophy, mild to moderate coronary atherosclerosis, and mild chronic portal inflammation of the liver. Staining of specimens from the heart and lung showed chlamydia pneumonia with a "massive" inflammatory infiltrate in both the heart and lung.

---

[143] *Id.* @ Chs 9, 10, 11, 12, 13, 14, 15, 16, and 17; in Multiple Sclerosis, *Id.* @ Ch. 14; in Alzheimer's Disease, *Id.* @ Ch. 15; in Inflammatory Arthritis, *Id.* @ Ch. 16; and in Asthma. *Id.* @ Ch. 17.

An analysis of animal models of myocarditis showed an "association" between chlamydia pneumonia and induced autoimmune murine (mice) myocarditis. When injected with chlamydia pneumonia, the mice developed autoimmune myocarditis, perivascular inflammation, fibrotic changes, and blood vessel occlusion in the heart, similar to what occurs in humans. The researchers did not attempt to treat the mice for chlamydia pneumonia, to attempt to determine the benefit of treatment.

Chlamydia pneumoniae Infection and Disease described studies of endocarditis. The authors reported endocarditis, in a fifty-nine-year-old male patient, who had a high titer to chlamydia pneumonia. The patient was given tetracycline and became afebrile in one week. He was discharged on doxycycline to prevent relapse. Three months later his aortic valve was replaced, and the valve material was thickened and fibrotic, with marked destruction and distortion of the valve. Pathology showed lymphocytes, plasma cells, eosinophils, and a few granulocytes, with large macrophages and active fibroblasts. The conclusion was chlamydia pneumonia caused the endocarditis.

A second report of ten patients, with endocarditis, and aortic valve and mitral valve damage, showed nine of ten patients had vegetations on the valve and fibrotic valves, with focal heavy infiltration of macrophages, plasmocytes, lymphocytes, and a few granulocytes. Seven cases had necrotic areas in the heart. The granulocytes tested positive for chlamydia pneumonia, and the conclusion was chlamydia pneumonia caused the endocarditis.

A third report was a patient with pneumonia and endocarditis, with disseminated intravascular coagulation and multi-organ failure, with a fatal outcome. Postmortem, the patient had an extremely high titer for chlamydia pneumonia, by PCR testing; and chlamydia was found in the lung. Fibrinous vegetations were found on the tricuspid, mitral, and aortic valves.

A fourth report was a fifty-four-year-old woman diagnosed with endocarditis, requiring a mitral and aortic valve replacement. PCR testing showed extremely high chlamydia pneumonia antibodies. Her heart valves showed marked destruction with calcification, fibrosis, and inflammatory infiltrate; and both valves were positive for chlamydia pneumonia, on pathology. The authors concluded chlamydia pneumonia caused the endocarditis and need for valve replacement, based on chlamydia pneumonia detected by PCR, and pathology of the resected mitral and aortic valves showing chlamydia pneumonia. Vegetation on the heart valves suggested longstanding chronic chlamydia infection and development of fungus.

Chlamydia psittaci and chlamydia trachoma infections were shown to be "associated" with endocarditis and myocarditis. The conclusion of the study was chlamydia species are epidemiologically linked to human heart disease.[144] Another report suggested endocarditis can be caused by psittacosis transmitted from a pet bird.[145] Psittacosis can be transmitted to humans from birds, or from any other pet or animal infected with psittacosis, including horses.

Dilated cardiomyopathy was reported in twenty-six patients. Dilated cardiomyopathy develops in some patients who have myocarditis, as the infectious process progresses. Serum concentration of fibrinogen was significantly higher in the dilated cardiomyopathy patients than in controls, indicating an ongoing inflammatory reaction to the chlamydia pathogens. Chlamydia pneumonia is known to cause an increase in fibrinogen, C-reactive proteins, and clotting factors. The conclusion was the etiology for dilated cardiomyopathy was persistent chlamydia pneumonia.

The patients with myocarditis, endocarditis, and dilated cardiomyopathy had extremely high titers to chlamydia pneumonia, and proof of chlamydia pneumonia infection was found in cardiovascular tissue. Some patients had negative PCR tests for chlamydia pneumonia; and chlamydia pneumonia was proven by analysis of tissue removed during surgery. Patients in these

---

[144] Penninger JM and Bachmaier K. 2000. Review of Microbial Infections and the Immune Response to Cardiac Antigens.The Journal of Infectious Diseases. 2000. 181(Suppl 3): S498–504. Infectious Diseases Society of America. Doi: 0022-1899/2000/18106S-0026$02.00.

[145] Shapiro DS, *et al.* 1992. Brief Report: Chlamydia Psittaci Endocarditis Diagnosed by Blood Culture. NEJM. 1992. Vol. 326(18):1192-1195. Doi: 10.1056/ NEJM199204303261805.

studies who were given a macrolide or doxycycline showed improvement or resolution of their disease. Patients given penicillin developed chronic fatigue or died. Dr. Merchant treated cardiomyopathy with macrolides, which improved cardiac function and significantly increased survival time. He treated aortic abdominal aneurysms, which are also "associated" with chlamydia pneumonia, with doxycycline and topical testosterone; and slowed the growth rate of the aneurysm and the patients survived.

Chlamydia pneumoniae Infection and Disease, reported studies involving treatment of cardiovascular disease with antibiotics.[146] In 1997, two pilot studies were done in the United Kingdom, by Gupta and colleagues, to study the treatment of cardiovascular disease with antibiotics. The study was done on sixty male survivors of acute heart attacks. One group was given azithromycin and the other a placebo. Dr. Gupta found a reduced risk of adverse cardiovascular events that lasted eighteen months, and a lowered C-reactive protein and fibrinogen, after a one-month course of azithromycin. The treatment group had a reduction in cardiovascular events at eighteen months, a reduction in inflammatory markers, and a reduction in chlamydia pneumonia titers, compared to the placebo group.

Another pilot study, involving treatment of cardiovascular disease, was done in Argentina, by Gurfinkel and colleagues. The study used roxithromycin for thirty days, and showed a reduction in severe recurrent angina, acute myocardial infarction, and ischemic death; however, the benefit decreased at three to six months, even though inflammatory markers remained lower than the control group. The Argentina study concluded longer-term treatment was necessary to give more lasting protective effects to the heart.

Forty male patients with endothelial dysfunction and congestive heart disease were studied; and patients treated with azithromycin had a reduction in chlamydia pneumonia titers and significant improvement

---

[146] Friedman H (Ed), *et al.* 2004. *Chlamydia Pneumonia* Infection and Disease. New York: Kluwer Academic/Plenum Publishers. Chlamydia pneumonia and Atherosclerosis—an Overview of the Association. (Neha J and Gupta S): Ch. 9.

in flow-mediated dilation of the brachial artery (improved endothelial function), as compared to the placebo group.[147]

In 2007, a study of patients with elevated IgA and IgG showed chlamydia pneumonia patients had a four to six-fold increase in coronary artery disease. Chlamydia pneumonia DNA was found in cardiovascular plaque, but not in normal tissue. An eight-year study found that people infected with common pathogens, including pathogens responsible for stomach ulcers and pneumonia (H-pylori and chlamydia) were more likely to have a stroke.

In 2009, a study reported one-hundred percent of patients with acute coronary symptoms tested positive for chlamydia pneumonia.[148] In 2010, chlamydia pneumonia was again identified in patients with acute coronary syndrome; and the authors concluded chronic chlamydia pneumonia may have a direct adverse effect on the arterial wall and endothelium, which may initiate or accelerate the atherosclerotic process.[149] Antibiotic susceptibility to chlamydia pneumonia strains recovered from atherosclerotic coronary arteries did not differ significantly from antibiotic susceptibility to chlamydia pneumonia isolates from respiratory strains.

Books and articles are definitive that chlamydia pneumonia is "associated" with cardiovascular disease.[150] In The Heart of the Matter, Dr. Salgo cites multiple references supporting the ability of chlamydia pneumonia to cause heart disease; and more than one study noted the decline in the deaths from heart attacks corresponded to macrolide treatment. Now scientists have noticed the incidence of macular degeneration is declining, which is also likely to be related to treatment with macrolides; because macular

---

[147] *See Id.* @ 125-129.

[148] Mancini F, *et al.* 2009. Characterization of the Serological Responses to Phospholipase D Protein of Chlamydophila Pneumonia in Patients with Acute Coronary Syndromes. Microbes Infect. Mar 2009. 11(3): 367-73. Doi: 10.1016/j. micinf.2008.12.015.

[149] Petyaev I, *et al.* 2010. Isolation of Chlamydia Pneumoniae from Serum Samples of the Patients with Acute Coronary Syndrome. Int J Med Sci. Jun 10, 2010. 7(4): 181-90. Doi: https://www.ncbi.nlm.nih.gov/pmc/articles/PMC2894221/.

[150] *See e.g.* The Heart Attack Germ; The Heart of the Matter.

degeneration is a vascular disease in the eye, similar to atherosclerosis, and also caused by chlamydia pneumonia. Treatment of chlamydia pneumonia for any reason would also treat vascular disease in the eye, and macular degeneration.

A 2006 editorial in Stroke asked, "Is There Anything Ever Learned From the Atherosclerosis and Cardiovascular Literature or Must We Start Over Again."[151] In 2010, editors of "Stroke" questioned, at what point do we move from association to causation, when patients have shown better outcomes with treatment? Our observation is that of these organisms, chlamydia pneumonia is the most important and has the most scientific basis, because it has been shown to cause endothelial dysfunction and inflammation in vessel walls, and be immunosuppressive to the immune system.[152] The research keeps being repeated and the associations and conclusions keep being confirmed; but no one reaches conclusions or offers theories of causation. Research fails to move toward research into treatment, which could benefit patients and confirm causation. The outcome of research is not reaching mainstream medical care or being converted into action, for the benefit of the patient.

Chlamydia pneumonia is well-established to have an "association" with heart disease and a variety of cardiovascular diseases, including stroke. Chlamydia pneumonia can become a chronic intracellular infection, in the cardiovascular system. Chlamydia pneumonia causes cardiovascular disease; and acute chlamydia pneumonia can be the precipitating event for both heart attack and stroke. Chlamydia pneumonia has been found in coronary arteries, cerebral arteries, femoral arteries, iliac vessels, and the brain. Macrolides extend life and prevent future morbidity and mortality in patients with cardiovascular disease. Heart conditions continue to improve the longer the patients are on macrolide treatment. It is time for

---

[151] Apfalter P. 2006. Chlamydia Pneumoniae, Stroke, and Serological Associations, Anything Learned from the Atherosclerosis-Cardiovascular Literature or Do We Have to Start Over Again? Editorial. Stroke. 2006. 37:756. Doi: doi.org/10.1161/01. STR.0000201970.88546.5e.

[152] Elkind S. 2010. Princeton Proceedings: Inflammatory Mechanisms of Stroke. Stroke. Oct. 2010. 41(10 Suppl): S3-8.

a coherent theory on the cause of heart disease, from the many studies showing chlamydia pneumonia is "associated" with heart disease and treatment benefits the patients in acute and chronic heart disease.

In 2007, scientists discovered soft plaque deposited in layers of the artery, leaving the same size lumen, but the artery had globs of cholesterol inside the layers of the arterial walls. The previous belief of medical science had been hard plaque only develops in the endovascular space, and decreases circulation in the arteries by making the lumen of the vessel smaller. Soft plaque and hard plaque can become infected with and harbor chlamydia pneumonia.

The immune cells fight the chlamydia pneumonia with biofilm, mucous, pus, inflammation, and fibrosis. The pus may not be completely flushed from the cardiovascular system, lung and brain; and may thin, spread, be flushed into the lymphatics and lung, or dry and harden in place. The immune cells create pus when attempting to attack the intracellular pathogen. The pus becomes soft plaque, and over time, the soft plaque becomes hard plaque. The vessel walls are stimulated to cover the pus with a cap of harder tissue, walling off the remnants of the battle against the infection and preventing the remnants of the immune battle from being flushed out of the vessels. The "thickening of the arteries" and "hardening of the arteries" is the result of soft plaque found inside the vessels and layers of the vessel walls, and in the lumen of the vessel, hardening over time and having been covered over with a harder cap.

In New Zealand, rabbits were infected with chlamydia pneumonia, and subsequently developed vasculitis, an inflammation of the blood vessels. The rabbits eating a normal diet developed atherosclerotic changes, in two to four weeks. The rabbits fed a high fat diet developed hard plaque, in four weeks. The rabbits given macrolides, twice a week for seven weeks, showed regression of the atherosclerotic changes and plaque. In another study, pigs were inoculated with chlamydia pneumonia and developed acute respiratory infection. In two weeks, the pigs developed endothelial dysfunction of the coronary arteries. Autopsies done on young soldiers returning from Vietnam showed grade III and grade IV atherosclerosis, comparable to what would be expected in a sixty-year old man, consistent with having acquired chlamydia pneumonia during deployment and developing atherosclerosis.

A new study found nearly a twenty percent rate of high blood pressure (hypertension) in young adults. Previous estimates suggested young adults had a four percent rate of hypertension. The primary investigator assumed the obesity epidemic was the cause of the epidemic of hypertension, in young adults. The rise in hypertension in young adults coincides with the growing refusal by pediatricians and primary care providers to prescribe antibiotics to treat acute infection, leading to chronic chlamydia pneumonia at a younger age, and cardiovascular disease and obesity at a younger age. Treating hypertension with anti-hypertensive medications is appropriate to lower blood pressure; however, it is important to recognize a pathogen is the cause of the increased rate of hypertension *and* the increased rate of obesity, in young adults.

Obesity has been "connected" to chlamydia pneumonia and toxoplasmosis. The epidemic of obesity and the high rate of hypertension in young adults could be caused by chlamydia pneumonia or toxoplasmosis; and an increased infectious burden in the population with immortal pathogens, parasites, and toxoplasmosis. Cardiovascular disease, stroke, cancer and obesity are increasing, consistent with the worldwide spread of undiagnosed and untreated acute and chronic chlamydia infections, and undiagnosed and untreated parasites.

Chronic cough is "associated" with persistent chlamydia pneumonia, and an increased risk of heart attack. A non-productive dry cough in the elderly is a poor prognostic sign. Chronic cough is known to increase the risk of cardiac events. Fibrinogen levels are higher in patients with a chronic cough, and chlamydia pneumonia causes elevated levels of thrombotic factors, which is fibrinogen. Chronic allergic rhinitis is caused by chronic chlamydia pneumonia; and chronic allergic rhinitis is "associated" with an increased risk of heart attack and stroke, which are also caused by chlamydia pneumonia.

Chlamydia pneumonia can invade the brain, via the bloodstream and immune cells; and can infect the sinus and spread to the eye and brain. In the brain chlamydia pneumonia generates inflammation, abnormal proteins, and plaque, creating a long-term risk for Alzheimer's disease and stroke. The plaque of Alzheimer's lesions and the plaque in the cardiovascular system are both caused by chlamydia pneumonia and the immune battle against the pathogen. Studies of the brains of Alzheimer's patients have repeatedly confirmed chlamydia pneumonia was at the bottom of the Alzheimer's lesions and tangles; and in tissue adjacent to the Alzheimer's lesions. The tangles in Alzheimer's are a neurovascular disease caused by chlamydia pneumonia.

Dr. Elkind, from the Departments of Neurology and Epidemiology, Columbia University and New York-Presbyterian Hospital, said atherosclerosis is a chronic inflammatory process, and several common bacterial and viral infections have been hypothesized to contribute to the inflammation of the vascular wall that leads to atherosclerosis. He said research provides evidence that inflammatory mechanisms play a central role in the pathogenesis and progression of atherosclerosis, plaque rupture, thrombosis, and stroke.[153] Dr. Elkind speculated no single infectious organism would be identified as the direct cause of atherosclerosis, although measures of multiple chronic infections (the "infectious burden"), have been associated with the risk of atherosclerosis and stroke affecting the carotid arteries.

Dr. Elkind suggested the aggregate burden of infections, which has been variably labeled "infectious burden" or "pathogen burden" may be associated with stroke, through mechanisms independent of atherosclerosis, including platelet aggregation and endothelial dysfunction. He suggested the overall infectious burden in a patient may contribute to inflammation of the vascular wall and atherosclerosis, and host factors may interact with the infectious burden to modify the risk of disease associated with

---

[153] Elkind M. 2010. Inflammatory Mechanisms of Stroke. Stroke. Oct 2010. 41(10 Suppl): S3-8. Doi: 10.1161/STROKEAHA.110. 594945.

these infections.[154] Dr. Elkind concluded if infectious burden plays a role in atherosclerosis or stroke, it is plausible that preventive anti-infective treatment, with vaccination or antibiotics, would reduce the risk of recurrent stroke. He concluded further studies are needed to determine whether an association between infectious burden and stroke exists, and whether infectious burden may be a target for intervention.

In epidemiologic studies, acute infections serve as triggers for heart attack and stroke. Any acute infection, in a patient with chronic chlamydia pneumonia, can trigger a heart attack or stroke. Acute chlamydia pneumonia should be recognized and promptly treated, to prevent triggering coronary events. Chronic chlamydia can also accelerate heart disease, due to the systemic effects of persistent infection, with a sudden initiation of infarction, caused by acute infection.[155]

In "Influenza-Like Illness as a Trigger for Ischemic Stroke", researchers studied the influence of acute "influenza like illness" on the occurrence of stroke.[156] The history of an "influenza-like illness" was obtained from the patient; rather than through diagnostic testing to confirm the type of prior acute infection. The true nature of the prior illness as influenza or chlamydia cannot be confirmed from self-reporting, because patients often do not know the correct diagnosis of influenza versus chlamydia.

"Influenza-Like Illness as a Trigger for Ischemic Stroke", reviewed 36,975 patients hospitalized for stroke, in 2009. The study found an acute

---

[154] Elkind M. 2010. Infectious Burden: A New Risk Factor and Treatment Target For Atherosclerosis. Infect Disord Drug Targets. Apr 2010. 10 (2): 84-90. PMID: 20166973. PMCID: PMC 2891124.

[155] Matthias M. 2000. The Potential Etiologic Role of Chlamydia Pneumoniae in Atherosclerosis: A Multidisciplinary Meeting to Promote Collaborative Research. J Infect Dis. 181 Suppl 3: S393-586. Jun 2000. Doi: 10.1086/512572. PMID 10950654. S449-S451; Matthias M. 2000. Detection of Chlamydia Pneumoniae within Peripheral Blood Monocytes of Patients with Unstable Angina or Myocardial Infarction. J Infect Dis. Vol. 181. 2000. Pp. S449-S451. Doi: 10.1086/315610. PMID: 10839736.

[156] Boehme A, *et al*. 2018. Influenza-Like Illness as a Trigger for Ischemic Stroke. Ann Clin and Transl Neurology. Apr 2018. 5(4): 456-463. Doi: 10.1002/acn3.545.

"influenza-like illness" was a trigger for stroke; and the risk of acute illness triggering a stroke increased with each decade of age. The greatest risk for stroke was within fifteen days after the acute illness, but the risk persisted for sixty days. The study also found a correlation between acute "influenza-like illness" in younger patients who suffered a stroke. Patients under age forty-five had the highest risk of stroke within fifteen days after an acute "influenza-like illness". The risk of stroke is particularly high after hospitalization for an acute "influenza-like illness". The authors refer to additional studies linking acute infection to stroke, and concluded one of the stroke mechanisms was "inflammation-mediated endothelial injury, or effects on the cardiac endothelium". The article states, "Infection has been identified as both a potential chronic risk factor and an acute trigger for stroke". The conclusions directly implicate chlamydia pneumonia as a cause of stroke and as a trigger for stroke.

The mean number of co-morbid conditions was higher in patients who had acute "influenza-like illness" prior to the stroke, than for those who had not had a prior acute influenza-like illness. The co-morbid conditions which occurred at a higher rate included congestive heart failure, peripheral vascular disorders, rheumatoid arthritis, and depression. The identified co-morbid conditions suggest chronic infectious etiology for the co-morbid conditions, and when chronic infection is followed by an acute "influenza-like illness", the acute illness can trigger a heart attack or stroke.

In a study of sixteen hundred Manhattan residents, with an average age sixty-eight, who tested positive for chlamydia pneumonia and were stroke free at the beginning of the study, sixty-seven percent experienced a stroke in the following eight years. The authors reported five pathogens were linked to the risk of stroke. In order of significance, the pathogens listed were chlamydia pneumonia, H-pylori, CMV, and herpes simplex 1 and 2. "Each of these common pathogens may persist after an acute infection and contribute to perpetuating a state of chronic infection". Dr. Elkind theorized chronic low-level infection attacked the vessel walls, causing inflammation and disease. The conclusion was infection may trigger inflammation that damages blood vessels and causes a stroke.[157]

Inflammatory biomarkers, such as a high-sensitivity C-reactive protein, have been identified as predictors of the first stroke, including atherosclerotic stroke, ischemic stroke, and lacunar stroke; and a predictor of the prognosis after stroke. Dr. Elkind reported a randomized clinical trial suggested the use of rosuvastatin therapy in otherwise healthy patients, with high C-reactive protein >2 mg/dL, can reduce the risk of a first stroke by fifty percent. He argued the prognostic role of C-reactive protein among patients after stroke is less clear, and other biomarkers, including lipoprotein-associated phospholipase A(2), may provide complementary information about the risk of stroke recurrence. Dr. Elkind argued no commonly accepted group of organisms or method of assessing infectious burden exists, and not all studies confirm an association between infection and stroke risk.[158]

Chlamydia pneumonia serology alone does not assist in identifying people who may benefit from antibiotic treatment. No single test in molecular biology or serology, including the micro-immunofluorescence (MIF), is consistently reliable in detecting the chlamydia bacterium. Even the specificity of MIF has been largely overestimated.[159] Prior use of penicillin use can cause a false negative PCR test for chlamydia pneumonia; even though chronic chlamydia pneumonia persists. The studies suggest relying on PCR testing for the conclusion chlamydia pneumonia is or is not the cause of heart disease and stroke are invalid, because PCR and MIF does not detect the pathogen in all patients with chronic chlamydia pneumonia infection.

---

[157] Elkind M, *et al.* 2010. Infectious Burden and Risk of Stroke: The Northern Manhattan Study. Arch Neuro. Jan 1, 2010. 67(1): 33-8. Doi: 10.1001/archneurol.2009.271.

[158] *Id.*

[159] Apfelter P. 2006. Chlamydia Pneumoniae, Stroke, and Serological Associations: Anything Learned from the Atherosclerosis-Cardiovascular Literature or Do We Have to Start Over Again? Stroke. 2006; 37:756–758. Doi: https://www.ahajournals.org/doi/abs/10.1161/01.str.0000201970.88546.5e.

Dr. Elkind alleged prior large scale randomized clinical trials of macrolide antibiotics for coronary patients showed macrolides were not effective in treating vascular inflammation and atherosclerosis. Dr. Elkind referred to studies that under-treated the chlamydia infections, and the patients likely had unidentified co-factors and co-infections. Many studies reporting on cardiovascular disease and patient outcomes failed to test patients for other immortal infections, or determine whether the patient was previously treated with penicillin, which could be confounding factors. Multiple antibiotic regimens were more effective than a single antibiotic, which demonstrates the need to test for all infections, because the infections causing heart disease and stroke can vary and require different antibiotic treatment. In other studies, treatment with azithromycin, clarithromycin, tetracycline or quinolones, for as short as one week, was shown to significantly reduce cardiovascular events, stroke, and death. The studies by Gupta and colleagues showed patients who had a heart attack and were given one month of azithromycin, had a reduced risk of heart attack and stroke.

In the academic study, "Azithromycin Coronary Artery Disease: Elimination of Myocardial Infection with Chlamydia" (AZACS), seropositivity to chlamydia pneumonia was not an inclusion criterion. Patients were given antibiotic treatment for three days in the first week, then one day per week for three months, which did not affect the cardiovascular outcome. After six months, the patients showed reduced inflammatory markers. Antibiotics did not necessarily affect IgG levels, but did reduce the mediators of inflammation and atherosclerosis. The patients showed improved end points, but the study was of insufficient duration and had insufficient numbers of patients, to reach a conclusion on cardiovascular events.[160]

---

[160] Anderson JL, *et al.* 1999. Randomized Secondary Prevention Trial of Azithromycin in Patients with Coronary Artery Disease and Serological Evidence for Chlamydia Pneumoniae Infection: The Azithromycin in Coronary Artery Disease: Elimination of Myocardial Infection With Chlamydia (ACADEMIC) Study. Circulation. Mar 1999. 30; 99 (12): 1540-7. Doi: https://doi.org/10.1161/circ.99.12.1540.

In the Wizard Trial, patients were given three azithromycin the first week, followed by one azithromycin per week for twelve weeks.[161] Azithromycin once per week, for persistent chlamydia infection, is illogical and not consistent with the scientific understanding of the microbiology of chlamydia pneumonia. Re-infection from monocytes and macrophages containing viable chlamydia pneumonia, during the antibiotic free period, may have caused re-infection, inflammation, instability of plaque, and increased cardiac events. The Wizard Trial did show that even with treatment of azithromycin only once per week, patients had a thirty-three percent reduction in the secondary end point of heart attack or death. Many cardiologists and neurologists falsely assumed from the Wizard Trial that macrolide treatment was not effective. The assumption is contrary to the improved end points in the Wizard Trial, and other studies which concluded longer term treatment was necessary to give more lasting protection against heart attacks.[162]

The ACES study, showed treatment with Azithromycin, once a week for a year, failed to prevent cardiovascular events, in patients with pre-existing advanced heart disease.[163] The ACES study did not change the recommendation for treatment of coronary artery disease with antibiotics, and questioned if the results in the study were due to use of too low a dose of antibiotic, insufficient duration of treatment, or because the heart disease was too advanced in study patients. The ACES study did not address primary prevention of cardiac events. The ACES study noted, in the study of animals, prompt treatment of chlamydia pneumonia after acute infection greatly reduced or eliminated the acceleration of atherosclerotic changes. Azithromycin has been shown to improve respiratory function,

---

[161] O'Connor C, *et al.* 2003. Azithromycin for Secondary Prevention of Coronary Heart Disease Events: The Wizard Study a Randomized Controlled Study. JAMA. Sep 2003. Vol. 290(11): 1459-1466. Doi: 10.1001/jama.290.11.1459.

[162] *See* Friedman H (Ed), *et al.* 2004. <u>*Chlamydia Pneumonia* Infection and Disease</u>. New York: Kluwer Academic/Plenum Publishers. Chlamydia pneumonia and Atherosclerosis—an Overview of the Association. (Neha J and Gupta S): Ch. 9.

[163] Grayston J, *et al.* 2005. Azithromycin for the Secondary Prevention of Coronary Events. NEJM. April 21, 2005. Vol. 352(16): 1637-1645. Doi: 10.1056/NEJMoa043526.

which aids in coronary artery disease, by improving delivery of oxygen to myocardial endothelium and muscle.

In 2012, a Tennessee study on Medicaid patients, reported an increased risk of cardiac events and even death, using azithromycin, in patients with pre-existing heart disease. In 2013, in response to the 2012 Tennessee study, the FDA issued a warning stating healthcare professionals should consider the risk of fatal heart rhythms with azithromycin, in patients at risk for cardiovascular events. In particular, the FDA warned of a QT prolongation. The FDA acted unusually fast, in issuing the warning, deviating from its normal slow response; and the warning for azithromycin in patients with pre-existing heart disease remains in effect. The 2012 study, on which the FDA warning was based, was seriously flawed. Cardiac patients benefit by macrolide treatment, and have a reduced risk of new cardiac events, shown in studies, before and after the 2012 study reported an increased risk of QT prolongation.

"Azithromax and Risk of Cardiac Events – An Updated View", explained why the studies treating cardiovascular disease patients with antibiotics were flawed.[164] Contrary to the 2012 study, "Association of Azithromycin with Mortality and Cardiovascular Events Among Older Patients Hospitalized with Pneumonia" reported on review of more than sixty-four thousand patients admitted to the Veteran's Administration Hospital for pneumonia, and found patients treated with azithromycin had a lower ninety-day risk of mortality and a small increased risk of heart attack, giving a net benefit to treating the patient with azithromycin.[165]

The Mayo Clinic published a review of chlamydia pneumonia and atherosclerosis, which included a summary of all trials using azithromycin for cardiovascular disease.[166] The Mayo Clinic reported, in acute coronary

---

[164] Wynn, R. 2014. Azithromax and Risk of Cardiac Events – An Updated View. Doi: wolterskluwercdi.com/dental-newsletters/azithromycin-and-risk-cardiac-events/.

[165] Mortensen E, *et al*. 2014. Association of Azithromycin with Mortality and Cardiovascular Events Among Older Patients Hospitalized with Pneumonia. 2014. JAMA. 311(21): 2199-2208. Doi: 10.1001/jama.2014.4304.

[166] Higgins J. 2003. Chlamydia Pneumoniae and Coronary Artery Disease: The Antibiotic Trials. Mayo Clin Proc. 2003. 78:321-332.

syndromes, the effect of antibiotics begins within five weeks, irrespective of chlamydia pneumonia serology; and that antibiotics do not affect IgG levels but do affect several mediators of inflammation and atherosclerosis. After a heart attack, short-term treatment with antibiotics in patients with positive chlamydia pneumonia serology and coronary artery disease did not significantly reduce cardiovascular events. In patients with acute coronary syndromes, no large and well-controlled studies have been done, but several studies showed a decrease in cardiac events with triple antibiotic regimens.

The Mayo Clinic offered hypotheses as to why prior studies did not show the benefit of treatment, including the period of antibiotic treatment was too brief, and the chlamydia pneumonia titers may be misleading. Chlamydia pneumonia serology alone does not identify those who benefit from treatment; and serology plus inflammatory markers are more important. Macrolides provide an anti-inflammatory effect; combination antibiotics may be superior to single antibiotic therapy; a longer duration of antibiotic therapy is necessary to achieve the anti-inflammatory benefit; and the overall infectious burden is important in designing therapy. The Mayo Clinic review of antibiotic trials did not report other pathogens found in patients.

In a large study in England, subjects who took tetracycline or quinolones for any reason, during the prior three years, had a lower risk for developing an acute myocardial infarction.[167] Treatments for as short as one week showed a benefit.[168] Patients treated with azithromycin or clarithromycin for any reason in the prior three years had a significant reduction in cardiac death and stroke; and continued treatment, even after years of treatment, provided continued benefit to the patient.[169] In a randomized,

---

[167] Meier C, *et al.* 1999. Antibiotics and Risk of Subsequent First-Time Acute Myocardial Infarction. JAMA. 1999. 281(5):427-431. Doi: 10.1001/jama.281.5.427.
[168] Elkind M. 2010. Infectious Burden: A New Risk Factor and Treatment Target for Atherosclerosis, Infect Disord Drug Targets. Apr 1, 2010. 10 (2):84-90. PMID: 20166973. PMCID: PMC 2891124.
[169] Friedman H (Ed), *et al.* 2004. *Chlamydia Pneumonia* Infection and Disease. New York: Kluwer Academic/Plenum Publishers. Chlamydia pneumonia and Atherosclerosis—an Overview of the Association. (Neha J and Gupta S): Ch. 9.

prospective, double blind placebo controlled trial of forty male patients with documented coronary artery disease and positive chlamydia pneumonia IgG antibodies, treatment with azithromycin for five weeks had a favorable effect on endothelial function, irrespective of antibody titer level.[170] In other studies, patients given azithromycin for six months had lower rates of heart attack and stroke.

Azithromycin and clarithromycin are effective against intracellular pathogens. Azithromycin and clarithromycin can neutralize chlamydia and/or keep the intracellular infection dormant; and may stabilize atheromatous plaque. Azithromycin improves endothelial function in coronary arteries; decreases interleukin 1, 6, and 8; decreases TNF-alpha; and decreases coagulation via decreased small cell von Willebrand factors. Azithromycin and clarithromycin have anti-inflammatory effects; and affect the production of cytokines and superoxide by activated lymphocytes, which improves vascular and coronary artery disease.

Azithromycin inhibited chlamydia pneumonia growth within monocytes; and caused significant decreases in neutrophil and monocyte trans-endothelial migration, due to inhibition of interleukin-8 and monocyte chemotactic protein-1 production. The positive effects of macrolide antibiotics on heart disease begin within five weeks of continuous therapy, and appear to benefit the patient, whether or not the serology is positive. Longer durations of antibiotic treatment are important in providing control of chlamydia pneumonia, reducing the inflammatory effects, and causing remission and regression of the damage done by a chronic chlamydia infection.

Dr. Merchant treated patients with chlamydia pneumonia and cardiovascular disease, with macrolides, for many years, observing the patient response to treatment. He observed patients benefitted from sustained low doses of macrolides; or continuous treatment, with periods in which treatment was stopped, based on the patient response. A patient with cardiomyopathy and completely clogged arteries lived five additional years

---

[170] Parchure N, *et al*. 2002. Effect of Azithromycin Treatment on Endothelial Function in Patients with Coronary Artery Disease and Evidence of Chlamydia Pneumoniae Infection. Circulation. 2002. 105:1298-1303. PMID: 11901039.

when given macrolides, despite the dire predictions of the cardiologists of imminent death. Another patient with cardiomyopathy and a low ejection fraction was treated with macrolides for many years, and his cardiac condition resolved. In patients with heart disease and arthritis, the co-morbid arthritis improved with treatment of chlamydia pneumonia.

Minocycline is effective in treating various forms of chlamydia, mycoplasma, and the chronic diseases caused by chlamydia and mycoplasma. Minocycline is a drug similar to tetracycline, and was effective at improving outcomes for strokes and multiple sclerosis, in animal models. Minocycline has a significant effect on the apoptotic cell-death pathway, including prevention of activated caspase-3 formation. Minocycline may extend stroke treatment windows, according to an open-label, evaluator-blinded study.[171] Minocycline provided a neuroprotective effect, which is further evidence of the infectious causes of stroke.

In heart disease patients, the diagnosis and treatment of chlamydia pathogens, and co-infections with H-pylori, should be considered. Prompt treatment of acute chlamydia pneumonia may prevent or minimize the risk of a heart attack or stroke. Treatment of chlamydia pneumonia in patients with cardiovascular disease and stroke could prevent future heart attacks and strokes; and aid in prevention of Alzheimer's disease, macular degeneration, and other co-morbid diseases caused by the same pathogens. The early diagnosis and treatment of chlamydia pneumonia will reduce the cost of acute heart events, and treating chronic cardiovascular disease; and can decrease the morbidity and mortality of cardiovascular disease and stroke.

Lung Disease

Chlamydia pneumonia has a predilection for attacking the lung, and specifically the endothelium in the lung. Chlamydia pneumonia has been "associated" with asthma, chronic pharyngitis (sore throats), and chronic obstructive pulmonary disease. Patients with asthma are infected with chlamydia pneumonia, and any respiratory infection can trigger wheezing.

---

[171] Lampl Y, *et al.* 2007. Minocycline Treatment in Acute Stroke. Neurology. 2007. 69(14):1404-1410. Doi:10.1212/01.wnl.0000277487.04281.db.

Chlamydia establishes itself inside endothelial cells, in the smooth muscle lining of the lung; and proliferates through smooth muscles and the vascular system, causing airway inflammation. Chlamydia pneumonia infects endothelial, mononuclear, and smooth muscle cells; and infected bronchial endothelial cells secrete TNF-alpha, and interleukin 1, 6, 7, and 10. The ability to bring oxygen into the cells is decreased; and nitric oxide production in the endothelial cells is increased. Endothelial cell dysfunction combined with increased nitric oxide production in the cells causes increased resistance to a methacholine challenge, which is the definition of asthma.

Chlamydia pneumonia induces abnormal apoptosis and a dysregulation of the immune response, in the lung. The presence of cytokines and TNF-alpha generated by chlamydia pneumonia are chemical markers diagnostic of asthma. Chlamydia pneumonia enhances the secretion of chemical mediators that cause airway remodeling, including MUC5AC production and gene expression, which is the biochemical basis of airway mucous hyper-secretion; and is significant in chronic respiratory diseases, bronchial asthma and COPD. Azithromycin, clarithromycin and telithromycin inhibit MUC5AC induction and mucous hypersecretion caused by chlamydia pneumonia, in airway endothelial cells.[172]

Twenty-four million people have asthma in the United States. Asthma is more prevalent in the United States than in some third world countries. Adult onset asthma has become common; and the incidence of childhood asthma, adult asthma, and COPD (chronic obstructive pulmonary disease) are increasing. Chlamydia pneumonia is causing asthma in younger and younger patients. Studies show asthma in children was preceded by respiratory infections, ear infections, bronchitis and pneumonia.

The incidence of asthma is increasing in tandem with the epidemic of undiagnosed and untreated chlamydia pneumonia; and the propensity of

---

[172] Morinaga Y, *et al.* 2009. Azithromycin, Clarithromycin and Telithromycin Inhibit MUC5AC Induction by Chlamydophila Pneumoniae in Airway Epithelial Cells. Pulm Pharmacol Ther. Dec 2009. 22(6): 580-6. Doi: 10.1016/j.pupt.2009.08.004. Epub. Aug 28, 2009.

United States doctors to prescribe penicillins for acute respiratory infections or deny antibiotics for severe acute respiratory infection. Penicillin can trigger chronic infections to become chronic disease, as it enlarges and changes the shape of the chlamydia reticulate bodies, causing further damage and confusion in the immune system. Failure to diagnose and treat acute chlamydia pneumonia causes a spread of the acute infection to additional host cells, and development of chronic infection; and spreads the chlamydia pneumonia within the family and in the community.

In 1992, Dr. Hahn showed patients with bronchitis and a positive culture for chlamydia pneumonia subsequently developed asthma. The symptoms, in all ten of Dr. Hahn's patients, resolved after prolonged courses of azithromycin. In 2003, Dr. Aries Gavino studied one-thousand children with asthma, ages two to eighteen. After a short course of azithromycin or clarithromycin, the children showed a sixty-four percent improvement in pulmonary function tests, and a thirty-one percent decrease in hospital admissions.

Scientific groups have reported prolonged remission of asthma after prolonged macrolide therapy. Many scientific papers have shown treatment with doxycycline, azithromycin, or clarithromycin, can control and improve asthma and COPD.[173] Recent reports showed clarithromycin and azithromycin treat asthma by decreasing and loosening mucous in the lung, and by adequate penetration of the lung tissue, to reach where the infection hides. Treatment improves pulmonary function, and gives clinical improvement.[174] The British Medical Journal reported, in six-hundred seven children with recurrent respiratory disease, the early use of azithromycin at the onset of acute symptoms may reduce the severity of wheezing.[175]

---

[173] *See e.g.* Saint S, *et al.* 1995. Antibiotics in Chronic Obstructive Pulmonary Disease Exacerbations: A Meta-analysis. JAMA. Mar 1995. 22-29; 273(12):957-60. Doi:10.1001/jama.1995.03520360071042.

[174] Emre U, *et al.* 1994. The Association of Chlamydia Pneumoniae Infection and Reactive Airway Disease in Children, Archives Pediatric Adolescent Medicine. 1994. 148:727-732. Doi:10.1001/archpedi.994.02170070065013.

[175] Wise J. 2015. Early Use of Azithromycin May Reduce Severity of Wheezing. BMJ. 351:h6153. Doi: doi.org/10.1136/bmj.h6153. *Published,* November 18, 2015.

At National Jewish Hospital, in Denver, patients with significant steroid-dependent asthma were treated with clarithromycin for eighteen months. The patients were able to reduce steroid dependence or stop the use of steroids, pulmonary function studies improved by thirty percent, and the patients continued to improve over time. The treatment of asthma with macrolide antibiotics was suggested to have an equal or greater effect on asthma than inhaled steroids.[176] Long-term treatment with clarithromycin was also shown to decrease the prednisone requirement in elderly patients, who had prednisone dependent asthma.[177] Low dose macrolide treatment has prolonged beneficial effects in mild and severe asthma, and COPD.

A Cochrane Collaboration concluded insufficient evidence existed to determine whether macrolide therapy was beneficial in asthma.[178] The Cochrane Collaboration acknowledges evidence treatment improved disease management and the patient's quality of life; and their findings were contradicted by the National Jewish Hospital findings, and many other scientific studies and reports.

The current standard of practice, in the United States, for patients with asthma, emphysema, and COPD, is inhaled corticosteroids (asmacort, pulmacort, vanceril, flovent), started early in the disease. Steroid inhalers and oral cortisone can delay, but will not prevent permanent lung damage caused by chlamydia pneumonia. Treatment of chlamydia pneumonia with steroids potentiates the ability of chlamydia to cause inflammatory changes, and causes further immunosuppression.

Dr. Merchant's experience is respiratory patients with asthma, COPD, and emphysema seldom need to be treated with steroids. Dr. Merchant treated asthma patients with azithromycin, clarithromycin or doxycycline; and observed with longer-term treatment the chronic respiratory conditions

---

[176] *Chlamydia Pneumonia* Infection and Disease. Ch. 17. p. 246.

[177] Garey K, *et al.* 2000. Long-term Clarithromycin Decreases Prednisone Requirements in Elderly Patients with Prednisone-Dependent Asthma. Chest. 2000. 118: 1826-1827. Doi: https://doi.org/10.1378/chest.118.6.1826.

[178] Cochrane Collaboration 2015. Systemic Review and Meta-Analysis. 2015. Chronic Disease Management for Asthma. Doi: cochrane.org/CD007988/EPOC_chronic-disease-management-for-asthma.

begin to reverse. Dr. Merchant also warned in the early 1980's that treating chlamydia pneumonia or mycoplasma with penicillin could cause asthma, which hypothesis was supported by the research reported, by Dr. Storz, in CHLAMYDIA AND CHLAMYDIA INDUCED DISEASES. The more appropriate and safer treatment for asthma is use of a macrolide antibiotic, which can also improve inflammation and co-morbidities. In retrospect, Dr. Merchant's asthma was likely caused by the penicillin he was given for pneumonia, at age three.

The FDA recently approved Oalizumub, for treatment of inflammation in eosinophilic asthma, in children over twelve and in adults. Oalizumub binds IgE to the body, which inhibits the body's ability to recognize cancer, and puts the patient at risk of developing cancer. Treatment requires an injection every two to four weeks. Oalizumub has side effects ranging from pain in the arm to triggering malignancies. The cost is $10,000 - $30,000 per year. Development and use of costly medicines rather than use of readily available and effective macrolides is a common theme in medical care. More testing for infectious pathogens, and more treatment with antibiotics directed at the pathogens causing asthma, is treating the cause safely, at less cost.

Sarcoidosis is a systemic inflammatory disease that causes granulomas throughout the body. Sarcoidosis is caused by chlamydia pneumonia and/ or chlamydia psittacosis; however, other forms of immortal pathogens may also cause sarcoidosis, alone or in combination. Chlamydia infections cause granulomas, which may also be called inclusion cysts. In sarcoidosis, granulomas start as a collection of inflammatory cells; and most often involve the lung, lymph nodes, eyes and skin. Patients with sarcoidosis have a higher risk of developing co-morbidities and "multi-morbidities", include coronary artery disease, congestive heart failure, arrhythmia, stroke, transient ischemic episode, arthritis, depression, diabetes, and a major osteoporosis fracture. Sarcoidosis treated with steroids causes steroid-induced complications, including diabetes and myocardial infarction.[179]

---

[179] Ungprasert P, *et al.* 2017. Increased Risk of Multimorbidity in Patients with Sarcoidosis: A Population-Based Cohort Study 1976 to 2013. Mayo Clinic Proceedings. Dec. 2017. Doi: doi.org/10.1016 /j.mayocp.2017.09.015.

A reasonable conclusion from existing scientific knowledge is sarcoidosis is a chronic lung infection of a type which causes granulomas. Chlamydia pneumonia and chlamydia psittacosis can infect the lung, cause pneumonia, create inclusion cysts, and become a chronic infection; however, the impact on the lung may vary based on the pathogen causing sarcoidosis.

Chlamydia pneumonia has been "implicated" in chronic runny nose, sinusitis, allergies, culture negative ear aches, and sore throats. A chronic runny nose (rhinitis) is a sign of chronic chlamydia pneumonia. Rhinitis patients are often sent to allergists, who do not find evidence of the classic manifestations of allergies. Most allergists are unaware of the relationship between chronic chlamydia pneumonia, allergies, and "allergy" symptoms. Patients are typically treated with symptomatic medication including steroids, which are a mainstay in an allergy practice. Long-term, steroids potentiate the infection, weaken the body's immune defense, and enhance the damage, increasing the risk of development of asthma and chronic lung disease.

Chronic chlamydia pneumonia increases the risk of lung cancer in smokers and non-smokers. Chlamydia pneumonia is prevalent in smokers; and further increases the risk of lung cancer. Children and the family of smokers are exposed to chlamydia pneumonia, and can be exposed and re-infected, through second-hand smoke. The smoking gauntlet, walking in and out of stores where employees are taking smoking breaks, expose a person to chlamydia pneumonia from inhaling the exhaled smoke. Chlamydia pneumonia causes chronic pulmonary inflammation; and the potential exists for lung cancer risk reduction, through treatments targeted at chlamydia pneumonia.[180]

Treatment of chlamydia pneumonia in lung disease could reduce morbidity, and improve patients' lung function and quality of life. Treatment of chlamydia pneumonia in lung disease could lead to a corresponding reduction in brain disease, eye disease, heart disease, arthritis, pain, aging, and death, which are caused by the same chlamydia pathogens.

---

[180] Chaturvedi A, *et al*. 2010. Chlamydia Pneumoniae Infection and Risk for Lung Cancer, Cancer Epidemiol Biomarkers Prev. Jun 2010. 19(6):1498-505. Doi: 10.1158/1055-9965.EPI-09-1261. Epub. May 25, 2010.

CHAPTER 11

CHRONIC INFECTION IN NEUROLOGIC DISEASES

Alzheimer's, Parkinson's and dementia have existed for thousands of years. Ancient Greek and Roman physicians associated old age with increasing dementia. Egyptian papyrus and Ayurveda medical treatises, the Bible, and Galen's writings described symptoms resembling Parkinson's disease; and diseases of aging were described in the 17th and 18th centuries. The infections causing Alzheimer's and dementia have, thus, also existed for thousands of years.

Alzheimer's disease and dementia are not genetic diseases. A genetic disease could not survive millennia, without being eradicated by the inherent genetic cost, even if the genetic cost per generation is low. Alzheimer's and dementia must have an infectious cause, because the diseases persist; and because the spouse and caretakers of patients with dementia and Alzheimer's disease, who have no genetic relationship, are at higher risk of developing dementia and Alzheimer's. The spouses and caretakers become infected with the underlying pathogens that caused the dementia and Alzheimer's disease, by close contact; and develop an independent course of chronic disease. Spouses and caretakers may also be exposed to the same pets, which can be vectors for chronic infections. Dementia and Alzheimer's are not contagious, but the infections pathogens causing dementia and Alzheimer's are contagious, and can cause chronic disease over a longer period of time.

Chlamydia species cause dementia and Alzheimer's; and also cause heart attack, stroke, macular degeneration, multiple sclerosis, and neurologic diseases. The development of dementia, Alzheimer's, and multiple sclerosis, may be dependent on the type of chlamydia pathogen, the susceptibility of the patient, and the duration of infection; triggered or potentiated by co-infections such as H-pylori, and other forms of chlamydia. Chlamydia pneumonia is "associated" with dementia and Alzheimer's disease; and H-pylori is "associated" with Parkinson's disease. Chlamydia pneumonia and H-pylori are likely pathogens, working independently or as co-infections, that cause dementia, Alzheimer's and Parkinson's.

Scientists now are starting to believe gut bacteria and dysbiosis play a role in Alzheimer's and Parkinson's disease, and propose a "gut-brain" connection, which further supports the role of intestinal pathogens and parasites in causing dementia, Alzheimer's and Parkinson's disease.

Alzheimer's Disease

In 1901, Alois Alzheimer, a German doctor, first described the mental decline and memory loss of Alzheimer's disease; and named the symptoms of mental decline and memory loss Alzheimer's disease. Dr. Alzheimer and his colleagues suggested microorganisms may contribute to the generation of senile plaque, found in Alzheimer's disease. However, science did not have the tools to identify the microorganisms, intracellular pathogens, or chlamydia, at the time Alzheimer's became a named disease.

Alzheimer's disease is a form of dementia; and has been associated with brain atrophy, the aggregation or accumulation of a cortical amyloid-B peptide plaque, and tangles of nerves, blood vessels, and proteins. Dementia is a direct result of neuronal damage and loss associated with accumulations of abnormal proteins in the brain. Chronic infections are frequently associated with amyloid deposits; and chlamydia pneumonia, has an "emerging role" in Alzheimer's disease.[181] Dr. Miklossy noted a spirochete, Treponema pallidum (syphilis), can cause the atrophic form of dementia; and bacteria or the poorly degradable debris are powerful inducers of cytokines, abnormal apoptosis, and amyloidogenesis. The

---

[181] Miklossy J. 2008. Chronic Inflammation and Amyloidogenesis in Alzheimer's Disease – Role of Spirochetes, Journal of Alzheimer's Disease. Apr 2008. Vol 13 (4): 381-391. Doi: 10.3233/JAD-2008-13404; Balin B, *et al.* 2008. Chlamydophila Pneumoniae and the Etiology of Late-Onset Alzheimer's Disease. Journal of Alzheimer's Disease. 2008. Vol 13 (4): 381-391. Doi: 10.3233/JAD-2008-13403.

process described by Dr. Miklossy is the same process caused by chlamydia pneumonia, in dementia and Alzheimer's disease. Doctors accept Treponema Pallidum can cause dementia, a sexually transmitted disease; but find it difficult to accept chlamydia pneumonia can cause Alzheimer's and dementia. Alzheimer's disease, dementia, and cerebral atrophy arise from common causes—chronic infection with immortal pathogens, which have spread to the brain.

In 1998, a study of post-mortem brain samples from Alzheimer's patients showed ninety percent had chlamydia pneumonia, as compared to 5% of control subjects. Chlamydia pneumonia was found in perivascular macrophages, microglia, astro-glial cells, temporal cortices, the hippocampus, the parietal cortex, and the prefrontal cortex. Electron microscopy identified inclusions containing chlamydia elementary bodies and reticulate bodies.[182]

In 2000, Brian Balin and Denah Appelt examined Alzheimer's brains, and searched for pathogens causing Alzheimer's, at autopsy. He examined nineteen brains of Alzheimer's patients and nineteen brains of control subjects. He found fragments of chlamydia pneumonia in seventeen of nineteen Alzheimer's brains. The control brains did not show fragments of chlamydia pneumonia. The seventeen Alzheimer's brains were positive for chlamydia pneumonia, and only one control brain was positive.[183]

In 2006, researchers at Wayne State University School of Medicine assessed the presence and characteristics of chlamydia pneumonia in brain-tissue samples from twenty-five patients, with late-onset Alzheimer's disease; and twenty-seven non-Alzheimer's disease controls.[184] Twenty of twenty-five Alzheimer's samples were PCR positive for chlamydia pneumonia, in multiple assays; and only three of twenty-seven control samples were PCR positive for chlamydia pneumonia. Culture of the chlamydia pneumonia

---

[182] *Chlamydia Pneumonia* Infection and Disease. *Id.* @ 213.

[183] Balin B and Appelt D. 2001. Role of infection in Alzheimer's disease. S2 JAOA. Vol 101. No 12. Supplement to December 2001. Part 1. PMID: 11794745.

[184] Gerard C, *et al.* 2006. *Chlamydophila* (Chlamydia) Pneumoniae in the Alzheimer's brain, FEMS Immunology & Medical Microbiology. Dec 2006. 48(3): 355-66. Doi: https://doi.org/10.1111/j.1574-695X.2006.00154.x.

organisms from brain tissue demonstrated the organisms were viable and metabolically active, even after the patient's death. Immunohistochemical analyses showed that astrocytes, microglia, and neurons all served as host cells for chlamydia pneumoniae; and infected cells were found in close proximity to both neuritic senile plaques and neurofibrillary tangles. The researcher's findings confirmed and significantly extended their earlier study, suggesting chlamydia pneumonia plays a role in the neuropathogenesis of Alzheimer's disease.[185]

In 2010, Brian Balin, Christine Hammond, and others, at Johns Hopkins and the Hahnemann School of Medicine, again reported a study of the brains of Alzheimer's patients.[186] They studied five Alzheimer's brains and five control brains, testing various areas of the brain typically associated with Alzheimer's. Researchers found chlamydia pneumonia at the site of the Alzheimer's lesions; and immunohistologic chemical analysis (stain) showed astrocytes, microglia and neurons all served as host cells for chlamydia pneumonia. Chlamydia pneumonia was concentrated in the areas of the brain affected by the complex biochemistry of Alzheimer's disease, in close proximity to both the neurotic senile plaques and neurofibrillary tangles. The researchers found damaged nerve cells, and chlamydia pneumonia inside and surrounding nerve cells; and found chlamydia in the middle of TAU proteins and beta amyloid. The researchers were able to grow chlamydia pneumonia in a culture, from two samples retrieved from the Alzheimer's brains. Chlamydia pneumonia pathogens were viably and metabolically active at autopsy; and like the Wayne State studies, showed chlamydia can live beyond the life of the host and is immortal.

Also in 2010, Italian researchers described chlamydia pneumonia as particularly important in Alzheimer's and multiple sclerosis. The study reported increasingly sophisticated testing methods have demonstrated

---

[185] Chlamydophila (Chlamydia) Pneumoniae in the Alzheimer's brain. FEMS Immunol Med Microbiol. 2006 Dec. 48(3):355-66. Epub 2006 Oct 18. PMID: 17052268. Doi: 10.1111/j.1574-695X.2006.00154.x.
[186] Hammond CJ, *et al.* 2010. Immunohistological Detection of *Chlamydia Pneumoniae* in the Alzheimer's disease Brain. BMC Neurosci. 2010. 11:121. Doi: 10.1186/1471-2202-11-121.

chlamydia pneumonia in a large number of people suffering from cardiovascular disease and central nervous system disorders. The study also confirmed monocytes infected with chlamydia were able to carry the infection across the blood-brain barrier.[187]

Alzheimer's is a chronic intracellular infection of brain cells that generates chronic inflammation, beta amyloid, and TNF-alpha. Chlamydia pneumonia increases inflammation, cytokines, interleukin 6 and 8, and TNF-alpha. Chlamydia pneumonia causes increased TNF-alpha, and the level of TNF-alpha is related to the quantity and chronicity of a persistent chlamydia pneumonia infection. TNF-alpha is a hallmark of Alzheimer's; and TNF-alpha, cytokines, and interleukins, are the clearest signal a patient is living with intracellular chlamydia pneumonia.[188]

High levels of TNF-alpha are "associated" with acute and chronic systemic inflammation; and escalated cognitive decline, among patients with mild to moderate Alzheimer's disease.[189] When the subjects in the study had an inflammatory event, they had a ten-fold increase in TNF-alpha levels. Plasma levels of TNF-alpha increase with age, particularly in dementia and atherosclerosis, in patients who are one-hundred years old.[190] Dr. Brunnesgaard's showed chronic chlamydia infections, which generate TNF-alpha and inflammatory cytokines, are a predictor of mortality.

---

[187] Contini C, *et al.* 2010. Review Article: Chlamydophila Pneumoniae Infection and Its Role in Neurological Disorders. Interdiscip Perspective Infect Dis. 2010. 273573. Doi: https://dx.doi.org/10.1155/2010/273573.

[188] Morimoto K, *et al.* Expression Profiles of Cytokines in the Brains of Alzheimer's Disease (AD) Patients, Compared to the Brains of Non-Demented Patients With and Without Increasing AD Pathology. J Alzheimer's Dis. 2011. 25(1): 59-76. Feb 24, 2013. Doi: 10.3233/JAD-2011-101815.

[189] Holmes C, *et al.* 2009. Systemic Inflammation and Disease Progression in Alzheimer's Disease. Neurology. 2009. 73(10): 768-774. Doi: https://doi.org/10.1212/WNL.0b013e3181b6bb95.

[190] Brunnesgaard H, *et al.* 2003. Predicting Death from Tumour Necrosis Factor-Alpha and Interleukin-6 in 80-Year-Old People. Clin Exp Immunol. Apr 2003. 132(1):24-31. Doi: 10.1046/j.1365-2249.2003.02137.x.

Chronic chlamydia pneumonia causes elevated C-reactive proteins, a marker of inflammation, which can damage the blood-brain barrier, making it easier for pathogens to cross the blood-brain barrier. Chlamydia pneumonia infects and replicates in monocytes, a subset of immune cells, which generate macrophages. Monocytes and macrophages attacking chlamydia pneumonia become infected with the pathogen; and infected macrophages carry chlamydia pneumonia across the blood brain barrier, spreading chlamydia pneumonia to the brain and central nervous system. Chlamydia pneumonia causes endothelial dysfunction in the brain and the nervous system, causing deterioration in brain cells. Chlamydia pneumonia causes DNA damage, impairs apoptosis, modulates enzyme activity and gene expression, and generates abnormal proteins. The immune battle against the pathogen generates inflammation and atrophy. The inflammation generated by the immune cells can harm adjacent brain cells. Abnormal proteins and debris from the immune battle against the pathogen create Alzheimer's plaque. As the prevalence of chlamydia pneumonia and overall burden of infectious disease increases with age, the risk of Alzheimer's disease and dementia increases.

Chlamydia pneumonia creates beta amyloid lesions, characteristic of Alzheimer's. Chlamydia pneumonia stimulates pro-inflammatory cytokines, which cause inflammation and decreased clearance of beta amyloid in the brain. Chlamydia pneumonia generates abnormal sticky proteins and causes the immune system to attack and generate pus that becomes plaque. Abnormal sticky proteins form a focus for Alzheimer's lesions and inclusions, which the immune system fights with an inclusion or plaque around the pathogens and abnormal proteins, to wall-off the pathogens and abnormal proteins. The build-up of plaque in the brain develops by the same mechanisms as plaque develops in the cardiovascular system and lung.

Everyone has beta-amyloid in the brain, but not everyone develops Alzheimer's disease. Plaque and tangles typical of Alzheimer's have been found in the brains of the elderly, who have no sign of cognitive decline. Researchers did not understand why some people with extensive signs of Alzheimer's are cognitively normal; and suggested it may be intellectual reserve, a mysterious process in these patients protected them from cognitive decline, plaque and tangles are not in critical memory parts of the brain, or genes protected the patients.[191] Researchers recently proposed beta-amyloid may be protective against Alzheimer's disease.[192]

Many studies examining the brains of patients who had Alzheimer's showed the overwhelming number of Alzheimer's patients had chlamydia pneumonia in the plaque, and in tissue adjacent to Alzheimer's lesions. Almost all people get chlamydia pneumonia in their lifetime, and all patients have plaque and tangles in the brain. The patients who progressed to Alzheimer's have chlamydia pneumonia in and adjacent to the plaque and tangles; and immune cells infected with chlamydia, in and around the Alzheimer's lesions. Chlamydia pneumonia and the immune battle against the pathogen creates the plaque and beta amyloid, reduces beta-amyloid clearance, causes endothelial dysfunction, creates an inflammatory reaction, and thereby causes Alzheimer's disease.

A doctor recently named another new type of dementia—"vessel dementia". Vessel dementia, also called vascular dementia, is not a new form of dementia—it is a description of endothelial dysfunction in the blood vessels of the brain, caused by chlamydia pneumonia. Research would show "vessel dementia" is merely an observation of endothelial dysfunction, caused by chlamydia pneumonia—chronic chlamydia pneumonia has spread to attack the vessels and endothelium, in the vessels of the brain, and in the brain.

Doctors are diagnosing frontal dementia, also known as frontal atrophy, in children! No doubt the doctors failed to investigate intracellular, community-acquired pathogens, and did not understand the impact of chlamydia pneumonia on the cardiovascular system in the brain. The doctors were not able to explain the patient's condition; and instead of

---

[191] Begley S. 2016. Their Brains Had the Telltale Signs of Alzheimer's: So Why Did They Still Have Nimble Minds? Doi: statnews.com/2016/11/14/alzheimers-brain-amyloid-plaque/.

[192] Johri S. 2018. New Alzheimer's Research: The Problem May Be the Solution. Doi: https://www.alliancehhcare.com/blog/. *Posted on:* April 6, 2018.

considering prior community outbreaks in schools, infections in the mother and father, and searching for any infectious cause, made a diagnosis that merely described the findings of brain atrophy and offered no hope to a child. Frontal dementia in a child should lead to immediate diagnosis and treatment of immortal pathogens known to attack the brain, including chlamydia pneumonia.

Appropriate treatment for chlamydia pneumonia with antibiotics that cross the blood brain barrier, penetrate the cell, and achieve adequate levels of medication in brain tissue, will cause the progression of Alzheimer's lesions to slow, and stabilize cognitive decline. Treatment of patients who have early dementia will improve or stabilize the condition. Treatment of patients who have Alzheimer's can stabilize symptoms and delay the progression of symptoms. Early treatment of chlamydia pneumonia may be the key to prevention of Alzheimer's and the progression of dementia.

A triple blinded controlled study was done to assess whether daily doses of doxycycline 200 mg. and rifampin 300 mg. had any beneficial effect on cognitive function, in Alzheimer's disease. The study found, with ninety-five percent confidence, the group treated with antibiotics had significantly less cognitive decline. The study proved rational treatment of chlamydia pneumonia can significantly reduce the morbidity and cost of care currently associated with Alzheimer's disease.[193] No long-term study of Alzheimer's disease has been done to examine patients who have consistently been treated with macrolides, for acute and chronic infections; or to determine if patients treated with macrolides for any reason, in prior years, had decreased risk for developing Alzheimer's disease.

Cardiovascular disease and Alzheimer's disease are common co-morbid conditions, supporting chlamydia pneumonia as a cause of Alzheimer's disease. Science knows the "association" and causal relationship between chlamydia pneumonia and heart disease, and chlamydia pneumonia and Alzheimer's disease. More and more doctors are suggesting Alzheimer's

---

[193] Loeb MB, *et al.* 2004. A Randomized, Controlled Trial of Doxycycline and Rifampin for Patients with Alzheimer's Disease, J Am Geriatr Soc. Mar 2004. 52(3):381-7. Doi: https://doi.org/10.1111/j.1532-5415.2004.52109.x.

may arise from infection; but the profession has barely touched on causes or treatment. Few doctors have the courage to say chlamydia pneumonia causes Alzheimer's, or to treat the patient with low-dose macrolides or doxycycline, to halt the cognitive decline.

Two well-known Harvard doctors recently claimed a novel theory that Alzheimer's is a response to infection, including chlamydia pneumonia, spirochetes, and HPV-1. Alzheimer's has been proposed as an infection since 1901, and chlamydia pneumonia has repeatedly been "associated" with Alzheimer's disease, since at least 1998. Chlamydia pneumonia may not be the only pathogen capable of causing Alzheimer's, and co-infections with immortal pathogens may act synergistically to cause Alzheimer's. However, the principle that chronic infection with one or more immortal pathogens causes Alzheimer's remains true, and the most consistent pathogen found in Alzheimer's brains, in many studies over the last twenty years, was chlamydia pneumonia. Chlamydia pneumonia is also known to cause the same cellular changes found in Alzheimer's disease.

Current testing to confirm Alzheimer's disease includes spinal taps, MRI's, PET scans, and scans with special dyes, to confirm the presence of plaque lesions. These methods are not suitable for screening large numbers of people or monitoring and treating Alzheimer's patients. Doctors now realize Alzheimer's can be diagnosed by examination of the eye, using retinal scans to evaluate blood vessels in the back of the eye. Retinal scans can detect beta amyloid and predict Alzheimer's, as much as twenty years before Alzheimer's symptoms develop. A retinal scan can also predict a heart attack, in the ensuing five years. An eye examination is far more practical and cost effective in diagnosing Alzheimer's and predicting a heart attack, than spinal taps, MRI's and PET scans. It is more appropriate and cost effective to use conventional, relatively sensitive serologic tests for chlamydia pneumonia, and combine the PCR tests with retinal scans, to identify the risk of Alzheimer's, and diagnose and monitor Alzheimer's; and to identify patients who are likely to benefit by treatment with low-dose macrolides.

Dr. Merchant believed Alzheimer's was caused by infection, based on experience and observation, long before studies proved chlamydia pneumonia causes Alzheimer's disease. Dr. Merchant acted on his belief and treated patients with macrolides; and observed Alzheimer's disease stabilize and improve. It became obvious the progression of Alzheimer's disease could be slowed or reversed with macrolide antibiotics. Treatment with macrolides, combined with the Memory Revitalizer, by William Sommers, M.D., gave far superior results in treating Alzheimer's.

Many studies confirmed chlamydia pneumonia in the brain of Alzheimer's patients; thus, it is time to develop a general theory of causation. It is time to acknowledge chlamydia pneumonia causes Alzheimer's, and treat patients, to prevent, delay, and mitigate Alzheimer's disease.

Parkinson's Disease

In 1817, Dr. James Parkinson, an English doctor, described the symptoms of shaking associated with Parkinson's disease; and the shaking symptoms were named Parkinson's disease. In 1912, Dr. Frederic Lewy described microscopic particles, in the brains of Parkinson's patients, and the particles were named Lewy bodies. Dr. Parkinson and Dr. Lewy did not have the tools to diagnose immortal infection, explain abnormal proteins, or identify the infectious cause of Parkinson's disease and Lewy bodies.

Parkinson's disease is a demyelinating disease, meaning the outer covering of the nerve, the epithelium of the nerve sheath, is being destroyed. Parkinson's disease is a chronic infection, and Parkinson's disease may be caused by more than one pathogen—any pathogen capable of getting into the central nervous system, causing demyelization of nerve cells, or causing damage to the surface sheath of the nerve. H-pylori, chlamydia trachoma, and chlamydia pneumonia have all been "associated" with Parkinson's disease. All three "associated" pathogens generate abnormally shaped proteins and inclusion cysts; and all three can invade the central nervous system. The effects of these pathogens are characteristic of neurodegenerative diseases and Parkinson's disease. It is likely any of these pathogens could cause Parkinson's, and H-pylori and chlamydia pathogens may co-exist, to cause Parkinson's disease. Dr. Merchant often saw H-pylori as a secondary infection, in patients with chronic chlamydia infections.

H-pylori is most strongly "associated" with Parkinson's disease. H-pylori attacks epithelium, including the epithelium in the stomach, on sheaths of nerves, and in the brain. Parkinson's disease is when the outer covering of the nerves in the brain, the epithelium of the nerve sheath, are damaged. H-pylori attacks the epithelium, then burrows deeper to attach to collagen; causing inflammation and generating abnormal proteins. The abnormal proteins known to be created by H-pylori look very similar or the same as "Lewy body" proteins. The abnormal proteins cause tissue to stick together, and when brain tissue sticks together it provides a focus for immune system attack and development of Parkinson's disease. Stomach ulcers are a common co-morbid condition in Parkinson's disease, and H-pylori is an accepted cause of stomach ulcers, further supporting the role of H-pylori in Parkinson's disease. Treatment of Parkinson's disease as an infection, with medications directed at H-pylori and other pathogens identified by PCR blood testing, is not ordinarily considered in the treatment of Parkinson's disease.

Researchers in Brazil studying mice recently found doxycycline at low doses can treat Parkinson's disease; and are hopeful the same result will be observed in humans.[194] The effectiveness of doxycycline supports an infectious cause of Parkinson's, which can be treated with doxycycline. Doxycycline is a treatment for H-pylori. No long-term study of Parkinson's has been done on patients who have been treated consistently with low-dose macrolides for acute and chronic infection, or who have been treated for H-pylori, to establish the effect of treatment on the risk of developing Parkinson's disease or the effect on existing Parkinson's disease.

The inability to sleep is often a precursor to Parkinson's disease. However, the inability to sleep and fatigue is a common complaint in *all* chronic disease, and is not unique to Parkinson's disease. The common symptom of inability to sleep across chronic diseases supports a common etiology

---

[194] Amparao F and de Sao Palo E. 2017. Antibiotic Doxycycline May Offer Hope for Treatment of Parkinson's Disease. Science News. May 17, 2017. Doi: sciencedaily. com/releases/2017/05/170503134119.htm.

and process causing chronic diseases. Chronic fatigue has also been linked to chronic infection; and fatigue is an underappreciated clue to chronic infection. The brain does not feel pain, and signals a problem with fatigue. The depletion of ATP in the cells, from immortal intracellular pathogens, causes patients to develop chronic fatigue at the cellular level.

Parkinson's disease is caused by chronic infection, which has reached the brain and caused the formation of proteins characteristic of Parkinson's disease. H-pylori is capable of invading the central nervous system, attacking the epithelium, creating abnormal proteins that resemble Lewy body proteins, infect and change the shape of neutrophils, and can become a chronic infection. H-pylori, alone or in combination with chlamydia pathogens, may create Lewy bodies, cause demyelization of nerve sheaths in the brain and central nervous system, and cause chronic diseases of the central nervous system. H-pylori and chlamydia, and the abnormal protein debris, are the primary causes of Parkinson's disease, alone or in combination.

Multiple Sclerosis

Parkinson's and multiple sclerosis are both demyelinating diseases of the central nervous system, meaning the outer covering of the nerve, the epithelium of the nerve sheath, is being destroyed. Parkinson's disease is similar to multiple sclerosis, but the infectious cascade occurs at different locations. Parkinson's disease occurs in the brain, and multiple sclerosis occurs in the central and peripheral nervous system. Chlamydia and H-pylori are capable of invading the central nervous system, attacking the epithelium, and becoming a chronic infection. Chlamydia and H-pylori, alone or in combination, can cause demyelization of nerve sheaths in the brain and central nervous system, and cause chronic diseases of the central nervous system.

Multiple sclerosis is caused by immortal infection in the nervous system. Chlamydia pneumonia, trachoma and psittacosis are all capable of invading the cerebral spinal fluid, attacking epithelium, and causing demyelinating diseases, including multiple sclerosis. All have been "associated" with multiple sclerosis. Toxoplasmosis is also capable of invading the central nervous system and causing demyelinating disease. Multiple sclerosis may be caused by specific types of chlamydia, or a particular combination of immortal infections and viruses. The lesions of multiple sclerosis proliferate along with the proliferation of the chronic infection. Patients with multiple sclerosis commonly have co-morbid conditions, including chronic fatigue, fibromyalgia, lupus, chronic lung disease, cardiovascular disease, inflammatory bowel disease, mental illness, and epilepsy, which are all "associated" with chlamydia infections or toxoplasmosis.

The "association" between multiple sclerosis and chlamydia infection has been known for decades. Chlamydia pneumonia was found in the CSF of ninety-seven percent of multiple sclerosis patients, and only eighteen percent of controls; and found in the CSF of newly diagnosed and relapsing-remitting muscular sclerosis.[195] Mothers who lose a child are at a fifty-percent greater risk of developing multiple sclerosis.[196] The increased risk for multiple sclerosis after loss of a child may not be solely caused by psychological stress. It may be infectious causes that contributed to the loss of the child also caused the multiple sclerosis, and the psychological stress triggered the chronic infection to become multiple sclerosis.

Multiple sclerosis can occur in clusters, which supports an infectious cause. In 1977, a New Jersey study of twenty-nine patients, from families with one or more cases of multiple sclerosis, found a strong correlation with small indoor pets (cats or dogs), owned in the ten years prior to the onset of the initial symptoms. When the multiple sclerosis group was compared to the control group, thirty three of forty-nine multiple sclerosis patients had a cat or dog in the house, within one year before onset of the first neurological symptom. Three families had more than one member who developed the initial symptoms of multiple sclerosis, in the same year, despite a wide variation in age. The study suggested exposure to small house pets may be "associated" with subsequent development of multiple sclerosis.[197] The

---

[195] Friedman H (*ed*), *et al*. 2004. *Chlamydia Pneumoniae Infection and Disease*. New York: Kluwer Academic/Plenum Publishers. Chlamydia Pneumonia as a Candidate Pathogen in Multiple Sclerosis. (Stratton C and Siram S). Ch. 14.

[196] Li J, *et al*. 2004. The Risk of Multiple Sclerosis in Bereaved Parents. Neurology. Mar 9, 2004. 65(5). Doi: doi.org/10.1212/01.WNL.0000113766.21896.B1.

[197] Cook S, *et al*. 1977. A Possible Association Between House Pets and Multiple Sclerosis. Lancet. May 7, 1977. 1(8019): 980-2. Doi: 10.1016/S0140-6736(77)92281-4.

New Jersey study also supports an infectious cause of multiple sclerosis, which can be transmitted by pets.

Owners of birds have higher rates of multiple sclerosis.[198] The fact multiple sclerosis is strongly "associated" with birds, suggests chlamydia psittacosis and other species of chlamydia transmitted from birds can cause multiple sclerosis. Birds transmit the infection to cats and dogs, who can then transmit the infection to owners. Although most cats acquire toxoplasmosis, not all cats acquire psittacosis; thus, research has led to inconsistent results in studies of cats and multiple sclerosis. Toxoplasmosis has also been implicated as a cause of neurodegenerative diseases.[199] Cats and dogs can acquire psittacosis from birds, and transmit the pathogen to members of the household; and cats are highly infected with toxoplasmosis, and can transmit toxoplasmosis to members of the household. One or both of these pathogens can cause multiple sclerosis.

Dr. Stratton and Vanderbilt University changed the direction of their chlamydia research laboratory toward neurology, and shifted the focus of research to multiple sclerosis; after he faced criticism for reporting his belief chlamydia pneumonia caused chronic fatigue. Dr. Stratton found almost one-hundred percent of multiple sclerosis patients, had positive tests for chlamydia pneumonia. He reported dramatic improvement in multiple sclerosis patients, who were treated for chlamydia pneumonia.[200] Treatment resulted in marked neurological improvement in multiple sclerosis, which was largely sustained for three years.[201] Dr. Stratton reported chlamydia infections very likely trigger multiple sclerosis, and an acute respiratory

[198] Brean J. 2002. Pet Birds Put Owners at Risk of Multiple Sclerosis. National Post. 2/22/2002. Doi: mult-sclerosis.org/news/Feb2002/PetBirdsMSRisk.html.

[199] Whiteman H. 2016. Toxoplasma Infection Might Trigger Neurodegenerative Disease. Medical News Today. June 2016. Doi: medicalnewstoday.com/articles/310865.php.

[200] Siram S, *et al.* 1998. Multiple Sclerosis Associated with *Chlamydia Pneumoniae* Infection of the CNS. Journal of Neurology. Feb 1, 1998. 50(2). PMID: 9484408.

[201] Friedman H (*ed*), *et al.* 2004. *Chlamydia Pneumoniae Infection and Disease*. New York: Kluwer Academic/Plenum Publishers. Chlamydia Pneumonia as a Candidate Pathogen in Multiple Sclerosis. (Stratton C and Siram S). Ch. 14.

infection often precedes a worsening of multiple sclerosis.[202] No long-term study has been done on patients who have been treated with macrolides for acute and chronic infection, to determine whether prior macrolide treatment prevented or delayed development of multiple sclerosis.

Despite knowledge multiple sclerosis is a chronic infection of the central nervous system, doctors fail to diagnose and treat infectious pathogens causing multiple sclerosis. Combination therapy with low-dose doxycycline and interferon are being tested for multiple sclerosis and relapsing-remitting multiple sclerosis, with some success; again, supporting multiple sclerosis is caused by an infection. Dr. Thibault and others studied ninety-one consecutive multiple sclerosis patients, and reported short duration antibiotic treatment insufficient; however, prolonged treatment of chlamydia pneumonia using a combined protocol of doxycycline and a macrolide antibiotic improved extra-cranial circulation, and benefited patients with both positive and negative chlamydia pneumonia serology, "betraying a lack of specificity" of the effect.[203] The patients may have had chlamydia pneumonia, but prior treatment caused a false negative test; or other pathogens caused the multiple sclerosis and were treated by the same medications.

Dr. Merchant treated patients with multiple sclerosis using azithromycin, ketolides, and synthetic tetracyclines (doxycycline and minocycline); and believes low-dose doxycycline can be used as the sole therapy. Low-dose doxycycline is well tolerated by patients. Treatment improved or halted the symptoms and progression of multiple sclerosis. He observed when the continuous macrolide therapy was interrupted, the lesions of multiple sclerosis would progress on the MRI scan.

Multiple sclerosis cannot likely be eradicated, because the pathogens causing multiple sclerosis are widespread in humans and animals, and difficult to eradicate. To eradicate the disease, would require a vaccine

---

[202] *Id.* @ 205.

[203] Thibault P. 2017. A Prolonged Antibiotic Protocol to Treat Persistent Chlamydophila Pneumonia Infection Improves the Extracranial Venous Circulation in Multiple Sclerosis. Phlebology. Doi: 10.1177/0268355517712884.

to protect against immortal pathogens causing multiple sclerosis. Until then, multiple sclerosis can be treated, by diagnosing and treating the immortal pathogens that cause multiple sclerosis. Treatment can reduce the infectious burden and cause the disease progression to slow or stop.

Other Neurologic Diseases

Whooping cough is a bacterium (Bordetella pertussis), which spreads as a community acquired infection. Immunization is protective in whole or in part; and after vaccination, the person can acquire whooping cough, but in a milder form. The vaccination must be repeated in adults, at least every ten years. Whooping cough starts with two weeks of a sore throat, then two weeks of a sinus infection, then two weeks of a lung infection; followed by four months of a whooping cough that causes wheezing and difficulty breathing at the end of bouts of coughing. When an infant acquires whooping cough, the infant has a seventy percent increased risk of developing epilepsy, by age ten. Doctors sometimes ignore the fact the whooping cough vaccination is only partially effective, or the prior vaccination was more than ten years ago; and that whooping cough outbreaks continue to occur in vaccinated and unvaccinated people. Whooping cough must be recognized and treated, to avoid triggering other chronic diseases, to avoid morbidity later in life, and to avoid transmission to vulnerable infants and adults.

Congenital toxoplasmosis creates severe disability in infants and children. Any child who acquires toxoplasmosis *in utero* or early in life is at risk of developing epilepsy months or years later, and at risk for a regressive developmental disorder. Toxoplasmosis may manifest in different ways, and as different forms of epilepsy, based on the location in the brain where toxoplasmosis invaded tissue, and the extent of the invasion. The severity of the epilepsy is dependent on the infectious burden of toxoplasmosis, the location of the toxoplasmosis infection in the brain, and amount of inflammatory damage and scar tissue from the immune battle against toxoplasmosis. Toxoplasmosis may be acquired months or years before the symptoms of epilepsy appear, or the toxoplasmosis may not cause any obvious symptoms; thus, toxoplasmosis is seldom investigated, in new cases of epilepsy.

Muscular dystrophy may be caused by chlamydia pneumonia, which spreads through smooth muscle tissue. Dr. Merchant treated a patient with progressive muscular dystrophy and a seizure disorder, using long-term macrolides. The treatment caused the muscular dystrophy to stabilize and the seizures to become well controlled. Any clinical problem that involves a progressive neurologic and/or muscular degeneration, including muscular dystrophy, multiple sclerosis, ALS, Alzheimer's, and Parkinson's, has an infectious cause which can be diagnosed and treated, to improve or stabilize the condition.

Streptococcus is a significant pathogenic bacterium capable of causing streptococcus-induced seizure disorders. Streptococcus has as many as eighty serovars, and some serovars are capable of damaging organs and infecting immune cells. Streptococcus type-M can cause heart and kidney damage, and may cause lupus and multiple myeloma. Chronic infection with streptococcus, and co-infections with other forms of chlamydia, may cause seizure disorders and may cause Tourette syndrome.

CHAPTER 12

CHRONIC INFECTION IN CANCER

Cancer has existed for at least 3,000 years. The remains of the aristocracy in Ancient Egyptian tombs show metastatic prostate cancer; and the remains of a Syrian king from the 7th Century BC also showed metastatic prostate cancer. Egyptian aristocracy were the first to have pets; and had close contact with cats, dogs, and pet monkeys, which were vectors for transmission of immortal animal pathogens capable of causing cancer.

The current image of cancer is as a malevolent doppelganger. A doppelganger is a tangible double of a living person that typically represents evil, a ghostly counterpart of a living person. Cancer is an expansionist disease, of fulminant, unstoppable growth, which develops when the body loses the ability to squelch its command for cells to grow. Normal apoptosis disappears and cancer transforms the cells into an indestructible, self-propelled automation of immortal replication. Cancer develops in one location, then metastasizes to new locations. The word metastasis, used to describe the migration of cancer from one site to another, is a mix of Latin words "meta" and "stasis", meaning "beyond stillness". Cancer is a disease that lurks inside us, waiting for the appropriate trigger to become cancer.[204]

Cancer is a single cell or group of cells (clone) infected by immortal pathogens. Cancer can develop from any cells infected by an intracellular pathogen; or from inclusion cysts that develop during the immune battle against the pathogen and abnormal proteins. The type of cancer may be determined by the type of pathogen, the predilection of the pathogen, the route of acquisition, the length of time the pathogen has persisted, co-infections, and triggers of cancer, such as low folic acid and environmental

---

[204] Mukherjee S. 2010. <u>The Emperor of All Maladies: A Biography of Cancer</u>. New York: Scribner.

carcinogens. Infection of immune cells impairs immune function and makes the patient vulnerable to new infections, and an increase in the infectious burden. Genetics, trauma, and social behavior can create a weak link for pathogens to attack. The intracellular pathogen invades tissue and then organs; becomes a chronic infection; migrates to adjacent tissue and organs; and metastasizes through the blood stream, immune cells, lymphatics, smooth muscles, vagus nerve, and interstitial spaces, to find new hospitable locations and weak links, which can become a focus for cancer.

Control of cell growth through apoptosis is an essential feature of normal cells. Cancer cells rely on growth in the most basic sense: the division of one cell to form two cells. Normal cells are programmed to die, and the process of cell death is regulated. Growth of cells is stimulated and arrested by specific signals. The loss of normal apoptosis and cancer are synonymous. Cancer is the failure of normal cells to die (loss of apoptosis), and rapid production of weaker infected cells. Cancer is unbridled growth not limited by apoptosis, giving rise to generation after generation of replicated infected cells that become cancer.

Clusters of cancer and rare cancer have occurred, supporting an infectious cause. It would be important to know whether the clusters of cancer occur after widespread community acquired infections with immortal pathogens; or after contact with specific pathogens existing within a cancer cluster. We know heart attack and stroke occur more frequently after a widespread community outbreak of immortal respiratory infections. It would also be important to known whether children or adults with newly diagnosed cancer had a recent community acquired infection, or had been treated for an acute infection with penicillin recently or in the past. Penicillin inhibits folic acid, changes the shape of the reticulate body released from the cell, and promotes yeast, which could promote cancer in patients with immortal infections.

Cancer is not contagious, but the infections and co-infections causing cancer are contagious. Caretakers and spouses of cancer patients are at higher risk of cancer, because they are exposed to the same infections and vectors for infection, in the household. Farmers have a higher rate of cancer, due to frequent close contact with domesticated animals, cats, mice, agriculture, and environmental toxins; and work in an environment that fosters cross-species transmission of chlamydia. Farmers are at greater risk of exposure to multiple types of chlamydia, in different animals; and exposure to parasitic infection from animals and soil.

In 1890, Dr. William Russell found "pleomorphic" microbes "wander" inside and outside the cancer. Pleomorphic microbes are microbes which have the ability to alter their shape and size, in response to environmental conditions. Dr. Russell observed pathogens and the immune cells fighting the pathogen, wandering inside and outside the tumor. The pathogens had the ability to infect and change the shape of the immune cells. In 1910, Frances Peyton Rous proved infection caused a specific type of cancer in chickens; and was criticized by his peers. Fifty-six years later, in 1966, Dr. Rous received a Nobel Prize for work he had done to prove the infectious cause of a type of cancer that occurs in chickens.

In the 1920's, Sydney Farber, M.D., at Children's Hospital in Boston, observed children would develop a severe sore throat, and within weeks the child would develop leukemia. The doctors observed pus was connected to leukemia, and leukemia was thought to be a "liquid" form of cancer, arising from pus in the white blood cells. Dr. Farber began treating childhood leukemia with folic acid antagonists. The anti-folate treatment briefly extended life, but the children died. Some children survived months longer than expected, at a time when childhood leukemia patients usually died shortly after their diagnosis. In children who had an infection that thrived on folic acid, treating leukemia with anti-folates had limited success.

Dr. Farber infuriated the administration at Children's Hospital with his first clinical trial using anti-folates, which was considered a failure. After the second clinical trial failed, the hospital staff voted to remove all pediatric interns from assisting with Dr. Farber's patients, because the staff believed the treatment was too desperate and experimental; and thus, not conducive to medical education. The staff argued it would be kinder and gentler to let the children die in peace. One clinician suggested Dr. Farber's novel chemicals be reserved only as a last resort for leukemia in children.

Dr. Farber responded, "By that time the only chemical you will need will be embalming fluid". Dr. Farber and his assistants then had to perform all the patient care themselves.

In 1921, a pathologist, Dr. James Ewing, identified bone sarcoma and it was named Ewing's sarcoma. Dr. James Ewing, Dr. William B. Coley, and Dr. Ernest Codman, treated bone sarcoma with a mixture of bacterial toxins. Dr. Coley observed occasional positive responses, but also unpredictable responses. Dr. Ewing opined cancer is a thousand diseases.

The work of Drs. Ewing, Coley and Codman never fully captured the attention of oncologists and surgeons. Instead plants, herb shops and churches were ransacked, by people seeking relief of cancer using Ewing's mixture. Cancer can be considered one disease—a disease of chronic immortal infection with intracellular pathogens, and the longstanding immune response battling the pathogens. Cancer can be considered many diseases, because different immortal pathogens can cause cancer, and can attack to cause cancer in many different ways.

In 1931, Dr. Otto Warburg proved the main property of cancer cells was low oxygen. His primary hypothesis was cancer is the consequence of replacement of respiration in normal cells with fermentation of sugar. He said cancer cells were generated mainly by anaerobic breakdown of glucose into fermentation; and believed cancer should be interpreted as a mitochondrial dysfunction. He believed cancer had one prime cause, replacement of oxygen in normal cells with fermentation and sugar.[205] Dr. Warburg unknowingly predicted chlamydia causes cancer, because we now know chlamydia pathogens cause mitochondrial dysfunction, consume ATP in the cell, consume sugar to cause fermentation, and impair oxygen transport into the cell. We also now know cancer cells consume and thrive on sugar, and abnormal sugar metabolism in the cells changes the microenvironment in the cell, and fosters the spread of the tumor.[206]

---

[205] Wikipedia. Warburg Hypothesis. Doi: en.wikipedia.org/wiki/Warburg_hypothesis.
[206] Mathupala S, *et al.* 2010. The Pivotal Roles of Mitochondria in Cancer: Warburg and Beyond and Encouraging Prospects for Effective therapies. Biochimica et Biophysica Acta 1797. 2010. 1225-1230. Doi: 10.1016/j.bbabio.2010.03.025.

Chlamydia induces fermentation and excess sugar, takes control of energy production, and changes the microenvironment.

In the 1940's, infection was postulated to be the cause of cancer, and some doctors reported success in treatment using antibiotics. In 1946, Dr. William Banbridge opined the search to eradicate this scourge was left to incidental dabbling and uncoordinated research.[207] The same concern is true today—the search for the cause of cancer has been a frantic and uncoordinated search for the small details of molecular biology and genes, hoping an answer will reveal itself. The search for cancer has been concentrated in the oncology specialty; and has not been coordinated among experts with the broad scope of knowledge necessary to recognize common patterns between intracellular pathogens and cancer cells, to discover the causes of cancer.

In September 1947, Dr. Farber tried aminopterin, an anti-folate drug, to treat childhood leukemia; and used pteroylaspartic acid to deliver his anti-folate drug. (Aminopterin was used off-label from 1953 to 1964 to treat psoriasis, causing dramatic improvement in psoriasis.) The second patient on whom he tried aminopterin had an unprecedented remission, in the history of childhood leukemia. Dr. Farber recruited more doctors and more leukemia patients for trials of his aminopterin anti-folate therapy. Farber's team treated sixteen childhood leukemia patients. Ten children had a temporary response; and five children remained alive, four to six months after diagnosis, which was an eternity, in 1947. Farber showed the anti-folates could drive leukemia cells down in some patients, even resulting in the complete disappearance of cancer cells—at least temporarily. Farber always confronted the same problem with anti-folates, after a few months of remission the cancer would return, even using the most potent anti-folate drugs. The remissions, even if temporary, were genuine remissions and historic in childhood leukemia.[208]

---

[207] Mukherjee S. 2010. The Emperor of All Maladies: A Biography of Cancer. New York: Scribner.
[208] Mukherjee S. 2010. The Emperor of All Maladies: A Biography of Cancer. New York: Scribner.

On June 3, 1948, Dr. Farber published a seven-page paper on his results treating childhood leukemia, with tables, figures, microscopic photographs, laboratory values, and blood counts. The paper was received by the medical community with skepticism, disbelief and outrage. In the summer of 1948, one of Farber's assistants performed a bone marrow biopsy on a child with leukemia, after treatment with aminopterin; and the assistant could not believe the results. The results looked so normal he wrote that one could dream of a cure. Dr. Farber went from being criticized and ridiculed for his work in childhood leukemia, to having his name on the Farber Medical Center at Harvard University.

In the 1980's, an Italian doctor, Tulio Simonchini, M.D., hypothesized yeast was the cause of cancer; and was criticized and persecuted for expressing his opinion. Fungus helps the pathogens survive and thrive, and hides the pathogens from the immune system. Yeast (fungus) is common in cancer, and depriving the infection and cancer of yeast may help treat cancer; but we must return to the question of why did the patient have yeast? Immortal intracellular animal pathogens and parasites cause fungus, in response to low oxygen and low ATP in the cell, and the pathogen consuming sugar and causing fermentation. By the time a patient develops a systemic fungal infection, the immortal infections have already become chronic, and the infectious cascade has progressed to cancer.

In the late 1990's, Dr. Ewald argued, as an evolutionary biologist, that most cancers must be infectious, and may be the result of co-infections acquired within the family. Dr. Ewald's observations are consistent with Dr. Merchant's long-held beliefs that chronic intracellular infection and parasites cause cancer; and chronic infection, plus low folic acid, plus time, will cause cancer. Co-infections, triggering events, and/or low folic acid may determine how quickly a person develops cancer.

In 2007, Dr. Andrew Dannenberg, Director of the Cancer Center at New York Presbyterian Hospital/Weill Cornell Medical Center, said infections cause many cancers, and up to one fifth of cancers are caused by chronic infection. Dr. Dannenberg said the magnitude of the link between cancer and chronic infection is grossly underappreciated; and that viruses, bacteria, and parasites trigger tumor development. He believed effectively treating infections has the side benefit of "preventing tumor development". The infectious causes Dr. Dannenberg identified were hepatitis B and C (liver cancer), HPV (cervical, throat and oral tumors), EBV (Burkitt's lymphoma), H-pylori (gastric cancer and MALT lymphoma), and schistosome parasites (bladder cancer). He also called on the medical community to develop improved vaccines and anti-invectives.

Eleven years after Dr. Dannenberg's insight, diagnosis and treatment of immortal infections and parasites has not been incorporated into oncology practice, or mainstream medical practice. Bias against infectious causes of cancer remain, and research into infectious causes continues to be underfunded. If the medical community will not listen to the head of the New York Presbyterian Hospital Cancer Center when he says some cancers are caused by an infection, what will it take to change medical thinking and medical practice? What will it take to break through the bias against infectious causes of cancer? What will it take for primary care doctors to treat acute and chronic infections with appropriate medications, and in doing so, prevent the development of cancer?

In 2018, researchers in Denmark studied the incidence of leukemia, lymphoma and brain cancer – the three most common cancers for children – in children who were hospitalized with pneumonia.[209] The study followed 83,935 Danish children (boys, n=47,650; girls, n=36,285), age zero to seventeen, who were diagnosed with pneumonia in an inpatient, outpatient, or emergency room setting, who had no prior history of cancer. A total of one-hundred sixty-eight cancer diagnoses occurred in the study population. Thirty-seven children were diagnosed within the first month, after the pneumonia diagnosis; and forty-three were diagnosed in the first six months. The absolute risk for developing leukemia, lymphoma, and brain cancer, within six months and five years after hospitalization for pneumonia, were 0.05% and 0.14%, respectively. The incident ratios

---

[209] Kitabjian A. 2018. Pediatric Patients Hospitalized for Pneumonia May have Elevated Cancer Risk. MSN. January 26, 2018. Doi: https://www.cancertherapyadvisor.com/lymphoma/pediatric-patients-pneumonia-higher-cancer-risk/article/739376/. *Originally published,* Pulmonology Adviser and BMJ.

were two-fold higher in children up to age fourteen; and were higher in girls, children diagnosed with immunodeficiencies, and children who had congenital malformations. The risk of developing lymphoid leukemia, myeloid leukemia, and non-Hodgkin's lymphoma was persistently higher in children up to five years post-pneumonia hospitalization, with higher than expected rates of non-Hodgkin's lymphoma and brain cancer found in children beyond the five years of follow-up. It would be important to know the pathogens causing the pneumonia; how many of the study subjects were treated with penicillin; and if children treated with penicillin had a greater incidence of cancer, in some or all risk groups.

In 2018, Facebook sponsored a study, which examined tissue adjacent to different types of cancer tumors. The study reported tissue adjacent to the cancer was not cancer, but was not normal. The tissue surrounding the tumor exhibited the same cellular properties as intracellular chlamydia. The tumor and adjacent cells were covered with immune cells, attempting to attack the intracellular infection, consistent with the findings of Dr. Russell. Chlamydia infected cells were found adjacent to Alzheimer's lesions; and polyps adjacent to cancerous polyps were also found not normal but not cancer. The finding proves a pattern in cancer and chronic disease, because the molecular findings match chlamydia pathogens, and tissue adjacent to cancerous tumors and adjacent to Alzheimer's lesions also have the same molecular findings as chlamydia.

The Facebook study found all cancers have similar genetic patterns. All cancers have similar genetic patterns because all cancers are caused by the same family of immortal animal pathogens. The variations in cancer DNA arises because different immortal pathogens, and combinations of pathogens, over time, can cause cancer. Chlamydia has the ability to alter genes, by generating abnormal sticky proteins that attach to genes and cause genetic abnormalities, reflected in DNA. Each form of chlamydia has many sub-types known as serovars, which may continue to mix and change when combined in a host with co-infections. Co-infections in humans can cause evolution of serotypes of the pathogens, into new or more virulent pathogens. The abnormal proteins and waste generated by the different species of pathogens can create evolving mutations in cancer DNA.

The cells adjacent to cancer showed cellular changes that match the cellular environment, in cancer and in chlamydia. Adjacent cells are infected with the same intracellular pathogen and continue to make new, weak, immortal and infected cells; disperse byproducts that add to the ball of debris that is forming the tumor; and continue to generate angiogenesis and an immune response to the pathogen. The immortal infection continues inside the tumor, in the weaker infected and immortal cells and in adjacent tissue, and the infected cells and damaged cell parts continue to send signals to the immune system to attack. As adjacent cells and pathogens in the tumor are attacked by the immune system, the tumor grows from the lack of apoptosis in the tumor cells and the continued accumulation of toxic byproducts from the ongoing immune battle.

Chlamydia-infected cells have the same molecular properties as cancer cells; and chlamydia is the only pathogen capable of causing the same molecular properties found in cancer cells. Chlamydia takes over control of cell function; damages apoptosis; and gives rise to rapid cell production of weaker infected copies of immortal cells. Chlamydia pneumonia induces interleukin 10, which stops programmed cell death. Chlamydia generates TNF-alpha, causes inflammatory cytokines, and C-reactive protein; and causes angiogenesis and impaired infected immune cells. Angiogenesis signals new vessel growth, which is a hallmark of both chlamydia and cancer; and one treatment for cancer has been to try to stop new blood vessels from growing, with anti-vessel growth drugs. Chlamydia depletes ATP and folic acid; consumes sugar and causes fermentation and fungus; and damages oxygen transport into the cell. Dr. Warburg proved the lack of oxygen transport into the cell is a hallmark of cancer. The chlamydia pathogen silences the signals of a normal tumor suppression gene, the KLF-6, from the liver and placenta, which is the gene intended to prevent tumor growth. Chlamydia also induces production of IL-8, an antigenic factor; and promoter of tumor growth in human non-small cell cancers.

Animal pathogens cannot ever merge peacefully into a human microbiome. The pathogens can only survive by living off the energy of the host, damage cell function and immune function, and set off an infectious cascade that ends in infinite replication of weak infected cells and cancer.

The pathogen takes control of the chemical messengers of the host cell, and acquires the capacity of limitless cell division and survival. The pathogen disperses abnormal sticky proteins, which provide a focus for a failed immune system attack, and the immune system attempts to wall-off the abnormal protein and pathogen, providing the focus for tumor development.[210]

Chronic intracellular infection and the immune system attack create a toxic mass, which is generated by the pathogen and immune battle, and becomes cancer. The toxic debris of infected cells no longer regulated by apoptosis, dead cells and cell parts, abnormal proteins, and byproducts of the immune battle, create a toxic mass of infected cells and debris that cannot be eliminated by the immune system, blood, or lymphatics. The pathogen changes the molecular properties of the adjacent cells, consistent with the molecular environment of cancer. Adjacent cells continue to foster the growth of the tumor, send signals to the immune system to attack, trigger angiogenesis, and continue to generate abnormal proteins and debris fostering growth of the tumor. The immune system continues to attack the infected cells in the tumor and adjacent to it.

Cancer is the toxic accumulation of cells infected with immortal pathogens, damaged cell parts, debris, abnormal proteins, and fungus, at the center of immortal infection. Cancer is the end result of a longstanding war between the pathogen and the immune system. Cancer is the end result of the infectious cascade caused by a chronic immortal infection. Chronic infection, plus time, plus a trigger for cancer such as low folic acid, environmental triggers, co-infections, or new acute infections, can trigger the infected cells to become cancer.

Viral infections, environmental triggers, chemicals, and/or drugs may join forces with chlamydia and other immortal pathogens to trigger cancer.

---

[210] *See* Kolata G, 2015. Brain Cancers Reveal Novel Genetic Disruption in DNA. New York Times (Health). Dec. 23, 2015. Doi: https://www.nytimes.com/2015/12/24/health/brain-cancers-reveal-novel-genetic-disruption-in-dna.html. (Sticky protein were found at the center of all gliomas in the brain and in numerous other types of cancer).

Non-infectious causes can exacerbate infectious causes of cancer. Exposure to carcinogens, poor diet, or infection with parasites, can combine with immortal pathogens or trigger cancer in patients with a chronic chlamydia infection. Studies in Africa, in areas where childhood cancer is endemic, identified EBV (mononucleosis) as also being endemic. EBV has been suggested as a cause of Burkett's lymphoma. Most people are infected with EBV in their life; and not all patients with EBV develop childhood cancers or Burkett's lymphoma. EBV may be a co-morbid chronic infection, which combines with chlamydia as a co-infection or bacteriophage, in a patient who has impaired immunity; and could be a trigger for cancer.

Scientists claim they have now "discovered" interstitial spaces, and are calling it a new organ and vehicle for cancer spread. They allege they had not previously see the collagen structures forming the interstitial spaces, because the fluid left the tissue when tissue was removed from the body and the spaces collapsed, prior to being sent to pathology. The existence of interstitial spaces is not new knowledge, but interstitial spaces and the collagen structure may be one vehicle for metastasis of some cancers. Chlamydia pneumonia damages endothelium, impairing fluid transport into the tissues. Chlamydia psittacosis is known to live and spread in the lymphatic system, and is a cause of some lymphomas and cancers. H-pylori is known to burrow below the epithelium and attach to collagen, and H-pylori is a known cause of cancer; thus, cancer involving spread through collagen likely involves H-pylori as a co-infection.

Intracellular pathogens have different manifestations in cancer, depending on the pathogen, duration of infection, and weak links. The type of chlamydia pathogen may determine the type of cancer. Chlamydia pathogens attack particular types of tissue, and spreads to weak links. Different co-infections may trigger different types of cancer. Different types of immune cells are programmed to attack different types of pathogens, and the type of immune cell attacking the intracellular pathogen may determine the type of blood cell that gets infected and the type of blood cancer that develops. Research could likely discover which particular infections and combinations of infections are common in different types of cancer, and different types of cancers in the immune cells.

Some forms of chlamydia are more virulent. Chlamydia pneumonia can have an insidious progression to cause chronic diseases, in the long-term. Chlamydia trachoma and chlamydia psittacosis are more virulent, and may be more likely to cause cancer. Chlamydia trachoma and chlamydia psittacosis have been "associated" with cancer. Chlamydia trachoma and psittacosis strains attack both the epithelium and the endothelium, causing a more rapid destruction of tissue; and/or the trachoma and psittacosis species are able to mix and exchange DNA with other pathogens, to evolve into more dangerous pathogens more quickly.

Trachoma is well-known to attack the reproductive tract to cause infertility, significantly increases the risk for ovarian cancer, and attacks the eye to cause blindness. Chlamydia trachoma doubles the risk of ovarian cancer; and powder has independently been "associated" with ovarian cancer. Powder can create a focus for inclusion cysts and ovarian cancer, and when a patient has chlamydia trachoma *and* uses powder in the vaginal area, the risk of ovarian cancer will be significantly greater; because chlamydia trachoma and powder can independently cause ovarian cancer.

Psittacosis has been "associated" with many types of cancer, including but not limited to melanoma, lymphoma, and eye cancer, in humans and birds. Psittacosis can rapidly mix phenotypes with other pathogens in animals, and evolve into new forms. Psittacosis is under diagnosed, and pet birds are considered a public health threat, because psittacosis causes chronic diseases, including cancer.

Currently, two clusters of a rare eye cancer are being investigated in Auburn, Alabama; and Huntersville, North Carolina. Students from Auburn University formed a support group for victims of melanoma of the iris, uveal tract and retina. Thirty-six patients, mostly women, in Auburn, including three students who lived in the same college dormitory; and eighteen patients in Huntersville, many who went to the same high school, have been diagnosed with a rare ocular melanoma, a cancer which ordinarily occurs in only six people per million per year. The first case of eye cancer in Auburn, was identified, in 1990. Recently some Auburn victims reported developing melanoma of the eye when pregnant; and development of liver, brain, and pancreatic cancer. The first identified case of eye cancer in Huntersville, leading to discovery of a second cancer cluster, was in 2009. Auburn and Huntersville have clusters of the same type of rare eye cancer, and the connection between the two cities is psittacosis from birds.

In 1972, Auburn University was overrun with pigeons. The pigeon population was destroying and defacing buildings, nesting in air ducts and air-conditioning systems, and depositing so many pounds of bird poop on roofs that the roofs were at risk of collapse. Auburn University conducted a "great pigeon extermination", in an effort to exterminate the pigeon population on campus. In 2015, the Birmingham Alabama Zoo had an outbreak of psittacosis in their avian sanctuary, and had to temporarily close the area to the public.

In 1973, a study was done inoculating fourteen rabbits intravenously, with psittacosis. The rabbits all developed keratoconjunctivitis, an eye infection caused by psittacosis. The study concluded the rabbit model was appropriate for the study of endogenous uveitis. The study also confirmed acute systemic infection with psittacosis can quickly spread to the eye, and become chronic uveitis, even without direct inoculation of the eye.[211] Fowl are considered the appropriate model for scientific study of eye cancer, because fowl get the same type of eye cancer as the victims in Auburn and Huntersville. Signs of psittacosis in birds include inflammation of the membranes around the eyes and lining the eyelids, squinting, and eye discharge; however, some infected birds may appear symptomatic.

The Southeastern Raptor Center is part of Auburn University, College of Veterinary Medicine. The Southeastern Raptor Center takes in hundreds of sick and injured birds of prey annually, then releases the birds thought

---

[211] Iversen JO, *et al*. 1974. Ocular Involvement with Chlamydia Psittaci (Strain M56) in Rabbits Inoculated Intravenously. Can. J. Comp. Med. July 1974. 38: 298-302. PMID: 277591. PMCID: PMC1319872.

healthy back into the wild. Raptors are infected with psittacosis worldwide, and have been known to eat pigeons that are infected with psittacosis. Caged and sanctuary raptors are most likely to have psittacosis.[212]

The Southeastern Raptor Center was a fertile location for birds to acquire and mix serovars of psittacosis, causing a more virulent strain in the raptors. Psittacosis is known to reconstitute its DNA by mixing with other pathogens, including mixing the DNA of psittacosis with the DNA with other serovars of chlamydia psittacosis and with chlamydia trachoma. The raptors could have brought new serovars of psittacosis to Auburn, and after release the raptors rapidly transmitted the new serovar of psittacosis to other local birds and to humans, in contact with or who inhaled particles of bird feces. The pathogen causing the eye cancer in Auburn may be a known strain of psittacosis, and/or endemic psittacosis in the local bird population; an unusual serovar or variant of psittaci introduced by the raptors at the Southeastern Center Raptor Center; and/or a recombination of the phenotypes of psittacosis and/or trachoma serovars in animals and humans. Psittacosis infection in pigeons and raptors in Auburn may have combined and reconstituted the phenotypes of psittacosis with other serovars of psittacosis, to form new variants. The psittacosis may also have combined with co-infections in birds or humans, to become more virulent and cause cancer.

The victims in Auburn could have been exposed through a contaminated environment; bird droppings in, on, and around the campus of Auburn University; or at the Southeastern Raptor Center. The Southeastern Raptor Center periodically has exhibitions open to the public, which could expose the population to psittacosis from the birds at the Southeastern Raptor Center.

In 2008, a raptor from the Southeastern Raptor Center, in Auburn, was transferred to the North Carolina Raptor Center, in Huntersville. In 2009,

---

[212] *See* Gerbermann H and Korbel R. 1993. The Occurrence of Chlamydia Psittaci Infections in Raptors from Wildlife Preserves. Tieraztl Prax. Jun 1993. 21(3):217-24. (85.1% of the one-hundred-twenty-one raptors tested were positive for psittacosis, and the birds showed no clinical signs of the infection). PMID 8346524; Fowler ME, *et al.* 1990. Chlamydiosis in Captive Raptors. Avian Dis. Jul-Sep 1990. 34(3):657-62. Doi: 10.2307/1591260. (41% of raptors tested were positive for psittacosis, and 35% were suspected psittacosis).

the first case of eye cancer in Huntersville was identified. The raptor from Auburn likely spread psittacosis to the raptors at the North Carolina Raptor Center, and to the local bird population; and infected the environment and the local bird population in Huntersville and at the North Carolina Raptor Center. The raptor from Auburn likely transmitted the psittacosis pathogen to local birds in Huntersville, causing transmission from birds to humans in Huntersville, and a new cluster of rare eye cancer. The North Carolina Raptor Center has a summer program for high school students; and although not confirmed, the high school in Huntersville attended by many of the Huntersville eye cancer victims, is believed to have had students who participated in the North Carolina Raptor Center summer program.

Chlamydia psittacosis, H-pylori, HPV, and trachoma, have long been "associated" with cancer of the eye. Of the pathogens "associated" with eye cancer, chlamydia psittacosis and H-pylori, are the most likely pathogens causing the eye cancer clusters, in Auburn and Huntersville. Both pathogens are "associated" with eye cancer and melanoma, alone or as co-infections; and psittacosis could have mixed and changed serovars to become more virulent in Auburn or in the patients who had co-infections with trachoma or H-pylori. Chlamydia psittacosis and H-pylori are attacked by neutrophils, and when neutrophils become infected the neutrophils show profound changes, including hyper-segmentation that resembles cancer. H-pylori may damage the ocular surface, allowing deeper invasion of psittacosis in the eye. H-pylori, chlamydia trachoma and/or ocular trachoma may be a co-infection with psittacosis, in some or all cases of eye cancer. The immune battle against the pathogens becomes a focus for cancer in the eye.[213]

---

[213] *See e.g.* Stefanovic A and Lossos I. 2009. Extranodal Marginal Zone Lymphoma of the Ocular Adnexa. Blood. 2009. Vol 114 (3): 501-510. Doi: 10.1182/blood-2008-12-195453; Ruiz A, *et al.* 2007. Extranodal Marginal Zone B-Cell Lymphomas of the Ocular Adnexa: Multiparameter Analysis of 34 Cases Including Interphase Molecular Cytogenetics and PCR for Chlamydia Psittaci. Am J Surg Pathol. May 2007. 31(5): 792-802. Doi: 10.1097/01.pas.0000249445.28713.88; Ferreri AJ, *et al.* 2004. Evidence for an Association Between Chlamydia Psittaci and Ocular Adnexal Lymphomas. Journal of the National Cancer Institute. 2004. Vol. 96 (8): 586-594. Doi: https://doi.org/10.1093/jnci/djh102.

Circumstantial evidence and scientific knowledge strongly suggests it was the birds! Chlamydia psittacosis is "associated" with eye cancer *and* melanoma; and with melanoma of the eye occurring during pregnancy. Pigeons, raptors, and caged raptors are heavily infected with psittacosis. Psittacosis is the most likely of the five pathogens "associated" with eye cancer, to jump from one town to a new town, five hundred miles away. The Huntersville cancer cluster began one year after a raptor was transferred from Southeastern Raptor Center to the Huntersville Raptor Center. The fact most of the Auburn and Huntersville victims were women, also implicates eye make-up as a vector for transmitting psittacosis to the eye and maintaining psittacosis on and near the eye. Psittacosis has been associated with ocular and follicular conjunctivitis; and twenty-seven percent of patients with chronic conjunctivitis tested positive for either chlamydia trachoma or chlamydia psittacosis.[214] None of the victims should be wearing eye make-up!

Italy has a high rate of eye cancer and lymphoma, caused by psittacosis from pigeons. Italy has high rates of rare cancers, lymphoma, and eye diseases such as retinitis pigmentosa; and higher rates of eye cancer, rare cancers, melanoma, and lymphoma.[215] Subclinical infection with chlamydia psittacosis was identified in patients with Sjögren's syndrome and parotid gland marginal zone B-cell lymphoma.[216] The higher rate of lymphomas and eye cancer in Italy, where psittacosis is common in the pigeons, and the population has frequent contact with pigeons, supports psittacosis as the likely pathogen in Auburn and Huntersville.

The Veteran's Administration recently noticed a high rate of eye cancer in Vietnam veterans, seventeen times higher than expected. The eye cancer in

---

[214] Lietman T, *et al.* 1998. Chronic Follicular Conjunctivities Associated with Chlamydia Psittaci or Chlamydia Pneumonia. Clinical Infectious Diseases. June 1998. 26:1335-40. Doi: 1058-4838/98/2606—0017$03.00.

[215] Buzzoni C, *et al.* 2016. Italian Cancer Figures – Report 2015: The Burden of Rare Cancers. Epidemiologia e prevenzione. Jan 2016. Doi: 10.19191/EP16.1S2.P001.035.

[216] Fabris M, *et al.* 2014. High Prevalence of Chlamyophila Psittaci Subclinical Infection in Italian Patients with Sjogren's syndrome, Parotid Gland Marginal Zone B-Cell Lymphoma, and MALT Lymphoma. Clin Exp Rheumatol. 2014. Jan-Feb; 32(1):61-65. PMID 2447326. Epub Jan 20, 2014. Doi: https://www.ncbi.nlm.nih.gov/pubmed/24447326.26.

Vietnam veterans is also likely caused by psittacosis acquired in Vietnam, combined with co-infections. Vietnam veterans suggested Agent Orange as a factor in the eye cancer, but Agent Orange was not in Alabama or North Carolina. Agent Orange may have been an environmental trigger in Vietnam; however, the Vietnam veterans likely acquired psittacosis in Vietnam, which was never diagnosed and treated. Years later, the psittacosis developed into eye cancer by endogenous spread or self-inoculation. Diagnosis of pathogens in Vietnam veterans with eye cancer will most likely uncover more than one co-infection, in the Vietnam veterans who developed eye cancer, which worked synergistically to cause eye cancer.

The clusters of eye cancer at Auburn University and in Huntersville provide an opportunity to identify the infectious causes of cancer; and to identify psittacosis as one of the most virulent forms of chlamydia, capable of causing cancer. Discovery of the infectious cause and common link, between the eye cancer in Auburn and Huntersville, can lead to discovery of the infectious cause of many cancers and recognition of the importance of examination and culture of cells adjacent to tumors. Moreover, some of the eye cancer victims have already developed new cancers, including but not limited to liver metastasis and pancreatic cancer. Psittacosis has been "associated" with both liver and pancreatic cancer. The psittacosis causing the eye cancer was not treated systemically, and has returned to cause cancer in other organs and systems. The victim of pancreatic cancer was told it was a new cancer, and not metastatic cancer from the eye; but the oncologist did not consider the psittacosis pathogen caused both cancers.

A $100,000 grant was planned, to investigate the connection and the cause of the cancer clusters in Auburn and Huntersville. The Health Department and head of the investigation did not consider infectious causes. The Health Department search of scientific research, for the initial phase of the investigation, did not list a single infectious pathogen as a potential cause needing investigation. The investigation was directed at non-infectious causes, like social connections, the environment, and genes. To date the money was spent tracking the geographic and social connections; and the next phase is planned to investigate genetic abnormalities. The investigation has made little progress in finding the cause of the eye cancer clusters, because no one is looking for infectious pathogens. The ophthalmologist in charge does not study infectious disease or cancer, the cancer specialist treating the patients has not considered infectious causes, and the Health Department is only interested in environmental causes. The oncologist investigating the Auburn cancer cluster reported she was at a loss as to the cause of the cancer cluster. The cause is environmental only in the sense bird feces contaminated the environment and spread psittacosis. The cause of the eye cancer clusters is psittacosis!

The first step to confirming the cause of the eye cancer cluster should be recognizing an infectious cause, and using reason to identify the most likely pathogen causing the eye cancer clusters. The second step should be testing the birds, including raptors in Auburn, the raptor sent to Huntersville from Auburn, the raptors at the North Carolina Raptor Center, and the local population of pigeons and raptors in Auburn and Huntersville, which were likely infected by the raptors from the Southeastern Raptor Center. Testing the raptors and pigeons in Auburn and Huntersville could confirm the presence of psittacosis, and the serovars of psittacosis in the birds.

The third step should be testing the victims for pathogens known to cause eye cancer, including chlamydia psittacosis, chlamydia trachoma, chlamydia pneumonia, and H-pylori, to determine what pathogens and combination of pathogens the victims harbor. Serovars of psittacosis in eye cancer victims can be compared to the serovars of psittacosis in the local raptors and pigeons; and common origins can be determined with advanced laboratory testing. Testing the victims for chlamydia psittacosis and other pathogens known to cause eye cancer, would provide the answer to the cause of the eye cancer cluster. Identifying the infectious causes of the eye cancer clusters can save lives, because patients with eye cancer caused by psittacosis, who were treated with antibiotics, had improvement or resolution of the eye cancer, and an improved prognosis, with or without enucleation.[217]

---

[217] *See e.g.* Stefanovic A and Lossos I. 2009. Extranodal Marginal Zone Lymphoma of the Ocular Adnexa. Blood. 2009. Vol 114 (3): 501-510. Doi: 10.1182/blood-2008-12-195453. (treatment response supported belief psittacosis was the cause of the diseases).

Doctors and patients in Auburn and Huntersville must recognize and treat respiratory psittacosis aggressively, and become aware eye cancer can be treated and the prognosis improved by treating psittacosis, even if it is in conjunction with enucleation of the eye and other forms of cancer treatment. Treatment may also protect the patients long-term from development of other psittacosis-related cancers, or improve the prognosis of victims who have had cancer develop in the liver and pancreas. Knowledge of the infectious cause of eye cancer will spread the warning of acquiring psittacosis from birds or cats; and protect new victims, who can be aware and be promptly treated for psittacosis. Residents can be made aware of the danger, and the need to avoid any hand-to-eye contact with birds or bird droppings.

The fourth step in the investigation should be finding the source of bird feces contaminating the environment, at Auburn University, on rooftops, in ventilation systems, at the raptor center, and on campus; and in Huntersville, at the high school, at the North Carolina Raptor Center, and in the community. Birds nesting on the rooftops can be a source of psittacosis contamination and transmission of psittacosis to humans. Identifying the infectious cause will direct the investigation to the source of contamination, and prevent new cases of eye cancer from the same vectors. The psittacosis serovar has already spread in the birds, and it may be difficult to eradicate the bird vectors for the serovar of psittacosis causing eye cancer.

New discoveries can be made in understanding cancer, by investigating psittacosis and other immortal pathogens as the cause of the eye cancer clusters. Where did the victims come in contact with the psittacosis? Was the psittacosis acquired as a severe respiratory infection, through airborne transmission and the pathogen attacked the eye systemically, or by direct eye-hand contact? Did the victims acquire ocular psittacosis, by self-inoculation of the eye, rather than through systemic spread of a respiratory infection? Did eye make-up play a role in spreading psittacosis to the ocular surface, to cause an eye infection and eye cancer? If psittacosis, alone or in combination with a co-infection of trachoma, H-pylori, and/or HPV, is shown to be the cause of the cluster of eye cancers; research could then diligently pursue infectious causes of cancer and the role of psittacosis and other immortal pathogens, in all types of cancer. H-pylori may be a co-infection, which attacked the ocular surface and provided a portal for psittacosis to invade the eye; and H-pylori alone is capable of causing cancer in other organ systems. The investigation could lead to profound and important discoveries in cancer research, including the infectious causes of many different types of cancer and the role of psittacosis and H-pylori in causing cancer.

Multiple immortal infections or immortal infections plus environmental triggers, can accelerate the progression of immortal infections to cancer. When a patient has more than one type of chlamydia or co-existing immortal pathogens, it is more likely the infections attack endothelium, epithelium and more than one type of host tissue, body system and organ. When the patient has more than one type of pathogen capable of causing cancer, more types of immune cells will attack and become infected, and the pathogens may be synergistic in causing and accelerating the development of cancer. The time course for development of cancer after acute infection may be weeks, months, years or decades, depending on the virulence of the infection, co-infections, environmental and chemical triggers, low folic acid, and possibly treatment with penicillin.

Long-term alcohol consumption increases the risk of cancer, and can be a trigger for cancer. Alcohol consumption depletes folic acid, in proportion to the amount of alcohol consumed; and low folic acid is a recognized trigger for cancer. Immortal pathogens and parasites deplete folic acid, and alcohol consumption independently depletes folic acid. The alcohol and chronic infection combined accelerate loss of folic acid and development of cancer. Low folic acid can interfere with mental stability, and increase the risk of alcohol addiction. Alcoholics require medical diagnosis, and folic acid and B12 supplements, to reduce the risk of cancer. A recent meta-analysis suggested the risk of drinking any alcohol is offset by the health risk of cancer, and the safest level of alcohol is none.[218]

---

[218] *See* 2018. GBD 2016 Alcohol Collaborators. Alcohol Use and Burden for 195 Countries and Territories, 1990-2016: A Systematic Analysis For the Global Burden of Disease Study 2016. The Lancet. 2018. Doi: 10.1016/S0140-6736(18)31310-2; *See also* 2018. No Safe Level of Alchol, New Study Concludes. ScienceDaily. Aug 24, 2018. Doi: https://www.sciencedaily.com/releases/2018/08/180824103018.htm. (three-million deaths globally related to alcohol, in 2016, and twelve percent of deaths in males ages fifteen to forty nine).

Blood cancers are caused by immortal infection in the immune cells. Immune cells are made in the bone marrow. The immune system includes many types of immune cells, including mast cells, which are the first to reach the pathogen; and leukocytes, which are white blood cells and include neutrophils, monocytes, macrophages, eosinophils, basophils, and lymphocytes. Lymphocytes include T-cells, B-cells, and natural killer cells. Plasma cells are immune cells called plasma B-cells, plasmocytes, or effector B-cells. Plasma cells make and secrete large quantities of antibodies to specific pathogens, at rates of one thousand antibodies per second. Plasma cells are transported by the lymphatic system to the pathogens.

Specific types of immune cells are programmed to attack specific types of immortal pathogens. The type of pathogen determines the types of immune cells signaled to fight the infection. The type of immune cell that attacks the pathogen and becomes infected by the pathogen will determine the type of blood cancer which develops; and is a clue to the type of infection causing the blood cancer. Chlamydia can infect all types of immune cells, can replicate in immune cells, and all forms of chlamydia cause blood clumping of the red or white blood cells, characteristic of some blood cancers and acute myeloid leukemia (AML). Research identifying immortal pathogens in blood cancer can lead to new discoveries regarding which infectious pathogens attack which types of immune cells, and new treatments directed at the pathogens in immune cells that cause blood cancers.

A team of immune cells attack the pathogen, in a series of programmed immune responses; and the team members engulf the pathogen, in a series of events, attempting to digest the pathogen and/or carry the pathogen to the plasma cells to be killed by antibodies made by plasma cells. For instance, mast cells and macrophages attack chlamydia pneumonia; neutrophils attack H-pylori and psittacosis; monocytes attack parasites; and plasma cells attack streptococcus with M-proteins attached. TNF-alpha is generated primarily by macrophages, but can be generated by any immune cell, and is a signaling protein involved in inflammation. The type of immortal infection will determine the type of immune cells that attack the pathogen, and whether TNF-alpha is generated to enhance the immune system attack. When the immune cells attack the pathogen, the immune cells become infected, and the pathogen continues to live intracellularly in the immune cells, where it can be spread wherever the immune cells can reach, and cause development of blood cancers.

Leukemia is caused by immortal pathogens infecting the white blood cells in the bone marrow. Leukemia may develop from acute co-infections, triggering an aggressive immune response, and rapid proliferation of large numbers of immune cells in response to the multiple acute infections. The immune cells are infected with the intracellular pathogens, causing the immune cells to misfire and rapidly reproduce by division. The immune cells lose apoptosis, and rapidly produce immortal white blood cells, which are weak replicas of white blood cells that are infected with the same pathogen. Leukemia, like many chronic diseases, can be caused by more than one pathogen, or combination of pathogens, infecting the immune cells—the point is, it is intracellular infection of the immune cells is the cause of leukemia.

Dr. Merchant treated a patient with leukemia, with Tequin, gamma globulin, and intravenous vitamin C, and the leukemia resolved. Tequin was later taken off the market due to complications of erupting infections that were life-threatening. Another type of mycin, salinomycin, has been used as an antibiotic to treat infections in chickens and cows, and is showing promise in the treatment of breast cancer and leukemia, by attacking infection in stem cells. Apoptosis can be restored or sensitivity increased with a mycin, which could improve the prognosis of the blood cancer.

Human parvovirus has been "associated" with childhood leukemia. Human parvovirus B19 is one of many serovars of parvovirus; and is believed different from the highly contagious parvovirus strain in dogs. Human parvovirus likely attaches itself to the immortal bacteria as a bacteriophage to cause cancer. Studies of childhood leukemia have also discovered children can have two rhinoviruses at the same time, increasing the virulence of viruses; and supporting co-infections are more dangerous than a single infection.

Multiple myeloma is cancer in the plasma cells. The plasma cells multiply and crowd the bone marrow; and the bone develops thin spots. Multiple myeloma cells produce large amounts of abnormal paraproteins, and in particular "M-proteins". Streptococcus and mycoplasma are the only known pathogens that have M-proteins on the surface, and the attack by the immune system can cause M-proteins to be released into the body and broken into fragments. The streptococcus and mycoplasma pathogens are attacked by macrophages. The macrophages act as scavengers in the body, cleaning up old dead cells, and engulf and digest bacteria and M-proteins on the surface of the pathogens. The macrophages die after attacking the M-proteins, and signal the immune system to an invader. The plasma cell starts as a B-cell, which encounters and digests the macrophage and remnants of the macrophage attack on the pathogen, internalizes the pathogen, and takes the pathogen to a T-cell, which triggers the B-cell to mature into a plasma cell. The plasma cell then creates thousands of antibodies per second, to attack the pathogen.

The process of the macrophage engulfing the pathogen and M-proteins, the B-cell digesting the pathogen, the B-cell taking the pathogen to the T-cell, and the T-cell maturing into a plasma cell, suggests the streptococcus type-M or mycoplasma pathogen can infect plasma cells and cause multiple myeloma. The correlation between M-proteins attached to specific streptococcus or mycoplasma serovars, and the diagnosis of cancer in the plasma cells based on the persistence of M-proteins, suggests investigation is needed into streptococcus or mycoplasma as a chronic intracellular infection in the plasma cells, causing multiple myeloma. Infectious causes of diseases in the immune cells and bone marrow, like leukemia, multiple myeloma, and aplastic anemia, may be detected by screening the blood for immortal pathogens.

Cancer of the lymphatics is caused by chlamydia, most likely chlamydia psittacosis. Chlamydia psittacosis has been "associated" with lymphoma, and is already known to cause MALT lymphoma in the eye.[219] Sjögren's syndrome, parotid gland marginal zone B-cell lymphoma, and MALT lymphoma patients were found to have a high rate of chlamydia

---

[219] *See* Decaudin D, *et al.* Ocular Adnexa Lymphhoma: A Review of Cliinicopathologic Features and Treatment Options. Review Article. Blood. Sept 11, 2006. Vol 108. No. 5. Doi: 10.1182/blood-2006-02-005017.

psittacosis.[220] Chlamydia psittacosis invades the lymphatics, directly or through the immune cells; and the byproducts of infection are deposited in the lymphatic system and joints. The lymphatics expel toxins in the body under the arm—next to sensitive, ductal soft tissue and breast tissue. Patients who had breast implants with rough surfaces have developed lymphoma, when psittacosis gained access to the implant through the lymphatics, and attached to the rough surface of the implant. Psittacosis has been shown to be "associated" with many types of cancer, but the medical profession has not accepted infectious causes of lymphoma, or psittacosis as a cause of cancer, and the information has not filtered down to the front-line practitioners, or to the patients.

H-pylori has also been "associated" with lymphoma. H-pylori is the most common infectious disease outside of the United States. H-pylori attacks the epithelium and the collagen layer under the epithelium; and can cause a gastric cancer, MALT lymphoma, non-Hodgkin's lymphoma, Hodgkin's lymphoma, and other diseases and syndromes. H-pylori creates abnormal proteins, and releases plasmids and fragments of nucleus, leading to an infectious cascade and focus for development of an immune battle that ends in cancer. H-pylori is attacked by neutrophils and then infects neutrophils. Neutrophils infected with H-pylori are less able to recognize H-pylori, change from three or four interconnected lobes to six or more segmented lobes, and the neutrophils secrete pro-inflammatory cytokines and cause toxicity in surrounding tissue. The hyper-segmentation of the neutrophils into lobules resembles characteristics found in tumor-associated neutrophils in mice.[221] The toxic secretions from the infected neutrophils

---

[220] Fabris M, *et al.* 2014. High Prevalence of Chlamyophila Psittaci Subclinical Infection in Italian Patients with Sjogren's Syndrome, Parotid Gland Marginal Zone B-Cell Lymphoma, and MALT Lymphoma. Clin Exp Rheumatol. 2014. Jan-Feb; 32(1):61-65. PMID 2447326. Epub Jan 20, 2014. Doi: https://www.ncbi.nlm.nih. gov/pubmed/24447326.

[221] Whitmore L, *et al.* 2017. Cutting Edge: Helicobacter Pylori Induces Nuclear Hypersegmentation and Subtype Differentiation of Human Neutrophils In Vitro. J Immunol. Mar 1, 2017. 198 (5): 1793-1797. Doi: doi.org/10.4049/jimmunol.1601292; Horrom T. 2017. Study Shows How H. Pylori Causes White Blood Cells to Morph. VA Research Communications. March 9, 2017. Doi: https://www.research.va.gov/ currents/0317-1.cfm.

damage surrounding tissue and help the H-pylori survive and spread; and the neutrophils do not die as quickly, because normal apoptosis in the neutrophils is destroyed. H-pylori can work synergistically with other pathogens, by damaging epithelium and providing a portal for other pathogens to invade deeper into tissue. Co-infection with H-pylori and chlamydia psittacosis damages the immune system, increases the overall burden of infections, and accelerates an infectious cascade and development of lymphoma, because each pathogen can independently cause lymphoma and the pathogens can work synergistically to cause cancer.

Brain cancers are caused by the immune battle against pathogens and abnormal proteins that gain access to the brain, which cause brain tissue to stick together. The brain is 90% glial cells (Latin for glue). The New York Times reported *every* case of glioma, a form of brain cancer, had sticky proteins between package-bow patterns of brain tissue.[222] Infectious pathogens generate abnormal proteins. Pathogens and abnormal proteins set off an immune response to fight the infection. Cancer forms where the tissue was stuck together, and the immune system fought to eradicate pathogens and abnormal proteins, and generated inflammation. CMV has also been "associated" with brain cancer, and may be an important co-infection with chlamydia and/or H-pylori in causing brain cancer.

Many studies have "associated" chlamydia pneumonia with lung cancer; and chlamydia pneumonia specific IgG and IgA antibodies are independently associated with the risk of lung cancer in non-smokers.[223] Smoking damages lung tissue, making the lung tissue more receptive to chlamydia pneumonia infection and spread; and development of cancer. Lung cancer is the end-stage in the infectious cascade caused by chronic chlamydia pneumonia. A study by the American Association of Cancer Research, co-sponsored by the American Society of Preventive Oncology,

---

[222] *See* Kolata G. 2015. Brain Cancers Reveal Novel Genetic Disruption in DNA. New York Times (Health). Doi: https://www.nytimes.com/2015/12/24/health/brain-cancers-reveal-novel-genetic-disruption-in-dna.html.

[223] Kocazeybek B. 2003. Chronic Chlamydophila pneumoniae infection in lung cancer, a risk factor: a case–control study. Journal of Medical Microbiology. 2003. 52:721-726. Doi: 10.1099/jmm.0.04845-0 04845.

suggested the potential for lung cancer risk reduction by treatments targeted at chlamydia pneumonia.[224]

Science has not identified immortal pathogens in breast cancer. In breast cancer typing, the difference between HER2-positive and HER2-negative breast cancer is the abnormal proteins attached to the outside of the tumor. The abnormal proteins are created by the underlying chronic infection, which continues in the tumor and in adjacent tissue; and attached to the outside of the tumor. Some scientists suggested rodent chlamydia could cause breast cancer; however, the role of chlamydia muridarum in breast cancer has not been studied and confirmed. Mice also develop heart disease from chlamydia pneumonia and can carry trachoma; and some speculate mice are an animal reservoir for trachoma. Any chlamydia pathogen from mice has the potential to cause chronic disease in humans.

The risk of breast cancer may be enhanced by shaving the armpits, because hair under the arms wicks away toxins expelled through the lymphatics. Immortal infection can cause an increase in body odor, as the body tries to flush the infection through the lymphatic system. Preventing the flushing of toxins keeps the toxins in the lymphatics, adjacent to breast tissue. Deodorant may be an environmental trigger for cancer; and particularly deodorant or antiperspirant containing aluminum, and antiperspirant used immediately after shaving under the arms. Deodorants and antiperspirants have never been tested for safety or for carcinogens, and some past and present products may contain carcinogens. An epidemiologic study is needed comparing the incidence of breast cancer around the world, and how the incidence of breast cancer compares to the practice of shaving under the arm and using deodorant. If body odor is present, or the patient has an increase in body odor, preventing perspiration is not the solution—encouraging perspiration and diagnosing and treating the infection is a better treatment.

---

[224] *See* Zhan P, *et al.* 2011. Chlamydia Pneumoniae Infection and Lung Cancer Risk: A Meta-Analysis. Eur J Cancer. 2011 Mar. 47(5) 742-7. Doi: 10.1016/j.ejca.2010.11.003. Epub 2010 Dec 29. PMID: 21194924. Doi: 10.1016/j.ejca.2010.11.003.

The Shoppe papilloma virus (SPV) was originally discovered in cottontail rabbits in the Midwestern United States, but can also infect brush rabbits, jackrabbits, snowshoe hares, and European rabbits.[225] SPV is known as cottontail rabbit papilloma virus (CRPV) or Kappapapillomavirus-2; and is a papillomavirus which infects leporids, causing keratinous carcinomas resembling horns. Human papilloma virus (HPV) is a form of the Shoppe papilloma virus (SPV), which evolved from rabbit SPV. HPV is a sexually transmitted disease, and an accepted cause of vaginal warts; and cervical, throat, and oral cancer. HPV may be a co-infection with chlamydia species, particularly chlamydia trachoma, which triggers and potentiates development of cancer.

Prostate cancer and cervical cancer can be caused by chronic chlamydia trachoma or HPV; or a combination of both infections. HPV probably also causes other types of cancers. Thus, it is reasonable to believe HPV can cause prostate cancer. Trachoma can cause ovarian cancer, and likely other types of cancers of the reproductive tract, and may also cause prostate cancer alone or in combination with HPV. The HPV vaccines were initially directed to young girls, in an effort to prevent cervical cancer; and only recently was the vaccine offered to boys, to curb the spread of HPV. Because of the delay in vaccination of boys, men now have HPV at six times the rate of women; and men are developing oral HPV at an alarming rate.[226] Chlamydia trachoma and HPV can cause prostate cancer, and co-infection with chlamydia trachoma and HPV could accelerate the development of prostate cancer.

Chronic hepatitis B and C are viruses known to cause liver cancer. Hepatitis is normally acquired through blood transfusions, sharing needles, or by sexual contact. Hepatitis B has been found in primates throughout Southeast Asia and Africa. Hepatitis C is thought to be a human virus; but has also been found in foxes, wolves and bears. An infected cat can

---

[225] Wikipedia. Shoppe Papilloma Virus. Doi: en.wikipedia.org/wiki/Shope_papilloma_virus.

[226] Markman M. 2018. Oral HPV Infection Rate Is Alarmingly High in US Men. 1/25/18. Doi: medscape.com/viewarticle/891633?src=WNL_infoc_180410_MSCPEDIT_TEMP2&uac=240405SY&impID=1602727&faf=1.

transmit hepatitis from animal-to-human, through a scratch. Chronic hepatitis creates a weak link for other pathogens to attack, and co-exists with immortal pathogens, to foster development of cancer. The difference between patients with hepatitis C who progress to liver cancer may be the presence of a co-infection with a chlamydia, the overall infectious burden, and the virulence of the hepatitis C virus.

Gastrointestinal pathogens cause cancer in the gastrointestinal tract and in abdominal organs. Gastrointestinal pathogens and parasites migrate to abdominal organs to evade acid in the stomach and find new hospitable locations for survival. Pathogens can migrate from the intestinal tract to the pancreas, gallbladder and liver; and become a focus for cancer. The tail of the pancreas is connected to the intestinal tract, on the left side, and accessed through the common bile duct. The liver and gallbladder are connected to the intestinal tract on the right side. Chlamydia pathogens and parasites have been found inside tumors in the pancreas, gallbladder, and liver. H-pylori has been "associated" with pancreatic cancer, and has been found in pancreatic cancer.

Crohn's disease is ulcers in the lower intestine, which can evolve into cancer. Crohn's disease and ulcerative colitis are virtually the same disease. H-pylori has already been identified as the cause of stomach ulcers; and some suggest treatment of H-pylori may cause the pathogen to migrate to the lower intestine, or that H-pylori may combine in the lower intestine with e-coli, to cause Crohn's disease and colon cancer. Christian Jobin, Ph.D., Professor at the University of Florida, College of Medicine, proposed a combination of microbes are the cause of colorectal cancer, and suggested that bacteroides fragilis and e-coli may combine to cause colon cancer.[227] He could not guarantee his hypothesis that a combination of microbes caused intestinal disease, as the holy grail of colon cancer; and urged doctors to diagnose the bacteria in the gut of patients undergoing colonoscopy. If H-pylori can cause ulcers and stomach cancer, and can reside in the lower intestine, it is reasonable to believe H-pylori can cause

---

[227] Arthur J, *et al.* 2014. Microbial Genomic Analysis Reveals the Essential Role of Inflammation in Bacteria-Induced Colorectal Cancer. Nat Commun. Sep 3, 2014. 5:4724. Doi: 10.1038/ncomms5724.

ulcers and colon cancer in the lower intestine, by the same mechanism of damaging the epithelium, invading the layers of the intestine, and creating a portal for other pathogens to enter the lining of the intestine.

In "Young Adult Cancer: Influence of the Obesity Pandemic", researchers compared obesity to the risk of cancer.[228] The author looked at thirteen types of cancer known to be increasing in frequency in young adults, including thyroid, breast, esophageal, gastric, colon, gallbladder, liver, pancreas, kidney, rectal, endometrial, ovary, myeloma, and meningioma. Obesity increased the risk of the thirteen types of cancers, and the highest incidence of cancers was in older adults. Obesity in young adults increased the risk for five of the thirteen types of cancer, including thyroid, breast, stomach, uterus, and ovary. The study did not consider the fact obesity and cancer were co-morbid conditions, caused by the same pathogens; or investigate whether the young adults with obesity had co-infections that cause cancer. An increased risk of cancer in obese patients is because obesity *and* cancer are caused by a chronic infection, and the pathogens have more than one manifestation, during different stages of the infectious cascade.

Childhood cancers were rare in Dr. Farber's time. Today, cancer in children is increasing worldwide. The increase in cancer in children is caused by an epidemic of unrecognized and untreated acute and chronic infection; and pediatricians prescribing penicillin derivatives for acute infection. Indirect evidence suggests use of penicillin to treat immortal chlamydia infections can trigger a chronic disease, including cancer. The refusal to diagnose and treat acute infections, and overuse of penicillin *in lieu* of macrolides and antiparasitics, has caused an increase in the rate of cancer and chronic diseases in children and young adults.

Pediatricians today are reluctant to prescribe antibiotics; and if prescribed, are likely to prescribe amoxicillin or broad spectrum cephalosporins—the most widely used antibiotics in the United States. As a group, doctors and pediatricians are pressured to avoid prescribing antibiotics, and trained that the initial antibiotic should be amoxicillin or a broad-spectrum antibiotic.

---

[228] Berger N. 2018. Young Adult Cancer: Influence of the Obesity Pandemic. Obesity April 2018. 26(4): 641-650. Doi:10.1002/oby.22137.

Pediatricians rarely recognize parasitic disease in children, or treat parasites in children. The refusal to give antibiotics and antiparasitics to treat acute immortal infections, and the excessive use of penicillin, corresponds to the rise in childhood cancer, cardiovascular diseases, and obesity, in children, teens and young adults. The professional pressure to avoid antibiotics and failure to diagnose and treat parasites in children, has led to the explosion in cancer and chronic disease in younger patients.

Treatment of underlying chronic infections can slow the progress of existing cancer. Antibiotic treatment of patients diagnosed with cancer has been shown to extend life, by as much as eight years. Mebendazole and albendazole are antiparasitic drugs, used to treat parasites and worms, which have been shown effective against some cancers, and stopped the progression and metastasis of some cancers. Regular treatment of worms and other parasites in children and adults was a common practice in past times, but the practice has been abandoned. The return to treatment of acute infection with appropriate antibiotics that are not penicillin or amoxicillin, and regular treatment of parasites in children and adults, would advance the overall health of the population, and could be life-saving, by preventing chronic diseases and cancers that are caused by immortal pathogens and parasites. Yet, oncologists do not acknowledge chronic infections cause cancer, try to determine which pathogens cause which types of cancer, or treat cancer patients for immortal infections. Yet, pediatricians continue to refuse to treat acute immortal infections and parasites in children, or refuse any antibiotic other than amoxicillin. Voluminous literature supports infection as a cause of cancer, and reasoning based on what is known about intracellular pathogens and parasites, should direct research and discovery to immortal infections that become chronic infections and can cause of cancer.

Oncologists use chemotherapy and radiation to kill cancer. Chemotherapy is a combination of toxic drugs that kill everything, with the hope the cancer is destroyed and the patient survives. Chemotherapy drugs previously included methotrexate, which inhibits folic acid; and is the same class of drugs known to induce secondary cancers many years later. When children with leukemia are treated with methotrexate, the children may develop secondary cancers anywhere in the body, in their twenties. When twenty to thirty-year old patients are treated for Hodgkin's lymphoma with chemotherapy and radiation, the patient can develop primary lung cancer twenty years later. Anti-folate medications were found to cause teratogenic effects, known as fetal amphoterin syndrome. Newer cancer treatments are moving away from mass destruction of cells with chemotherapy, toward targeted therapy using monoclonal antibodies.

Anti-vessel growth drugs (Avastin) were approved for gastrointestinal cancers, and the indications subsequently expanded to lung cancers and other types of cancer. The anti-vessel growth medications cut off the blood supply to cancerous tumors, hoping to retard growth of the cancer. Anti-vessel growth drugs are expensive, at $30,000 per dose; and have severe unintended side effects on normal adjacent tissue. The use of Avastin in multiforma glioblastoma caused a shocking loss of brain function. In the eye, Avastin is diluted and packaged into smaller injectable doses, to treat wet macular degeneration, by stopping new blood vessels from growing on the retina. A smaller molecule anti-vessel growth drug that is more compatible with the eye (Lucentis) is approved for wet macular degeneration; but is less used because of the significantly higher cost of Lucentis, versus diluted and pre-packaged Avastin sold off-label. Chlamydia pathogens induce angiogenesis (the formation of new blood vessels). Medications that block new blood vessels are attempting to stop the angiogenesis caused by the chlamydia pathogen, and may slow cancer development; but do not address the root cause of angiogenesis or the root cause of cancer.

A valuable and long-overlooked treatment for cancer is imiquimod, which is a topical TLR-7 agonist. The trade name of imiquimod was Aldera, prior to the expiration of the patent. Imiquimod is a crème applied to the skin, and wherever it is applied the crème attracts the body's immune cells to the location. Imiquimod was initially approved for treatment of warts, and all types of facial and skin cancers. Imiquimod is now being tested in hundreds of cancer clinical trials. New forms of TLR agonists are being developed, in pellet form, which can be used at the time of cancer surgery. Stronger versions of imiquimod have now been developed, known as TLR-8 and TLR-9; and are being used to treat a variety of cancers.

The most recent study of lymphoma in mice showed resolution of the cancer at the primary and metastatic sites, by injecting a combination of two drugs, a TLR-9 agonist in combination with an anti-vessel growth drug. TLR-7 and TLR-8 were reported to be suitable substitutes for TLR-9. The NIH called imiquimod an old drug for a new purpose, in treating breast cancer and metastatic breast cancer. Imiquimod used for breast cancer can fight cancer at the primary site, reduce the size of the tumor, reduce metastasis, and eradicate cancer at metastatic sites. Application of imiquimod during radiation can make radiation more effective.

All TLR drugs bring the white blood cells to the location of the primary cancer, and re-program immune cells to reduce the confusion in the immune system and allow the immune system to attack metastatic cancer; which is the only way imiquimod crème applied at the primary cancer site could eradicate metastatic cancer. The body's own immune cells are attracted to the primary cancer and re-programmed to recognize the cancer; and thereby become effective at attacking cancer at metastatic cites. Imiquimod is a simple, available, relatively inexpensive, and helpful treatment for cancer; but it is seldom utilized by practicing oncologists.

Scientists are now studying yeast analogues and structures, which are thought to suppress the biochemical basis of cancer. Forty years after Dr. Simonchini suggested cancer was caused by fungus, and was ridiculed for his opinion, scientists are studying fungus to develop new cancer treatments. We have moved from the development of penicillin from mold by Alexander Fleming, to some of the most promising new anti-cancer drugs being derivatives of mold. Treating fungus may interrupt the progression of immortal infections causing cancer, and slow the infectious cascade; and may be one way to deprive cancer and parasites of the environment needed for survival, to improve the prognosis.

Cancer doctors and cancer researchers have an inherent bias against infectious pathogens causing cancer, which is impeding discovery. Oncologists continue to think of cancer as miscues of the genetic code, setting off an irrevocable series of molecular events—but for the 15-20% of cancers proven to be "associated" with infections. Cancer doctors research small details in cell biology, Cluster Differentiations, abnormal proteins, C-reactive proteins, cytokines, TNF-alpha, genes, the proteinbiome, inflammasomes, apoptosomes, etc.; and fail to look at a bigger picture over a longer period of time, to deduce and discover the cause of cancer. Spending money on research into genes and small details in cell microbiology has not given an answer to the cause of cancer; and research findings and conclusions are confused because immortal infections can cause genetic abnormalities.

The cause of cancer will not be discovered by cancer doctors alone, because the answer to the cause of cancer cannot be found within the cancer specialty, or within any one specialty. The cause of cancer cannot be discovered by cancer doctors, because cancer is caused by intracellular animal pathogens, acquired long before the cancer diagnosis. Oncologists do not study immortal infections or parasites as a cause of cancer; do not diagnose the infectious causes of cancer; do not treat infection, but for serious infections developing during chemotherapy; have not focused research on infectious causes in cancer; and do not consider the prior twenty-year infectious cascade that became cancer. Oncologists do not have patients over a long period of time, to know the patient's history of infectious pathogens or how the acute infections have been treated, which is critical to understanding the cause of cancer. Oncologists must search for immortal pathogens in every type of cancer, to gain understanding of the causes of cancer. Oncologist must accept more than one type of pathogen can cause cancer, and different pathogens may cause the same or different types of cancers. Oncologists will have to look outside their specialty, explore the infectious pathogens in cancer patients, and compare the pathogens found to different types of cancer, to discover the cause of cancer.

Chlamydia is a slow moving pathogen that in time can become cancer. Chlamydia is the only bacteria that causes molecular changes identical to cancer. The body responds to chlamydia as if it was a form of cancer, with TNF-alpha, angiogenesis, and loss of apoptosis. Understanding the root cause of cancer to be infectious, and understanding the infectious cascade, can lead to new discoveries and new ways to attack cancer, by attacking chronic infection at points along the infectious cascade. Treatment to interrupt the infectious cascade could potentially forestall cancer or improve the prognosis in cancer; and supplementing standard cancer treatment with treatment of immortal pathogens could improve the outcomes in cancer. Knowledge immortal pathogens cause cancer can inform how to avoid cancer, and direct treatment of acute and chronic infections to prevent cancer. Replacing nutrition could fight cancer; and a good diet and fitness could avoid cancer triggers, by increasing the ability of the host to fight cancer.

In the South Valley, Dr. Merchant said water borne parasites were causing chronic disease and cancer. He said chronic infection and an increased infectious burden, plus time, plus low folic acid caused by chronic parasitic infection, caused cancer. Dr. Russell proved cancer tumors had microbes inside and outside of the tumor; and Dr. Warburg proved cancer cells had low oxygen and excess fermentation. Dr. Marshall proved ulcers were caused by H-pylori; and H-pylori is now a known cause of cancer. The thinking of many before and after our own confirmed our unwavering belief that intracellular pathogens are the cause of chronic diseases, including cancer.

Tools did not exist in 1864, 1890, 1910, 1920, 1931, and 1948, to identify intracellular animal pathogens causing chronic infection and cancer. Today many more scientists and thinkers are starting to believe and report cancer is caused by chronic infection. Cancer is the end-stage of the infectious cascade, and war between the pathogens and the immune system.

CHAPTER 13

CHRONIC INFECTION IN AUTOIMMUNE DISEASES

Rheumatologists treat arthritis and autoimmune diseases. Twenty-five-years ago scientists suggested arthritis was caused by an infection; and fifteen-years ago scientists recognized infection causes some types of arthritis. Rheumatologists are not interested in diagnosis and treatment of infectious causes of arthritis or autoimmune diseases. Rheumatologists prescribe anti-inflammatories, muscle relaxants, pain medications, steroids, and TNF-alpha inhibitors. TNF-alpha inhibitors are expensive and potentially harmful, because TNF-inhibitors potentiate the underlying immortal infection by interfering with the normal immune response of TNF-alpha, trigger pathogens to become a chronic disease, and cause serious complications.

Arthritis is a non-specific diagnosis of pain and stiffness in joints. Arthritis is considered an autoimmune disease; and like many other diseases, has been divided into multiple forms. Arthritis includes osteoarthritis, degenerative arthritis, rheumatoid arthritis, and inflammatory arthritis. Arthritis is caused by immortal pathogens that infect joint tissue, by direct migration or circulating immune cells, and deposit abnormal proteins and debris from the immune battle in the nearest joint. Infectious pathogens deposited in the joint cause reactive pain and inflammation. Arthritis refers to the symptom of joint pain, and patients are treated symptomatically, without diagnosis and treatment of the immortal pathogens causing arthritis. Symptomatic treatment will not cure arthritis, and increases the risk of death from other chronic diseases, such as heart attacks from anti-inflammatory medications; diabetes from steroids; and development of cancer and other chronic diseases, from TNF-inhibitors.

Autoimmune diseases are a category of diseases of "unknown origin". Purportedly the immune cells attack healthy cells and organs. Autoimmune diseases include lupus, fibromyalgia, chronic fatigue, and reduced immunity to infection. Autoimmune disease can cause inflammation anywhere in the body, and reduce immunity. Reduced immunity from intracellular infection of the immune cells, and the infectious cascade, cause secondary bacterial, viral, parasitic and yeast infections. Inflammation is the body's natural defense to infection, and a sign of an immune system battle to eradicate the pathogens and debris. When the immune cells are unable to eradicate the pathogen, an aggressive immune response, generating TNF-alpha, will cause greater inflammation, indicating a more significant and longstanding chronic infection.

Reduced immunity is caused when immortal pathogens infect the immune system, impairing and confusing the immune response. The immune system is not attacking healthy tissue, the immune system is responding to signals to attack intracellular pathogens. The immune system may attack or damage healthy tissue when the immune system is confused, or when TNF-alpha inflammation generated by the immune cells inadvertently damages adjacent cells. Chlamydia, parasites, the overall infectious burden, and the infectious cascade cause arthritis, lupus, fibromyalgia, chronic fatigue, and reduced immunity.

Arthritis and autoimmune disease have inflammation in the joints, can have reduced immunity, and have common and overlapping co-morbid conditions. Patients with "inflammatory diseases", such as rheumatoid arthritis and lupus (SLE), have a higher risk of atherosclerosis. Patients who have SLE are nearly four times more likely to have subclinical atherosclerosis. Patients with rheumatoid arthritis, psoriasis, and psoriatic arthritis have very high inflammatory markers, including high TNF-alpha. Chlamydia infection and the immune system generate TNF-alpha, to fight intracellular infection. Atherosclerosis is a co-morbid condition and well-established to be caused by immortal infections, and the co-morbid conditions known to be cause by immortal pathogens support arthritis and autoimmune diseases are also caused by immortal pathogens.

The specific pathogen(s) causing arthritis and autoimmune diseases have not yet been definitively identified, because arthritis and autoimmune disease can be caused by more than one pathogen. Science reports only an "association" between the disease and pathogens, and different scientists have found different pathogens in "association" with the arthritis and autoimmune diseases. Scientists look for one pathogen at a time in chronic disease, and do not ask what infectious pathogens are found in the patients with arthritis and autoimmune diseases, to confirm an infectious cause.

Historically, soldiers who took anti-malarial medicines noticed their rheumatoid arthritis and lupus symptoms improved. The effectiveness of anti-malaria drugs against rheumatoid arthritis and lupus supports the underlying cause of rheumatoid arthritis and lupus is an immortal bacteria and/or parasite, which can be treated with the medication used to treat malaria. Anti-parasitic drugs may be directed at one pathogen, and also kill other pathogens susceptible to the same type of medication. Antiparasitics drugs have been shown helpful in treating lupus; and lupus and rosacea can also be treated with doxycycline. The effectiveness of antiparasitics and antibiotics against both SLE and rosacea support these diseases are caused by chronic infection that is susceptible to treatment with antiparasitic drugs and appropriate antibiotics. Historical evidence of improvement in rheumatoid arthritis and lupus, by using anti-malarial medications, which are also effective against other parasites, may have provided a basis for Dr. Blount to believe a limax amoeba was a cause of rheumatoid arthritis.

In the 1930's, before antibiotics, when people got a urine infection, the urine infection progressed to arthritis, and then chronic fatigue. The progression from urine infection to arthritis and chronic fatigue is an example of an infectious pathogen that becomes chronic, and when untreated transforms into a chronic disease. Urine infections were the initiating cause of both arthritis and chronic fatigue. Acute urine infections can refer pain to the nearest joints, and cause pain in the knees or hips. When an acute urine infection ascends to the kidney, it can refer pain to the back.

Dr. Blount and Dr. di Fabio said arthritis, multiple sclerosis, and brain diseases are caused by an infection. Dr. Blount tried to tell the medical community rheumatoid arthritis and many other chronic diseases were caused by a limax amoeba; and was persecuted for his opinions, despite his experience in curing himself and thousands of patients. In Rheumatoid Diseases: Cured at Last, 1982, the authors reported the limax amoeba had been found in tissue in over one-hundred different diseases. In the second edition of Rheumatoid Diseases: Cured at Last, 2017, Dr. di Fabio reports other infectious pathogens are also now recognized to cause arthritis and chronic disease, meaning more than one pathogen can cause the same disease. Whether Dr. Blount cured arthritis by treating amoebas; cured other types of parasites; or cured immortal infections such as trachoma, psittacosis, and toxoplasmosis, which can cause arthritis, by using an anti-parasitic drug that treats amoebas and also treats these immortal pathogens, cannot be determined. Dr. Merchant saw patients with positive rheumatoid factor, whose rheumatoid factor turned negative; and complaints of fatigue, myalgia and joint pain improved, with treatment with azithromycin or clarithromycin.

Scientists have long suggested the connection between arthritis and sexually transmitted diseases, meaning primarily chlamydia trachoma. Chlamydia trachoma has been "associated" with rheumatoid arthritis, and debris from chlamydia trachoma has been found in arthritic joints.[229] *Chlamydia Pneumonia* Infection and Disease, Ch. 16, reports the chlamydia trachoma found in arthritic joints was both viable and metabolically active in the joint.[230] Some have suggested ocular trachoma is even more likely to cause arthritis.[231]

---

[229] Friedman H (*ed*), *et al.* 2004. Chlamydia Pneumonia Infection and Disease. New York: Kluwer Academic/Plenum Publishers. Chlamydia Pneumonia as a Candidate Pathogen in Multiple Sclerosis. (Stratton CW and Siram S). Ch. 14. p. 230.

[230] Friedman H (*ed*), *et al.* 2004. Chlamydia Pneumonia Infection and Disease. New York: Kluwer Academic/Plenum Publishers. Chlamydia Pneumonia and Inflammatory Arthritis. (Whittum-Hudson J, *et al*). Ch. 16.

[231] Gerard H, *et al.* 2010. Patients with *Chlamydia*-Associated Arthritis Have Ocular (Trachoma), Not Genital, Serovars of C-Trachomatis In Synovial Tissue. Microb Pathog. Feb 2010. 48(2):62. Doi: https://doi.org/10.1016/j.micpath.2009.11.004.

Chlamydia pneumonia was also found in arthritic joints, but at a lower rate than chlamydia trachoma.[232] Studies showed chlamydia pneumonia elicits an inflammatory reaction, and inflammation of the synovial fluid, in the joint, causing reactive arthritis. Researchers have identified both chlamydia pneumonia and chlamydia trachoma in fluid from an arthritic knee; and scientists have suggested chlamydia psittacosis is a cause of temporomandibular joint pain and disease (TMD). Some studies identified other immortal pathogens, including mycoplasma and pseudomonas, in arthritic joints; and feline mycoplasma was reported to cause sudden onset arthritis. Rheumatoid arthritis is caused by chronic chlamydia pneumonia, chlamydia trachoma, or chlamydia psittacosis infection; and can also be caused by other immortal pathogens, mycoplasma, feline mycoplasma, and hospital acquired pathogens.

Chlamydia pneumonia and chlamydia trachoma were reported as the cause of undifferentiated spondylo-arthritis (arthritis in the spine).[233] Seventy patients with either reactive arthritis or undifferentiated oligoarthritis were studied. During the study, three had symptomatic upper respiratory infections; and five developed acute reactive arthritis, after infection with chlamydia pneumonia. In these patients, specific lymphocyte proliferation, in the white blood cells, in the synovial fluid, and high specific antibody titers, suggested an acute infection with chlamydia caused the arthritis.[234]

Researchers found chlamydia pneumonia DNA in muscles and joints, spread by monocytes, macrophages and mast cells. The immune cells attack the pathogen and the immortal pathogen infects immune cells, impairing the immune system and allowing the pathogen to spread and become an autoimmune disease. Chlamydia also spreads in the smooth muscles, and the immune system and smooth muscles spread the chronic infection in soft tissue throughout the body, causing widespread pain and fatigue.

---

[232] Friedman H (*ed*), et al. 2004. <u>Chlamydia Pneumonia Infection and Disease</u>. New York: Kluwer Academic/Plenum Publishers. Chlamydia Pneumonia and Inflammatory Arthritis. (Whittum-Hudson JA, et al). Ch. 16. p. 32.

[233] Carter J, *et al*. 2009. Chlamydiae as Ethologic Agents in Chronic Undifferentiated Spondyloarthritis. Arthritis Rheum. May 2009. 60(5):1311-6. Doi: 10.1002/art.24431.

[234] *Id.*

The temporomandibular joint (TMJ) is a complicated joint. The TMJ is the only joint required to both rotate and translate. The TMJ is required for many ordinary activities of daily living, such as breathing, talking, eating, and swallowing. The TMJ is subject to stresses equal to or greater than a hip joint, and is used almost continuously. Temporomandibular joint disease (TMD) is pain and loss of range of motion in the TMJ.

The treatment of TMJ pain and TMD was relegated to dentists and oral surgeons, rather than medical doctors trained in infectious disease, or rheumatologists trained in arthritis. Dentists are not trained in infectious causes of arthritis, or trained and licensed to diagnose and treat systemic immortal infections. Dentists and oral surgeons fail to diagnose infections in the head and neck, which can refer pain and cause TMJ pain. Dentists and oral surgeons treat TMJ with anti-inflammatories, pain medications, splints, braces, and TMJ surgery. TMJ implants were marketed as a way to solve TMJ pain and TMD; but did the opposite—TMJ surgery and TMJ implants were a downward spiral to more surgeries and universally failed, causing extreme pain, loss of range of motion in the TMJ, and morbidity. The TMJ is never a good place for surgery, or a medical implant, absent a catastrophic injury or cancer. Dentists and oral surgeons will never discover the cause of TMD—dentists and oral surgeons only treat TMJ/TMD, and do not diagnose pathogens that can cause joint pain or TMD.

Chlamydia psittacosis has been "associated" with TMJ pain and TMD; and some scientists believe chlamydia psittacosis is the cause of TMD. Psittacosis can inhabit the lymphatics and the immune cells in the lymphatics, and move from the lymphatics to the TMJ. The infection and its byproducts invade the TMJ joint, deposit debris from the infection and the immune battle, and cause inflammation and damage to the joint and cartilage. TMJ pain is more frequently diagnosed in women; and women are more likely to be exposed to psittacosis through ownership and interaction with pet cats and pet birds, and have exposure to psittacosis through gardening. TMJ patients are known to have a multitude of co-morbid conditions, caused by the same underlying immortal pathogens causing the TMJ pain; and psittacosis is not likely to be the only pathogen which can cause TMJ.

TMJ sufferers formed the TMJ Association, a centralized advocacy and support group seeking "a cure" for TMD. The TMJ Association holds conferences, engages in advocacy, and solicits funds for research. Carolyn tried for years to convince the TMJ Association to direct research toward infections, co-infections, and co-morbid conditions, but no one wanted to change the direction of the research. TMJ pain and TMD is the same as pain and degeneration as occurs in any other arthritic joint, but for it occurs in a complicated and frequently used joint that sustains a high level of stress. The TMJ should be treated like any other arthritic condition—diagnose and treat the underlying infections, which are causing inflammation and pain, in the TMJ.

Small misalignments in the spine or joints can cause pain, even if the misalignments are dismissed or too small to be noticed by doctors on x-rays or scans. Shoes with high heels worn over a lifetime can cause degeneration of the foot, knee and hip; and all too often, later in life, cause patients to submit to surgery for hip and knee replacements. Patients with co-morbid cardiovascular disease are at risk of emboli following hip implant surgery. Wear shoes that avoid joint degeneration later in life. Avoid injuries to joints that haunt us later in life. Don't make joints a weak link, and a target of chronic infection.

Chronic disease in vital organs adjacent to the skeletal system can refer or radiate pain to the back. How and where the patient puts a hand or hands to describe the pain, often corresponds to the organ causing the pain. Conditions such as blocked arteries, cardiovascular events, stomach pain, gastrointestinal disease, gallbladder disease, liver disease, pancreatic disease, kidney stones, kidney infection, urinary tract infection, etc., can all cause back pain. Any and all of these medical conditions are reported as co-morbid conditions in arthritis patients, because these chronic diseases originate from the same infectious causes as the arthritis. Back pain from arthritic conditions and back pain from chronic disease in vital organs must be distinguished, for diagnosis and formulating a treatment plan.

The usual symptomatic treatments of arthritis, by rheumatologists, are steroids, or a non-steroidal anti-inflammatory (NSAID), to reduce inflammation. Steroids are sometimes injected directly into the joint. Steroid drugs suppress the immune system; and eventually cause a worsening of the chronic disease, by weakening the immune system and potentiating the underlying immortal infections. Steroids accelerate degeneration of the joint, increase blood sugar, and can trigger or worsen diabetes. Chronic use of steroids causes muscle wasting, atherosclerosis, diabetes, osteoporosis, cataracts, weight gain, and can worsen degeneration of the arthritic joint. Joint injections with steroids, and joint implants, lead to a downward spiral of joint degeneration, surgery, worsening pain, and in some cases chronic infection in the implant.

NSAID drugs increase the patient's risk of developing a chronic disease and death. An NSAID can cause joint degeneration, destruction of cartilage, cardiac events and kidney damage. A meta-analysis of thirty-one studies, covering 116,000 patients, found significant risk of cardiovascular events among patients who take non-steroidal anti-inflammatories. A study of patients taking celecoxib and Diclofenac, compared to a placebo, showed a four times greater risk of cardiac death in patients taking NSAID drugs. When last checked, Google had 941,000 citations for rofecoxib side effects; and 2,860,000 citations for Ibuprofen side effects. NSAIDs can cause gastric bleeding; kidney failure; severe allergic reactions; depression; mood changes; sudden or unexplained weight gain; and diabetes. The NSAIDs cause edema (swelling), which the patient and doctor then assume is from arthritis, then more NSAIDs are prescribed, creating a vicious cycle of worsening inflammation from infection and higher doses of NSAIDs. If a patient drinks alcohol while taking an NSAID, the alcohol increases the risk of kidney damage from an NSAID; and many patients are unaware of the risk of drinking alcohol when taking an NSAID.

In autoimmune disease, chlamydia, H-pylori, and other pathogens and parasites have become chronic and widespread, and damaged epithelial and endothelial function throughout the body. Autoimmune disease is often caused by co-infections with immortal pathogens, parasites and viruses. Chlamydia hosts other bacterial and viral pathogens; and can hide inside parasites, inclusion cysts, and spongy tissue, throughout the body. Wherever chlamydia or its infectious byproducts hide is another target for immune system attack, and confusion by the immune system in what cells to attack.

Autoimmune disease is the immune cells attacking intracellular infection and the abnormal byproducts of the infection. Specific types of immune cells are programmed to attack specific types of infections, and the immune system works on pattern recognition. Chlamydia and H-pylori infect the immune cells targeting the infection and can replicate in immune cells, and immune cells can further spread the pathogen in the body. Infected immune cells are altered in size and shape by the pathogen, and have impaired immune response, causing reduced immunity and vulnerability to new acute infections.

When the patient has unexplained reduced immunity and inflammation, the medical community assumes the professional immune cells are attacking normal organs and tissue, joints, the brain, and other organs. The immune system is not attacking healthy tissue, the immune system is attacking the immortal intracellular infection, abnormal proteins, and infectious byproducts. The immune system attack causes inflammation in the tissue, and failure to eradicate the infection causes a more aggressive immune system attack and greater inflammation.

In autoimmune disease, the chronic infection has spread to host cells throughout the body, including the immune cells and smooth muscles. Chlamydia pneumonia spreads through the blood vessels, smooth muscles, and immune cells, causing endothelial dysfunction. As the infection proliferates, more host tissue and professional immune cells become infected, and more and more cells are robbed of the ATP energy and the oxygen necessary to function and to thrive. The intracellular chlamydia depletes the energy in the cell, and causes fermentation of sugar. Endothelial function becomes impaired, and the endothelium cannot keep the tissue properly hydrated, causing both dehydration and edema. The impaired immune system can become confused by the abnormal protein shapes on the surface of pathogens and intracellular infection in the immune cells, and molecular mimicry can cause a mistake in which cells to attack. The immune battle causes inflammation, and failure to eradicate the pathogen causes the immune system to release TNF-alpha, causing a greater degree of inflammation. A high level of inflammation can cause collateral damage in healthy adjacent tissue. The patient develops pain and fatigue, as a greater number of cells become infected, a greater number of cells are deprived of the energy and oxygen necessary to make the cell function, and endothelial function is more widespread. Autoimmune diseases have been successfully treated with antibiotic and antiparasitic medications.

In autoimmune disease, the pathogen and the immune system battle generate new infectious elementary bodies; and disperse abnormal proteins and byproducts, such as fragments of cells, nucleus, and plasmids, that trigger an immune response, wherever deposited. Abnormal proteins attached to or generated by the pathogen and the immune battle cannot be killed, are sticky, and get stuck in tissue, which impairs passive function, damages feedback loops that regulate bodily functions, and may be another source of pain. The immune system may mount an exaggerated white blood cell attack, with TNF-alpha, against the abnormal proteins, and flush the proteins into the lymphatics or encapsulate the infection with fibrous tissue. Abnormal proteins can become the focus for formation of inclusion cysts. Some refer to encapsulation of the abnormal protein or pathogen as a giant cell reaction, others as an inclusion cyst; and both giant cell reactions and inclusion cysts are common in autoimmune disease and in immortal intracellular infections.

Reiter's and Sjögren's syndromes are autoimmune diseases, which have overlapping symptoms. Reiter's syndrome is the combination of arthritis, conjunctivitis and urethritis; and is a subset of reactive arthritis. Sjögren's syndrome includes swollen glands in the neck, dry and irritated eyes, dry mouth and difficulty swallowing. Reiter's and Sjögren's patients have symptoms of arthritis, and dry red eyes. Chlamydia trachoma has long been "associated" with the development of Reiter's syndrome; and the role of chlamydia pneumonia was still being studied, in 2004.[235] The

---

[235] *Chlamydia Pneumonia* Infection and Disease. (Whittom-Hudson JA *et al.*). Ch. 16. p. 228-229.

commonality in these diseases suggests common underlying pathogens, such as chlamydia trachoma, psittacosis, pneumonia, and/or parasites, cause the autoimmune syndromes.

An Italian study found patients with Sjögren's syndrome, parotid gland marginal zone B-cell lymphoma, and MALT lymphoma, had a high rate of chlamydia psittacosis.[236] *All* of the psittacosis patients were rheumatoid factor positive; suggesting a strong correlation between psittacosis and autoimmune disease. Italy has also an unusually high rate of rare cancers, including eye cancer; a high rate of lymphoma; and an increasing rate of melanoma, which have all been "associated" with chlamydia psittacosis.

Rheumatologists treat Reiter's and Sjögren's syndromes symptomatically, which suppresses the immune system, and potentiates the infection. The long-term outlook for patients with Sjögren's who are treated with immuno-suppressant drugs is an increased risk of lymphomas and B-cells cancers, caused by the same pathogens that cause Reiter's and Sjögren's syndromes; and the same pathogens that cause lymphoma. Chlamydia induced reactive arthritis has been identified as a co-morbid condition in Sjögren's syndrome.[237] B-cell lymphoma can mimic multiple myeloma. B-cells mature into plasma cells, which are the cells involved in multiple myeloma; thus, infected B-cells can become plasma cells, infected with the same intracellular pathogen causing cancer. In a meta-analysis, high level of neutrophils, and a high ratio of neutrophils to lymphocytes are a prognostic sign for B-cell lymphoma,[238] further supporting psittacosis and H-pylori as a cause of the cancer, because both psittacosis and H-pylori are attacked by and infect neutrophils, and change the shape of the neutrophils to resemble cancer. H-pylori may be synergistic in lymphoma, by allowing

---

[236] Fabris M, *et al*. 2014. High Prevalence of Chlamyophila Psittaci Subclinical Infection in Italian Patients with Sjogren's Syndrome, Parotid Gland Marginal Zone B-Cell Lymphoma, and MALT Lymphoma. PMID: 2447326.

[237] Chang H, *et al*. 2008. Korean J Intern Med. Concurrence of Sjögren's Syndrome in a Patient with Chlamydia-induced Reactive Arthritis; An Unusual Finding. June 2008. 21(2): 116-119. Doi: 10.3904/kjim.2006.21.2.116.

[238] Wang J, *et al*. 2017. Prognostic Significance of Neutrophil-to-Lymphocyte Ratio in Diffuse Large B-cell Lymphoma: A meta-analysis. PLoS One. Apr 25, 2017;12(4):e0176008. Doi: 10.1371/journal.pone.0176008. eCollection 2017.

other pathogens to invade deeper into tissue, attacking epithelium, and changing the shape of neutrophils. Chlamydia trachoma and chlamydia psittacosis both likely cause Reiter's and Sjögren's syndrome.

Lupus is considered an autoimmune disease, which does not have a known cause. Lupus is defined by symptoms, and a positive ANA blood test showing antibodies to nuclear material. The symptoms of lupus overlap with rheumatoid arthritis (RA), Sjögren's, scleroderma, fibromyalgia and Raynaud's. Lupus patients have a butterfly rash on their face, similar to rosacea. Lupus can damage the immune system, brain, nerves and blood vessels in the eyes, and the nervous system, lung, kidney, joints, and skin. Lupus can cause mouth sores, light sensitivity, fatigue and fevers; and exacerbate ulcerative colitis, pancreatitis, and liver conditions, resulting in nausea, vomiting, recurring and persistent abdominal pain, bladder infections, and blood in the urine. Lupus can cause swelling in the joints, legs, hands and feet; and fingers and toes may turn white or blue, consistent with Raynaud's phenomenon. Symptoms of lupus may also be different in women and men. The overlapping and co-morbid conditions, symptoms, and phenomenon of lupus, and the fact lupus may have a sudden onset or a slow progression, and may be temporary or permanent, strongly support an infectious cause and common infectious causes, in all of these autoimmune diseases of unknown origin.

One study compared fifty lupus patients with fifty normal control patients, and found toxoplasmosis antibodies were significantly more common in lupus patients. The lupus patients also had particularly high titers of toxoplasmosis. The authors of the study advised doctors not to ignore toxoplasmosis infection in lupus patients.[239] Cats and dogs owned by lupus patients are also at higher risk of developing lupus, again supporting an infectious cause of lupus.[240]

---

[239] Wilcox M, *et al*. 1990. Toxoplasmosis and Systemic Lupus Erythemmatosus. Ann Rheum Dis. Apr 1990. 49: 254-257. Doi: https://www.ncbi.nlm.nih.gov/pmc/articles/PMC1004049/.

[240] Chiou SH, *et al*. 2004. Pet Dogs Owned by Lupus Patients Are at Higher Risk of Developing Lupus. 2004. 13(6):442-9. Doi: 10.1191/0961203303lu1039oa.

Lupus causes kidney damage, in approximately fifty percent of patients and is called "lupus nephritis", describing an inflamed kidney in a patient with lupus. Trachoma causes urethritis in Reiter's syndrome, which supports the role of chlamydia trachoma in lupus. Trachoma can ascend the urinary tract and damage the kidney. Lupus nephritis may be caused by pathogens in the urinary or the reproductive tract; which are capable of ascending the urinary tract to damage the kidney. The pathogens may be transmitted or migrate to the urinary tract and to the kidney, from the gastrointestinal tract or reproductive tract. When the pathogens ascend upwards to the kidney, the infection and abnormal proteins cause inflammation, clog filtration in the kidney, damage the kidney, cause blood in the urine, and can cause kidney failure. The difference between lupus, and lupus with kidney failure, is that the underlying infections or co-infections have ascended from the urinary tract to the kidney; or the immortal pathogens have directly attacked the kidney.

When a pathogen is found, in lupus, the assumption is the cause was not found, because the pathogens found are not consistent across all lupus patients. Doctors need to look for all of the pathogens capable of causing autoimmune disease, alone or in combination, not search for one at a time. Finding all the causes begins with routine laboratory testing for immortal pathogens, in autoimmune disease patients.

Antibiotics and antiparasitics have been used to treat lupus; and to treat rheumatoid arthritis, juvenile arthritis, rosacea, and autoimmune diseases. The success of treatment with antibiotics and anti-parasitics, suggest the pathogens causing lupus are susceptible to treatment with antibiotics or antiparasitics; and the pathogens and parasites causing lupus, and the combination of pathogens, may differ in different patients. Lupus is most likely caused by chlamydia, probably chlamydia trachoma or chlamydia psittacosis; parasites, including toxoplasmosis; and may be caused by more than one pathogen or combination of these pathogens. Lupus may occur due to a combination of co-infections, and particularly when the co-infections include toxoplasmosis.

Streptococcus-M is another pathogen capable of causing kidney damage in lupus patients. Lupus nephritis and multiple myeloma are co-morbid conditions. Multiple myeloma is likely caused by mycoplasma or streptococcus type-M, because mycoplasma and streptococcus-M are the only bacteria that have M-proteins on the surface of the pathogen, and M-proteins define the diagnosis of multiple myelomas. Henoch-Schoenlein Purpura (HSP) and glomerulonephritis are kidney damage and kidney failure, known to be caused by streptococcus type-M. Streptococcus type-M may play a role in causing lupus nephritis and multiple myeloma, independently; or as a co-infection with chlamydia trachoma, chlamydia psittacosis, and/or parasites. Doctors do not routinely investigate infectious pathogens causing lupus, or lupus nephritis; consider a pathogen and/or a parasite when diagnosing lupus; or consider a second separate streptococcal or chlamydia trachoma infection, in lupus nephritis.

HSP is an autoimmune disease, and the syndrome can be confused with lupus.[241] HSP was named after Dr. Edward Henoch, and his teacher Dr. Johann Schoenlein, in the 1860's, before science had the ability to diagnose pathogens. Previous doctors described HSP, in 1802, and 1808; however, the prior name "Heberden-Willan Disease" is no longer used. Dr. Schoenlein "associated" HSP with skin manifestations, arthritis, and gastrointestinal involvement. Dr. Henoch and Dr. Schoenlein described the symptoms of HSP; and both wanted credit for describing the syndrome causing kidney damage. In 1914, William Osler, MD, proposed an allergic mechanism for HSP.

HSP is also called IgA vasculitis, anaphylactoid purpura, and purpura rheumatic, which all describe inflammation in the kidneys, vessels, skin and joints. The symptoms of HSP include nephropathy and glomerulonephritis, meaning a swollen and inflamed kidney. In HSP, the kidney filtering system becomes inflamed, and abnormal proteins become stuck in the kidney. HSP may cause a skin rash, pain in the abdomen, joint inflammation, and systemic vasculitis (inflammation of the blood vessels); and causes M-proteins and blood in the urine. Streptococcus and

---

[241] Wikipedia. Henoch-Schoenlein Purpura. Doi: en.wikipedia.org/wiki/Henoch%E2%80%93Sch%C3%B6nlein_purpura.

mycoplasma are the only pathogens which have M-proteins on the surface. HSP is known to develop after infections with streptococci (β-hemolytic, Lancefield group A), hepatitis B, herpes simplex virus, parvovirus B19, Coxsackie virus, adenovirus, H-pylori, measles, mumps, rubella, mycoplasma and numerous other pathogens. Any vasculitis can also be caused by chlamydia.

HSP has the same symptoms as another well-known kidney disease— post-streptococcal glomerulonephritis, which is known to be caused by streptococcus-M. In post-streptococcal glomerulonephritis, antibody complexes containing immunoglobulin-A are found in the blood vessels. The pathogen causing HSP and post-streptococcal glomerulonephritis is streptococcus type-M. Streptococcus type-M, acquired as an acute urine infection, can migrate upwards to the kidney and cause kidney inflammation, systemic inflammation of the blood vessels, and high levels of M-proteins in the urine. Nephrologists fail to consider infectious causes of HSP; or the fact the same symptoms arise in HSP and post-streptococcal glomerulonephritis. Lupus nephritis, HSP, and acute glomerulonephritis have similar or identical symptoms.

A teenage acquaintance developed a kidney disease, after a summer traveling in Europe. During the trip, the mother and father reported getting a horrible sore throat, but did not report whether the teenager also got the sore throat, or if any of them sought treatment. Shortly thereafter, while in Turkey, she and her mother spent the day in the hotel swimming pool. When the family returned home, the child was taken to the hospital on more than one occasion, and diagnosed with HSP. A "pediatric nephrology specialist" did extensive and invasive medical procedures, including a kidney biopsy, on a child with a history of spending a day in the hotel swimming pool, in Turkey; and likely had a history of a severe sore throat prior to the development of the HSP. The specialist did not consider or try to diagnose an infectious cause of HSP. Once the triad of symptoms named HSP was identified; further diagnostic efforts to find infectious pathogens and treat the pathogens were not pursued. The mother thereafter developed "kidney stones", for the first time in her life; which likely arose from the same pathogen. The most likely pathogen causing the HSP and the new onset of a kidney stone was streptococcus-M, based on the circumstances just prior to the onset of the disease.

Turkey has more than eighty different serovars of streptococcus, some of which invade the urine, migrate up the urinary tract, and cause chronic kidney infections, kidney stones, kidney inflammation, glomerulonephritis, and kidney failure. Streptococcus-M is endemic in Turkey, and is known to cause heart valve damage, kidney damage, and glomerulonephritis; and to generate abnormal M-proteins in the urine. Streptococcus-M is also a likely cause of Bechet's disease, a blistering skin condition, first identified in Turkey. Streptococcus type-M throws off abnormal proteins that damage the kidney, just as streptococcus type-M damages the heart; and causes blood and M-proteins in the urine. Knowledge of pathogens in an endemic area and in a foreign country, knowledge of which pathogens have M-proteins attached, knowledge of the effect of streptococcus-M on the kidney, and the fact HSP is diagnosed by M-proteins in the urine, support an infectious cause, and the infectious cause is likely streptococcus type-M.

Lupus, HSP, and glomerulonephritis are all caused by infectious pathogens, and deposits of abnormal M-proteins. The distinction is likely based on the specialty and interest of the doctor diagnosing the disease. Modern technology, including PCR testing and high-throughput sequencing, is needed to identify the infectious causes of HSP, lupus, and many autoimmune diseases.

Fibromyalgia is widespread pain with chronic fatigue. Fibromyalgia is an "inflammatory" process in the muscles, joints, bowel, and brain. Inflammation, pain, depression, and fatigue are the definition of fibromyalgia; and are also the hallmarks of a chronic intracellular infection. Fibromyalgia is caused by multiple chronic infections, spread to cells and smooth muscles throughout the body, causing widespread endothelial dysfunction, impairment of cell function, and pain. Patients with fibromyalgia have co-morbid conditions of arthritis, sleep and mood disturbances, recurrent infections, imbalance in hormones, and malabsorption of nutrients, caused by the same pathogens causing fibromyalgia. Co-infections may cause fibromyalgia, based on the impact on diverse organs and systems.

Fibromyalgia can be caused by chlamydia pneumonia; and may also be caused by chlamydia trachoma, and/or chlamydia psittacosis, independently or as co-infections. Patients with fibromyalgia and chronic fatigue have higher PCR levels of chlamydia pneumonia. The high PCR levels confirm the cells are not getting sufficient energy or oxygen on a cell-by-cell basis. Chlamydia pneumonia attacks the endothelium and smooth muscle and spreads through smooth muscle; and causes increased cytokines and TNF-alpha, markers of inflammation. Chlamydia trachoma, chlamydia psittacosis, and H-pylori can attack epithelium and endothelium, and get into the central nervous system and attack nerve sheaths and nerves. Chlamydia and the immune battle against the pathogen cause inflammation, and generate byproducts that impair passive function. The immune system attacks the infection wherever the chronic infection or its byproducts are found, and causes inflammation in the muscle fiber layers and adjacent tissue and in the central nervous system.

Fibromyalgia has been hypothesized by others to be caused by infection, injury, or stress. Fibromyalgia has been described as nerve cells sending messages of pain, and/or as the failure of the mitochondrial cells to make the energy necessary. The fibromyalgia website and Dr. Teitelbaum suggest when cells do not work effectively to meet the energy demands of the cells and carry out cellular activity, it causes an inflammatory response, which researchers confirmed is especially true in muscle cells. The description of the nerve cells sending pain messages suggests damages to the nerve sheaths, by a pathogen that attacks the epithelium, similar to development of demyelinating diseases caused by chlamydia and H-pylori. Chlamydia pneumonia attacks endothelium and smooth muscle cells, causing dehydration of tissue from loss of the endothelial pump. Chlamydia takes over the cell function, deplete cell energy, causes loss of oxygen in the cells, and triggers an inflammatory reaction. Chlamydia causes what others described as "mitochondrial dysfunction", and chlamydia causes the same molecular changes postulated by Dr. Teitelbaum as the cause of fibromyalgia.

Fibromyalgia has recently been sub-divided into another sub-category, named small nerve peripheral neuropathy. Small nerve peripheral neuropathy is a description of pain caused by the pathogen(s), not an independent diagnosis or a separate disease. If fibromyalgia damages small nerves, it is similar or the same as other central nervous system diseases like multiple sclerosis, Parkinson's, and Alzheimer's; but is occurring in the peripheral nerves rather than in the central nervous system. In "peripheral small nerve neuropathy" the chlamydia pathogens have attacked the outer nerve sheath in the small peripheral nerves, causing pain. An Israeli study showed hyperbaric oxygen caused a seventy percent reduction in symptoms of fibromyalgia[242], which supports depletion of oxygen in the cell by chlamydia as a cause of fibromyalgia. Dr. Merchant used hyperbaric oxygen as one treatment for fibromyalgia.

Chronic fatigue has been called autoimmune, rheumatologic, orthopedic, and an internal medical problem of unknown origin. Chronic fatigue is not a diagnosis—it is a description of a symptom, which occurs in virtually *all* chronic diseases. Chronic fatigue patients suffer chronic inflammation; and have dysbiosis, fungal infection and malabsorption of nutrients. Authors have noted a correlation and overlap between chronic fatigue and infectious disease, which to date has only been called a "coincidence". Chronic chlamydia depletes energy from the cells, and impairs oxygen from getting into the cells; and when it becomes widespread causes chronic fatigue.

The differential diagnosis in chronic fatigue includes polymyositis, polymyalgia rheumatic, rheumatoid arthritis, lupus, cancer, Lyme disease, and chronic hepatitis B or C. All of the diseases are caused by immortal pathogens; and the pathogens may manifest differently in different patients, or manifest differently at different points in the infectious cascade. Chronic fatigue is caused by multiple chronic infections with immortal bacteria, viruses, and parasites; and a high infectious burden.

---

[242] Efrati S, *et al.* 2015. Hyperbaric Oxygen Therapy Can Diminish Fibromyalgia Syndrome – Prospective Clinical Trial. PLOS One. May 26, 2015. Doi: doi. org/10.1371/journal.pone.0127012.

Dr. Merchant treated a patient with chronic fatigue, who had seen more than twenty doctors. Treatment with a macrolide resolved the chronic fatigue. He also treated a patient with chronic fatigue, who had high blood pressure, coronary artery disease, two prior strokes, chronic depression and chronic pain; and after treatment of immortal infections with macrolides, the chronic fatigue improved and stabilized.

TNF-alpha is one of the key inflammatory mediators used to diagnose autoimmune disease, and chlamydia is known to cause an increase in TNF-alpha. TNF-alpha is a cell-signaling cytokine expressed by white blood cells, to fight and destroy small tumors in the body. The immune cells fighting the chlamydia infection release TNF-alpha cytokines and interleukin cells, which cause inflammation and pain. When TNF-alpha is over-expressed, it drives inflammation, which can damage the lung, cartilage, bone, bowel, and nervous system tissue. TNF-alpha has been found in numerous chronic diseases caused by immortal chlamydia pathogens, which are defined by inflammation. High levels of TNF-alpha were found in the reproductive tract of patients with chlamydia trachoma; and in the cerebral spinal fluid in patients with autism. The chlamydia infection is causing the TNF-alpha and inflammation; and high levels of TNF-alpha are now recognized to exist in many different chronic diseases. The level of TNF-alpha may be determined by the type of chlamydia infection, the persistence and duration of the chronic infection, and the overall infectious burden. More virulent forms like psittacosis and trachoma may cause higher levels of TNF-alpha.

Any condition caused by an underlying intracellular infection will be adversely impacted by TNF-inhibitors. TNF-inhibitors reduce the clinical evidence of TNF-alpha, without treating the chronic infections that caused the increase in TNF-alpha; and allows the chronic infections to proliferate. TNF-alpha inhibitors interfere with the TNF-alpha immune defense, potentiate the underlying infection, and substantially increase the risk of secondary infections. TNF-alpha inhibitors inhibit the action of macrophages and their movement (chemotaxis) into areas where needed to fight infections. TNF-inhibitors may cause low white blood cell counts, leading to serious infection or bleeding. TNF-inhibitors destroy T and B cells, which results in leucopenia, a shortage of white blood cells; putting patients at risk for fatal infections, cancer and death.

Warnings for TNF-inhibitors include development of respiratory infection, tuberculosis, cancer, leukemia, lymphoma, and death. Complications include serious infections, septic arthritis, infected joint replacements, pneumocystis pneumonia, and tuberculosis. TNF-inhibitors can trigger pan-cytopenia, aplastic anemia, and aggravation of congestive heart failure. People given TNF-inhibitors develop new heart failure, worsening heart failure, new or worsening psoriasis, allergic reactions, lupus like syndrome, autoimmune hepatitis, liver failure, tuberculosis, bacterial sepsis, invasive fungal infections such as histoplasmosis, and death. TNF-inhibitors can trigger demyelinating disorders, multiple sclerosis, seizures, and optic neurosis; and increase the incidence of lymphoproliferative diseases, leukemia, and lymphoma. Use of a TNF-alpha inhibitor has been linked to a rare type of lymphoma. TNF-alpha inhibitors increase the risks of all malignancies and recurrence of cancer in patients with prior malignancies. TNF-inhibitors should not be used for arthritis, psoriatic arthritis, and autoimmune disease; and will potentiate the underlying immortal infection, by interfering with the immune system attack on the pathogen.

TNF-alpha inhibitors include Enbrel, Humira, and Remicade. Treatment with TNF-inhibitors cost a minimum of $18,000, per year; and can cost as much as $50,000, per year. The cost of treatment with macrolides and cyclines (doxycycline, tetracycline, minocycline), is less than $2,000 per year, including blood monitoring. The better way to attack arthritis and autoimmune disease is to attack the pathogens that are causing the promotion and expression of TNF-alpha and inflammation, and causing the arthritis.

Rheumatologists and endocrinologists refuse to acknowledge arthritis and autoimmune diseases are caused by chronic infection, and continue to treat patients symptomatically for inflammation, pain, and elevated TNF-alpha. The attack by the immune system causes inflammation, the inflammation can increase when the immune system generates TNF-alpha, and adjacent normal tissue can be damaged by the inflammation. The pathogens spread and deposit debris that interferes with passive function, and cause pain in joints and muscles. The immune system is impaired, and can be confused by intracellular infection, abnormal proteins, and molecular mimicry which cause the immune system to attack healthy tissue or damage adjacent tissue with inflammation from high TNF-alpha. The pathogens set in motion a cascade of inflammation, inclusion cysts, a more extensive and aggressive immune system attack, and ultimately autoimmune disease.

All chronic diseases are essentially autoimmune disease, because virtually all chronic disease arises from infectious pathogens, and the battle of the immune system against the pathogens. It is time to recognize inflammation—redness, heat, swelling and pain—is caused by chronic infection; and infection is causing the inflammation and pain, depletion of energy in the cell, and the autoimmune disease! The body does not attack itself—it attacks intracellular pathogens and debris from the intracellular pathogens. When the attack is unsuccessful, the immune system generates a higher level of inflammation with TNF-alpha, causing a worsening of the autoimmune disease, damage to adjacent cells, and a greater level of pain.

CHAPTER 14

CHRONIC INFECTION IN ENDOCRINE DISEASES

Endocrinologists treat endocrine diseases arising from the endocrine glands, which include the thyroid, pituitary, pancreas, adrenal, and reproductive glands. The endocrine glands work together to secrete hormones and send signals, to other endocrine glands and to organs, in a feedback loop, to help the body function and remain in balance. The endocrine glands are spongy and porous, and hospitable to infection with immortal chlamydia pathogens. Intracellular infections, and/or H-pylori and parasites, can damage and block the functioning of the endocrine glands, causing a deficiency or excess in hormone secretion and endocrine gland signals.

Diabetes occurs when the pancreas fails to produce sufficient insulin. The pancreas is a spongy and porous endocrine gland, which is attached to the gastrointestinal tract. Diabetes is an endocrine disease because it involves failure of an endocrine organ; an autoimmune disease because diabetes causes reduced immunity; and an inflammatory disease because diabetes causes inflammation. Medicine assumes diabetes is caused by the immune system attacking cells in the pancreas, causing loss of cell function, inflammation, and impairing the ability of the pancreas to produce sufficient insulin.

The characterization of diabetes as a chronic inflammatory disease or an autoimmune disease leads to the obvious question of what is causing the inflammation and impaired immunity—it's the immortal infection! The body attacks the intracellular infection which creates the inflammation; and the infected immune cells create reduced immunity and can mistakenly attack or damage healthy cells. When the immune system attack is not successful, the immune system generates TNF-alpha, a more potent inflammatory trigger. The infection and inflammation cause direct injury to cells, can damage adjacent cells, and causes damage to passive function. When the immune system attacks the pancreas, the immune system is attacking intracellular infections and/or parasites; and byproducts of the pathogens hiding in immune cells, inclusion cysts, and biofilm.

Chlamydia pathogens gain entry into the gastrointestinal tract from sinus drainage and lung mucous; and finds favorable host tissue along the gastrointestinal tract. Common parasites begin as an intestinal infection, and can migrate to the pancreas, gallbladder and liver, from the intestine. The organs along the gastrointestinal tract hide and protect pathogens from stomach acid. Pathogens and parasites and can cause damage and mechanical obstruction in the pancreas, biliary tract, and common bile duct; and immortal pathogens and parasites have been found in the pancreas, and in pancreatic cancer. H-pylori is another gastrointestinal pathogen which has recently been "associated" with pancreatic cancer. Immortal pathogens and parasites can migrate to the liver and gallbladder, providing a focus for immune system attack, stones, cysts, and organ damage.

Diabetic patients often develop a larger belly, or a wide-belly shape, consistent with dysbiosis, metabolic syndrome, and leaky gut syndrome. A large belly is almost synonymous with intestinal parasites, including giardia, cryptosporidiosis, and worms. Diabetic patients have reduced immunity, caused by pathogens infecting immune cells, excess sugar and altered pH; and are, thus, vulnerable to secondary parasitic disease, metabolic disease, and loss of nutrition. Parasites can migrate to the pancreas, and create blockages and damage function. Chronic parasitic infections can cause weight gain, and a craving for sugar, which can predispose the patient to diabetes.

Diabetes is caused by immortal infections, combinations of infections, and parasites, inhabiting the gastrointestinal tract. More than one pathogenic bacteria, parasite, and virus, alone or in combination, can cause or trigger diabetes, by more than one mechanism. Immortal pathogens attack the pancreas, and damage and weaken epithelial and/or endothelial cells, depending on the type of chlamydia. Chlamydia depletes the pancreatic cells of the ATP energy needed to function; and makes pancreatic cells less able to make insulin. Infectious byproducts create abnormal proteins and plasmids, and create inclusion cysts, which clog and impair functioning of the pancreas. Fungus develops from reduced oxygen in the cells and fermentation, caused by the cell consuming sugar. An increased pH makes the person more susceptible to urinary tract infection from intestinal pathogens and pathogens in the reproductive tract. Parasites can also migrate to the pancreas and block passive functions, and provide a focus for chronic disease. The medical establishment assumes infections follow diabetes; however, it is reasonable to consider whether diabetes follows infection. More than four-million references appear when searching Google for "chlamydia and diabetes".

Diabetes is a disease of excess sugar in blood and tissue. When the islet cells in the pancreas do not make insulin, as in juvenile diabetes; or does not make sufficient insulin, as in adult-onset diabetes, the body cannot rid itself of excess sugar in blood and tissue. When the cells in the pancreas are weakened by intracellular infection, it is difficult for the pancreas to produce insulin. Chlamydia reverses the energy charge in the cell, needed to move sugar across the cell membrane and into the cell. The sugar stays in the bloodstream and interstitial spaces instead of supplying energy to the cells. The chlamydia pathogen consumes sugar, when ATP is depleted, causing fermentation; damages the cell wall and reverses the energy charge, making the cells less able to bring sugar into the cell; and leaving excess sugar in the bloodstream and interstitial spaces.

Diabetes has been divided into different forms, depending on the age of onset and manner in which the pancreas fails. Type-1 diabetes is juvenile diabetes, which develops in childhood. Juvenile diabetes is considered an autoimmune disease, in which the immune system attacks the islet cells in the pancreas, and the islet cells can no longer make sufficient insulin. Juvenile diabetes is known to develop after a severe acute infection. It requires an inquiring doctor to discover the acute infection that preceded the development of juvenile diabetes, and prior infections with immortal bacteria and parasites, as the inciting event triggering juvenile diabetes. The child who develops juvenile diabetes may already have a weakened immune system, damaged by chronic immortal infection. The reduced immunity and co-infections with immortal pathogens allows chlamydia and viral infections to trigger juvenile diabetes; particularly in a patient who has a genetic predisposition. Children with juvenile diabetes have co-morbid conditions, including juvenile rheumatoid arthritis, suggesting chlamydia pathogens capable of causing rheumatoid arthritis are also a cause of juvenile diabetes; and chlamydia pathogens are also causing the co-morbid conditions.

The scientific literature postulated juvenile diabetes is caused by a viral infection, of an enterovirus type. An enterovirus cannot be the entire explanation, because not every child who gets an enterovirus develops juvenile diabetes. Another scientific article postulates Coxsackie virus B3, in juvenile diabetes. Many people get the Coxsackie viruses; and yet, not all patients with Coxsackie virus B3 get diabetes. Some postulate a rotavirus, cytomegaly virus, mumps, or rubella are triggering events for diabetes; yet, not every child who gets these viruses develops juvenile diabetes. The enterovirus, or the Coxsackie virus B3, may attach to the intracellular pathogens and/or parasites, allowing the pathogen access to the pancreas; and work as co-infections to damage the pancreas and cause juvenile diabetes. The child may have acute co-infections, with more than one virus, chlamydia or mycoplasma and a virus, two immortal bacterial infections; or chlamydia and parasites; and acute co-infections trigger diabetes.

Type-2 diabetes develops in adults, and is also known as adult-onset diabetes. Type-2 diabetes results from the failure of the pancreatic cells to produce sufficient insulin, and failure of individual cells in the body to bring sugar across the cell wall and into the cells. Type-2 diabetes is consistent with intracellular chlamydia infection, which deprives the pancreatic cells of energy to make insulin, and deprives the cells in the body of energy and oxygen, and the ability to bring sugar into the cell. Adult onset diabetes is caused by a long-term chronic infection, with organisms that cause endothelial dysfunction and inflammation in the pancreas, consistent with the known effects of chlamydia pneumonia. In mice, acute chlamydia infection has been shown to cause the development of diabetes, and accelerate insulin resistance. Acute infection in an adult diabetic patient triggers a need for more insulin to control sugar.

Juvenile and adult onset diabetic patients have multiple chronic infections, and a high infectious burden. Diabetic patients have many co-morbid conditions, including cardiovascular disease, recurrent urinary tract infections, and kidney disease. Diabetic patients are at higher risk for heart attack, stroke, and Alzheimer's disease. Cardiovascular disease and stroke are caused by chlamydia pneumonia, which damages the endothelium in the cardiovascular system and creates plaque in the vessels. Chlamydia causes angiogenesis, the formation of new blood vessels; and in the eye, diabetics develop new blood vessels on the retina, which are fragile and bleed easily. H-pylori has been implicated as a pathogen "associated" with cardiovascular disease, which is present in the gastrointestinal tract and has been "associated" with pancreatic cancer. The co-morbid conditions of diabetes, kidney disease, cardiovascular disease, and Alzheimer's, are all caused by the same pathogens and the same parasites. Diabetic patients may have the same infections or combinations of infections, or different infections and different combinations of infection, in different patients.

Diabetics have a higher risk of cancer, including cancer of the pancreas, liver, breast, colon, rectum, bladder, and female reproductive tract. All of these organs are susceptible to invasion by immortal pathogens from the intestine, and breast cancer is susceptible to pathogens in the lymphatic system and immune system. Sugar feeds cancer; thus, high sugar caused by diabetes can feed cancer. The same pathogens causing diabetes can cause cancer, when the infectious cascade is longstanding and the infectious burden is high. Metformin is used to lower blood sugar in diabetics; and in Europe, Metformin has been used to fight cancer. Cancer is caused by immortal pathogens, which feed on sugar after depleting the ATP in the cells, and depriving cancer of sugar may be one method to interrupt the development of cancer.

Some propose sub-dividing diabetes into a third form of the disease. Diabetes type-3 is alleged to be caused by a defective gene, APOE 4, which interprets how the brain processes beta-amyloid, an Alzheimer's plaque. In other words, diabetes causes a change in epigenetic signals, preventing the body from clearing beta amyloid in the brain, causing Alzheimer's disease. Chronic intracellular infection can alter genes and gene expression, and the abnormal gene can be inherited from a parent. The APOE 4 gene may be a marker suggesting a diabetic patient will develop Alzheimer's disease; but the gene marker "associated" with diabetes and Alzheimer's is caused by immortal infection or was inherited from a parent with the same immortal infection.

Chlamydia pneumonia in the brain damages endothelium in the vessels and brain, and reduces the ability of the body to remove plaque from the brain. Diabetics are at higher risk for Alzheimer's disease, cardiovascular disease, and kidney disease, because all are caused by the same pathogens or combination of pathogens. Alzheimer's disease is caused by chlamydia pneumonia; and Alzheimer's disease is a well-known co-morbid condition with diabetes. Diabetes type-3 is not a new or independent disease, and merely describes a condition in which the chlamydia pneumonia has proliferated and invaded the brain through the cardiovascular system, damaged endothelium, and formed Alzheimer's plaque in a diabetic patient.

Diabetics often have or develop co-morbid kidney disease. Urinary tract infections are caused by cross contamination from the gastrointestinal tract, when the pH of the urine has been increased, by excess sugar and fermentation; and/or an impairment of the ability of the kidney to lower the pH of the urine. The pH of the urine must be lower than the pH in the intestinal tract, to prevent gastrointestinal pathogens from infecting the urinary tract. The kidney converts the pH in the urine from 7.4 to 6.0, so that intestinal pathogens cannot survive in the urine. A chronic chlamydia infection in diabetics can increase the pH through sugar and fermentation; or infection with chlamydia or other pathogens can cause kidney damage, making the kidney less effective in lowering the urine pH. Pathogens in the urinary tract have the potential to ascend upwards to the kidneys, damaging the ability of the kidneys to maintain a lower pH in the urine and increasing the risk of new urinary tract infections and kidney infections.

Low potassium is "associated" with diabetes. Potassium supplementation has been shown to help prevent or delay development of diabetes. The body maintains the balance of salt and potassium in the body, through filtration in the kidneys, guided by an endocrine feedback loop. When the kidneys have endothelial dysfunction, inside the filtration tubules, the kidney fails to maintain the necessary balance of sodium and potassium. The effect on the filtration system of the kidney suggests chlamydia pneumonia is the cause or a co-infection in diabetes.

All chlamydia infections cause inclusion cysts. Inclusion cysts can create clogging and a focus for immune system attack in the pancreas, and in the kidney. Chlamydia and/or its byproducts of abnormal proteins and debris have been found inside kidney stones. Patients with kidney stones should be tested and treated for immortal pathogens and all forms of streptococcus. In some cases, iatrogenically acquired pathogens, from prior treatment, surgery, and hospitalization, like klebsiella or pseudomonas, can also cause kidney stones. Kidney stones should be considered an unrecognized immortal infection, leading to a thorough investigation of the immortal infectious pathogens causing the disease and kidney stones.

Doctors would have a better understanding of the infectious causes of diabetes if all diabetic patients were tested for chronic infections and parasites, and given appropriate treatment for infectious pathogens and parasites. Newly diagnosed diabetic patients are not tested for immortal pathogens, because doctors who treat diabetes view the pancreas as a segmented, malfunctioning body part, without consideration of systemic immortal infections, gastrointestinal disease, co-morbid conditions, or the whole patient. A history of acute infections before the onset of the diabetes, a longer-term history of immortal infections, and a history of contact with pets and other domesticated animals, should be obtained from any newly diagnosed diabetic patient. A history of prior antibiotic treatment with penicillin is necessary, to evaluate whether the use of penicillin used to treat acute infection triggered the diabetes or caused false-negative tests. If immortal pathogens are found, we likely already have drugs to treat, or at least mitigate, the infections causing diabetes.

In 1855, adrenal insufficiency was named "Addison's disease", after Dr. Thomas Addison. Addison's disease is most associated with President John F. Kennedy. Patients with Addison's disease and diabetes have almost four times the rate of mortality, as compared to patients who have only diabetes. In 1912, an excess in adrenal hormones (ACTH) was named Cushing's disease, by Dr. Harvey Cushing. The adrenal gland works with the pituitary gland, and the endocrine system can malfunction from improper signals from the pituitary gland or the adrenal gland. Cushing's disease can arise from a benign pituitary tumor, causing an endocrine signal to secrete excess ACTH from the adrenal gland. Pituitary tumors assumed to be asymptomatic are frequently found on autopsy.

The thyroid is an endocrine gland, in the neck. Thyroid disease may cause low levels of thyroid hormones (hypothyroid), high levels of thyroid hormone (hyperthyroid), or alternating high and low thyroid hormones. Hashimoto's thyroiditis is considered an autoimmune disease, which is also called chronic lymphocytic thyroiditis. Hashimoto's refers to chronic inflammation in the thyroid, causing a low level of thyroid hormones. Low thyroid causes dry skin and a feeling of being cold. High thyroid causes the eyes to bulge forward, due to periorbital swelling behind and around the eye; and can cause mental instability and aggression. High thyroid may precede low thyroid, in Hashimoto's thyroiditis.

Thyroid disease is most likely caused by chlamydia or H-pylori. Thyroid disease may be caused by different immortal pathogens in different patients; and it may be a specific pathogen, a combination of pathogens, or different pathogens in different people. H-pylori may be an independent cause or co-infection in thyroid disease. Co-morbid conditions for thyroid disease include virtually every organ system, including eye diseases, cardiovascular diseases, kidney diseases, gastrointestinal diseases, orthopedic degeneration, lowered immunity to infection, mental illness, and reproductive issues relating to fertility. The co-morbid conditions give clues to the underlying infectious pathology causing thyroid disease; and all of the co-morbid conditions are "associated" with chlamydia and H-pylori.

Thyroid disease is caused by an intracellular pathogen that triggers the immune system to create antibodies, in a pattern specific to the pathogen. Thyroid anti-bodies attacking the infection in the thyroid also fit a lock and key pattern inside the eye. Thyroid orbitopathy is swelling of the soft tissue around the eye, causing the eye to bulge forward; and compression of the optic nerve behind the eye, damaging the optic nerve in a manner similar to what occurs from glaucoma. Surgery on the eyes of a patient with pre-existing high levels of thyroid antibodies, has the potential to cause thyroid eye disease and thyroid orbitopathy, when surgery creates a portal that allows the thyroid antibodies enter the eye. Subsequent eye surgeries, in a patient with thyroid orbitopathy, can cause periorbital swelling in the fellow eye, which was untouched by surgery.

The connection between thyroid antibodies and thyroid eye disease suggests the thyroid antibodies are antibodies to H-pylori. H-pylori can damage the cornea, anterior chamber angle, and retina. Neutrophils and other immune cells that fight H-pylori can become infected, and carry the H-pylori pathogen to the eye. A sub-clinical dose of doxycycline was shown to improve or resolve Graves's orbitopathy (high thyroid causing swelling around the eye and protrusion of the eyeball).[243] Low dose doxycycline treats a chronic H-pylori infection and other chronic diseases caused by H-pylori, such as Parkinson's disease. Improvement in thyroid orbitopathy with doxycycline supports and infectious cause of thyroid disease, and thyroid eye disease.

Thyroid eye disease patients are often steroid responders, meaning the intraocular pressure increases when the patient is treated with steroids. In eye surgery, steroids are injected in the eye, and patients are prescribed steroid drops after surgery, to treat the inflammation caused by surgery. The injected steroids used at surgery and steroid drops after surgery can affect the surgical eye and the fellow eye, although steroid drops have a weaker response and take longer to have a noticeable response in the fellow eye. Steroid drops are more likely to impact the fellow eye in a patient with thyroid eye disease. Steroid induced high pressure can cause damage similar to glaucoma. The steroids injected and given as drops after surgery worsen underlying chronic infections, by potentiating and changing the infection and raising intraocular pressure.

---

[243] Lin M, *et al*. 2015. Efficacy of Subantimicrobial Dose Doxycycline for Moderate-to-Severe and Active Graves' Orbitopathy. Int J Endocrinol. 2015: 285698. Doi: https://dx.doi.org/10.1155/2015/285698.

The reproductive system is dependent on a well-functioning endocrine system. The endocrine glands, particularly the pituitary, adrenal and ovary, must be coordinated, using signals and a feedback loop; and be in balance to send the endocrine signals at the correct time, to create the release of an egg and the environment necessary to become pregnant. A failure of the endocrine system to function in a balanced and coordinated feedback loop can result in the lack of ovulation and infertility.

Diseases affecting the endocrine glands can affect almost any organ, cause a variety of chronic diseases, and reduce fertility. Any endocrine disease should be investigated with a search for pathogens and parasites causing the endocrine diseases.

CHAPTER 15

CHRONIC INFECTION IN REPRODUCTIVE DISEASES

Sir William Osler described syphilis (Treponema Pallidum) as "The Great Imitator", because syphilis mimics so many other diseases and syndromes, as it moves through various stages of the syphilis infectious cascade. Syphilis, like Lyme disease and H-pylori, is a spiral bacterium, which makes the bacteria more difficult to eradicate; because spiral pathogens become tangled in the epithelial and collagen layers of tissue.

Chlamydia species, like syphilis, can evolve into a chronic systemic disease, with variable symptoms during the infectious cascade. Acute chlamydia infections can become chronic infections, and can migrate or metastasize to other parts of the body, through the bloodstream, lymphatics, smooth muscle, and by direct migration to adjacent tissue; and as a Trojan horse of the immune system. In chronic chlamydia, the symptoms change over time, and cause diverse chronic diseases, depending on the organ and system attacked, as the pathogens proliferate and attack weak links.

The reproductive system is a portal for immortal pathogens. Sexually transmitted diseases can infect the reproductive tract and spread to the urinary tract and kidney. Intestinal pathogens can contaminate the reproductive and urinary tracts, and ascend upwards to cause reproductive disease and kidney disease, particularly if the pH is altered. Vaginal yeast arises from chronic infection, or from treatment of recurrent urinary infections, changing the pH of the vagina and making the urinary and reproductive system more vulnerable to infection, with pathogens from the gastrointestinal tract.

Chlamydia trachoma is the most common sexually transmitted disease. Ninety-two million new cases of trachoma are diagnosed each year. Chlamydia trachoma can damage the endothelium and epithelium, expanding the potential host sites in the body. Chlamydia trachoma can infect the mouth, urethra, cervix, and rectum, in women; and the urethra, prostate, mouth, and rectum, in men. Sexually transmitted pathogens acquired through the reproductive tract, cause reproductive system disease, systemic disease, disease in a sexual partner, and disease in a fetus. The greater the number of sexual partners, the greater the chance of acquiring a sexually transmitted disease. The cultural norm of one sexual partner may have developed because centuries of observation demonstrated those with many sexual partners developed poor health and had an early demise.

In women, sexually transmitted chlamydia trachoma causes a variety of reproductive diseases, including pelvic inflammatory disease (PID), endometriosis, infertility, tubal pregnancies, recurrent miscarriages, and prematurity. Chlamydia trachoma ascends up the reproductive tract, causing ectopic pregnancy and infertility.[244] Chlamydia trachoma can cause damage to a fetus, including birth defects. Chronic chlamydia trachoma can cause chronic disease in the urinary tract, and the kidney. In the urinary tract, chlamydia trachoma may be named "interstitial cystitis" to describe the effects of the pathogen and inflammation in the urinary tract. When a woman presents with reproductive problems, doctors should test the mother for immortal pathogens, to determine an infectious cause.

A mouse biovar of chlamydia trachoma is considered a more virulent form of trachoma, and can invade both the urine and reproductive tract. In mice, after inoculation vaginally with chlamydia *suis* in group one, and chlamydia trachoma in group two, chlamydia *suis* and chlamydia trachoma were isolated from both the uterus and fallopian tubes, weeks after inoculation.[245] Long term, sexually transmitted chlamydia trachoma

[244] Morre S, *et al.* 2006. Description of the ICTI Consortium: An Integrated Approach to the Understanding of Chlamydia *Trachomatis* Infection. Drugs of Today. 2006. Vol. 42. Suppl A107-114. Doi: https://www.ncbi.nlm.nih.gov/pubmed/16683050.

[245] Donati M, *et al.* 2015. A Mouse Model for Chlamydia *Suis* Genital Infection. FEMS Pathogens and Disease. 2015. 73:1–3. Doi: 10.1093/femspd/ftu017.

has the potential to cause cancer; and chronic diseases like arthritis, multiple sclerosis, fibromyalgia and chronic fatigue.

PID describes infection in the reproductive organs and in the pelvis; which causes inflammation, scarring, pain, and infertility. Ninety percent of the cases of PID are caused by chlamydia trachoma. As the infection spreads, it causes inflammation and scarring in the uterus and fallopian tubes; and obstruction in the fallopian tubes, inclusion cysts, and a sticky environment, which hampers the proper release of an egg from the ovaries, and implantation of a fertilized egg in the uterus. Patients with PID can be treated with antibiotics; however, damage to the fallopian tubes and uterus may be irreversible. Chlamydia trachoma also causes endometriosis, which is when the tissue lining the uterus grows outside the uterus, causing pain.

Chlamydia trachoma, chlamydia pneumonia, chlamydia psittacosis, and toxoplasmosis in the mother, can be transmitted to the fetus through the placenta or blood stream. Intracellular pathogens have been found in the placenta. Chlamydia abortus has also been shown to cause miscarriages, placenta previa, and late-term fetal demise. Pathogens transferred to the fetus, *in utero,* may be aerobic or anaerobic pathogens; however, oxygen levels *in utero* are low, with the only oxygen coming from the mother's bloodstream. Thus, only pathogens capable of surviving in a low oxygen environment, or without oxygen, can survive *in utero.*

Chlamydia trachoma, chlamydia pneumonia, chlamydia psittacosis, and toxoplasmosis, can infected a fetus *in utero* and be devastating to the fetus. Immortal pathogens can cause abnormalities in fetal development, and the earlier in the pregnancy the pathogen is acquired, the greater the potential damage to the fetus. Babies infected *in utero* and/or early in infancy have a lifetime for pathogens to proliferate and become a chronic disease. A newborn does not have an established immune system for the first two years of life, and the earlier a child is infected, the longer the child's immune system will have to fight the chronic infection. Over a long period of time, immortal infections will become chronic disseminated infection, and infection of the immune cells. Infections acquired *in utero* will combine with diseases acquired in childhood and other immortal infections over the life of the child, acquired as immortal co-infections, which can trigger or cause chronic disease.

The type of pathogen in the mother affects the type of damage to the fetus, based on the predilection of the pathogen for specific tissue. Any infection with a predilection for a particular type of tissue or organ in an adult or an animal, will have the same predilection in the fetus; but will be more destructive to a fetus because of the vulnerability of the developing fetus and lifetime duration of the chronic infection. Chlamydia pneumonia attacks cardiovascular tissue, lungs and brain; and will affect development of the heart, cardiovascular tissue, and/or brain, in the fetus. Trachoma and psittacosis can attack the eye and central nervous system of an adult, and may similarly attack a fetus and cause blindness years later, or central nervous system disease. Toxoplasmosis can attack the brain, eyes and central nervous system of an adult, and similarly can attack the brain, eyes and central nervous system of a fetus. If the mother is malnourished from gastrointestinal disease or chronic immortal infection, the fetus will be deprived of nutrients, including folic acid, critical for fetal development and avoidance of spinal abnormalities, in the fetus.

Acute immortal infections can impact the fetal development, and in some cases chronic immortal infection in the mother can impact the fetal development. For some pathogens which can impact fetus development, it unknown if the immortal infection must be an acute infection, or if chronic infection presents the same or a greater risk to a fetus. When an infant is born or develops a chronic disease, doctors should test mothers and infants for immortal pathogens capable of crossing the placenta and infecting the fetus, to determine if an infectious cause in the mother caused the chronic disease and morbidity in the fetus. Doctors should test mothers and infants for immortal pathogens when the fetus shows any problem anatomically or in cognitive function.

Cystic fibrosis is a disease of unknown origin, believed to occur in infants with a biochemical defect. In cystic fibrosis, the cells in the lung are thought to be immunologically impaired and produce copious amounts of mucous. Cystic fibrosis is be caused by pathogens acquired *in utero*, that attacks the lung. Cystic fibrosis is an impairment of the pulmonary endothelial cells; and chlamydia pneumonia, trachoma and psittacosis can attack endothelial cells in the lung. Cystic fibrosis may also be caused by less commonly known types of chlamydia; and may be from combined infection. Children with cystic fibrosis are treated symptomatically, suffer for a lifetime, may require a lung transplant, and have a shortened lifespan.

Chlamydia trachoma or chlamydia psittacosis are likely causes of cystic fibrosis, because the presentation in cystic fibrosis matches the presentation of a respiratory trachoma and respiratory psittacosis infections. Chlamydia trachoma is relatively common in women and pregnant women, whereas the rate of infection with psittacosis is not known. Cystic fibrosis presents in infants in the same way trachoma or psittacosis respiratory infections present in adults. Cystic fibrosis presents with copious thick mucus, pus, and sputum clogging the lung; consolidation of pus in the lower lung; inclusion cyst formation; and low oxygen levels. Cystic fibrosis causes scarring in the lung, which is typical of trachoma and psittacosis.

Chlamydia pneumonia was found in cystic fibrosis patients, and significant benefit was observed with continuous macrolide therapy, which was assumed to provide an anti-inflammatory effect.[246] However, macrolide therapy was only beneficial when continued long-term. The effectiveness of macrolides in treating cystic fibrosis supports cystic fibrosis is a chronic lung infection; and the persistence of the infection with long-term macrolide therapy suggests it is an immortal infection, and may be more than one immortal infection. If cystic fibrosis is caused by infection with chlamydia trachoma or psittacosis, it explains why macrolide treatment was effective, but required continuous long-term therapy. Macrolides reduced inflammation and partially treated the infection. Drugs effective against trachoma and psittacosis, alone or in combination with a macrolide, may be more effective treatment for cystic fibrosis.

---

[246] Friedman H (*ed*), *et al*. 2004. *Chlamydia Pneumoniae* Infection and Disease. New York: Kluwer Academic/Plenum Publishers. Role of Chlamydia Pneumonia as an Inducer of Asthma. (Hahn DL). Ch. 17. P. 245-246.

Newborn infections with chlamydia trachoma can be identified by gram stain of the conjunctivae or nasopharynx, and a PCR test for chlamydia. Newer swab testing may be particularly useful in detecting pathogens in infants. IgM may be elevated in infants, representing an infection that has been present for weeks or months during pregnancy. Antibiotics like penicillin, the go-to drug of pediatricians, given to patients with cystic fibrosis for an acute infection, will not treat the underlying condition and have the potential to make the cystic fibrosis worse.

Cerebral palsy is a disease of the central nervous system, which can be caused by immortal pathogens acquired *in utero* or early infancy. Some forms of chlamydia and toxoplasmosis attack the central nervous system, and cause multiple sclerosis in adults. Toxoplasmosis has been hypothesized to cause cerebral palsy, if acquired by the fetus *in utero*. When chlamydia trachoma or toxoplasmosis is acquired by the fetus, it is reasonable to believe that a fetus could develop similar neurologic and central nervous system problems as adults, from the same immortal pathogens.

Autism has been dramatically increasing in the United States. Prior studies suggested ninety percent of autism cases were caused by defective genes. If autism was caused by defective genes, autism would be phased out of existence, in a few generations. The high genetic cost of autism suggests defective genes alone cannot be the cause of autism.

As scientific research advances, a greater percent of autism cases have been shown to *not* be genetic. Twins have been studied, because twins are presumed to have the same genetic predisposition and are affected by the same intrauterine environment. The rate of autism is higher in twins than in two siblings who are not twins, suggesting the conditions the twins shared in the womb contributed to the development of autism. Mathematical modeling of autism in a twin study showed only thirty-eight percent of the cases could be attributed to genetics. In two articles from the "Journal of Psychiatry", authors suggested environmental factors in the womb, not genetic factors, are at work in fifty-eight percent of autism cases. The experts were surprised to find fifty-eight percent of the cases of autism in twins were not caused by genetic defects. The experts failed to state what environmental factors were at issue, or the role of acute or chronic infections during pregnancy.[247]

Some attributed an increase in autism to an increase in C-sections. C-sections may play a role in autism, but cannot be the entire explanation. Antibiotics given during and after C-sections may damage the microbiome of the mother and child, or transform infectious pathogens into a chronic disease. If C-sections are a potential cause autism, one has to ask why doctors have not done more to reduce the rate of C-sections, which can be as high as fifty percent in some hospitals. The rate of C-sections in the hospital can be attributed to doctors not being available throughout labor, and get worried and impatient for the delivery. Doctors assume C-sections are a safer alternative for them than waiting, because the doctor believes he is less likely to be sued doing a C-section than waiting patiently for nature to deliver the baby. If C-sections cause autism, one answer is less C-sections and more direct involvement of medical practitioners during labor and delivery.

Midwifes doing home births have a rate of C-sections less than five percent; and the infant is not exposed to hospital pathogens. The fetus has antibodies to household pathogens through the mother's bloodstream, but lacks any immunity to hospital pathogens. Infants born at home, vaginally, have the most diverse and healthy microbiome. Infants born by C-section are at higher risk for developing a number chronic health problems, and scientists are investigating treatment of the infant's microbiome, by inoculation with the mother's bacteria during the first two months of life.

Some have attributed autism to vaccines, or some component or combination of vaccines. In recent vaccine litigation, the plaintiff proved autism was caused by giving multiple vaccines at the same time; and the conclusion of experts and the court was the risk of autism from multiple vaccines occurs in children with "mitochondrial disorder". Mitochondrial disorder is a description in microbiology, not a diagnosis. Mitochondria

---

[247] *See e.g.* Wong CC, *et al.* 2014. Methylomic Analysis of Monozygotic Twins Discordant for Autusm Spectrum Disorder and Related Behavioural Traits. Molecular Psychiatry. 2014. 19: 495-503. Doi:10.1038/MP.2013.41.

make the energy inside the cell, and "mitochondrial disorder" refers to malfunction of the mitochondria—the cell does not have enough or make enough intracellular energy. Mitochondrial disorder is describing the effect of chlamydia on the cell, in that the pathogen hijacks the energy making ability of the cell and depletes ATP inside the cell. The finding suggests that if a vaccine causes autism, it occurs in the presence of a child with a chronic chlamydia infection, acquired *in utero* or after birth.

Autism and autism spectrum disorders are caused by chronic infection in the mother; or acute infection during pregnancy that was not treated and was transmitted to the fetus, *in utero* or at birth. Autism is recognized to have co-morbid conditions, including gastrointestinal dysbiosis and immune dysfunction, leading to a conclusion immortal pathogens and parasites cause autism. The rate of autism has increased because doctors fail to diagnose and treat immortal infections in pregnant mothers, including chlamydia infections and toxoplasmosis.

Doctors are beginning to hypothesize infectious causes of autism. In mice, treatment with antibiotics was shown to reduce or eliminate autism in the fetus; and prevented autism in subsequent births. If antibiotics prevented autism in mice, then bacterial pathogens are the cause of autism, not genes and not a virus. Studies also showed high levels of TNF-alpha in the spinal fluid of autism victims, and high levels of cytokines in the blood plasma, suggesting immune dysfunction.[248] TNF-alpha in the cerebral spinal fluid and a high level of cytokines in the blood, and co-morbid gastrointestinal disease, strongly support immortal pathogens were transmitted to the fetus, and caused autism. Studies have connected infection during pregnancy to autism, and the fetal abnormalities and the findings of TNF-alpha in cerebral spinal fluid and cytokines in the blood in autism are consistent with immortal chlamydia pathogens acquired by the fetus during pregnancy.

---

[248] Patterson PH. 2011. Maternal Infection and Immune Involvement in Autism. Trends Mol Med. Jul 2011. 17(7): 389-394. Doi: 10.1016/j.molmed.2011.03.001; Chez MG, *et al.* 2007. Elevation of Tumor Necrosis Factor-Alpha in Cerebrospinal Fluid of Autistic Children. Pediat Neurol. 2007. 36: 361-365. Doi: 10.1016/j. pediatrneurol.2007.01.012.

Toxoplasmosis acquired during pregnancy can cause severe brain damage in a fetus. Toxoplasmosis in the brain of a fetus causes regressive developmental disorders, which are also called childhood disintegrative disorders. Regressive developmental disorders occur in a child who was normal at birth, and begins to regress mentally and physically months or years after birth. The child may have regression of intelligence, loss of physical abilities, and development of seizures. Regressive developmental disorders have been incorporated into a larger category of autism spectrum disorders, and have as many as a dozen different sub-categories of named syndromes, including Aicardi Syndrome, Angelman Syndrome, Rett Syndrome, Ring Chromosome 20 Syndrome, or Sturge-Weber Syndrome. The named regressive developmental disorders have the same signs and symptoms as congenital toxoplasmosis.

Regressive developmental disorders have been attributed to genetic defects, which again cannot be the complete answer. If genes cause regressive developmental disorders, we would no longer have regressive developmental disorders; and would not have a dozen different names for minor variations in regressive developmental syndromes. It is unknown whether regressive developmental disorders occur only after acute toxoplasmosis infection during pregnancy, or whether chronic toxoplasmosis in the mother can also damage a fetus; because symptoms of toxoplasmosis are dismissed or the infection is not diagnosed in infants, children and adults.

Toxoplasmosis acquired *in utero* can cause epilepsy in infants and children. Childhood epilepsy also has many different diagnostic categories, based on the nature and frequency of the seizures. Childhood seizure disorders, also known as childhood epilepsy syndromes, include benign Rolandic epilepsy, juvenile myoclonic epilepsy, infantile spasms or West syndrome, Lennox-Gastaut syndrome, and Dravet syndrome or Severe Myoclonic Epilepsy of Infancy. Some epilepsy syndromes are called "idiopathic" or do not fit within diagnostic categories. Toxoplasmosis in the brain can have different manifestations in different people, related to the age at which the infection was acquired (*in utero* or infancy), the location of the infection in the brain, the duration of infection, and the total infectious burden.

Toxoplasmosis attacking the motor control sections of the brain will cause the most violent seizures.

The differential diagnosis in childhood epilepsy syndromes is dependent on the bias and specialty of the examiner, and name given to the seizure disorders by that specialty. Seizures occur in regressive disability syndromes, and regressive disability disorders occur in childhood epilepsy syndromes. The symptoms of seizure disorder syndromes overlap with the symptoms of regressive disability syndromes. The diagnosis of seizure disorder syndromes versus regressive developmental disorder may be dependent on the specialty evaluating the child and the most significant presenting symptoms.

Antibiotics used to treat chlamydia and other immortal infections, in the fetus, are showing promising results in helping "fragile X" disability. Fragile X disability is part of autism spectrum disorders. Minocycline is seemingly able to reverse some of the fragile X disability and improve behavior. With enough perseverance, and targeted antibiotics, the antibiotics should continue to help the fragile X patient to improve over time. Based on the success of antibiotic treatment in fragile X disability, indicating infectious pathogens play a role in the disease, diagnosis and treatment should be extended to other developmental disabilities and regressive developmental disabilities, in infants and children. Infants who develop epilepsy should be tested for infectious immortal pathogens, particularly chlamydia pathogens and toxoplasmosis.

Cavernous sinus malformation has long been assumed to be a genetic disease, common in Hispanics in Northern New Mexico. Cavernous sinus malformation is a cluster of malformed and tangled blood vessels in the brain. Cavernous sinus malformation causes neuronal degeneration, glial cell proliferation, neurofibrillary tangles, and sclerosis in the hippocampal cells. Babies with cavernous sinus malformation have long-term health problems ranging from headaches to epilepsy, and in some cases, cavernous sinus malformation can cause death.

In 2017, the University of Pennsylvania reported research in mice, showing acute intestinal infection acquired in pregnancy caused cavernous sinus vascular malformations. The multistate study involving thirty doctors, in a study of mice, found acute infection during pregnancy caused cavernous sinus malformation—not genetics. The study showed acute and untreated infections with gram-negative bacteria, present in the intestine, and acquired by the mother during pregnancy, caused cavernous sinus malformation in the fetus. However, the type of infection thought to cause cavernous sinus malformation was not stated. Chlamydia are gram negative bacteria, which can infect and reside in the intestine.

Cavernous sinus malformation is a tangle of abnormal blood vessels in the brain, similar to tangles in the brain that form in Alzheimer's disease. The similarity of tangles in the brain, between cavernous sinus malformation and Alzheimer's disease, suggest a common infectious etiology. The connection between an acute gram-negative bacterial infection during pregnancy and development of cavernous sinus malformation suggests a chlamydia pathogen is the cause of cavernous sinus malformation. Chlamydia pneumonia is a gram-negative bacteria, can attack vessels and the brain, can cause Alzheimer's, and Alzheimer's and cavernous sinus malformation have similar tangles in the brain. When acute chlamydia infections are acquired during pregnancy, the fetus is at greater risk of damage to the vascular system and brain development. Chronic chlamydia pneumonia causes Alzheimer's disease; thus, is likely involved in or contributes to the development of cavernous sinus malformation.

One family reported four children had cavernous sinus malformation, which may have been from chronic infection or re-infection in the mother, during pregnancy, from the same vector. We will not know until doctors begin to test mothers of children born with cavernous sinus malformation for immortal infections, and learn more about the proper functioning of the microbiome and the pathogens within it.

Chlamydia pneumonia causes cardiovascular disease, lung disease, Alzheimer's disease and multiple sclerosis; and chlamydia pneumonia, trachoma and psittacosis cause Parkinson's disease, multiple sclerosis, neurologic diseases, and arthritis. Any of these infections in the mother, acquired in pregnancy, can migrate to the brain and adversely impact the neurologic and vascular development of a fetus, alone or in combination with co-infections.

The Zika virus was identified as a cause of microcephaly in infants. Chlamydia trachoma and toxoplasmosis can invade the central nervous system; and Zika can attach to trachoma or toxoplasmosis as a bacteriophage, and move with other pathogens into the brain to cause microcephaly. Brazil has one of the highest rates of sexually transmitted disease, and one of the highest rates of toxoplasmosis, in the world. Brazil has a high rate of pet ownership, of cats and dogs, and fecal waste is left on the sidewalks and in parks. The pets in Brazil are highly infected with toxoplasmosis; thus, the population of pet owners is highly infected with toxoplasmosis. Underlying immortal infections with chlamydia trachoma and toxoplasmosis likely allowed Zika to attach to the trachoma or toxoplasmosis, as a bacteriophage, and be carried to the fetal brain to cause microcephaly.

Chronic parasitic infection from contaminated water and animals, and the infectious cascade of malabsorption in the mother, can also deprive the fetus of proper nutrition during pregnancy, including folic acid. Any patient drinking contaminated water at any time is at risk of parasitic infection, which causes a greater infectious burden with parasites and greater malabsorption of folic acid and B12, over time. Low folic acid is "associated" with spina bifida, and can contribute to early and late medical problems and chronic disease in the infant. Pregnant women are now advised to take supplemental folic acid; and in mothers with chronic diseases that deplete folic acid, supplementation of folic acid has been shown to help normal fetal development.

Infection with chlamydia pneumonia, *in utero*, is the likely cause of premature cataracts in infants and children. Chronic chlamydia pneumonia infections are known to cause premature cataracts in adults. Dogs with cataracts and treated with antibiotics or anti-inflammatory drugs had resolution or improvement of premature cataracts.

CMV (cytomegalic virus) includes eight separate species. CMV has been found in rhesus monkeys and primates. Once CMV is acquired, it becomes a chronic infection. CMV is related to the herpes viruses, and can be devastating to the fetus. CMV acquired *in utero* can lead to loss of eyesight or loss of hearing in a child, five to seven years after birth. By the time loss of eyesight or hearing occurs, infectious causes are not considered. Whether the loss of eyesight is CMV alone, or CMV as a co-infection and bacteriophage, is not known.

In utero infections with chlamydia and other immortal pathogens and parasites cause a variety of abnormalities in the fetus, including birth defects, autism, cystic fibrosis, cerebral palsy, loss of vision or hearing, epilepsy, regressive developmental disorders, vascular abnormalities, damage to mental health, cavernous sinus malformation, ADHD, and many others. In order to discover the cause of fetal abnormalities, doctors must test the mother for immortal infections; determine if the infection was acute or chronic during pregnancy; and determine, if possible, how long the mother had the infections and the overall burden of infections. Test infants and children for immortal pathogens, and recognize treatment of the infections may help treat or prevent chronic disease. Consistent testing and diagnosis of infections in adults, pregnant and new mothers, newborns, and infants, will help the medical community find an answer on how to prevent morbidity and mortality in mothers, fetuses and infants.

When an immortal pathogen is found, in an infant with a fetal abnormality or disease, or in the mother of the infant, treatment of the infection may avoid or reduce the long-term suffering and morbidity from chronic disease. Treatment during pregnancy or early in life presents a risk to a fetus or infant; however, the risk must be weighed against the benefit of treatment in preventing a lifelong disability and chronic disease, in the child. After the studies on autism and cavernous sinus malformation, and the finding of TNF-alpha in the spinal fluid of children with autism, obstetricians should stop fearing treatment of pregnant mothers and instead fear *not* treating pregnant mothers for acute infection. Penicillin should be avoided in pregnant mothers, because penicillin may have the same damaging effect in the fetus it causes in an adult, when used to treat acute immortal infection.

Men develop chronic reproductive diseases from the same immortal pathogens that cause chronic reproductive disease in women. The prostate is an endocrine gland in men, and a spongy organ that can harbor chlamydia trachoma and other sexually transmitted diseases. The prostate hides the infections, until years later, when the chronic infection becomes prostate cancer. Men get HPV, and HPV is a known cause of cervical cancer; thus, it is reasonable to believe HPV may also cause prostate cancer. HPV and trachoma may act synergistically to cause prostate cancer.

Men can harbor and chlamydia trachoma and HPV infections in the prostate, which can be transmitted to sexual partners. Chlamydia trachoma has been found in semen, including in the semen of donors at fertility clinics.[249] Sexually transmitted pathogens can infect the prostate and urinary system; and undiagnosed and untreated, chlamydia trachoma causes reproductive, prostate, urinary and kidney diseases. Men can have recurrent urine and kidney infections, as the prostate enlarges and the infection spreads in the urinary tract. Men need investigation and diagnosis of chlamydia trachoma and HPV when the male or female have a reproductive, urinary or kidney disease. Failure to treat both sexual partners when pathogens are diagnosed leads to failed therapy, re-infection, a greater infectious burden, and chronic disease; and may also contribute to the development of other chronic diseases, such as heart disease and arthritis.

Peyronne's disease is a syndrome in which the erect penis has a curve, arising from scar tissue inside the penis. Peyronne's disease is thought to

---

[249] Pannekoek Y, *et al*. 2003. Assessment of Chlamydia Trachomatis Infection of Semen Specimens by Ligase Chain Reaction. Journal of Medical Microbiology. 2003. 52:777-779. Doi: 10:1099/jmm.0.05187-0.

be a connective tissue disorder, involving the growth of fibrous plaques. The connective tissue damage, fibrous plaque, and scar tissue in the penis developed from spread of the chlamydia trachoma infection and is causing the curvature, just as scar tissue forms in women who develop PID or endometriosis. Co-morbid conditions with Peyronne's disease include heart disease and diabetes, and high cholesterol may exacerbate Peyronne's disease. The co-morbid conditions support chronic infection causes Peyronne's disease, and that sexually transmitted trachoma may also cause other chronic diseases.

CHAPTER 16

CHRONIC INFECTION IN EYE DISEASES

The eyes are the window to the soul—and the eyes are a window into health. The eyes reveal current health, can reveal systemic disease, and can predict future health. The eye is a microcosm of what is happening inside the body. The eyes can predict and identify chronic disease, and give clues to the pathogens involved in chronic disease. The iris can even potentially predict cancer, metastatic cancer, and the organs affected by cancer.

Vision affects how a person sees and interacts with the world. Vision loss affected the art of many impressionist painters. Claude Monet had well-documented visual problems. Edgar Degas lost central vision in one eye, in his thirties; and in the other eye in his fifties. Mary Cassatt was diabetic, suffered from diabetic retinopathy and cataracts, and underwent multiple operations on her eyes. She reported her vision becoming dimmer, but was able to paint with oils using more vibrant colors, in the later years of her life. George DuMaurier had retinal problems and was blind in his left eye. The vision impairments of famous impressionist painters may have been inspired by poor vision. The impressionist art reflects loss of the artists' ability to see details, and may reflect how the impressionist painters saw the world with impaired vision.

Carolyn's thirty-five-year legal career was defined by eye litigation. She spent decades studying eyes, in every field of eye care, which gave her a broad perspective on eye issues, and extensive knowledge of the eye. She represented many hundreds of clients with eye injuries, and became known nationally as the eye lawyer. Each eye case expanded her knowledge and insight into the eyes and eye diseases. She can discern a lot about a person's health by merely observing the appearance of their eyes, and knowing their eye history. She saw many vision disasters caused by eye care professionals who failed to recognize immortal infection, before proceeding with eye surgery or procedures, or dismissing the importance of symptoms.

Chlamydia pathogens will emerge as the cause of many non-traumatic eye diseases and syndromes. Chlamydia pneumonia, chlamydia trachoma, chlamydia psittacosis, H-pylori and toxoplasmosis can attack the eye, and cause damage similar to the damage caused by the same pathogen in other organs and body systems.

To understand the impact of immortal infection in the eye, one must first understand the structures in the eye and the normal eye. The front of the eye is the clear cornea. The cornea, like other tissue in the body, has five layers. The front outer layer of the cornea is epithelium, and the underside of the cornea is endothelium. The stroma is the middle collagen layer of the cornea. Bowman's membrane and Descemet's membrane separate the epithelium and endothelium from the stroma, to create a barrier to protect the stroma from infection and inflammation. The corneal epithelium and stroma are separated by Bowman's membrane; and the corneal endothelium and stroma are separated by Descemet's membrane.

Corneal epithelial cells regenerate in a centripetal pattern, as the epithelium marches in a spiral up to the dome of the central cornea. The corneal epithelium is approximately one-tenth the thickness of the total cornea, and can vary in thickness, as regeneration of the epithelium fills in peaks and valleys on the surface if the cornea. Corneal epithelium can be thicker over low spots, and thinner over high spots, because as the epithelium regenerates it smooths an irregular surface. Varying thickness on the corneal epithelium can initially mask an irregular corneal shape and a thinning disease.

The iris is the colored part of the eye; and the pupil in the center of the iris adjusts larger or smaller to allow more or less light into the eye. The flat iris and dome of the cornea form an angle inside the eye, called the anterior chamber angle. The anterior chamber angle controls fluid movement in and out of the eye, and maintains proper intraocular pressure. The natural lens inside the eye is behind the iris, and separates the front and back portions of the eye. The natural lens is inside a posterior capsule, and the natural lens and capsule are similar in size and relationship to an M&M candy. The lens is like the chocolate candy inside, and the capsule is like the candy coating. The natural lens and capsule is suspended by zonules, which adjust the lens to give clear vision at all distances. With age, the zonules stiffen, and do not adjust focus as well, creating a need for reading glasses for close vision.

The vitreous is a gel-like fluid which fills the inside of the eye, between the iris and the retina, and keeps pressure on the retina to remain attached. A vitreous detachment occurs when the vitreous pulls away from the retina, due to trauma, chronic dehydration, or infection. When a vitreous detachment occurs, the vitreous can pull a piece of retina with it, causing a floater. Small floaters can reabsorb in time; however, vitreous detachment suggests a problem in the retina and increases the risk of a retinal tear, hole, or detachment.

The retina is the back surface of the eye, and has layers, like other tissue in the eye and the body. The inner most layer of the retina is epithelium. When fluid gets in between the layers of the retina, from retinal tears or holes, the retina can partially or fully detach. The macula is the central most part of the retina, representing the central one degree of vision that gives the clearest vision. The optic nerve sends the images from the macula to the brain.

Ophthalmologists are surgeons—and are not trained nor directed to diagnose infections. Ophthalmologists take a medical history, but only examine the eyes and only consider eye diseases. The ophthalmology patient is a body part—an eye in a bed, for which the ophthalmologist prescribes drops, and on which the ophthalmologist does procedures and surgery. Eye procedures and surgery are the mainstay of ophthalmology. Procedures and surgery attract cytokines (immune inflammatory markers), monocytes and lymphocytes; and infected immune cells and inflammatory markers can enter the eye through the portal created by the surgery. Steroids given during and after all eye surgeries reduce inflammation, but can potentiate infection in the eye and trigger elevated eye pressure.

Despite many scientific articles "associating" immortal infection to eye diseases, ophthalmologists do not generally consider infectious causes of chronic eye disease. Chlamydia species and H-pylori have been linked to ocular surface disorders, glaucoma, and retinal disorders; and toxoplasmosis has been linked to retinal disease and blinding eye diseases. Chlamydia psittacosis causes MALT lymphoma (lymphoma in the eye), Waldenstrom syndrome, and has been "associated" with other forms of lymphoma. Chlamydia pathogens can have other bacterial and/or viral pathogens attached to them on the inside or outside of the pathogen, which are carried to the eye with the chlamydia pathogens, to cause chronic disease.

Ophthalmologists do not often recognize the need for diagnosis and treatment of immortal pathogens, and are not trained to recognize the importance of co-morbid conditions. Ophthalmologists do not recognize co-morbid medical conditions as relevant to eye disease, or caused by the same pathogens; thus, do not coordinate with primary care doctors or refer patients for treatment of infection. Cardiovascular disorders and stomach disorders are common co-morbid conditions in eye disease—so common the co-morbid conditions may be dismissed as unimportant or "not my concern". Heart disease and Alzheimer's are common co-morbid condition in patients with eye disease involving the vessels of the eye, particularly macular degeneration and stroke in the eye. Stomach disorders and retinal disease are common co-morbid conditions. Ophthalmologists need to routinely recognize and diagnose immortal infections in eye diseases; and be prepared to treat these pathogens aggressively or coordinate care with someone who can diagnose and treat immortal pathogens.

Chlamydia pneumonia causes endothelial dysfunction, in the cornea and internal structures, of the eye. Chlamydia pneumonia can cause corneal thinning diseases; vascular damage in the eye causing reduced blood flow to the macula, and macular degeneration; and strokes in the eye. Chlamydia pneumonia can cause inclusion cysts, restricting blood flow in the eye and causing a stroke in the eye. Chlamydia pneumonia has been "associated" with premature cataracts, cataracts, iritis, uveitis, glaucoma, macular degeneration and retinal disease. Chronic chlamydia pneumonia can cause cataracts to develop at a younger age; and may cause cataracts in infants. Chlamydia pneumonia damages the endothelial pump, which damages the ability to move fluid in and out of the layers of the cornea.

Chlamydia pneumonia attacks the endothelium inside of the blood vessels in the eye, just as occurs in cardiovascular disease. Chlamydia pneumonia can clog and cause constriction of the small vessels in the eye sooner than the larger vessels in the cardiovascular system, reducing the blood supply to the macula and optic nerve. Endothelial dysfunction, clogging of the vessels with plaque, and narrowing of the vessels, cause reduced blood flow to the macula and macular degeneration. New fragile blood vessels can form on the retina, as chlamydia stimulates angiogenesis, and the body tries to restore blood flow to the macula to restore nutrition to the macula and optic nerve.

Cardiovascular disease and Alzheimer's are common co-morbid conditions in patients with macular degeneration, and macular degeneration arises from the same type of damage chlamydia pneumonia causes in the cardiovascular system and brain, which supports chlamydia pneumonia as a cause of macular degeneration. Moreover, vessels in the back of the eye can predict cardiovascular disease, heart attack, and stroke, even before cardiovascular disease is diagnosed. The vessels in the eye can predict Alzheimer's years before development of Alzheimer's disease.

Chlamydia trachoma, chlamydia psittacosis, and H-pylori, can cause corneal thinning and loose surface tissue; and when the same pathogens reach the retina, cause loose tissue on the surface of the retina. Chlamydia pneumonia and H-pylori have been linked to glaucoma. The severity of glaucoma has been "associated" with high chlamydia titers. Chlamydia pneumonia and H-pylori can cause retinal disease. H-pylori can cause loose surface tissue, retinal thinning, damage to the internal layers of the retina; and retinal holes, tears or detachments.

Chlamydia trachoma is considered the leading cause of blindness worldwide. Sexually acquired trachoma can be spread from the reproductive tract to the eye, by self-inoculation. Chlamydia trachoma has a predilection for attacking eyes and reproductive organs. Chlamydia trachoma can be spread by intimate contact, and by close contact within the family. At Ellis Island, immigrants waiting to enter the United States were screened for trachoma, using the same dirty eye hook on every patient. The dirty eye hook would have spread trachoma and other infectious pathogens in the eye to immigrants, defeating the purpose of the screening.

Ocular trachoma is caused by a different serovar of chlamydia trachoma, which attacks the eye directly. Ocular trachoma can be transmitted by a particular type of fly that migrates across the United States and feeds on trachoma secretions. The fly lands on the face of an infected person, and then transfers the trachoma to the next person's face. Pictures of children in Africa whose faces are covered with flies, are an indication of ocular trachoma. Arthritis is a common co-morbid condition in patients with ocular trachoma, and ocular trachoma is known to be "associated" with arthritis. Ophthalmologists know ocular trachoma causes misdirected eyelashes; yet, do not diagnose trachoma in patients with misdirected eyelashes.

Ophthalmologists should be able to diagnose and treat trachoma and psittacosis in the eye; and H-pylori. Ophthalmologists seldom recognize the wide variety of symptoms caused by trachoma, or the need for oral medication to treat trachoma. When treatment for trachoma is prescribed, ophthalmologists may use too short a course of antibiotics or less effective antibiotics. Ophthalmologists seldom diagnose chlamydia psittacosis, even in patients with diseases and syndromes known to be caused by psittacosis. Ophthalmologists do not consider or attempt to diagnose chlamydia or H-pylori, in ocular surface disease, glaucoma or retinal disease.

CORNEA, *Fundamentals, Diagnosis and Management*, is a fundamental text for corneal specialists.[250] CORNEA, at Ch. 51 (Singal N, Rootman D), discusses chlamydia pneumonia, trachoma and psittacosis in conjunction with eye disease.[251] CORNEA recognizes chlamydia organisms cause a

---

[250] Krachmer J, Mannis M, and Holland E (*eds*). CORNEA, *Fundamentals, Diagnosis and Management*. 2nd Ed. 2005. Philadelphia: Elsevier Mosby. (Singal N, Rootman D). Ch. 51.

[251] *Id.* @ Ch. 51.

variety of eye diseases, and gives numerous ophthalmology names for the many eye diseases and syndromes caused by the chlamydia pathogens. Chlamydia trachoma is known to cause inclusion cysts around the eye, and ophthalmologists name of the inclusion cysts caused by trachoma "lymphogranuloma venereum conjunctivitis". The text describes adult inclusion conjunctivitis, lymphogranuloma (trachoma), and psittacosis; and the conclusion is, "Chlamydia is responsible for a large spectrum of human ocular infections."[252] Chlamydia trachoma causes lymphogranuloma venereum, which ophthalmology named a separate disease. The name describes a symptom and finding of ocular trachoma, rather than the cause.[253] Treatment for trachoma is recommended, to wit: azithromycin, doxycycline, and tetracycline, based on the infection; for a duration that varies from one day to three weeks.

CORNEA, *Fundamentals, Diagnosis and Management*, addresses a myriad of diseases called "itis", such as conjunctivitis, iritis, or uveitis; and numerous syndromes named for doctors who first described the syndromes, such as Fuchs corneal dystrophy, Stephens-Johnson syndrome, and Cogan's syndrome (which is not an all-inclusive list of diseases and syndromes of the eye). Infectious agents like streptococcus, staphylococcus, acanthamoeba, herpes, and sexually transmitted diseases are mentioned; but little mention is made of chronic chlamydia infection as a cause of chronic eye disease, or as a cause of any of the "itis" diseases and syndromes of unknown origin. No mention is made of treatment for the many "itis" syndromes and diseases of unknown origin.

In Atlas of CLINICAL OPHTHALMOLOGY, the discussion of chlamydia is limited to five pages, and is primarily directed at ocular surface disease, inclusion bodies, and conjunctivitis; and to chlamydia trachoma.[254] Atlas of CLINICAL OPHTHALMOLOGY states anterior and posterior uveitis are from unknown causes; and are associated with

---

[252] *Id.*

[253] *See* Pannekoek Y. 2006. Inclusion Proteins of Chlamydiaceae, Drugs Today (Barc). Mar 2006. 42 Suppl A:65-73. PMID: 16683046.

[254] Spatin D, *et al. (eds)*. 2005. Atlas of CLINICAL OPHTHALMOLOGY. 3rd Ed. Elsevier Limited.

multiple sclerosis, sarcoidosis, and Behcet's disease[255]—all diseases caused by immortal pathogens that attack the eye. Toxoplasmosis is noted as a rare cause of posterior uveitis and scleritis (inflammation of the white surface of the eye); and may be involved in "Fuchs Heterochromic Iridocyclitis" (FHI), a condition of unknown origin, in which the iris disintegrates and disperses particles in the anterior chamber and precipitates on the underside of the cornea.[256] Patients with FHI are predisposed to glaucoma and cataracts because chronic infection in the iris causes inflammation, which can accelerate cataracts; and the pathogen causes disintegration of the iris and dispersion of iris particles that clog the anterior chamber angle, causing pigment-dispersion glaucoma. Toxoplasmosis from cats and toxocara from dogs are described as pathogens that invade the retina, causing posterior inflammation and leaving lesions that cause loss of vision.[257] Considering Atlas of CLINICAL OPTHALMOLOGY discusses pathogens acquired from cats and dogs as a possible cause of sight-threatening eye disease, the history of contact with pets should be part of the history and evaluation of all ophthalmology patients.

H-pylori has been "associated" with blepharitis, rosacea, glaucoma, "idiopathic" central serous chorioretinopathy (ICSR), and other eye diseases. H-pylori can invade the eye, by migrating from the stomach to the eye; or by self-inoculation. H-pylori can migrate from the cornea to the inner structures in the eye, down the iris, into the anterior chamber angles, into the vitreous, and ultimately to the retina. H-pylori causes ocular surface disease, and in patients with glaucoma, treatment of ocular surface disease helps control intraocular pressure.[258] Treatment of H-pylori has also been reported to be helpful in patients with rosacea;[259] which is

---

[255] *See Id.* @ Ch. 10. Intraocular Inflammation (Stanford M and Spalton D). p. 300-308.

[256] *Id.* @ 298.

[257] *Id.* @ 309-311.

[258] Batra R, *et al.* 2014. Ocular Surface Disease Exacerbated Glaucoma: Optimizing the Ocular Surface Improves Intraocular Pressure Control. J Glaucoma. Jan 2014. 23(1)56-60. Doi: 10.1097/IJG.0b013e318264cd68.

[259] Dakovic Z, *et al.* 2007. Ocular Rosacea and Treatment of Symptomatic Helicobacter Infection: A Case Series. Acta Dematoven APA. Vol 16. 2007. No. 2. PMID: 17992465.

consistent with H-pylori being a cause of ocular surface disease, glaucoma and rosacea.

H-pylori has been "associated" with corneal ulcers, which is consistent with the predilection of H-pylori to attack epithelium, and the ability of H-pylori to cause ulcers, in the gastrointestinal tract. H-pylori attacks the epithelium, and burrows downward, causing disintegration of Bowman's membrane and a loose corneal surface; and attaches to collagen. The damage to the epithelium by H-pylori can provide a route for other pathogens to enter the eye. As H-pylori moves deeper, the stroma becomes inflamed and starts to atrophy, causing corneal thinning, from loss of the collagen structure and fluid within the collagen structure, and inflammation created by the pathogen.

When H-pylori attacks the anterior chamber angle, it causes loss of intraocular pressure control and glaucoma. H-pylori can migrate deeper in the eye to attack the retina, causing damage to the retinal epithelium, and the inner layers of the retina. The literature is replete with reports "associating" H-pylori with retinal diseases, including lattice degeneration, vitreous detachment, RPE (loose epithelium), ICSR, retinal holes or tears, and retinal detachment. H-pylori damages the retinal epithelium, causing loose tissue on the surface of the retina and retinal disease, and allows other pathogens to invade the retina. Any patient with retinal disease should be tested for intestinal pathogens and H-pylori, to preserve vision in the damaged eye and prevent vision loss in the fellow eye.

Toxoplasmosis is a parasite transmitted to humans from cats, and can cause sight threatening disease. A cat scratch on the cornea can cause blindness. Toxoplasmosis on the retina will eat away at the retina, leaving de-pigmented areas, decreased vision, and ultimately cause blindness. When a patient has de-pigmented lesions on the retina, particularly a cat owner or person in contact with cats, toxoplasmosis should be considered in the differential diagnosis. Caution around cats, and caution around cat litter boxes, is the best means to avoid toxoplasmosis; and contact with cats should be disclosed to the ophthalmologist and considered in the differential diagnosis of chronic retinal disease.

Veterinarians know pets transmit infectious pathogens to their owners, and know cats transmit toxoplasmosis to owners. Veterinarians known owners can transmit pathogens to the pets. Veterinarians know horses get psittacosis, and get the same psittacosis and fungal eye infections as people. Unfortunately, ophthalmologists do not make the connection between animal pathogens and chronic eye disease of "unknown origin". Ophthalmologists should routinely inquire into pets, particularly cats, birds, dogs, horses and other livestock, as part of the medical history.

The NIH reports more than eighty intestinal pathogens can migrate into the eye, including giardia, amoebas, and worms. The pathogens can migrate along the vagus nerve, from the gastrointestinal tract to the sinus, from the sinus to the eye, and from the sinus or eye to the brain. Stomach pathogens can migrate through the blood or lymphatics to the eye, transferred by the immune system, or be transferred to the eye by self-inoculation. Pathogens in the sinus and eye can migrate along the optic nerve to the brain, and can cause meningiomas on the optic nerve or the surface of the brain.

Stomach disease is a common co-morbid condition in patients with eye disease and with retinal disease; and co-morbid stomach disease suggests H-pylori, chlamydia, toxoplasmosis, or parasites are causing the eye disease. Ophthalmologists seem unaware gastrointestinal pathogens can get into the eye. Gastroenterologists knew fifty years ago that intestinal bacteria and parasites had extra-intestinal effects on the body, and intestinal pathogens could cause eye disease. Today, gastroenterologists and ophthalmologists seem to have forgotten the connection between gastrointestinal disease and eye disease.

CORNEA, *Fundamentals, Diagnosis and Management*, has a chapter on Inflammatory Bowel Disease and Other Systemic Inflammatory Diseases of the Cornea. Chapter 66 recognizes the co-existence of intestinal diseases and the role of inflammation in the cornea.[260] Co-morbid conditions are

---

[260] Krachmer J, Mannis M, and Holland E *(eds)*. CORNEA, Fundamentals, Diagnosis and Management. 2nd Ed. 2005. Philadelphia: Elsevier Mosby. (Singal N, Rootman D). Ch. 51. (Stolar GL, *et al. eds*). Ch. 6

divided into primary, secondary and coincidental co-morbid conditions. Crohn's disease and IBS are discussed as co-morbid conditions in corneal disease. Rheumatoid arthritis is identified as a co-morbid condition.[261] Arthritis has long been "associated" with chlamydia trachoma—the most important pathogen in blinding eye diseases. CORNEA, *Fundamentals, Diagnosis and Management* discusses neutrophil dysfunction, the type of immune cell that attacks H-pylori and chlamydia psittacosis; and discusses endothelial dysfunction, which is caused by chlamydia species; but fails to recognize immortal infections have infected the immune cells and caused the neutrophil dysfunction and endothelial dysfunction. CORNEA, *Fundamentals, Diagnosis and Management* fails to recognize the same immortal infections are causing the eye disease, stomach disease, and arthritis; and causing the cellular and tissue changes identified as various eye diseases.

We have a critical gap in eye care as it relates to immortal pathogens causing eye disease, because no eye care specialty is trained to diagnose and treat the immortal infections and parasites causing chronic eye diseases. Ophthalmology has a narrow focus; and is not concerned with knowledge in other ophthalmology sub-specialties, other medical specialties, or the knowledge of veterinarians. Ophthalmologists are not seeking to understand why chronic eye diseases are occurring, or trying to curb eye disease at an earlier stage. No one asks why a community would have a higher rate of particular eye diseases, or tries to identify a vector for the increased rate of eye diseases in a community. An ophthalmologist may be brilliant in eye surgery; but unable to shift their focus from surgery to using medical diagnosis and treatment for eye diseases, or reasoning to discern the cause of the eye diseases treated in ophthalmology. Ophthalmologists approach eye diseases with, "it's there, let's treat it"; and the options are drops, surgery and lasers.

The vast majority of ophthalmologists are not aware chronic immortal intracellular pathogens from animals are a cause of eye disease; and do not consider immortal pathogens in diagnosing eye disease. None of the ophthalmology specialties are trained in a medical approach to eye

---

[261] *Id.* Juvenile Arthritis. (Tauber J). Ch. 116.

disease; and few are trained or have comprehensive knowledge of immortal infections and parasites in eye diseases. They do not take a history of contact with pets and domesticated animals, even when the risk from animals is reported in ophthalmology texts. Ophthalmologists do not consider co-morbid conditions as clues to the infectious causes of eye diseases, do not understand co-morbid conditions are caused by the same pathogens as the eye disease, and do not consider co-managing patients with primary care physicians who are able to diagnose and treat immortal infections. Ophthalmologists need to recognize chronic infection causes eye disease, and establish co-management relationships with knowledgeable primary care doctors who are able to diagnose and treat immortal infections that are outside the scope of ophthalmology.

Primary care doctors have little interest in eye diseases, and are even afraid to diagnose and treat eye disease; thus, refer all patients with eye complaints to an ophthalmologist. Optometrists are not medical doctors and are not physicians, even though called "doctor". Medicare refers to optometrists as "optometric physicians" so they can be paid when co-managing cataract patients with ophthalmologists. Optometrists scope of practice in limited to vision correction, and the diagnosis and treatment of some eye diseases, with prescription drops. Optometrists tend to prescribe broad-spectrum and combination antibiotic drops, as a shot-gun treatment for eye infections. Optometrists have no training in surgery, including refractive surgery; and are not trained in immortal infection or systemic diseases. Optometrists perform preoperative screening and post-operative care for refractive surgery patients, without adequate training and knowledge to do so; or based on misguided training, administered by vested interests, and demands for a high approval rate.

Ophthalmology cannot solve the mysteries of eye disease, because ophthalmologists do not diagnose immortal pathogens; the research questions into infectious causes of eye disease are framed too narrowly; or the answer lies outside their specialty. Research asked the question, "Does chlamydia pneumonia cause glaucoma?" The outcome of the study is only one third of the patients have positive chlamydia pneumonia PCR tests, so it is called an "association". The researcher moves on to the next study and asks, "Does chlamydia trachoma cause glaucoma?" Only one third of the patients are positive for chlamydia trachoma. The researcher does another study and starts with the question, "Does H-pylori cause glaucoma?" Only one third of the patients have H-pylori, so again it is called an "association". The researchers are unwilling to state causation, to avoid potential criticism or any accusation of a non-scientific conclusion. No one takes as step back to look at bigger questions or asks, "What infections do the patients have in glaucoma?" No one asks, "What co-morbid conditions do patients have with glaucoma, and are they caused by the same pathogen causing the glaucoma?" The research seldom proceeds to determine if treatment of the pathogens helped the glaucoma; and conclusions helpful to diagnosis and treatment seldom reach the front-line practitioner. No one says to the front-line practitioner to go forth and treat!

Ophthalmologists should focus on diagnosis of infectious causes of eye disease. Ophthalmologists need to engage in preventive medicine; and stop focusing on end stage of eye disease; and treatment with expensive, uncomfortable, and sometimes harmful drops, injections, lasers and surgeries. Oral and topical azithromycin are the standard treatment for eye diseases across the world, and have significantly reduced the rates of blindness, in Africa. Doxycycline is recognized as treatment for patients with eye disease and rosacea. Observation and wisdom guided therapy throughout the world, proves treatment of chronic infections in the eye can cure eye diseases and prevent blindness.

Vision Correction, the Normal Eye, and Learning to Read

The most common reason for patients to see an eye care professional is to get a refraction (prescription) for glasses or contact lenses. Clear vision is determined by anatomy—the shape of the cornea, the clarity of the natural lens, and the distance between the cornea and the retina. The cornea should be a smooth dome, which is not too steep or too flat, has no uncorrectable irregularities (higher order aberrations), and has no unusual areas of thinning or bulging. The shape of the cornea determines where light focuses in the back of the eye, and if the focus is on the macula, in front or behind the macula, or at two points behind the eye. When the cornea has a very irregular surface with multiple focal points, regular glasses will not correct vision, and contact lenses may be needed for best vision.

Glasses and contact lenses adjust where the images coming through the cornea and pupil focus on the retina, to adjust the focal point onto the macula. When the focal point is in front or behind the macula, the patient is nearsighted or farsighted, and has blurry vision. Myopia is the ability to see near but not far. Hyperopia is the ability to see far but not near. When a person has two focal points the patient has astigmatism, which causes double vision or distorted vision.

Presbyopia is the need for reading glasses in middle age, which are needed when the zonules become stiff and the lens no longer adjusts as needed to see near. Myopia, hyperopia, astigmatism and presbyopia are not a disease!

Snellen Visual Acuity is a crude measure of visual acuity, first developed during the Civil War. Snellen Visual Acuity measures acuity or blur—specifically how well a person sees black images on a white background, at a distance of twenty feet. The ability to read a Snellen chart is only one component of good vision, and people can read a Snellen chart with impaired quality of vision. Quality of vision is important in activities of daily life, and has as many as twenty components, including vision at all distances, vision in all lighting, contrast sensitivity, glare, distortion, multiple images, ghosting, depth perception, color vision, sun sensitivity, night vision, vision fluctuation, binocularity (the eyes work together), visual field, and comfort.

Vision impacts a child's ability to read successfully. The failure to acquire the ability to read in early grades leads to reduced self-esteem, adverse social consequences among peers, and development of adaptive personality disorders. Successful reading requires binocularity (both eyes work together), without deviation in either eye. A fixed gaze that gives the ability to maintain focus to scan smoothly across a line on a page. A child's lack of binocularity or deviation in gaze may be too small to be noticed by an eye care professional; yet significant enough to impact reading.

Several visual tools are available to help the child who has difficulty learning to read. First, children in kindergarten through second grade should have class contests staring at each other, trying not to blink. The winner will likely be the best reader in the class. The contest is fun and helps develop the fixed gaze necessary to successfully read. Second, the child should be checked for any deviation in the direction of gaze, in either eye, no matter how small, including an evaluation for amblyopia or lazy eye and lack of binocularity. Any child with a minor deviation in gaze in one or both eyes and a reading problem should be prescribed the most expensive lenses available in their glasses. The newest computer-generated glasses allow clear vision across the entire lens, and not just at one focal point, which can compensate for minor eye deviations, and improve a child's ability to read. Third, no matter the age, any child having difficulty reading should complete the EyeQ program. The EyeQ computer program was initially developed to improve reading speed; but works well for children who are having difficulty reading, by strengthening eye muscles, improving fixed gaze, and improving smooth scanning across the page, using fun computer games.

Chronic Eye Diseases

The average thickness of a healthy central cornea is approximately 550 microns (mcns), which is slightly more than half a millimeter. By comparison, a credit card is 700 mcns thick. The center of the cornea should be the thinnest point, and corneal thickness should uniformly increase toward the periphery. The cornea of a person who has a central corneal thickness of 520 mcns may be normal, or an early sign of a corneal thinning disease. The cornea of a person who has central corneal thickness of 580 mcns may be normal; or a sign of swelling and dehydration over the course of a day, and an evolving corneal thinning disease. Thick corneas can be healthy, or caused by failing corneal endothelium, which causes swelling in the cornea, and causes the cornea to be measured thicker. Rigid contact wear can thin the cornea; and toric contacts for astigmatism can cause thinning inferiorly, because the weighted bottom of a toric contact lens can rock back and forth, leaving a skirt pattern of thinning on the inferior cornea.

The age at which a child first needs glasses is an important clue to the diagnosis of corneal thinning diseases. Most children need vision correction for myopia (see near but not far) in elementary school, after someone notices the child cannot see the board in the front of the class. The child's myopic refractions may change every year or two, until the child is grown. Once the child is grown, the vision should remain stable for decades; until reading glasses are necessary in middle age. Some children in the early grades may have perfect vision or be hyperopic (see far but not near), and as the child grows the hyperopia will disappear and the child will not need glasses.

When a person has a corneal thinning disease, the person does not need glasses until their late teens or early twenties, and thereafter requires frequent changes in their refractions for distance or astigmatism, over the next two decades. The refraction may increase or decrease, the astigmatism may increase, and the refractive error in the eyes may become more different from one another, causing difficulty in depth perception. The late onset need for glasses, then changing refractions, indicates the shape of the cornea is changing to become steeper and/or more irregular; and suggests the patient has an immortal infection attacking the surface of the eye.

Corneal "thinning disease" is a description of a symptom or finding. Keratoconus is a catch-all term used to refer generally to five different types of corneal thinning diseases, including keratoconus, pellucid margin degeneration, keratoglobulus, endothelial dystrophy, and Fuchs corneal dystrophy. The family of corneal thinning diseases are characterized by endothelial dysfunction, thinning of the cornea, and an abnormal corneal shape. Corneal thinning diseases cause high spots and thin spots on the cornea, with decentered thinness and bulging in the thin spots. Corneal thinning diseases may start on the front surface or on the underside of the cornea. The initial attack on the ocular surface or underside of the cornea, and type of thinning and steepening pattern, determines which thinning disease is diagnosed. Corneal thinning diseases are often preceded by an eye infection and inflammation, and by endothelial dysfunction causing edema and artificially thick corneas.

Keratoconus is a thinning disease in which the cornea is steepening and thinning; and bulging forward in a cone shape, causing high spots called a "cone". The process of corneal regeneration may initially cause variable epithelial thickness, which conceals an early "cone". The eye passively smooths an irregular surface, making the epithelium thicker in low spots and thinner in high spots. The regularity or irregularity of the surface is measured by corneal topography. Keratoconus beginning on the posterior cornea, the endothelium of the cornea, can be seen on corneal topography.

Corneal thinning diseases are caused by immortal pathogens. When the epithelium is irregular, or the surface is loose, it may be H-pylori. When the cornea has signs of endothelial dysfunction, on the posterior surface, it is likely caused by chlamydia pneumonia. Band keratopathy and pellucid margin degeneration are inferior corneal surface abnormalities, caused by infection or traumatic injury from toric contact lenses, or chlamydia trachoma. When two chronic infections, one attacking epithelium, and burrowing deeper to destroy Bowman's membrane and attach to collagen; and one attacking endothelium and migrating upward to destroy Descemet's membrane, the pathogens will synergistically accelerate thinning diseases. Invasion of immortal pathogens into the collagen and stroma of the cornea causes loss of hydration, inflammation, and stromal thinning. When the thinning disease is advanced the patient can form hydrops, which are fluid bubbles that develop deeper in the corneal layers and pop, causing pain and cloudiness in the cornea. The bubbles are an indication the infection has penetrated the epithelium or the endothelium; and any effect on tissue involving bubbles should include testing for H-pylori and streptococcal pathogens. H-pylori and streptococcus can cause bubbles.

In 2014, scientists discovered patients with mitral valve prolapse had a significantly higher rate of keratoconus.[262] The authors described both mitral valve prolapse and keratoconus as "idiopathic" non-inflammatory conditions, meaning they do not know the cause and cannot explain the cause beyond it is something unique about the patient. The co-morbid

---

[262] Akcay E, *et al*. 2014. Impaired Corneal Biomechanical Properties and the Prevalence of Keratoconus in Mitral Valve Prolapse. Journal of Ophthalmology. Vol 2014. Article ID 402193. Doi: https://dx.doi.org/10.1155/2014/402193.

finding of mitral-valve prolapse and corneal thinning disease support a common infectious cause of the mitral-valve prolapse and corneal thinning disease, and a possible relationship to streptococcal infections known to cause mitral-valve prolapse. Chlamydia pathogens are also known to damage the heart, and the mitral valve; and chlamydia has been found in tissue from resected mitral valves. It may be chlamydia pneumonia, chlamydia trachoma, chlamydia psittacosis, H-pylori, or sub-clinical streptococcus-M; or a combination of pathogens causing corneal thinning disease.

Ophthalmologists do not understand corneal thinning diseases; thus, blame patients with keratoconus for rubbing their eyes, alleging eye rubbing is damaging the collagen structure and changing the shape of the cornea. Eye rubbing is one method to self-inoculate pathogens into the eye, which can cause thinning diseases. Patients rub their eyes to relieve symptoms of itching and irritation, which may contribute to contour abnormalities on the ocular surface; but eye rubbing is not the reason patients develop thinning diseases and abnormally shaped corneas. Chronic infection causes both the eye rubbing and corneal thinning disease. Eye allergies—it is marketing! An allergy is a default diagnosis that should not be used until infectious causes have been excluded. Moreover, allergies have also been "associated" with chlamydia pneumonia.

Fuchs Corneal Dystrophy is in the family of thinning diseases, first named by an Austrian ophthalmologist, Dr. Ernst Fuchs (1851-1930). During the 1920's, Drs. Kraupa, Vogt, Graves and Fridenwalds proved Fuch's Corneal Dystrophy was an endothelial disease. In 1925, Dr. Fridenwalds told the New York Academy of Medicine that Fuchs endothelial changes preceded epithelial changes, and that Fuchs dystrophy may be the late sequel to a "deeper affliction". Fuchs Corneal Dystrophy, also called Fuchs Endothelial Dystrophy, is defined by endothelial dysfunction, just as chlamydia pneumonia is defined by endothelial dysfunction. The first signs of Fuchs Corneal Dystrophy are blurry vision in the morning, followed by profuse watering of the eyes. The cornea swells and becomes thick at night, and the eye waters profusely in the morning as the swelling subsides. As the disease progresses the patient develops a thin cornea and reduced vision, from the ebb and flow of swelling, the spread of the pathogen, and inflammation. The endothelial dysfunction in Fuch's dystrophy is caused by chlamydia pneumonia, which is well-known to cause endothelial dysfunction, in tissue throughout the body.

No refractive surgery should ever be done on a patient with a corneal thinning disease. LASIK cuts and weakens the cornea, and removes tissue, further thinning and weakening the cornea. PRK surgery may be suggested by refractive surgeons for patients who have a thin cornea, deemed too thin to have LASIK; and the doctor does not recognize early keratoconus, or seeks to provide any refractive surgery the doctor can justify, rather than warn the patient of the true nature and risks arising from a possible thinning disease. After PRK the thinnest point of the cornea is even more weakened, Bowman's membrane is destroyed and no longer protects the stroma, and the epithelium has to regrow in an abnormal pattern to re-smooth the corneal surface. If PRK is recommended, it is a *per se* admission the patient is not a good candidate for any refractive surgery.

Pterygium are an abnormal lesion on the sclera, which is the white surface of the eye. Pterygium are caused by infection, and surgery to remove pterygium often makes the pterygium worse. Antibiotics used during and after surgery can treat the infection but can also cause the pathogen to become more antibiotic resistant. The pterygium can return in an even more aggressive form. A surgeon cannot easily cut out an infection, and surgery on any infection creates a high risk the infection will spread to new tissue or return. Patients with pterygium should be treated with antibiotics eye drops and ointment, as needed; and if drops and ointment are not sufficient, and surgery is required, it should be in conjunction with antibiotic drops and medications, before and after the pterygium surgery.

Blepharitis is when the eyelid margin is inflamed and not producing sufficient fluid or poor-quality fluid, necessary to mix with other eye fluids and maintain the health of the corneal surface. Fluid produced by the eye is a natural barrier to a corneal infection. Blepharitis is not a diagnosis, it is a description of inflammation, labeled as "itis". Blepharitis is a chronic infection of the eyelid margin, and a common cause of chronic dry eye. Blepharitis may be dismissed as unimportant or a mild irritation; however, chronic dry eye can lead to vision problems, vision fluctuation, less resistance to infection on the ocular surface, and make contact lens wear difficult. Chronic blepharitis can cause ocular surface disease; and shed pathogens across the cornea from the base of the eyelashes, which can invade the cornea if the epithelium is damaged. Blepharitis may be caused by a number of different pathogens, including H-pylori, chlamydia pneumonia or chlamydia trachoma; or may be caused by from p-acnes, a type of bacteria that lives on the skin and can become pathogenic when it invades an anaerobic environment, at the base of the eyelashes. Blepharitis predisposes a patient to thinning diseases, and other ocular surface diseases, by making the ocular surface more hospitable to pathogens and less protected by healthy fluid.

Women are particularly prone to blepharitis and "dry eye syndrome" because women wear eye make-up. Eye make-up presents a risk to eye health, particularly mascara or any eye make-up containing sparkles or powder. Sparkle and powder are indigestible materials, and the immune system will create an inclusion or scar tissue around the indigestible particles. Ophthalmologists do not warn eye make-up can transfer infection to the base of the eye lashes, and cause chronic blepharitis and dry eye.[263] Patients with any ocular surface disease should stop wearing all eye make-up.

No eye make-up has ever been tested for safety! The FDA is required to monitor cosmetics; however, a grandfather clause, in the Food Drug and Cosmetic Act, of 1938, allowed all cosmetics already on the market to remain on the market, without testing for safety. Any new eye make-up is approved under the grandfather clause, without testing for safety, based on substantial equivalency to cosmetics which were sold, prior to 1938.

Cataracts is considered a disease of aging. Cataracts is when the natural lens inside the eye becomes cloudy. Cataracts has three major forms—posterior

---

[263] *See* Wang M, *et al.* 2018. Investigating the Effect of Eye Cosmetics on the Tear Film: Current Insights. Clinical Optometry. 2018. 10: 33-40. Doi: doi.org/10.2147/OPTO.S150926.

sub-capsular cataracts (lens becomes cloudy), cortical cataracts (spokes of cloudy material move from the periphery of the lens toward the center), and nuclear sclerotic cataracts (yellowing of the lens caused by long-term sun exposure). In cataract surgery, the front of the posterior capsule around the lens is removed to allow removal of the natural lens, and a clear manufactured intraocular lens is implanted inside in the posterior capsule. Excess tension on the retina during cataract surgery can cause a horseshoe shaped retinal tear.

After cataract surgery, the back portion of the capsule can become cloudy, reducing vision, and ophthalmologists perform YAG laser surgery to remove a portion of the cloudy capsule from behind the lens. After a YAG laser surgery, the posterior capsule is open in front and behind the implanted intraocular lens; and the posterior capsule no longer separates the front and back of the eye. YAG laser surgery increases the risk of retinal detachment by four-hundred percent; and forty-percent of all retinal detachments occur in post-cataract surgery patients.

Premature cataracts is when cataracts develops in a younger patient. Premature cataracts are "associated" with chronic chlamydia pneumonia. Patients with multiple chronic infections, and people who have had refractive surgery, are more likely to develop premature cataracts. When cataract surgery is done on younger patients, the long-term risk of sight-threatening complications is greater; because the patient has more years to live after the surgery, in which to develop complications from the cataract surgery. The younger cataract patient is more likely to need YAG laser surgery, and has more years in which to develop a retinal detachment. Whether cataracts in the elderly or premature cataracts could be prevented or delayed by treatment of chronic infections is unknown, and could be the subject of further research and meta-analysis.

Occasionally, babies are born with cataracts or found to have cataracts shortly after birth. The ophthalmologists' solution is to operate on the infant and implant a manufactured intraocular lens, to improve vision and prevent developmental delays. If an infant or child has premature cataracts, the child and parents should be tested for immortal infections, particularly chlamydia pneumonia. Cataracts in young dogs have been treated and cured by treating inflammation and chronic infection, in the eye, suggesting premature cataracts and cataracts occurring in infants could be similarly treated prior to defaulting to surgery on the eyes of an infant or to delay the need for the first eye surgery. Even if treatment gives only temporary improvement, it could allow the child to grow before the first eye surgery and reduce the total number of eye surgeries needed, in the child's lifetime.

"Clear lens extraction" is cataract surgery done for refractive purposes, on a healthy eye. Clear lens extraction is a dangerous choice for younger patients, because younger patients have many years to develop complications from cataract surgery; may develop other eye diseases in the future, which are complicated by the intraocular lens implant. In younger patients, the risk of needing a YAG laser surgery is greater, which increases the risk of retinal detachment and sight-threatening complications, in their lifetime. If a patient subsequently develops other eye diseases, such as cataracts, glaucoma, or retinal disease, the intraocular lens is a complicating factor making it more difficult to successfully treat the eye diseases. If the refraction changes in the ensuing years, the only choice is to return to glasses or contacts, or have another surgery. The clear lens extraction patient will likely need additional surgeries in their lifetime that can subject the patient to sight-threatening complications, as the patient ages.

Glaucoma is an eye disease in which the intraocular pressure becomes high enough to damage the optic nerve, and cause a measureable loss of peripheral vision. Ocular hypertension is thought to be a precursor to glaucoma. Ocular hypertension is high intraocular pressure, without damage to the optic nerve or loss of peripheral vision. Glaucoma and ocular hypertension are descriptions of a finding of high intraocular pressure, damage to the optic nerve, and visual field loss—not a diagnosis of the cause of glaucoma or ocular hypertension.

Glaucoma has five or more forms, each describing the findings observed in the patient. The most common form of glaucoma is "primary open angle glaucoma" (POAG). In POAG, the intraocular pressure is high, but the anterior chamber angle remains open. POAG is a description of high intraocular pressure, without an objective explanation. High titers of chlamydia pneumonia have been associated with POAG, without systemic disease.[264] POAG is caused by endothelial dysfunction in the anterior chamber angle, which is caused by chlamydia pneumonia. A second type of glaucoma is closed angle glaucoma, which is when sticky material and scarring close or partially close the anterior chamber angle, reducing the ability of the eye to control intraocular pressure. Chlamydia trachoma and H-pylori can attack epithelium, clog the anterior chamber angle, and cause sticky residue, creating closed or partially closed angles.

A third type of glaucoma is pigment dispersion glaucoma, which is when iris particles disperse into the anterior chamber angle, clogging the angle, and causing high intraocular pressure. Toxoplasmosis can attack the iris, and cause disintegration of the iris and pigment dispersion into the anterior chamber angle. A fourth type of glaucoma is inflammatory glaucoma, which is a description of inflammation in the eye thought to be causing high pressure. Infections in the eye with one or more immortal pathogens can cause inflammatory glaucoma and/or mixed glaucoma. A fifth type of glaucoma is mixed glaucoma, which is when the patient has more than one type of glaucoma.

Different types of glaucoma may be caused by different pathogens and by different mechanisms. Chlamydia pathogens that have been "associated" with glaucoma include chlamydia pneumonia, chlamydia trachoma, and chlamydia psittacosis. H-pylori has also been "associated" with POAG. H-pylori has been found in the aqueous humor of patients with POAG,

---

[264] Yuki K, *et al*. 2010. Elevated Serum Immunoglobulin G Titers Against Chlamydia Pneumoniae In Primary Open-Angle Glaucoma Patients Without Systemic Disease. J Glaucoma. Oct-Nov 2010. 19(8): 535-9. Doi: 10.1097/IJG.0b013e3181ca7868.

and reported to be strongly "associated" with it, and may be a cause of glaucoma.[265]

Glaucoma can be caused by more than one pathogen or parasite that migrates inside the eye and into the anterior chamber angle, damaging the ability of the eye to maintain pressure control. Chlamydia pneumonia can migrate or metastasize to the anterior chamber angle, and damage endothelial function. The reduced endothelial function in the anterior chamber angle impairs the pumping of fluid in and out of the eye, and causes loss of control of intraocular pressure and POAG. Chlamydia trachoma and psittacosis damage the cell functioning in the anterior chamber angle, and clog the drainage system with sticky material and debris; and can damage the epithelium or endothelium. H-pylori damages epithelium on the surface of the eye, the iris, the anterior chamber angle, and the retina. When H-pylori migrates into the anterior chamber of the eye, H-pylori damages epithelial function, causing glaucoma. Toxoplasmosis can attack the iris, causing disintegration of the iris and pigment dispersion glaucoma. Any or all of the pathogens, alone or in combination, can cause inflammatory glaucoma and mixed glaucoma.

The cause glaucoma is not known, in part because ophthalmologists are not looking for infectious causes. Ophthalmologists do not diagnose immortal chronic infections by PCR testing, treat glaucoma as an infection, or refer patients for diagnosis and treatment of systemic chronic infection. Even when research reveals an infection is "associated" with a glaucoma, the research seldom moves to treatment of the infection, in animals or humans, to determine the benefit of treatment. The most famous ophthalmology researcher, in Japan, published infection was "associated" with glaucoma. He was contacted to ask if he tried treating any of the patients in his study, based on his findings. The answer was "no", he went on to the

---

[265] Deshpande N, *et al.* 2008. Helicobacter Pylori IgG Antibodies in Aqueous Humor and Serum of Subjects With Primary Open Angle and Pseudo-Exfoliation Glaucoma In A South Indian Population. J Glaucoma. Dec 2008. 17(8):605-10. Doi: 10.1097/IJG.0b013e318166f00b. PMID. 19092454; Kountouras J, *et al.* 2001. Relationship Between Helicobactor Pylori Infection and Glaucoma. Ophthalmology. Mar 2001. 108(3): 599-604. PMID: 11237916. Doi: https://doi.org.10.1016/S0161-6420(00)00598-4.

next research project. Subsequent researchers showed glaucoma patients benefited from treatment of immortal infections; but the information has not filtered down to the routine practice of "glaucoma specialists".

More than twenty-five articles have "associated" both H-pylori and chlamydia pneumonia to glaucoma; and despite the abundance of literature supporting infectious causes of glaucoma, the entire Atlas of Glaucoma failed to mention chlamydia, H-pylori or other immortal pathogens, in the discussion of glaucoma.[266]

Treatment of glaucoma is symptomatic reduction of intraocular pressure with drops; use of lasers to make holes in the iris, to relieve pressure; surgery to reduce intraocular pressure; and surgical implantation of glaucoma devices, to control pressure. Glaucoma devices have a high five-year failure rate, can make the patient worse, and can cause corneal damage from touch on the underside of the cornea, leading to blindness and even enucleation. Glaucoma specialists should shift the focus to identifying the pathogens causing glaucoma, and effective treatment of chronic infections in the eye; and not rely solely on descriptions of the types of glaucoma and symptomatic reduction in intraocular pressure, using drops, lasers, surgery and implantable devices.

The Atlas of CLINICAL OPHTHALMOLOGY discusses glaucoma and its pathogenesis.[267] The text described the pathogenesis of POAG as an abnormal composition of the extracellular matrix, changes in the endothelium of the trabecular meshwork, cells in the cytoskeleton, and accelerated cell death and collapse of the trabecular beams.[268] In angle closure glaucoma, the pathogenesis is described as a cellular problem, with neovascularization (rubeotic glaucoma), endothelial dysfunction, and epithelialization of the anterior chamber.[269] Pigment dispersion glaucoma

---

[266] Choplin N, Traverso C (*eds*). 2014. Atlas of Glaucoma, 3rd Edition. Boca Raton, FL: CRC Press.

[267] Spatin D, *et al.* (*eds*). 2005. Atlas of CLINICAL OPHTHALMOLOGY. 3rd Ed. Elsevier Limited. Primary Glaucoma. (Garway-Heath D, Foster P, and Hitchings R). Ch. 7. p. 187-220.

[268] *Id. @* 192.

[269] *Id. @* 233.

is described as a generalized basement membrane disorder; and fails to mention toxoplasmosis, H-pylori, or other infectious pathogens as a cause of disintegration of the iris and pigment dispersion.[270] The descriptions of the pathogenesis of glaucoma describes findings not causes; however, the descriptions do confirm numerous types of immortal pathogens cause glaucoma. The description of the pathogenesis of glaucoma coincides with the effects of chlamydia pneumonia, H-pylori, toxoplasmosis, and other immortal chlamydia pathogens, which attack the endothelium or epithelium, damage the collagen matrix, impair normal apoptosis, and cause angiogenesis (formation of new blood vessels).

Low-pressure glaucoma is damage to the optic nerve and loss of peripheral vision, in an eye with normal intraocular pressure. Low pressure glaucoma is not true glaucoma. Thyroid eye disease causes swelling behind the eye, compression of the optic nerve, and loss of visual field which appears identical to the damage and visual field loss in glaucoma. Thyroid disease is a common co-morbid condition in eye diseases and low-pressure glaucoma, but is not part of the specialty of ophthalmology. Low thyroid can cause ocular surface disease, including dry eyes; and high thyroid can cause swelling in the soft tissue behind the eye, compressing the optic nerve, and causing the eyes to bulge forward. Lowering pressure in low pressure glaucoma does not stop optic nerve compression behind the eye, and surgery to relieve optic nerve compression is a drastic neurosurgery. The pathogens causing low pressure glaucoma may include H-pylori, which is also likely causing the thyroid disease. Attack on the pathogens causing thyroid disease may help in the treatment of low pressure glaucoma.

Surgery on the eye presents a higher risk to patients with thyroid disorders. Anti-thyroid antibodies and inflammatory cells attack the eye through an open portal at surgery. Invasion of anti-thyroid antibodies and cytokines (inflammatory markers) cause inflammation and periorbital swelling in and around the eye, setting off the cascade of thyroid eye disease and thyroid orbitopathy (periorbital swelling causing the eye to bulge), and compression on the optic nerve. Surgery on either eye can cause prolonged periorbital swelling, and damage to the surgical eye and the fellow eye,

---

[270] *Id.* @ 243.

damaging the optic nerves from swelling behind the eye, and transient rises in intraocular pressure. Patients with thyroid disease and thyroid eye disease are particularly susceptible to steroid-induced elevation in intraocular pressure; and treatment with steroids during and after surgery, can cause elevated intraocular pressure in the treated and fellow eye, worsening optic nerve damage.

A leading thyroid eye disease researcher wrote numerous publications over the course of a decade, describing thyroid eye disease, at a cellular level. He reported thyroid inflammatory markers and cytokines, including anti-thyroid antibodies, matched the lock and key mechanism in the eye; and when cytokines and inflammatory markers invade the eye it causes thyroid eye disease and thyroid orbitopathy. Ten years after he began publishing his research, he wrote a review article of his own published articles, citing himself almost fifty times, for the proposition his ten years of research confirmed his initial hypothesis that thyroid antibodies matched the lock and key mechanism in the eye and cause thyroid eye disease. No doubt his research is correct at a cellular level, but why did it happen? Cellular explanations about CD40 and CD154, and cytokines do not explain a root cause of thyroid eye disease. The researcher did not consider infectious causes of inflammation and the cytokines that attacked the eye. H-pylori is associated with both CD40 and CD154, the same Cluster Differentiations reported to be attacking the eye in thyroid eye disease. H-pylori can attack the thyroid, and the thyroid antibodies attacking the eye may actually be antibodies to H-pylori. H-pylori can cause thyroid disease and thyroid eye disease.

Despite the absence of discussion, in CORNEA, *Fundamentals, Diagnosis and Management*, and the Atlas of Glaucoma; and the limited discussion in Atlas of CLINICAL OPHTHALMOLOGY. which devolved into a discussion of symptoms, findings, and syndromes, ophthalmology literature and texts support infectious causes of many chronic eye diseases. The microbiology literature for chlamydia and H-pylori support infectious causes of eye diseases, based on known targets of the pathogens and tissue damage caused by the pathogens. Ophthalmology literature supports infection can migrate from one part of the eye to another. Atlas of <u>CLINICAL OPHTHALMOLOGY</u> warns cats and dogs can transmit pathogens that cause eye disease. Yet, ophthalmologists cannot accept infection can penetrate the cornea to damage the inner layers of the cornea; migrate to the inside of the eye, causing more damage; and reach the retina and inner layers of the retina. They do not inquire into a history of contact with animals. They do not consider immortal pathogens in chronic eye disease—they are surgeons.

Age related macular degeneration (AMD) is the most common cause of vision impairment in developed countries. The macula is the central point on the retina, and sends signals to the brain through the optic nerve. The macula provides the central and most clear vision, in the visual field. Macular degeneration can be dry macular degeneration (no bleeding of the vessels in the back of the eye), or wet macular degeneration (bleeding from vessels in the back of the eye). When vessels bleed in the back of the eye, dry macular degeneration becomes wet macular degeneration. Macular degeneration can eventually cause loss of central vision. Late stage AMD includes neovascularization and blood vessels on the retina that are fragile and can bleed into the back of the eye, cause separation of retinal layers, and a retinal detachment. Chlamydia pneumonia, H-pylori, and CMV have been correlated with the wet form of macular degeneration; and the "association" has been made between H-pylori and ICSR (idiopathic central serous chorioretinopathy).[271] Scientists recently linked chlamydia pneumonia to AMD, but still "remain cautious".

Macular degeneration is a cardiovascular disease in the retinal vessels, causing a restriction in blood supply to the macula. Chlamydia pneumonia causes narrowing of the vessels in the eye and plaque, reducing blood supply to the macula; and causes angiogenesis during the infectious cascade. Patients with macular degeneration have co-morbid heart disease, cardiovascular disease high cholesterol, and high blood pressure. Patients with macular degeneration have an increased risk of myocardial infarction, because heart disease and macular degeneration are both caused

---

[271] Camelo S. 2014. Potential Sources and Roles of Adaptive Immunity in Age-Related Macular Degeneration: Shall we Rename AMD into Autoimmune Macular Disease? Review Article. Autoimmune Diseases. Vol 2014. Doi: doi.org/10.1155/2014/532487.

by chlamydia pneumonia, which causes endothelial dysfunction in blood vessels in the cardiovascular system and in the eye.

AMD and Alzheimer's are common co-morbid conditions. Chlamydia pneumonia causes plaque in the vessels of the eye, just as chlamydia pneumonia causes plaque in the heart, just as chlamydia pneumonia causes plaque in the brain. People at risk for Alzheimer's disease are at twice the risk for falls, due to visual spatial abnormalities, including reduced visual acuity, spatial sensitivity, motion perception, contrast sensitivity, visual field, depth perception, and color discrimination. Poor vision and falls cause Alzheimer's patients to seek help from an ophthalmologist.

Alzheimer's disease can be predicted, diagnosed, and monitored, with a retinal scan, based on the degree of damage to the retinal vessels in the back of the eye. Researchers examined pictures of retinal vessels to detect Alzheimer's; and found the vessels in the back of the eye had the same level of plaque as the Alzheimer's brain. Physicians in Germany are working to develop diagnostic testing for Alzheimer's by looking in the patient's eyes; and it has been hypothesized a high-quality image of retinal vessels could diagnose Alzheimer's twenty years before the disease develops. Another scientist found the width of certain blood vessels on the retina were significantly different in people with early Alzheimer's, as compared to healthy controls. The blood vessels on the retina had plaque deposits of beta amyloid, an Alzheimer's related protein, similar to those in the brain of Alzheimer's patients. A retinal scan is an easier and cheaper method for early detection of Alzheimer's, and can predict Alzheimer's decades before development of Alzheimer's. A retinal scan and a PCR blood test for chlamydia pathogens, and for chlamydia pneumonia in particular, could predict Alzheimer's with even greater specificity and determine which patients would most benefit by early treatment.

The rate of macular degeneration is reported to be decreasing in the population, most likely because of increased usage of macrolide antibiotics. Treatment with macrolide antibiotics could delay the development of macular degeneration, and prevent progression to wet macular degeneration. If cardiologists, ophthalmologists and other specialties recognize and treat chlamydia pneumonia early in the course of acute and chronic disease, other chronic diseases like macular degeneration, heart disease, heart attack, stroke, Alzheimer's, arthritis, and multiple sclerosis, which are caused by chlamydia pathogens, could potentially be prevented, delayed, or reduced in severity.

Chlamydia pneumonia can cause strokes in the eye, blocking the blood supply to the optic nerve, by the same mechanism chlamydia pneumonia causes strokes in the cardiovascular system or the brain. In ophthalmology, a stroke in the eye is named NAION (non-arteric anterior ischemic optic neuropathy), or AION (anterior ischemic optic neuropathy), a description of restricted blood flow to the optic nerve caused by a clot. Patients *with* NAION were found to have higher levels of chlamydia pneumonia IgG titers.[272] Vein or artery occlusions in the eye are mini-strokes, caused by clots in small vessels of the eye, caused by chlamydia pneumonia and inclusion cysts or plaque. New blood vessels start to grow in the back of the eye, as chlamydia generates angiogenesis and the body tries to restore blood flow around the stroke blockage.

Medical practice for wet macular degeneration and vessel occlusion (stroke) in the eye, is injections in the eye, directed at stopping new blood vessels from growing on the retina, and preventing new fragile blood vessels from bleeding. The injections in the eye are with Avastin or Lucentis. Patients are given injections of anti-vessel growth drugs every month, for wet macular degeneration, and more frequently for retinal vein occlusions. Any disease which includes increased vascular growth factors and increased angiogenesis, is caused by chlamydia pneumonia. If ophthalmologists insist on injections, perhaps oral treatment or injections directed at the immortal infection in the eye should also be considered. Any patient with cardiovascular disease and macular degeneration should be treated with long-term azithromycin, which can improve the prognosis for the disease and delay loss of vision.

---

[272] Weger M, *et al*. 2002. Chlamydia pneumoniae Seropositivity and the Risk of Nonarteritic Ischemic Optic Neuropathy, Ophthalmology. 2002. 109:749-752. Doi: doi.org/10.1016/S0161-6420(02)-1031-4.

Avastin was developed for gastrointestinal cancers, based on the theory stopping blood vessels to the cancer would kill or slow the growth of cancer. Avastin was incorporated into ophthalmology by compounding pharmacies, which diluted the Avastin into smaller units in prefilled injections, and sold the pre-filled injections for "off-label" for treatment of AMD and vessel blockage. Lucentis is an anti-vessel growth drug, approved for treatment of AMD and vessel blockage, which has smaller molecules than Avastin and is more compatible with the eye. The most recent drug approval for Lucentis makes the connection between endothelial dysfunction and vessel growth on the retina, in macular degeneration, which supports chlamydia pneumonia as the cause of the eye diseases. Lucentis was FDA approved before Avastin; however, injections in the eye with off-label Avastin cost substantially less to the ophthalmology practice and Medicare, i.e. $100 versus up to $2,000 for Lucentis, which is what drove the use of Avastin off-label to become the standard over Lucentis, and later be approved by the FDA for macular degeneration and vessel occlusions. Avastin and Lucentis have become a profit center for retinal surgeons, who inject Avastin into eyes all day long, and can make $10,000 a day or more, giving Avastin shots to patients with macular degeneration.

Retinal pigment disorders and geographic atrophy are retinal disorders that can be caused by chlamydia pneumonia's direct effect on the small blood vessels of the eye; or by H-pylori attacking the retinal pigment epithelium and collagen. H-pylori is recognized to damage retinal epithelium, and cause geographic atrophy; and similar ocular surface disorders and atrophy appear on the cornea, when H-pylori attacks the corneal epithelium and collagen.

H-pylori can cause RPE (retinal pigment epithelium not well attached to the retinal layers below), lattice degeneration, retinal holes, retinal tears, and retinal detachments. H-pylori attacks the retinal epithelium, and burrows downward to attack collagen; and the retinal surface loses adherence to the inner tissue layers. H-pylori attaches to collagen and inner layers of the retina, causes inflammation; causes thinning, pitting, and atrophy; and ultimately causes retinal holes, tears and detachments. (Chlamydia trachoma and chlamydia psittacosis are also known to attack retinal epithelium and endothelium.) Chronic infection with H-pylori and/or chlamydia, can cause thinning and stretching of the retina, and lattice degeneration. In lattice degeneration, the retina thins and stretches to the point it develops holes or thin spots, at the peripheral edges of the retina. Retinal tissue can only expand to its limits, before the tension from stretching creates holes, to release the stress from stretching. Chronic infection with toxoplasmosis can also cause retinal degeneration, with depigmented areas on the retina, and ultimately loss of vision.

H-pylori can cause idiopathic central serous chorioretinopathy (ICSR) and chorioretinitis, which refer to inflammation in the middle layers of the retina. Idiopathic always means the doctor does not know the cause, and blames the disease on something unique about the patient. ICSR was previously considered an idiopathic blinding disease, before discovery ICSR was caused by H-pylori. H-pylori has been known to cause ICSR, since at least 2014.[273] In ICSR, the patient develops fluid bubbles in the layers of the retina, and the bubbles float to the retinal epithelial surface and pop, causing localized loss of vision where the bubble formed. As the number of bubbles increase, more vision is lost, and the patient develops micro-retinal detachments and eventually blindness. The bubbles forming in the layers of the retina seem similar to the bubbles which form in the layers of the cornea, in advanced keratoconus, known as hydrops and described as fluid-filled bubbles. H-pylori can cause ocular surface disease and keratoconus, and can cause diseases of the retina involving the surface and inner collagen layers, with similar manifestations of loose surface tissue, thinning and pitting, and hydrops. Treatment of H-pylori has been shown to improve, stabilize, or resolve ICSR.

Seventy percent of children born with toxoplasmosis, who were not treated within the first year, developed new lesions on the retina during the next

---

[273] *See* Mateo-Montoya A, *et al.* 2014. Helicobacter Pylori as a Risk Factor for Central Serous Chorioretinopathy: Literature Review. World J Gastrointest Pathophysiol. Aug 15, 2014. 5(3):355-358. *Published online.* Doi: 10.4291/wjgp.v5.i3.355.

decade.[274] The lesions on the retina were similar to chorioretinitis, and similar to ICSR. Any patient who has lost any or all of their vision in one eye due to retinal disease or detachments, should be referred and evaluated for H-pylori and toxoplasmosis, to prevent further damage and damage to the fellow eye.

Retinitis pigmentosa is considered a retinal dystrophy (thinning and degeneration of tissue), which causes a gradual loss of vision and ultimately blindness. Dr. Merchant treated a thirty-five-year-old patient who had been diagnosed with retinitis pigmentosa, and was told by her retinal specialist she would be blind in five years. Dr. Merchant did blood testing, which showed H-pylori and psittacosis. After treatment of H-pylori and psittacosis, the patient had a dramatic improvement and stabilization of her vision. She significantly improved in Snellen visual acuity and contrast sensitivity vision testing; and was able to return to normal activities of daily living, driving, and even driving at night. Her vision has remained stable for three years.

Italy has the highest rate of retinitis pigmentosa in the world. Italy has high numbers of pigeons infected with psittacosis, and a significant amount of close contact with pigeons. The high rate of retinitis pigmentosa, in Italy, and the success treating a patient with retinitis pigmentosa who had psittacosis, supports that retinitis pigmentosa is caused by chlamydia psittacosis. Any person or child diagnosed with retinitis pigmentosa should be tested for immortal infections, including H-pylori and psittacosis, and given treatment for immortal infections, rather than dismissed without hope for saving their vision.

Optic neuritis is a description of a finding of inflammation in the optic nerve, an unexplained disease. Optic neuritis is a chlamydia pneumonia infection in the central nervous system. Dr. Pohl reported on a patient with three attacks of optic neuritis, within five months, and a positive chlamydia pneumonia test in the cerebrospinal fluid, who after treatment

---

[274] Phan L, *et al.* 2008. Longitudinal Study of New Eye Lesions in Children with Toxoplasmosis Who Were Not Treated During the First Year of Life. Am J Ophthalmol. Sep 2008. 146(3):375-384. Doi: 10.1016/j.ajo.2008.04.033.

with rifampicin had resolution of the attacks for six years.[275] Dr. Merchant treated a patient who had been diagnosed with optic neuritis, after recurrent episodes of waking up blind in one eye. She saw a neurologist, and an MRI of her brain showed white spots, similar to what occurs in multiple sclerosis. Dr. Merchant treated the patient for chronic infections, and the optic neuritis disappeared. Moreover, the white spots on her MRI disappeared, which was considered impossible! The patient had no further episodes of optic neuritis, and the only explanation for the success of treatment is infectious pathogens caused both the optic neuritis and the white spots in the brain, on MRI.

Ophthalmologists are now incorporating TNF-inhibitors for retinal disease, to treat inflammation, rather than diagnosis and treatment of the root infectious cause of retinal disease. Retinal disease and retinal degeneration are caused by chronic infection, which is sub-clinical and undiagnosed. Diagnosis of pathogens and treatment of pathogens is a better and safer course of treatment, than the alternatives now being used.

Chlamydia pneumonia, H-pylori, and toxoplasmosis are known to cause retinal diseases; however, retinal patients are not offered diagnosis or treatment for chlamydia pneumonia, H-pylori, or toxoplasmosis. Chlamydia pneumonia causes endothelial dysfunction and angiogenesis, and macular degeneration. H-pylori and toxoplasmosis attack the surface of the retina, cause loose surface, and penetrate to deeper layers of the retina. Retinal specialists do not recognize the immortal infections attack the retina or that immortal pathogens "associated" with corneal disease and glaucoma can migrate to the retina, and attack the retina and vascular system in the eye. H-pylori and toxoplasmosis are rarely considered in diagnosing retinal disease, or treated to prevent a worsening of retinal disease. History of contact with cats and litter boxes is not a routine part of the retinal patient history. Treatment for animal pathogens and for intestinal pathogens can improve the prognosis for the retina in the affected eye, and protect the fellow eye from retinal damage. Diagnosis

---

[275] Pohl D. 2006. Recurrent Optic Neuritis Associated with Chlamydia Pneumonia Infection of the Central Nervous System. Developmental Medicine & Child Neurology. 2006. 48:770-772. Doi: 10.1017/S00121622060011642.

and treatment of immortal pathogens and parasites should be part of the diagnosis and treatment of all retinal patients, and particularly in patients with co-morbid stomach disease or other chronic diseases.

Ophthalmology is riddled with syndromes and descriptions of symptoms and findings. The syndromes and findings were named after the doctor who first described the symptoms, findings, or refer to a constellation of symptoms and findings. Syndromes and descriptions of symptoms and findings were named as diseases, before technology was available to diagnose infectious causes. Ophthalmology is focused on diagnosing syndromes, symptoms, and findings; and treatment with drops, lasers and surgery—not on diagnosis of systemic immortal infections that cause chronic eye disease. Optometrists are focused on correcting vision with glasses and contact lenses, and are not trained in diagnosing and treating systemic infections or chronic disease. Eye care professionals have the approach to eye disease of, "I see it...I do it". They see a finding and treat it symptomatically, they see a refractive error and prescribe glasses or contacts. They do what they were trained to do, and what they always do.

A list of some of the syndromes, symptoms and findings in ophthalmology, and named a disease, include but are not limited to endothelial dystrophy, Fuchs corneal dystrophy, glaucoma, macular degeneration, RPE, ICSR, and retinal detachment. Syndromes include but are not limited to Waldenstrom syndrome, Wegener's syndrome, Stargardt syndrome, Cogan syndrome, and Stevens-Johnson syndrome. Eye diseases can be defined by endothelial dysfunction, epithelial dysfunction, inflammation, or inclusion cysts, rather than the root infectious causes. Syndromes, symptoms, and findings, and eye diseases of unknown origin, should be considered immortal infections, until proven otherwise.

Fuchs Corneal Dystrophy is defined by endothelial dysfunction, and is caused by chlamydia pneumonia. Glaucoma is chlamydia pneumonia and/or H-pylori damaging the anterior chamber angle, causing loss of intraocular pressure control. Closed angle glaucoma is caused by immortal pathogens generating sticky substances and sticky abnormal proteins, and cause scarring and tissue to stick together, in the anterior chamber angle.

Wegener's syndrome is characterized by granulomas and inflammation in the blood vessels of the eye, characteristic of chlamydia infections. Granulomas (inclusion cysts); inflammation in the eye; and inflammation in blood vessels, are all consistent with immortal chlamydia infection. Waldenstrom syndrome is a "hyper-viscosity disease". MALT lymphoma is lymphoma of the eye, and has been "associated" with psittacosis and with H-pylori; as have other forms of lymphoma. Waldenstrom syndrome and MALT lymphoma (lymphoma in the eye) are caused by chlamydia psittacosis infection in the eye, and/or H-pylori.

Stargardt syndrome is the development of macular degeneration in a young patient, assumed to be caused by genetic defects. Stargardt syndrome is most likely caused by chlamydia pneumonia, which damages the vascular system in the eye, *in utero* or in a young child. Chlamydia pneumonia causes macular degeneration in an adult, and in an infant or young child the vessels to the macula are smaller and can clog more easily and more quickly. The child may also have a genetic abnormality, from pathogens present in the parents or child and altering genes. Stargardt syndrome, ICSR, and retinitis pigmentosa may also, in some cases, be caused by H-pylori or toxoplasmosis; or combined infection with immortal pathogens. Investigation into the cause of Stargardt syndrome should include testing the parents and the child for immortal pathogens. Macular degeneration in a young patient requires aggressive treatment of chlamydia pneumonia and any other immortal pathogens diagnosed, to prevent disabling vision impairment and improve the prognosis.

Cogan syndrome is a rare disorder characterized by recurrent inflammation in the front of the eye (the cornea), and often accompanied by fever, fatigue, weight loss, episodes of dizziness, and hearing loss. Cogan's syndrome can lead to deafness or blindness. Any pathogen attacking epithelium, particularly H-pylori, can attack the front of the eye and move downward to cause recurrent inflammation, in the front of the eye. Chlamydia trachoma or psittacosis can attack epithelium and endothelium, causing corneal inflammation. The pathogens attacking the cornea can migrate downward to the iris. CMV and other viral pathogens may play a role in Cogan syndrome, because infection with CMV *in utero* is known to cause blindness and hearing loss, five to seven years after birth. The patient with Cogan syndrome likely has multiple co-infections, working synergistically to cause harm; and the symptoms common in Cogan syndrome could be caused by various forms of immortal infection, alone or in combination.

The diagnosis and treatment of syndromes, symptoms and findings in the eye, *in lieu* of diagnosing infectious causes, often leads to surgery, procedures, and treatment with steroids. Steroids are frequently prescribed in ophthalmology, during and after intraocular surgery, and after laser treatments, to control inflammation. The steroids provide symptomatic relief and lessen inflammation, but can also potentiate immortal infections and cause a rise in intraocular pressure. Any use of steroids should be limited, and intraocular pressure monitored closely during steroid use, because patients with chronic infections may respond to steroids with increased intraocular pressure and secondary systemic effects, not routinely evaluated by an ophthalmologist. Steroid drops used in the eye for a long enough period of time can induce systemic side effects and systemic disease.

Refractive Surgery

Refractive surgery is an elective cosmetic surgery on the eye, intended to eliminate the need for glasses. Refractive surgery is a surgery—*not* a procedure! Refractive surgeons refer to themselves as refractive "surgeons". Refractive surgery is an elective surgery, because the need for glasses is not a disease. Refractive surgeons generally choose to wear glasses rather than undergo the refractive surgery they perform. Refractive surgeons know the risks, and are not willing to subject themselves to the same risk they impose on patients. Refractive surgery has already caused substantial morbidity, and will cause substantial morbidity in the future to millions of people. Refractive surgery is an evolving public health crisis that will cause chronic eye diseases and morbidity in patients, for years to come. Refractive surgery makes healthy eyes sick, and sick eyes sicker!

Refractive surgery is referred to as a "procedure" to serve vested interests who gain from the patient having the surgery. The use of "procedure" is intended reduce patients' fear, make patients believe the surgery is less risky, and to avoid regulation and oversight that arises if LASIK is called a surgery. Any subsequent refractive surgeries to fix poor vision from the initial surgery are referred to as enhancements, touch-ups, or little touch-ups! The nomenclature for surgeries to fix problems created the first refractive surgery is again intended to convince the patient second surgeries are minor, routine, and any problems with the initial surgery can be fixed with a minor second procedure. No refractive surgery has ever withstood the test of time!

All refractive surgery is a surgery of subtraction—tissue is removed from the cornea, taking away part of the fixed amount of corneal tissue a person needs to last a lifetime. The cornea is approximately one-half millimeter thick, and refractive surgery can only be performed on the front half of the cornea, which is only one-fourth of a millimeter thick. The front one-fourth millimeter of the cornea provides corneal stability. All refractive surgery weakens the cornea; disrupts the organization of the cells; and creates a barrier of fibrous tissue blocking fluid transport from the endothelium to the corneal surface.

All refractive surgery equipment has a standard deviation, leaving several sources of deviation, and making all refractive surgery a best guess on tissue one-fourth of a millimeter thick. The surgeon uses a formula for removing tissue that removes approximately twelve microns per diopter—two percent of the cornea is removed per diopter, and one hundredth of a millimeter or less can be the difference between success and failure, which leaves little room for a mistakes or standard deviations. The surgeons make their best guess, and hope the patient is happy with the results or never understands how they were deceived.

Refractive surgery cannot be fixed or undone. Many patients have significant side effects and complications immediately, and others are initially "happy" with the outcome and develop complications and poor vision over time. Quality of vision can be reduced, ranging from mild to severe; future eye health is put at risk; work-life can be impaired; quality of life permanently damaged. Visual impairment causes cognitive impairment, as the patient ages and vision declines. Treatment of eye diseases later in life is more difficult and more likely to have a poor outcome. Many patients with poor outcomes require some form of specialized contact for useful vision; and as vision declines or the patient ages, contact wear can become more difficult. Refractive surgery is a long-term crisis of visual impairment, cognitive decline, and increased demand for corneas to perform corneal transplants. Eventually, the need for corneal transplants could exhaust the supply. What will society do when millions of patients need corneal transplants, because of refractive surgery done decades earlier?

In LASIK surgery, a blade or laser slices the front of the cornea, into two pieces, creating a flap. Under the flap, in surgery for myopia, the laser removes a layer of tissue in a circular pattern across the corneal surface, and the flap is replaced over the residual bed of cornea. In astigmatic LASIK, tissue is removed in an oval pattern, often over the myopic treatment. In hyperopic LASIK, the laser creates a circular trench in the periphery of the cornea, to artificially steepen the central cornea. During enhancements, which come in many forms ranging from retreating the eye with a laser, to a flap lift to try straighten folds, to removing epithelial ingrowth under the flap, or to treat inflammation under the flap. Particularly abhorrent is a LASIK enhancement on a prior radial keratotomy patient, because as one of the original participants in LASIK studies and obtaining FDA approval said, "LASIK on top of RK turns the eye into a pizza pie".

The cornea never regains its original shape or state of health. The corneal nerves are cut, which are necessary to provide a feedback loop to generate fluid production in the eye from the lacrimal gland; which can lead to chronic dry eyes and in some cases chronic nerve pain. If the patient already has dry eye due to blepharitis, after LASIK, two-thirds of the mechanisms that trigger production of fluid to the ocular surface are damaged and the weakest mechanism of the three, goblet cells on the ocular surface, is all that remains. Subsequent surgeries can make complications worse, and enhance long-term dry eye.

The left eye is particularly vulnerable to complications, from LASIK surgery, whenever a flap cut was made with a keratome blade. Practitioners did not change keratome blades before cutting the flap in the second eye, to reduce cost and speed surgery times. Re-use of the same keratome blade can cause epithelial cells from the first eye to be deposited under the flap of the second eye, and can also cause damage to the flap edge because the blade is duller. Epithelial cells under the flap and a damaged flap edge can cause irritation and inflammation, which are a focus for complications.

Some patients may be satisfied initially, or even for many years, before developing disturbing visual complications and anatomical abnormalities years later. Reports have already surfaced of patients who were initially satisfied developing sight-threatening and painful complications, even ten and fifteen years after LASIK, including iatrogenic ectasia and a split in the layers of the cornea. Flap separation and ectasia may occur from long-term dry eye, caused by the original and any subsequent surgeries. Many patients are harmed immediately by LASIK surgery, and the over promise and under deliver mentality of refractive surgeons and their agents. Once LASIK is done, the cornea never returns to normal, and the patient is never in the clear, in terms of developing complications, including sight-threatening complications.

PRK is ordinarily not done, unless the patient's cornea is too thin for LASIK surgery. Refractive surgeons agree corneas thinner than five-hundred microns should not have LASIK surgery, because a thin cornea is an early sign of a thinning disease; and agree the residual bed on the cornea under the refractive surgery treatment must be at least three-hundred microns thick, for the cornea to remain stable. PRK is only suggested when the cornea is too thin for LASIK surgery; and the mere fact a surgeon or optometrist suggests PRK is an indication the patient is *not* a good candidate for any refractive surgery! The surgeon and optometrist promote PRK as an alternative to LASIK, to avoid losing the patient and the income from refractive surgery, because many have no other source of income than new patients wanting refractive surgery.

In PRK surgery, the epithelium is manually scraped off the surface of the cornea, rather than creating a flap. After scraping off the epithelium, corneal stroma is ablated with a laser in the same manner as in LASIK surgery. PRK destroys the separating membrane between the epithelium and stroma, and removes stroma. PRK is seldom done because it takes longer to perform, and the patient will suffer significant pain and light sensitivity for five to nine days, while the epithelium regenerates over the ocular surface. The patient risks irregular regeneration of the epithelium and dangers created by the permanent loss of the separating membrane.

One-hundred seventy complications of LASIK have been identified, and patients are not informed of the large number of potential complications, the magnitude of harm caused by the complications, the patient will likely suffer multiple complications at the same time, and the complications can be permanent and life-changing. Complications of LASIK include development of cells, inflammation and chronic irritation between the flap and the underlying corneal stroma, particularly in the left eye, referred to as "diffuse lamellar keratitis". Diffuse lamellar keratitis is a name describing the symptom of chronic inflammation, "itis", between the flap and the underlying corneal tissue. Some patients develop corneal melt, most likely from pathogens already in the eye and released or potentiated, by refractive surgery. LASIK causes fibrous tissue between the flap and the underlying cornea, which never heals and is not as strong as the original cornea. The fibrous scar tissue can be broken with any impact, in sports, a car accident with airbag deployment, a punch in the eye, a fall, or even running into the cabinet handle with an eye. Flap rupture is a catastrophic, vision threatening complication.

Patients are told of possible risks of refractive surgery, which the patient may or may not understand; but never told the degree of risk or that all or a number of these risks can and do occur, and can occur at the same time, be permanent, be severe, and nothing can be done to restore good vision and healthy eyes. Patients are not told of pre-existing problems in their eyes, or the worse the eye health prior to refractive surgery, the more likely the patient will have complications. When patients ask about risks, they are often given a "yes, but" answer, as in "yes, the surgery has risks, but don't worry"; "yes the surgery has risks, but that does not happen here"; "yes the surgery has risks, but the complications are temporary and will fade in a few months"; and "yes the surgery has risks, but we can fix problems with an enhancement or little touch-up".

Patients are not told of the alarming rate of complications in patients, the true rate of complications in the left eye, or that refractive surgery seldom, if ever, provides perfect vision in both eyes or good vision for a lifetime. Patients are not told refractive surgery can cause symptoms and complications that impair work, and activities of daily living; and in some cases have caused severe depression, suicidal ideation, and suicides. Surgeons delegate informed consent to optometrists and non-medical staff, who are not allowed to explain risks, beyond what is written on the consent form. Delegation to staff gives the surgeon more time to make money, and allows the surgeon to avoid concealing the risks directly to patient's face, giving the surgeon plausible deniability the surgeon deceived the patient. After the fact, refractive surgeons do not see the patients, allowing or causing them to ignore complications caused by the surgery and deny complications exist or occur frequently.

Patients are not told refractive surgery seldom works as intended, and is a best guess. Surgeons are hoping the surgery will get close to the desired correction and reduce, but not eliminate the need for glasses, without causing new visual problems which are intolerable to the patient and cannot be corrected. Refractive surgery is not based on an accurate assessment of what is needed for perfect vision or what amount of tissue is actually removed.

The best the patient can hope for is to avoid a disaster in either eye, and find "happiness" without glasses, despite permanent loss of quality of vision, ongoing dry eye, and the likelihood the patient will need glasses or contacts in the subsequent five years. Very few patients are able to achieve perfect vision, with no refractive error in either eye, even if the surgery is considered a complete success. In a best-case scenario, no refractive surgery can give better vision than the patient's corrected vision before surgery. Vision can only stay the same or get worse. Virtually all patients lose quality of vision, in one form or another. The lucky patient is happy with the initial result, but few patients maintain good vision for a lifetime.

More than half of the refractive surgery patients require glasses within five years; and after refractive surgery, the glasses do not work well at correcting vision because the refractive surgery created an irregular corneal surface. Visual aberrations are common, and "higher order aberrations" (an irregular pattern that causes loss in the quality of vision) cannot be corrected with glasses and may or may not be correctable with contact lenses. The cells of the cornea no longer line-up like a perfect igloo, impairing healthy regeneration of corneal tissue, causing quality of vision loss, including streaks and flares in vision that the patient may see as starbursts, halos, and glare. The patient may need contact lenses, and even hard contact lenses or scleral lenses, to force the eye into a smooth shape and compensate for the irregular surface, to regain functional vision.

After refractive surgery, the refractive surgeon does not want to hear visual complaints, and does not always believe patients who report visual complaints. Desperate patients have said to their doctor they cannot see, and the refractive surgeon response was, "yes you can". When the patient says they can't see, the patient means they are "having great difficulty with their vision"; and the refractive surgeon hears "I don't have any vision". The refractive surgeon or optometrist may deny the patient has their reported vision problems, because the patient read some of a Snellen chart; and many ophthalmology and optometry offices do not even own a contrast sensitivity chart, to measure quality of vision loss; yet, deny the patients' vision loss to the patients.

The surgeon's endless excuses then begin, from "you knew the risks" to "we can fix this" with more surgery, more drops, specialized contact lenses or collagen cross linking, which at best mitigate the visual difficulties and iatrogenic damage. The refractive surgeon wants to believe if the patient can wear a hard contact lens or a scleral lens, no matter how uncomfortable or inadequate; or appears to have "reasonable" vision on a Snellen chart, even though reduced as compared to before surgery, with correction, and the patient has loss of quality of vision—"no harm no foul!" You were warned! You took the risk! No, that is not true! The surgeon took the risk, by not informing the patient of facts that would have dissuaded the patient from refractive surgery.

After refractive surgery, the refractive surgeon and their agents continue to conceal; and try to convince the patient any adverse consequences of surgery can be handled, to be patient for problems to resolve, or the patient is "reminded" they were warned before surgery. The refractive surgeon and their agents will allege the symptoms are not that bad; or allege no harm no foul because uncomfortable and expensive specialty contact lenses give "adequate" vision. When the patient has obvious complications, which the surgeon cannot deny, the patient may be told they were warned, "too bad for you, it can happen", and "you took the risk". It may take two years or more for the patient to realize the surgery caused harm, and by that time the refractive surgeon is no longer caring for the patient.

The latest excuse by refractive surgeons for poor outcomes is, it was you! It was your genes, or your unpredictable response, that we could not have known in advance. No, that is not true! Genes are used as an excuse for their lack of judgment in performing the refractive surgery. It was bad judgment, the equipment, the standard deviation in cuts and lasers, and their attempt to find excuses to do surgery rather than heeding warning signs found in preoperative screening. It was concealing risks from the patients for profit. It was a fundamental flaw in the concept of refractive surgery. The excuse of "anything but me" is no longer credible, and blaming genes and the patient is wrong and cruel.

Refractive surgery clinical studies did not use nor provide objective measurements of success. Refractive surgeons evaluated the success of the refractive surgery based on the patient's "happiness" immediately after surgery, rather than final vision after healing or objective measures of good visual acuity and quality of vision. From the refractive surgeon's point of view—if the patient is happy when they arose after surgery then the surgery was a success, which was and is referred to as "20/happy". The refractive surgeon ignores the fact the happiness and immediate elation will fade, and turn into regret and longstanding problems with the patient's eyes and vision. Happiness wanes, as vision problems impact the quality of life; but by that time the refractive surgeon is not available or in denial the surgery could cause problems.

The refractive surgeons and manufacturers measured success by comparing the uncorrected Snellen visual acuity before surgery, with the uncorrected Snellen vision after surgery, to allege success; and obtain approvals from the FDA to sell or market refractive surgery devices. The same argument is also often made during lawsuits against refractive surgeon for negligence. Comparison of uncorrected visual acuity prior to surgery, to uncorrected visual acuity after surgery, is a false equivalency. Snellen visual acuity is a crude measurement of visual acuity, which does not represent the visual needs of a person, in activities of daily living. The world does not exist in black and white at twenty feet, in perfect lighting. The goal of surgery is to have good visual acuity without vision correction—not poor and uncorrectable vision after surgery. The refractive surgeons and manufacturers allege success, even when the uncorrected vision after surgery is insufficient to give functional vision, requires vision correction, vision correction is difficult or impossible, or vision cannot be corrected to the pre-surgery level of visual acuity and the patient lives with visual aberrations. The industry advertises success based on false equivalency, ignoring the most important components of good vision, and knowing the surgery seldom gives perfect vision in both eyes.

The goal of too many refractive surgeons is to get away with it, the patient never finds out what was done to them, it will be too late for the patients to bring a lawsuit, or the damage done is "not significant" enough to justify bringing a lawsuit. The laser equipment manufacturers hope the patient will never discover their negligence; or any lawsuit against manufacturers will be barred by the judiciary, based on a false interpretation of the Medical Device Amendment, of 1976, alleged to "preempt" any lawsuits by patients—meaning patients have no right to sue manufacturers for injuries caused by refractive surgery devices, or the false marketing of refractive surgery. No reasonable patient would agree to refractive surgery, knowing the true risks, the true long-term risks, the deceit involved in marketing refractive surgery, and the difficulty of obtaining any remedy for the injuries caused by refractive surgery.

Early in the course of LASIK surgery, refractive surgeons were getting lung disease and lung cancer, from breathing the plume of tissue lasered off during refractive surgery. The pathogens in the eye were likely vaporized during the refractive surgery, and the doctor inhaled the pathogens and broken parts of pathogens. Refractive surgeons now protect themselves from inhaling the plume created by the laser, but the patient is not protected from breathing the pathogens from the plume from their own eyes, into their own lung.

Refractive surgery frequently causes dry eyes, which can last for months, years, or become permanent. Refractive surgery will worsen pre-existing dry eye, and in patients with pre-existing dry eye, refractive surgery can cause severe and permanent dry eye. Creation of a LASIK flap cuts corneal nerves, and creates a fibrous scar across the cornea that impairs fluid from the endothelium crossing the barrier created by the fibrous scar, to reach the front surface of the cornea. Some patients have dry eyes so severe it causes pitting on the surface of the cornea, called superficial punctate keratitis or SPK. Dry eyes make the eyes more vulnerable to infection, and can cause discomfort and vision problems for a lifetime. Reports have surfaced of flap separation ten years after LASIK, and late onset ectasia, which may be caused by chronic dry eyes and dehydration of the cornea. Dry eyes and lack of fluid transport in the cornea makes the tissue weak and dry, and no longer able to hold the flap and underlying cornea together and the cornea stable.

Many refractive surgeons ignore blepharitis, and do not diagnose infection at the eyelid margin; or warn patients considering surgery of the danger of refractive surgery in a patient who has blepharitis. Some refractive surgeons will pre-treat blepharitis with antibiotic drops, which cannot assure the blepharitis will not cause complications, or return to cause complications after surgery, when drops are discontinued and the pathogens causing blepharitis are shed across the cornea cut by LASIK. Preexisting blepharitis creates a risk of severe and permanent dry eyes after refractive surgery. Refractive surgery also creates a potential portal and weakened corneal surface that can make the cornea vulnerable to invasion by pathogens.

Refractive surgery requires extreme intraocular pressure when the corneal flap is cut; and can cause premature and iatrogenic cataracts. The pressure inside the eye during the flap creation is extreme, and the extent of harm from an acute extreme pressure spike is unknown. Some have reported vitreous detachments, floaters, retinal tears, and retinal detachments. The Professional Use Manual and Operator's Manual for refractive surgery equipment contain strong warnings to avoid directing the laser into the eye. Patients getting refractive surgery are getting a laser directed straight into their eye. Refractive surgery can induce premature cataracts, from the laser damaging the natural lens; and reports have been made of iatrogenic cataracts after refractive surgery. Patients nearing the age of presbyopia will require reading glasses sooner, after having refractive surgery.

As the person ages and develops cataracts, treatment is more complicated and greater risk, after refractive surgery. LASIK causes a thinner and unstable cornea, which is unpredictable in cataract surgery. The correct intraocular power to use in cataract surgery is less predictable, and the patient can have a "power miss", when the dome of the cornea collapses or changes unpredictably during cataract surgery. When a person develops hyperopia from the dome collapsing in cataract surgery, vision correction for reading becomes more difficult and the reading correction more extreme.

LASIK causes a thinner cornea, which artificially reduces intraocular pressure measurements. The diagnosis of glaucoma can be delayed because thinning of the cornea artificially lowers the intraocular pressure measurement; and treatment of glaucoma may become more complicated. When patients develop high intraocular pressure later in life, thin spots on the cornea can become weak spots, and develop into bulges or hydrops. Development of glaucoma can aggravate the problem of an abnormal or changing corneal shape, and vision fluctuation. Thin spots on the anterior or posterior cornea before refractive surgery, caused by chronic infection, are made even thinner and weaker by the surgery. The barrier of scar tissue across the cornea, from the flap cut, may also impair absorption of glaucoma drops into the eye intended to reduce intraocular pressure.

Refractive surgery does not ordinarily cause blindness, but can cause blindness in rare instances. Complications of refractive surgery, efforts to rehabilitate vision, and subsequent development of eye diseases, can lead to sight threatening complications, later in life. Refractive surgeons do not consider refractive surgery a "sterile procedure"; thus, take few sterile precautions and some do not even wear gloves. Aggressive bacterial and fungal infections can cause blindness, in the short term; and sub-clinical infections can cause long-term complications. Loss of visual acuity and loss in the quality of vision can lead to falls and accidents. Some patients are dependent on ophthalmologists for life, or require corneal transplants, creating huge medical expenses; and a risk of repeat corneal transplants causing secondary cataracts and glaucoma, and loss of vision at the end of life. Secondary complications and procedures, and surgery to repair the damage from refractive surgery, can become sight threatening.

Patients with preexisting H-pylori and/or trachoma may have bands of scar tissue across the cornea and an increase in blood vessels on the sclera, both of which make refractive surgery more dangerous and the prognosis for a good outcome poor. If the patient needs a corneal transplant to rehabilitate iatrogenic keratoconus or other complications after refractive surgery, the infection and blood vessels on the cornea can cause premature failure of the corneal transplant; the need for repeat corneal transplants; and ultimately low vision or loss of vision at the end of life.

Keratoconus patients seek refractive surgery at twice the rate at which keratoconus occurs in the population, because keratoconus patients become frustrated with changing refractions and poorly corrected vision. Patients with corneal thinning diseases are the ones most likely to have chlamydia and/or H-pylori attacking their eyes; and most likely to have a sight-threatening or life altering complication caused by refractive surgery. The FDA labeling states "signs of keratoconus" are a contraindication, meaning if the patient has *any* signs of early keratoconus they should not have refractive surgery, because of the risk of an iatrogenic, sight-threatening injury, outweighs any potential benefit. Some refractive surgeons have asked, "How many signs" of keratoconus are needed to reject the patient for surgery. The answer is, "If you have to ask, it is too many".

High volume refractive surgeons as a group, in conjunction with the American Academy of Ophthalmology, began calling "signs of keratoconus", as opposed to "full-blown" keratoconus that has progressed to hydrops, a "relative contraindication". The group wrote articles in the refractive surgery journal and American Academy of Ophthalmology Journal, to protect refractive surgeons who were sued for ignoring signs of keratoconus and causing injuries to patients. A "relative contraindication" is a non-sequitur because a contraindication is a contraindication, and the term has nothing "relative" about it. A relative contraindication more appropriately falls in the category of the patient should be warned, but refractive surgeons rarely warn the patient with signs of keratoconus, before proceeding with surgery. Refractive surgeons try to ignore signs suggesting a corneal thinning disease, and find any excuse to justify refractive surgery, because they only make money if the patient agrees to have refractive surgery. The high volume refractive surgeons banded together to protect each other, rather than protecting the vision of patients, which led to more surgeons defying or being confused by accepted standards for refractive surgery candidacy and more patients being harmed. Neither LASIK nor PRK is safe when the patient has *any* signs of *any* corneal thinning disease.

Refractive surgery patients have a high rate of suicidal ideation and suicide. When the refractive surgery outcome is not what was planned, promised, or expected, the patient eventually realizes nothing can be done to restore good vision or improve the comfort in their eyes and vision. Patients feel betrayed by doctors who made grandiose promises of happiness and vision without glasses; who did not fully inform the patient of the risks, or the risks were not understood. The patient blames themselves for having the surgery, sees only misery ahead, has impairment in daily activities, impairment in work, becomes depressed, and engages in suicidal ideation or suicide.

Refractive surgery has been so profitable to ophthalmology, it spawned an industry of corporate chains and itinerant refractive surgeons, who push the limits for "safe" refractive surgery, to expand the number of eligible patients and expand income. Itinerant surgeons seldom personally evaluate the patient's candidacy before surgery; and only see the patient at surgery and for a short visit on post-operative one day. Optometrists are not trained as surgeons, may have little understanding of refractive surgery standards, and often have secondary gain in approving of patients for surgery, which is the income from preoperative and post-operative co-management visits, or incentives for approving more patients. An Inspector General Report, "Itinerant Surgery", April 1989, reported a significant increase in risk and complications with itinerant surgery in cataract surgery[276], but no similar study has been done for refractive surgery. Some consider the practice of itinerant refractive surgery unethical.[277] Itinerant surgery has been normalized by the refractive surgery industry, without proof of safety for patients.

High volume and itinerant refractive surgeons and their optometry agents may be trained by their employers and expected to exceed standards for candidacy. The itinerant surgeon and their optometry agents may ignore corneal topography showing steep spots and thin spots on the cornea, particularly thin spots on the posterior (underside) cornea. Some do not know how to interpret corneal topography to identify contraindications and high-risk factors for refractive surgery, even though topography is the most important screening tool before refractive surgery. Thin and steep spots on the surface of the cornea may be disguised by abnormally thick epithelium; and thin spots on the underside of the cornea are an important sign of a thinning disease, and of chlamydia infection attacking the endothelium. Thin spots anywhere on the cornea, will become even thinner spots after surgery, which are weaker than the rest of the cornea and likely to bulge over time. Refractive surgery done on a patient with corneal thinning disease will cause progressive and accelerated thinning and steepening, and will become iatrogenic ectasia, an accelerated form of keratoconus. Iatrogenic ectasia is a significant complication that can lead to a corneal transplant and sight-threatening complications.

---

[276] Kusserow RP, Inspector General. 1989. Itinerant Surgery. Office of Inspector General, Office of Analysis and Inspections.

[277] *See* 2009. EyeNet. American Academy of Ophthalmology. Ask the Ethicist: The Itinerant Surgeon. Nov/Dec 2009.

Collagen cross linking is being promoted as a way to stabilize or control adverse complications of refractive surgery, specifically the ongoing thinning and bulging of the cornea into an abnormal and irregular shape, known as iatrogenic ectasia or iatrogenic kerectasia. For collagen cross linking, the surgeon props the eye open with instruments, scrapes off the epithelium, puts riboflavin drops in the eye, and exposes the eye to ultraviolet light for up to thirty minutes. After the cross linking, the patient has significant pain and uses antibiotic drops, for five to nine days, until the epithelium regrows over the cornea. The reason collagen cross linking may work, in slowing ectasia, is because the chronic infection causing a thinning disease has invaded the stroma; and by scraping off the epithelium and exposing the stroma to ultraviolet light, then applying antibiotic drops directly on the stroma, for five to nine days, the underlying infection in the stroma is more effectively treated, and the infectious burden decreased. Some ophthalmologists are now trying "epi-on" collagen cross linking. Antibiotic drops may not be as effective in treating the ectasia when the epithelium is intact, because the epithelium may prevent penetration of the drops to the underlying layers of the stroma.

The FDA only reviews the devices used in refractive surgery, not the refractive surgery itself. Refractive surgery itself has never been reviewed or approved by any government agency or authority. State authorities only supervise facilities performing surgery, not medical offices performing "procedures"; and the FDA does not review "procedures" at all.

The first time LASIK/PRK was reviewed by the FDA, the Ophthalmic Devices Panel voted 9-0 *not* to approve the devices for use in refractive surgery. It was only after political pressure was brought to bear, and the FDA requested reconsideration and approval of the devices, to try to control what was already being done, that a new Ophthalmic Device Panel was convened to approve LASIK/PRK. Morris Waxler, former Director of Medical Devices when LASIK was approved, has now petitioned the FDA for a new review of LASIK and to reject approval of refractive surgery, because the dangers of refractive surgery were fraudulently concealed to gain approval.

The FDA never developed a list of adverse events for refractive surgery; thus, even if a patient has an adverse event, and even if the doctors know the patient had an adverse event, the doctor may not know the adverse event is reportable or may choose not report the adverse event. When adverse events are reported, the manufacturer is an intermediary, and in almost all instances chooses to blame the doctor or patient rather than the devices, and conceals the report of an adverse event from the FDA. The marketing, the failure to define of complications and adverse events, the lack of reporting, and the money to be made, has made refractive surgery a free-for-all. Every time refractive surgery fails, the doctors and manufacturers represent to the FDA and the patients, "Sorry we did not know, but now we have something better". To date, that has never been true and the better version always also fails. *No refractive surgery has ever withstood the test of time!*

A desire for refractive surgery, to get rid of glasses and contacts and find happiness, can create a lifetime of regret. Few attain the goal of good vision without glasses, and virtually no one attains the goal of good vision in both eyes, or in both eyes for a lifetime. If you don't like your glasses, buy more expensive glasses; and if you want to see the clock at night, buy a projection clock that projects large numbers on the bedroom ceiling. If some people are lucky enough to have done well after refractive surgery, good for them. Too many people do not do well, or their vision and eye anatomy deteriorates over time. Many patients wish for their old glasses and contacts. Long-term many refractive surgery patients will view the decision to have refractive surgery as one of the worst decisions of their life.

Refractive surgeons wear glasses! Refractive surgeons know the short and long-term risks, even while denying and concealing the true extent of the risks to patients! A few refractive surgeons and other medical and dental professionals had refractive surgery, and regretted their decision; and in some cases, refractive surgery ended their careers.

Some ophthalmologists are now promoting new types of refractive surgery, as the public becomes more aware of the risk and interest in LASIK fades. One is called SMILE, in which a pocket is created in the cornea and the laser removes tissue inside the pocket, instead of cutting a flap and using the laser under a flap. SMILE will fail like all other refractive surgeries, as patients develop haze over the central cornea from opposing layers of fibrous scar tissue, across the cornea. Some manufacturers and ophthalmologists dreamed up a titanium mesh corneal inlay, with eight-hundred holes, which is implanted in a pocket between layers of corneal tissue, to provide reading vision without glasses. The idea of a titanium implant in the cornea, for reading vision, is absurd. A metal foreign body in the middle of the layers of the cornea that blocks passive fluid transport and creates fibrous scar tissue, is not likely to be successful long term.

Refractive surgery has been a profitable business for ophthalmologists and a public health nightmare for patients and society. Refractive surgery is selling hope and happiness, without any defined measures of success or accepted list of adverse events or complications. Patients who most desire refractive surgery are the most likely to have a poor outcome. Refractive surgery causes healthy eyes to become sick, and makes unhealthy eyes sicker. Refractive surgery is a disgrace to the eye care profession, and a fraud on the public. Refractive surgeons and their agents have deceived patients about risks, filled their pockets with cash, and created hundreds of thousands of patients with visual impairment and at risk for low vision at the end of life. Refractive surgery causes a chronic eye disease, by damaging the structure of the eye; becomes an origin of disease; and causes a lifetime of eye problems and regret for the patient.

CHAPTER 17

CHRONIC INFECTION IN SKIN DISEASES

The skin is our largest organ, in total volume. The skin protects us from most pathogens, unless the skin is broken by a wound or surgery. Touching a doorknob or another person will not transmit infection, unless after touching the contaminated surface or exposure to a sick person, one touches the eyes, nose, mouth, or other open portal to the body. The skin cannot protect us from all pathogens, and infections can be acquired on the skin and through the skin.

The skin can be a clue to immortal infections inside us, if we observe and investigate. Skin abnormalities can arise from self-inoculation, from the nose and mouth; and from hands and/or cell phones contaminated with biofilms from the nose and mouth. Biofilm is a slime that covers and harbors immortal infections and supports the growth of fungus. Biofilm from the nose and mouth harbors pathogens, which can be deposited on the skin and create sub-clinical infection with immortal bacteria and/or fungus. Biofilm may also contain undiscovered nano-particles and nano-bacteria, the pathogenesis of which is not known.

Chlamydia pneumonia infections, and fungus generated by pathogens, can spread from the nose and mouth, to the skin; and cause a variety of brown spots. Brown spots develop on the hands, forearms, and face, where hands, fingertips and devices contaminated the skin with biofilm. Brown spots may develop where fingers often touch skin when the arms are crossed, and on the forehead from hats contaminated with bacteria or fungus. The brown spots of bacteria or fungus on the skin may appear in a pattern consistent with the vector contaminating the skin. Modern cell phones spread pathogens to the skin in the form of brown spots on the face, which follow the pattern of the cell phone touching the face.

Immortal bacteria and fungus come out the mouth and nose and onto the cell phone or landline, in the form of biofilm; and the biofilm is transferred to the face on contact, causing brown spots or localized pimples. Brown spots are a low-grade infection, with a bacterium, nano-bacterium, or fungus, transferred to the arms, hands and face by hand (finger-tip) contact, and to the face by cell phone contact. Brown spots on the skin are diagnostic clue suggesting an immortal infection has been transferred from the body to the skin.

Brown spots can be treated and significantly improved in appearance with prolonged application of topical antibiotics and/or antifungals, depending on whether the sub-clinical infection is bacterial or fungal. Sun damage may cause the skin to be more susceptible to low grade infections and fungus, because excessive sun exposure creates a weak link. However, sun damage alone would not leave a specific pattern of brown spots that match the pattern of cell phone contact or hand contact, unless phone contact already created a weak link on the skin, in a specific pattern.

Pimples and acne are localized infections of the skin, often arising from hand-to-face contact, or phone-to-face contact. Pimples can be caused by skin contact with dirty hands, contaminated devices, or anything else touching the face, particularly if the method of contact includes biofilm. Old style landline phones spread pathogens to the chin, where the mouthpiece touched the face, causing pimples. Acne is a more serious, deeper, and widespread eruption of pimples. Acne can arise from systemic infection transferred to the skin, chronic infection erupting on the skin; or excessively touching the face with hands, fingertips and devices. Acne and pimples can be treated with antibiotic cream topically, or in more severe cases are treated systemically with an antibiotic. A single pimple can be treated with a small amount of imiquimod, to help the body expel the pimple naturally. In all cases, patients with acne and/or pimples should be educated in face hygiene, and to keep their hands and devices clean and away from the face. Acne warrants evaluation of the habits causing pimples and acne, and investigation into immortal pathogens.

Eczema and psoriasis are skin conditions of unknown origin, which cause rashes. The distinction between eczema and psoriasis is determined by the location of the rash and the appearance of the rash. Eczema is a red, itchy, patchy rash; for which patients are given topical, symptomatic treatment. Eczema has been proposed as a chronic skin disease, caused by an allergic reaction triggering a hypersensitive reaction.

Psoriasis is a thick patch of white scales on the skin, thought to be from an autoimmune reaction causing an overproduction of skin cells. Psoriasis is considered a more significant chronic disease than eczema. Psoriasis is thought to be a systemic disease that ignites inflammation in the body, including in blood vessels and joints. Psoriasis typically attacks between ages fifteen and thirty-five. More than one immortal pathogen may cause psoriasis; and the pathogen causing psoriasis may be different, in different patients.

A national study linked psoriasis to an increased risk for cardiovascular disease, high blood pressure, diabetes, sleep disorders, depression, obesity, Crohn's disease, and autoimmune diseases. Psoriasis patients have co-morbid conditions, which include higher rates of heart attacks, strokes, painful and swollen joints, high blood pressure, diabetes, sleep disorders, depression, obesity, Crohn's disease, inflammatory bowel disease, diarrhea, bloody stools, and cancer; including lymphoma, squamous cell cancer, and sarcoma. The co-morbid conditions for psoriasis suggest the skin disorder and the co-morbid conditions are linked by immortal infection or combinations of immortal infections, during different stages of the infectious cascade.

Psoriasis may be caused by chlamydia pneumonia, which is strongly linked to cardiovascular disease. Co-infections, and/or chlamydia trachoma or chlamydia psittacosis, may also cause psoriatic arthritis, based on the typical age of onset, the presence of arthritis as a co-morbid condition; and the "association" of trachoma and psittacosis with arthritis and cancer. Psoriasis is most likely caused by chlamydia pathogens; however could be caused by more than one type of chlamydia. Psoriasis patients likely have co-infections, and suffer fungal infections as part of an infectious cascade, which combine to cause skin rashes that are dry and scaly.

Psoriatic arthritis describes a patient with two co-morbid diseases—psoriasis and arthritis. Whether psoriatic arthritis differs from psoriasis with arthritis as a co-morbid condition is unclear, and may be dependent on the specialty of the doctor making the diagnosis and severity of the joint involvement. In the patient with psoriatic arthritis, the pathogens causing psoriasis have attacked the joints, to cause swollen and painful joints. Chlamydia pneumonia causes cardiovascular disease; and chlamydia trachoma, chlamydia psittacosis, and mycoplasma, can cause arthritis and joint degeneration. The use of TNF-inhibitors for psoriatic arthritis can potentiate the chlamydia infection, transform reticulate bodies into a larger form, and cause chronic chlamydia infection to become a more serious chronic disease or evolve into a new chronic disease.

Rosacea is a skin disease, and the name describes the characteristic redness and rashes on the face, often in a butterfly pattern—not the cause of the disease. A rosacea rash on the face appears similar to a lupus butterfly rash. Rosacea has numerous co-morbid conditions, including eye disease, intestinal disease, and joint disease; and ocular rosacea can be sight-threatening. Chlamydia trachoma and chlamydia psittacosis cause numerous eye diseases and sight-threatening eye disease; chlamydia pneumonia, trachoma, and psittacosis cause arthritis; and all chronic infections can cause joint pain. H-pylori causes intestinal disease, thyroid disease, and eye disease, including glaucoma and retinal disease. Rosacea may be caused by any of these pathogens, or a combinations of pathogens, which are known to cause various eye diseases and systemic diseases related to rosacea.

The treatment of rosacea with antibiotics and/or antiparasitics must be based on diagnosis of the type of immortal pathogens, which are causing the rosacea. Rosacea has been successfully treated with antibiotics (doxycycline) and antiparasitics. Low-doses of doxycycline have been shown to benefit rosacea and acne[278], and to improve ocular rosacea and

---

[278] Bikowski JB. 2003. Subantimicrobial Dose Doxycycline for Acne and Rosacea. Sinkmed. 2003. July-Aug; 2(4) 234-45. PMID: 14673277.

glaucoma. Doxycycline can cause rosacea to virtually disappear, along with many systemic effects caused by the same pathogens. A rosacea rash appears similar to a lupus butterfly rash; and antibiotics and antiparasitics have also been effective in treating lupus. The success of antibiotic and antiparasitic treatment for rosacea and lupus, and the similarity of the butterfly rash, suggests the same pathogens are causing rosacea and lupus, and the diseases may be the same disease at different stages of an infectious cascade.

Impetigo is a streptococcal infection on the skin. Impetigo often occurs on the face, around the mouth. Impetigo is highly contagious, and creates a linear spread of blisters, followed by a cluster of blisters. Patients with impetigo ordinarily seek care from a doctor, because the seriousness of the skin infection is obvious and disfiguring. Oral antibiotics are likely needed. Streptococcal infection should be considered in any patients with signs of bubbles or blisters, in any tissue, in any part of the body.

Behcet's syndrome is a dermatologic condition that causes blistering skin rashes, erupting from every orifice. Behcet's syndrome is thought to be a rare condition that occurs in Vietnam and the Middle East, Vietnam, Turkey and Greece. The Behcet's syndrome rash looks like streptococcal blisters, and/or impetigo. Patients in the United States are given expensive TNF-inhibitors, for unexplained inflammation, instead of diagnosis of chronic infections. Behcet's syndrome is a disease in desperate need of investigation into the root infectious causes of the disease.

The first description of Behcet's disease was by Hippocrates, who also documented and described streptococcus. Behcet's syndrome was attributed to Hulusi Behcet, a Turkish dermatologist, who described and named the blistering skin disease. In the 1940's, Dr. Behcet described blisters on the skin, which formed around virtually every orifice; but did not have the capacity to diagnose the specific pathogen causing Behcet's syndrome. The erupting skin rashes appear similar or the same as impetigo, which is known to be caused by streptococcal infection. No one considered disseminated infection caused Behcet's disease, or tried to treat Behcet's syndrome as an infection. Behcet's syndrome is likely caused by disseminated systemic streptococcal type-M infection, which escapes from orifices in the body onto the skin, and forms blisters; just as impetigo erupts when biofilm from the mouth contaminates the skin.

The regions where Behcet's disease is most common is exactly the geographic regions known to have endemic streptococcus type-M. Turkey has eighty serovars of streptococcal infection; yet, no one ever questioned Behcet's syndrome as an infection, or tried to treat Behcet's disease as a disseminated streptococcal infection. Neither Dr. Behcet nor anyone after him considered that Behcet's syndrome could be caused by endemic streptococcus-M pathogens, which are known to cause heart disease (rheumatic fever), kidney disease (glomerulonephritis) and impetigo. Behcet's disease still remains a syndrome of unknown origin.

Behcet's disease/syndrome is a disseminated blistering skin infection, which has also been described as a systemic vascular disease affecting multiple organs. Behcet's disease can cause systemic vasculitis, meaning inflammation in the vessels; and "inflammatory" eye disease and blinding events. Streptococcus type-M may become disseminated due to an underlying weakness in the immune system caused by undiagnosed co-infections with chlamydia and parasites; by intracellular invasion of streptococcus pathogens and byproducts; or may be only one pathogen, a particularly virulent form of untreated streptococcus. TNF-inhibitors will never cure the infection and can only make the infection worse, by further weakening the immune system and potentiating the underlying infection causing Behcet's disease.

Mosquitoes transmit viral pathogens through the skin, by a bite, including hemorrhagic fevers, Zika virus, and West Nile virus. If a virus is causing the acute or chronic illness, and is transferred to the skin by coughing or contact with secretions, where the skin is broken, a wart may develop. Some parasites can invade through the skin, including shistomiasis, and leishmaniosis; and parasitic worms, which reside in the small intestine, like hookworm and roundworm. Hookworm can be acquired by walking barefoot in an area contaminated by animal feces. Some worms can be acquired through the skin, by the bite of a specific fly that transmits worms from cattle to people.

Scabies is an under-recognized parasitic skin disease, caused by a common parasitic mite that burrows into the skin, and causes intense itching with heat. Scabies, like other parasites, become more active at sunset and sundown, causing the itching to become more intense. Scabies mites create an itchy linear pattern of scabs, referred to as a track. Scabies can live in the hair, in which case the bites will follow a pattern along hairlines, or along hats or helmets. Scabies can evolve into moles, as the immune system attacks and tries to expel the skin parasite. Imervectin is an oral medication, can treat scabies, and is very safe; however, Imervectin is grossly underutilized.

Morgellons disease is a skin disease, in which lesions develop on the skin and hairy filaments project out of the skin lesions. Morgellons was previously considered a psychosomatic illness; and many doctors alleged Morgellons was a self-reported skin condition arising from delusional parasitosis and compulsive scratching. It is unclear why Morgellons disease would ever be considered psychosomatic, when hairy filaments are projecting out of the skin that cannot be imagined. Recently, the CDC identified Morgellons disease as a real disease, arising from an unknown cause. The CDC suggested it may be caused by bacteria that are part of the normal flora of human beings. The hairy filaments on the skin were thought to be a "protein expression of some sort". A "protein expression", appearing as a hairy filament, suggests a pathogen causes Morgellons.

The cause of Morgellons disease has been proposed to be an anaerobic bacterium that lives harmlessly on the skin; and burrows into the skin where the pathogen can thrive in an anaerobic environment. Morgellons has been proposed to be caused by a spiral anaerobic bacterium, in the intestine, for which treatment has not been determined. Whatever pathogen is causing Morgellons is proposed to be throwing off scat that appears as hairy filamentous projections coming out of the skin. Morgellons may also be a parasite that invades subcutaneous tissue and lives under the skin, and causes intense itching.

Morgellons disease patients have co-morbid intestinal disease, which supports Morgellons disease is some variant of H-pylori infection. H-pylori is a spiral anaerobic bacterium in the intestine, which burrows through epithelium and attaches to collagen. The H-pylori pathogens may have attacked the epithelium on the skin, and invaded the collagen below the skin. Morgellons disease patients have more intense itching at sundown, which supports Morgellons disease is some form of parasitic infection. Morgellons may be caused by a parasitic roundworm, spread by black flies and mosquitoes; or roundworms transmitted by dogs and cats. Roundworms (toxocara) are the most common parasitic infection in dogs and can also infect cats. Morgellons has been treated with a prolonged course of doxycycline, which will also treat H-pylori; and been treated with potent third and fourth generation antibiotics and antiparasitics, with success.

Parasitic roundworms can attack the collagen, in subcutaneous fat layers under the skin, causing intense itching, and filamentous projections from the skin. Parasitic roundworms can also invade the lymph system and lymph nodes. Subcutaneous filariasis is caused by the Loa worm, the streptocerca worm, or the Onchocerca volvulus worm, which are types of worms that invade the subcutaneous layers of the skin. Subcutaneous filariasis also occurs in cattle, horses, and dogs. Could the diagnosis of Morgellons be confused with filariasis, because filariasis is rare in the United States; or could Morgellons be a late stage of untreated scabies or filariasis? Filariasis has been reported in the United States; and the diagnosis of Morgellons may reflect observed and reported symptoms, by a medical provider who is not familiar with filariasis. Filariasis is treated with albendazole and Imervectin in combination; and Imervectin helped Dr. Merchant's patients suffering from Morgellons.

Miasma creates de-pigmentation, or brown patches on the skin. Miasma is sometimes referred to as the mask of pregnancy. Miasma can cause both excess pigmentation and de-pigmentation. Miasma can occur in men or women, and is often caused by a fungal infection on the skin. Miasma in pregnancy is thought to be induced by hormonal changes that stimulate melanin in the body. In pregnant patients, the fungal infection may be preexisting, and the pregnancy reduces immune function, allowing the fungal infection to manifest itself. Excess pigmentation or de-pigmentation in the skin can often be treated with antibiotics or antifungal crème, and does not need to be burned off or cut off, except as a last resort. Widespread skin disease may justify systemic treatment with antibiotics or antifungal medication.

Baldness is thought to be genetic, although hair loss in women can occur and is named alopecia. Baldness may be caused or precipitated by chronic infection with bacteria, fungus, and/or parasites that invade the base of the hair follicles. By observation, baldness is often caused and spread by wearing baseball caps that are sweaty or dirty. The more the baseball caps are worn, the sweatier and dirtier the baseball caps, the more likely baldness will spread over the scalp. Baseball caps aggravate existing baldness, as the caps are used to cover baldness, and spread the pathogens and fungus with heat and sweat, to more hair follicles of the scalp. If baseball caps are necessary or you love them, buy new clean ones and frequently wash the baseball caps.

Alopecia is alleged to be an autoimmune disease, and can occur in humans or animals. It is proposed to be an autoimmune disease, or infection in the hair follicles with bacteria, viruses or parasites. An autoimmune disease is an attack by the immune system, by an infectious pathogen.

Skin cancer comes in three major forms, basal cell, squamous cell, and melanoma. Skin cancer can be caused by underlying chronic infection, weak links, or persistent infection at the location of the skin cancer. Melanoma does not necessarily occur in sun-exposed areas, and has been "associated" with chlamydia psittacosis. The usual response of the medical system is to burn or cut off skin cancer. Burning and cutting may be required, depending on the type of skin cancer, how far and how deep the skin cancer has spread, and the location and type of skin cancer. Imiquimod, a TLR7 inhibitor, is one of the most effective treatments for early skin cancer, particularly basal cell skin cancer. Imiquimod applied to the skin attracts the patient's own white blood cells, to attack the cancer. Imiquimod can cure warts and superficial skin cancers, and is particularly useful for skin cancer on the face. Melanoma treatment and prognosis may be improved by a TLR7 inhibitor, and treatment of psittacosis. Imiquimod is now being widely used in cancer clinical trials, alone and in combination with other cancer drugs.

Imiquimod has been vastly underused, by front line practitioners and oncologists for skin cancer and for all types of cancer. Imiquimod has been shown to prevent or slow metastatic breast cancer, and eradicate breast cancer at metastatic sites. Imiquimod combined with anti-vessel growth drugs have cured metastatic lymphoma. Imiquimod and treatment of psittacosis, or any other pathogen diagnosed, combined with traditional cancer treatment, could improve the prognosis for melanoma. Imiquimod may be a targeted treatment for cancer, in which the imiquimod attracts immune cells, and creates natural antibodies to the cancer. Reprogramming of immune cells is the only explanation for how application of a crème at the primary cancer site could eradicate metastatic cancer at a remote site. Imiquimod is an old drug now being repurposed and used for many new indications, and to program the immune system to make anti-bodies to cancer.

CHAPTER 18

CHRONIC INFECTION IN MENTAL ILLNESS

Dr. Merchant observed the connection between chronic parasitic infection and mental illness, while working in the South Valley. He observed patients who had mental instability, belligerence, and mental health problems, including alcohol and opioid use, who also had low folic acid and B12. The 1988 giardiasis article reported parasites caused malabsorption of nutrients, specifically folic acid and B12, which caused mental instability and a tendency toward belligerence and aggression. We suggested testing and treating patients with mental illness for parasitic infection, and for low folic acid and B12. Low folic acid and B12 has since been "associated" with mental illness and decreased cognitive function; and treatment with folic acid and B12 has been shown to improve mental health.

Recently, doctors noticed that patients with mental illness had unusual pathogens in the gut, and suggested pathogens in the gut (or byproducts of these pathogens) are causing mental illness—"the gut-brain connection". Mental illness can start with infection in the gut, and cause loss of nutrients needed for stable mental health. Pathogens in the gut can spread to the brain, sinus, or eyes, by migrating from the stomach along the vagus nerve, or through the immune system and lymphatics. Immortal pathogens affect mental stability directly and indirectly, by depleting the energy in the cell, dispersing abnormal proteins and debris, and by competing for nutrients. Immortal pathogens consume folic acid and B12; and parasites block the absorption of folic acid and B12 absorption and consume folic acid and B12. Multiple immortal infections and parasites increase the infection burden, accelerate malabsorption and loss of folic acid and B12, and increase the risk of mental illness.

Mental health is a multifaceted problem, which is complicated by pharmaceutical mismanagement with psychiatric drugs. Chronic infection destroys the patients' sense of well-being, destroys normal social interaction, and leads to abnormal thought patterns. Poor mental health can be caused by medical illness, and by an adaptation to the consequences of medical illness. Mental health patients need medical diagnosis and treatment for chronic infection; and not just mental health care and psychiatric drugs. A patient should never be labeled a mental health patient, prior to a complete medical work-up and diagnosis of immortal pathogens that can damage mental health and cause cognitive decline. All mental health patients should be tested for all types of chlamydia infections and other immortal pathogens and parasites that are known to affect mental health; and treated for chlamydia, parasites, fungus, and any other infection diagnosed. They should be given folic acid and B12 supplementation to replace nutrition lost by chronic infections, to stabilize their mental health and restore mental health.

Depression has been "associated" with "inflammatory diseases", including heart attack, heart disease, stroke, cancer, Alzheimer's, Parkinson's, diabetes, arthritis, lupus, multiple sclerosis, ALS, fibromyalgia, hypothyroid, chronic pain, and HIV. "Association" with other diseases, rather than causes, means the other diseases can be co-morbid conditions. Patients with depression have high levels of TNF-alpha, IL-1B (interleukin), and IL-6, which impair cognition. Studies showed patients with symptoms of depression and coronary artery disease have higher levels of chlamydia pneumonia IgG, TNF-alpha, and IL-1B. Chlamydia pneumonia induces the production of TNF-alpha and IL-6. Toxoplasmosis has also been shown to cause depression and a wide variety of other mental illnesses, including but not limited to bipolar disorder, unreasonable anger and reckless behavior. The co-morbid conditions are caused by the same pathogens causing inflammation and depression.

Chronic inflammation is the body's reaction to infectious pathogens—redness, heat, swelling and pain are the hallmarks of infection. Depression is an early manifestation of chronic chlamydia invading the brain, causing inflammation. Chronic depression has also been "associated" with a higher

ACES score, reflecting childhood trauma. The ACES score is important. However, mental health professionals should consider whether the person who inflicted the childhood trauma may have been infected with immortal pathogens, and transmitted immortal pathogens to the child, which cause or aggravate ongoing depression and situational depression.

Psychiatrists prescribe psychiatric drugs for depression, which cause serious side effects. Psychiatric drugs are symptomatic treatment for depression, which can make the patient worse, suicidal, violent toward others, or homicidal. Five of the top ten drugs most likely to induce violence are anti-depressant drugs, including Prozac, Paxil, Luvox, Effexor and Pristiq. The violent five anti-depressants are SSRI drugs that cause an increased rate of suicidal ideation and suicide; and homicidal ideation and homicide. SSRI drugs are highly addicting, and the risk of suicide and violence is greatest when starting the drug, changing the dose, and attempting to withdraw from the drug.[279] The SSRI drugs cause significant withdrawal symptoms, which can last for an extended time, and during withdrawal the SSRI drugs can induce suicide, violence, and homicide. Good medical care, diagnosis and treatment of chronic infections, and supplementation of nutrition, is a better and safer treatment for depression than symptomatic treatment of depression with addicting SSRI drugs.

Manufacturers sell SSRI drugs, and doctors prescribe SSRI drugs, while concealing the dangerous side effects, including addiction, withdrawal, and violence toward self and others. In 2011, mental health professionals prescribed fourteen million Paxil prescriptions, and more than twenty-five million Prozac prescriptions. The rate of suicides and violence toward others has increased, corresponding to the increased use and availability of SSRI drugs. SSRI drugs are a billion-dollar industry, sold without warnings the drugs are highly addicting; and lead to suicide, violence, homicidal ideation and homicides. SSRI drugs are a shortcut to care, *in lieu* of medical diagnosis and treatment, and *in lieu* of collaborating with doctors capable of diagnosing pathogens known to cause mental illness.

---

[279] *See* Horgan J. 2013. Did Antidepressant Play a Role in Navy Yard Massacre? Scientific American. Sep 20, 2013. Doi: https://blogs.scientificamerican.com/cross-check/did-antidepressant-play-a-role-in-navy-yard-massacre/.

The clinical trials for Prozac, the first SSRI drug, were manipulated by the manufacturer to gain approval; and adverse events were concealed. Prozac was the predicate drug on which to base approval of other SSRI drugs, like Paxil. Peter Breggin, M.D. reported he personally examined FDA documents from the original clinical studies of Prozac; and found the manufacturer gave clinical subjects Valium, when the subjects developed a high rate of anxiety and agitation taking Prozac. The manufacturer also manipulated the statistical analysis to make the suicide rate appear higher in the placebo group; to conceal an increased rate of suicide in the Prozac treatment group. The manufacturer received FDA approval, without disclosure of the use of Valium in clinical studies, to control anxiety and agitation caused by Prozac; or the higher rate of suicide in the treatment group. The FDA did not approve Prozac, they unwittingly approved the combination of Prozac and Valium, without disclosure to prescribing doctors. The SSRI drugs cause a higher risk of suicide and violence toward others—and the risk applies to teenagers and adults, not just teenagers; and to men and women, not just to men, as the manufacturers would like anyone with knowledge of the risks to believe. The drugs do not work and are dangerous![280]

In a study by the Drug Safety Research Unit in Southampton, Professor Healy reported that one in two-hundred-fifty patients, who took Paxil or Prozac, were involved in a violent episode. In the study of 25,000 people, violence included thirty-one assaults and one homicide. Subsequent studies showed higher rates of suicide on the SSRI drugs than when patients were given placebos; and anti-depressants increase the risk of death from all causes, by thirty-three percent.[281] Depressed patients on SSRI drugs have a higher rate of death because they have a higher rate of suicide, a higher rate of committing violent crimes, and chronic medical conditions which are not being diagnosed and treated.

---

[280] Breggin P. 2013. <u>Psychiatric Drug Withdrawal, A Guide for Prescribers, Therapists, Patients, and Their Families</u>. New York: Springer Publishing Company.
[281] Brooks M. 2017. Antidepressants Tied to a Significantly Increased Risk for Death, Medscape Family Medicine. Sept 21, 2017. Doi: medscape.com/viewarticle/886015.

The FDA and the manufacturers have known, since before 2004, that SSRI drugs cause violence toward others and homicides. Advocacy groups sought a warning on homicidal ideation, homicides, and violence toward others, in 2004, which manufacturers strongly resisted. The FDA refused to require the warning on homicides and violence toward others. A Dear In 2006, a "Dear Doctor" letter was sent by the manufacturer warning of an increased risk of suicide at all ages. Other countries around the world have required warnings of aggression, hostility, agitation, hallucinations, confusion, altered mental status, impulsive and disturbing thoughts, violence toward others, homicidal ideation, and homicide, on the labeling for the SSRI drugs, starting in 1991, and have continued to add warnings thereafter.[282]

In 2016, Dr. Peter Gotzche reviewed clinical studies and published trials in Europe and the United Kingdom, and reported SSRI drugs increase the risk of suicide and violence in all ages, increase the risk of suicide attempts, and increase aggression in children and adolescents. He also reported when Paxil was given to healthy adults, the drug also lead to suicide and violence. His conclusion was "it can no longer be doubted that antidepressants are dangerous and can cause suicide and homicide at any age."[283] Despite an international warning for violence toward others, homicidal ideation, and homicide for SSRI drugs, the doctors, investigators, and public are not generally aware of the risk of violence toward others or homicides, and doctors have not given the warning in practice.

The FDA documented an 840% higher risk of violent acts when a patient takes or withdraws from SSRI drugs, and has documented over *fifteen-thousand violent acts* related to SSRI drugs.[284] It is well accepted in the

---

[282] International Warnings on Psychiatric and Other Drugs Causing Hostility, Aggression, Homicidal and Suicidal Behavior/Ideation. Doi: //files.ondemandhosting. info/data/www.cchr.org/files/International_Warnings on Psychiatric Drugs Suicide Homicide.pdf.

[283] Gotzche P. 2016. Antidepressants Increase the Risk of Suicide and Violence at All Ages. Nov 16, 2016. Doi: https://www.madinamerica.com/2016/11/antidepressants-increase-risk-suicide-violence-ages/.

[284] Breggin P. Psychiatric Drug Facts: What Your Doctor May Not know. Doi: https://breggin.com/psychiatry-has-no-answer-to-gun-massacres/.

industry the FDA receives reports of less than one percent of adverse events, which means SSRI drugs could be responsible for more than one and a half million violent acts toward others. Doctors prescribing SSRI drugs are not aware of the risks of violence and homicide, and even the Office of the Medical Investigator may not be aware, despite the astounding amount of violence and homicides caused by SSRI drugs.

All countries now warn of the risk of suicide, when taking SSRI drugs. In 2007, after many years of public advocacy, the FDA required a black box warning on SSRI drugs for suicide. The FDA continues to refuse to require a black box warning for violence toward others and homicides, which warnings have been blocked by politicians and manufacturers, and concealed from doctors and the public, by the manufacturers and the FDA.

The United States has the highest rate of anti-depressant usage and the highest rate of gun ownership in the world—a deadly combination. Anti-depressants given to males can increase testosterone, and trigger violent episodes toward self and others. Peter Breggin, M.D. calls it "medication madness" causing mayhem, murders, and suicides.[285] Dr. Breggin describes the shooters on SSRI drugs as being in a fugue-like state, disassociated from normal controls over behavior. The SSRI drugs cause the shooter's mental health to decline, and the shooter to be more depressed and angry, agitated, confused, and filled with rage against anyone and everyone. The shooter wants to die, and wants revenge for the injustices suffered over their lifetime, against perpetrators of the injustice and innocent people. The mass shooters are committing a "revenge suicide". SSRI drugs can turn boys and men into revenge mass murders. Lives are lost and families of the victims and the killers are destroyed by suicide, violence, and homicide, induced by SSRI drugs. SSRI medications to treat depression in patients with chronic chlamydia in the brain and/or toxoplasmosis in the brain, is a dangerous combination.

Virtually *every* mass shooter in the United States has been linked to troubled boys and men who were prescribed SSRI drugs. Reports confirmed at

---

[285] Breggin P. 2008. Medication Madness, the Role of Psychiatric Drugs in Cases of Violence, Suicide, and Crime. New York: St. Martin's Griffin.

least thirty-five mass shooters were taking or withdrawing from SSRI drugs, including Columbine, Virginia Tech, the Aurora Movie Theater, the Pulse nightclub, the Navy Yard, and Parkland High School. The Las Vegas shooter was given diazepam, another drug with the potential to induce violence toward others, for a psychiatric condition and sleep, three months before the shooting. The Las Vegas shooter may have been in a state of confusion and agitation from the medication, or withdrawal from it. In New Mexico, one of the least populated states, at least six mass shootings and untold violence and suicide have been caused by SSRI drugs, or withdrawal from SSRI drugs; and in one case, days before the shooter murdered five people, including two policemen, the doctor who prescribed the SSRI medications dismissed complaints by the patient he was having unusual thoughts of homicide as "it will pass". SSRI drugs increase agitation, anxiety, and confusion; worsen any or all preexisting symptoms; and can create a "medication madness".

The revenge-suicide mass shooters on SSRI drugs have commonalities in their countenance. They all look sick! The shooters look gaunt; their eyes look sunken; they have dark circles under the eyes; they have red and irritated eyes; and they have bulging eyes. Adam Lanza, James Holmes, Stephen Paddock and Omar Mateen all had darkened circles under their eyes, suggesting undiagnosed and untreated chronic disease. Adam Lanza and James Holmes were gaunt with bulging eyes, which is a sign of high thyroid and chronic disease; and high thyroid is also caused by infectious pathogens and has been "associated" with mental instability. Stephen Paddock looked sick, and told friends he felt sick all the time. He reported he had chronic fatigue, and was in pain all the time, prior to the Las Vegas shooting. Apparently, no one observed Stephen Paddock's countenance; and he was prescribed valium for anxiety and sleep instead of diagnosis and treatment of the medical conditions that made him feel sick all the time, gave him chronic pain, and made him unable to sleep. No one recognized the countenance of mass shooters that suggested a chronic disease. The shooters were all prescribed SSRI medications and anti-anxiety medication as a shortcut, *in lieu* of medical diagnosis and treatment.

The Parkland, Florida high school shooter, Nikolas Cruz, is a frightening example of what can happen when mental health professionals ignore medical illness; and prescribe psychiatric medications *in lieu* of medical diagnosis. Nicholas Cruz had an autism spectrum disorder, was identified at age three as developmentally disabled, and had a misalignment of his eyes that would make reading and interpreting the world difficult for a child. He likely developed behavioral problems in response to his disability, and his difficulty reading and interpreting the world. He was sad, bullied, and an outcast among outcasts. He was socially awkward, immature, and pushed away from social circles, because he was verbally aggressively and had violent outbursts. His internal and external anger accelerated over his life, as he experienced rejection and bullying. He engaged in self-mutilation and cruelty to animals. He was expelled from three schools for violent outbursts. He had intermittent explosive disorder with recurrent impulsive, problematic outbursts and violent and physical aggression, disproportionate to the situation. Police were called to his home *thirty-nine times* prior to the shooting, because of his explosive outbursts of anger and rage.

Nicholas Cruz was reported to have seen a mental health professional a year before the Parkland High School shooting, and may have gotten "medications" for his depression. We do not know what medications he was given, if he took the medications, or if he was withdrawing from the medications at the time of the shooting. Paxil is commonly prescribed by mental health professionals, in the circumstances presented by Nicolas Cruz. Shortly after seeing the mental health professional, Cruz began posted homicidal ideation online, stating he wanted to become a professional school shooter. During the next year, his girlfriend broke up with him and he self-mutilated in response to the break-up. He was expelled from school for getting into a fight with his prior girlfriend's new boyfriend. His adopted mother died, and he was orphaned, and without a stable home. He was disconnected from society, with no anchor, no future, and no hope; and likely disconnected from the mental health professional who had prescribed his medication for depression. His homicidal ideation started when he was given psychiatric drugs, and evolved into a mass murder on Valentine's Day, when he was overwhelmed by the effect of the SSRI drugs, his medical conditions, and situational depression.

Nicholas Cruz' mental health problems were consistent with longstanding toxoplasmosis, acquired from cats. Toxoplasmosis causes schizophrenia, depression, anger, aggression, disproportionate anger, violent outbursts, self-mutilation, explosive violence, and intermittent explosive disorder. We do not know Nicholas Cruz's exposure to cats *in utero*, before his adoption, or growing up with his adopted parents; however, after his mother's death, two months prior to the shooting, he moved in with a family with six cats. The exposure to six cats, and possibly kittens, may have caused acute re-infection and exacerbation of his toxoplasmosis, at a point in time when he had particularly high situational stress; although, the toxoplasmosis infection was likely longstanding. The SSRI drugs worsened his depression, anger and anxiety; and triggered homicidal ideation and worsening of his intermittent explosive disorder.

Nicholas Cruz's countenance suggests immortal pathogens were acquired *in utero,* causing autism and developmental disorders; and toxoplasmosis acquired *in utero* or after birth, causing mental illness. He likely had toxoplasmosis, which was causing numerous mental disabilities and mental illnesses, was given SSRI drugs, and had access to guns. He had prior episodes of intermittent explosive disorder, and the SSRI drugs caused homicidal ideation and explosive rage that led to the mass shooting at Parkland High School.

Investigation into the motives of mass shooters do not include a medical investigation of pathogens causing mental illness, or the drugs given by mental health professionals that induce violence and homicide. Investigators are not generally aware of the potential for SSRI drugs to cause homicides and mass shooting. Investigators seldom report whether the shooters owned cats or were exposed to cats or other animals that could transmit pathogens known to impact mental health and cause explosive rage, homicidal ideation, and homicide. A pet history and diagnosis of toxoplasmosis and other pathogens causing mental illness is rarely considered when investigating mass shootings. Adam Lanza had a cat in his household, and before the Sandy Hook mass murder demanded the cat not come near him. Stephen Paddock had cats. James Holmes had a dog, and other pets cannot be determined. Nikolas Cruz had two dogs, and was cruel to animals; and moved in with a family with six cats. One of the mass murders in New Mexico is confirmed to have been committed by a person who was chronically ill, depressed, had three cats, and was given Paxil, instead of medical diagnosis and treatment.

Common patterns in mass shooters emerge, which could be used to identify potential school shooters and mass shooters. We need to empower doctors, mental health professionals, families, friends, schools, workplaces, and the point of access to guns, to identify potential school shooters and mass murderers. A point system could be used to identify potential school shooters and mass shooters, which could include SSRI drugs; pets, particularly cats; undiagnosed physical complaints; depression; social isolation; anger; aggression; self-mutilation; killing of animals; violent outbursts; domestic violence; stalking; and access to guns. SSRI drugs plus some or all of these factors should trigger an investigation that empowers authorities, administrators, and families to remove all guns from the household, and prevent access to purchasing guns or ammunition.

Schools should be notified of students who are prescribed SSRI drugs; advocate for medical evaluation of those on SSRI drugs; report concerning events in children taking SSRI drugs; and investigate adverse circumstances in the home of children who bully others, that would cause the child to be a bully or act out violently. We need to identify potential mass shooters, prevent access to guns by those who have the common patterns of all prior mass shooters, and help potential shooters obtain the necessary medical evaluations and learn to calm their anger. Schools need to work to deter bullying; promote early training in conflict resolution and ways for students to calm anger, before the person becomes an angry man with a gun.

We need to train and empower families; and school administrators, counselors, and teachers, to look for and address these triggers in potential school shooters, and empower fellow-students of potential shooters to recognize and report the danger. The community needs to be educated about the astounding amount of violence caused by SSRI drugs, and the fact SSRI drugs induce suicide, homicide, and revenge suicide. We need legislation to remove guns from those taking SSRI drugs, and those who meet the criteria of potential mass shooters.

Angry violent men with a gun are the most dangerous among us. The angry and violent men with guns, who take SSRI drugs, are the ones who commit mass shootings. Yet, angry violent men with guns are not defined as mentally ill, even though angry violent men are most likely to need mental health counseling, to learn to calm and diffuse their anger.[286] We need to implement a new diagnostic category in mental health, for angry, violent men, with guns, particularly if prescribed SSRI drugs, so they can receive treatment to diffuse their anger and violence, and be taught to cope with their anger without violence. Males prescribed SSRI drugs should be put on a registry that prohibits gun purchases, and allows confiscation of guns for the duration of SSRI treatment and withdrawal. We need to remove guns from angry men with guns who take SSRI drugs. Any patient on an SSRI drug must be restricted from access to guns and from purchasing guns!

Society cannot stop mass-murder revenge-suicide until the mental health system recognizes the infectious causes of mental illness, diagnoses medical illnesses in mental health patients, and stops giving SSRI drugs to depressed boys and men with access to guns. Specialized training and licensing should be required for psychiatrists before they are allowed to prescribe any of the violent five psychiatric drugs; and patients should be subject to special monitoring when taking SSRI drugs. The mental health system must stop relying on SSRI medications, *in lieu* of diagnosis of medical illness causing depression, in patients of all ages. No mental health professional should prescribe SSRI drugs, until the patient has had a complete medical evaluation, including screening for pathogens; medical diagnosis and treatment immortal infections and parasites; and efforts have been made to diagnosis and treat toxoplasmosis. When SSRI medications are prescribed, mental health professionals must take

---

[286] Hayes L. 2018. Anger Isn't a Mental Illness. Can We Treat it Anyway? Slate Magazine. Apr 16, 2018. Doi: https://slate.com/technology/2018/04/anger-isnt-a-mental-illness-but-we-should-still-treat-it.html.

responsibility to warn of the risk of addiction, withdrawal that can last many months, suicidal ideation and suicide, aggression and violence toward others, homicidal ideation, and homicide. The mental health professional must take responsibility to inquire as to the SSRI patient's access to guns and assure all guns are secured in the home. Warnings must be given to the patient, the family, and to schools, whenever a patient is prescribed SSRI drugs.

Mental illness is a symptom of medical illness! The major problem in the mental health system is mental health professionals have little or no training in diagnosing medical conditions, chronic infections, or even chronic infections and parasites known to be "associated" with mental illness. Mental health professionals do not attempt medical diagnosis, and have abdicated their responsibility to diagnose medical conditions. Psychiatrists do not do medical diagnosis, and seldom work with other doctors who can do medical diagnosis and medical treatment of psychiatric patients. Psychologists are not allowed to do medical diagnosis, nor trained in medical diagnosis. In the mental health system, the patient gets counseling and psychiatric drugs. Psychologists do the counseling, and the psychiatrists prescribe psychiatric drugs.

The mental health patient is left without anyone who can and will diagnose their medical illness. The psychologist needs to become part of the team, seeking clues to the cause of medical illnesses in their patients, particularly animal contact; and provide the information to the psychiatrist or medical provider, who can diagnose and treat the patient. The psychiatrist needs to evaluate every patient for medical causes of mental illness, or refer patients to doctors who can evaluate medical causes of mental illness. Every mental health patient needs and deserves an extensive medical evaluation for immortal pathogens and parasites. A history of pets, and particularly cats, should be part of any effort to diagnose the root cause of any mental illnesses. Yet, mental health professionals fail to consider prior exposure to cats or toxoplasmosis, or other medical causes of mental illness; and prescribe SSRI medications for a variety of mental health conditions known to be caused by toxoplasmosis.

The Veteran's Administration Hospital in Albuquerque reported the fourth highest rate of suicide among veterans, in the country.[287] The veterans return from war with immortal infections and parasites that go unrecognized, undiagnosed, and untreated; and the patients are referred to psychiatry for their report of a mental health concern. The Veteran's Administration does not diagnose and treat medical illnesses in mental health patients; and the default position of psychiatrists at the Veteran's Administration Hospital is to prescribe Paxil. The Veteran's Administration prescribes Paxil, then leaves patients without access to doctors for extended times between visits; and when the patient develops strange thoughts of suicide or homicide, or the patient is experiencing withdrawal, the veteran is unable to reach a doctor or unable to make a timely appointment. The psychiatrists at the Veteran's Administration ignore medical conditions, and use SSRI drugs as a shortcut to diagnosis and care, causing a higher rate of suicide among veterans. Dr. Merchant treated Vietnam veterans who suffered from post-traumatic stress disorder (PTSD), by treating chronic infections and supplementing folic acid and B12, which significantly improved their mental health.

Patients subjected to difficult conditions in military deployments are at greater risk of acquiring parasites and immortal infections; and unusual pathogens common in other parts of the world, such as leishmaniosis, shistomiasis, and unusual forms of streptococcus. The Veterans Administration should establish a special permanent department to evaluate returning veterans for infectious pathogens and parasites. Veterans returning from any foreign deployment should be given a routine screening to diagnose and treat immortal infections and parasitic disease, to prevent ongoing and future chronic disease. Returning veterans complaining of mental health problems in particular should be given a complete medical examination and testing for immortal pathogens and parasites. The Veterans Administration ignored a parasitic infection in Vietnam veterans for forty years, and the Vietnam veterans are now developing liver cancer; ignored infectious pathogens that are now causing a higher rate of eye

---

[287] Hayden M. 2017. NM is 4th in U.S. for Suicide Rate Among Veterans. Albuquerque Journal. Oct 1, 2017. Doi: abqjournal.com/1071713/ nm-ranks-high-in-veteran-suicides.

cancer; and ignored medical illness causing mental illness, prescribed SSRI drugs, and now observes a high rate of suicide among veterans.

Scientists reported mothers taking SSRI drugs during pregnancy, and during the year before delivery, have an increased risk of having a child with autism. It is probable underlying immortal infections caused depression in the mother, which led to prescribing an SSRI drug. The chronic infection made the mother depressed, and the chronic infection caused maternal depression *and* autism in the fetus. The infectious cause of autism was present in the mother during pregnancy and transmitted to the fetus; and/or the anti-depressant medications combined with chronic infection to caused autism in the fetus. Autism has also been linked to infection *in utero*, and infants with autism have high TNF-alpha in the spinal fluid and co-morbid gastrointestinal disease. A recent study of the brains of fetuses exposed to SSRI drugs in pregnancy showed alteration in brain development, in areas of the brain leading to anxiety and depression later in life.[288] SSRI drugs can increase anxiety and depression in adults, and cause the same effect in the brain of a developing fetus.

The Editor-in-Chief of the "Psychiatry Journal", Joseph Coyle, called two studies on SSRI use before and during pregnancy game changers.[289] Conditions in the womb were found to be as important, or more important than genes, in causing autism. The twin study author said much more emphasis needs to be directed to prenatal conditions and autism susceptibility; and environment in the womb is more important than genes. The environment in the womb includes fetal exposure to SSRI drugs, and underlying immortal pathogens in the mother, which cross the placenta and cause both depression in the mother and autism in fetus. Untreated infection in pregnancy has been "associated" with autism,

---

[288] Lugoo-Candelas C, *et al.* 2018. Associations Between Brain Structure and Connectivity in Infants and Exposure to Selective Serotonin Reuptake Inhibitors During Pregnancy, JAMA Pediatr. April 9, 2018. Doi: 10.1001/jama pediatrics.2017.5227. Doi: jamanetwork.com/journals/jamapediatrics/fullarticle/2676821.
[289] Tarkan, L. 2011. New Study Implicates Environmental Factors in Autism. New York Times. July 4, 2011. Doi: https://www.nytimes.com/2011/07/05/health/research/05autism.html.

regressive developmental disorder, and cavernous sinus malformation. Prenatal care and woman considering pregnancy, who want to reduce the risk of autism in their child, should not take SSRI medications; and should be tested and treated for chlamydia, toxoplasmosis, and other immortal infections that cause depression and can cause autism. Doctors fear treating pregnant women for infections, because of fear the treatment may be harmful to a fetus; when doctors should fear *not* treating a pregnant woman with acute or chronic infections, because the risk of damage to the fetus from the pathogen may be greater than the risk of treating infections.

We frequently hear the United States has an opioid crisis. We have more opioid use in the United States than any other country in the world. The average number of people in this country who have an opioid prescription is sixty-six out of one-hundred people. One county in Arizona had more opioid prescriptions than people, at a rate of one-hundred twenty-six prescriptions per one-hundred people.[290] The opioid crisis arises from both mental health and medical health. The patient may have had a trauma, surgery, or cancer that justified pain medications. Justified pain prescriptions are not causing the opioid crisis. The opioid crisis is a multifaceted problem.

First, "Why are patients having so much pain?" The patients should be evaluated for chronic infections, as a possible explanation for the pain, before defaulting to opioid prescriptions. Second, medical boards and insurance companies arbitrarily penalize doctors who prescribe opioids to a patient. Doctors are required to check state computer programs monitoring opioid prescriptions, for every pain prescription. After an opioid is prescribed, medical boards and insurance companies pressure the doctor to limit or restrict pain medication, without offering the patient an alternative treatment for pain or medical diagnosis. Some patients feel obtaining pain prescriptions from doctors is too difficult, or the doctors refuse to prescribe pain medications, causing patients to hoard opioids in the medicine cabinet or seek opioids on the street. Adults use and

---

[290] Alltucker K. 2018. Ariz. County Had More Opioid Rxs Than People. Jan 29, 2018. Doi: https://www.azcentral.com/story/news/local/arizona-health/2018/01/29/opioid-crisis-hit-arizona-mohave-county-hardest/1069801001/.

hoard opioid medications, in case they need them and cannot find a doctor willing to prescribe pain medications when needed. Children and adults take opioids from medicine cabinets, become addicted, and when the supply is restricted, seek opioids on the street. Third, pressure to deny opioid prescriptions to patients has caused the prescribing of opioid pain medications to be concentrated in a few doctors, who specialize in anesthesiology or pain. Pain doctors are not trained in medical diagnosis and treatment; and do not consider medical diagnosis and treatment of chronic infection as part of their responsibility.

We have approximately sixty-eight million cats and sixty-two million dogs in the United States.[291] The United States has the highest rate of depression, the highest rate of SSRI usage, the highest rate of opioid prescriptions, one of the highest rates of pet ownership, the highest rate of gun ownership, and the highest rate of mass shootings. The issues are connected to each other, because chronic disease, mental illness, and chronic pain are often undiagnosed and untreated immortal pathogens that have been transmitted to humans, from animals.

Medicare pays for an average of twenty-three million opioid pills per day. States allowing medical cannabis had a fourteen percent drop in opioid prescriptions, which converts to three-million-seven-hundred-thousand less opioid pills dispensed per day. States allowing homegrown cannabis for medical use saw a drop of one-million eight-hundred-thousand opioid pills prescribed per day. Cannabis can be effective for pain, be a step-down drug for opioid addictions, and can be an effective treatment for post-traumatic stress disorder.

SSRI drugs and opioids are shortcuts to doing the work necessary to diagnose a chronic infection. Treating depression with SSRI drugs worsens mental health; makes all pre-existing symptoms worse; and leads to suicidal ideation, suicide, violence toward others, homicidal ideation, and homicide. Treatment of pain using opioid medication instead of treating the root cause of the pain, leads to dependence on opioids, desperation by patients

---

[291] Rabinowitz P, *et al.* 2007. Pet Related Infections. American Family Physician. Nov 2007. 76(9): 1314-1322. Doi: www.aafp.org/afp/2007/1101/p1314.html.

who hold onto opioids for future needs, and more addiction. Diagnosing and treating the root cause of the mental illness, understanding why the patient needs opioid drugs, and finding less harmful alternatives to relieve symptoms, are better and safer for the patient.

Too many children are labeled as ADHD, and diverted into the mental health system, when they have a medical problem causing their lack of attention and focus. Attention deficit disorder may be caused by pathogens, parasites, dysbiosis, lack of nutrition, and lack of sleep. Parasites compete for critical nutrition required for mental focus, cognitive function, and mental stability. An immortal infection or parasite can rob the brain of nutrition needed for brain development, focus and calm; and impair sleep needed for cognitive function and focus. Toxocara (roundworm) has been associated with decreased cognitive function, decreased learning, and lower IQ. No one asks if ADHD children have co-morbid stomach issues, or immortal infections, even when adults complain of disruptive burping. No one has investigated the biochemical and PCR test results for children with ADHD; or done studies to determine how many ADHD children have parasites and benefit by treatment of parasites. The mental health system does not diagnose medical diseases! Children with ADHD, who Dr. Merchant treated with antibiotics, antiparasitics, and probiotics, showed improvement in ADHD. Any child or adult with ADHD should be evaluated for intestinal pathogens, parasites, dysbiosis, and sleep disorders.

Eating disorders are characterized as a psychiatric problem. Eating disorders are a medical disease. Eating disorders are caused by chronic gastrointestinal infection, including chlamydia infections, parasitic infections, and worms, alone or in combination, causing dysbiosis. A patient with parasitic disease can be too thin or too fat, anorexic, nauseated, and/or bloated. Intestinal infections reduce appetite and the desire to eat, cause nausea, make food unappealing, and cause a decline in mental health. As the infections worsen, the malabsorption worsens, causing further decline in mental health. The patients with eating disorders are inducted into the psychiatric system; then given psychiatric drugs instead of medical diagnosis and treatment for immortal pathogens and parasites.

Psychiatric drugs, prescribed for symptoms without medical diagnosis, are causing a nation of people addicted to drugs who are committing violent acts toward self and others. All mental health professionals must understand the role of immortal infection with chlamydia and parasites; and learn to diagnose and treat chronic infection. Psychiatry and psychology, and pain specialists, cannot find the cause of mental illness, opioid addiction, ADHD, or eating disorders, because they do not look for medical illness or chronic infection. Psychiatrists have no idea about medical causes of mental illness, or the root cause of mental illness, even when infectious pathogens have been proven to cause mental illness. Any mental illness is a complex medical problem in need of medical diagnosis and treatment, and nutritional supplements to replace nutrition lost from chronic infection and causing mental instability. Psychiatrists must become informed as to immortal pathogens and parasites causing mental illness. In any chronic disease involving mental health, medical causes need to be identified and treated. Psychiatric patients deserve the same careful medical diagnosis and treatment as every other patient.

CHAPTER 19

CHRONIC INFECTION AND AGING

The Neanderthal and Denosovans cultures disappeared from earth, more than 40,000 years ago. Scientists have shown both cultures were heavily infected with pathogens and "viroids". Viroids are the smallest known infectious pathogens, composed of a short strand of single-stranded RNA, without a protein coat. The viroids identified were likely remnants of immortal pathogens; and the finding of a high level of infectious pathogens and viroids in ancient remains suggests infections within the culture were a possible explanation for extinction of the culture. Clusters of chronic diseases have been reported in close-knit communities, when immortal infections have proliferated in the community. Clusters of childhood leukemia, rare cancers, and eye cancer have been reported in close-knit communities. Infectious pathogens can spread and cause clusters of chronic disease, which could devastate a culture as the infection is passed among community members, causing infection and re-infection, and ultimately chronic disease and a genetic cost. The genetic cost of a culture being heavily infected with immortal infections may have contributed to the extinction of the Neanderthal and Denosovans.

Today, animal species are going extinct because of a high burden of infectious disease. The koalas are known to be highly infected with immortal pathogens, which is harming the fertility and lifespan of the koala, and threatens the koala species with extinction. Tasmanian devils are so heavily infected with immortal pathogens that when they bite each other, during courting or battle, they transmit an aggressive form of cancer; and the Tasmanian devils are also becoming extinct.

Aging occurs at the cellular level. As the person ages, inflammatory markers increase and immune system function decreases. Cells that have finished their proliferative life span *in vitro*, and reached a terminal, post-mitotic state, are called senescent cells. Senescent cells no longer divide. The definition of senescent cells originated from the belief the irreversible non-dividing state has a relationship to aging.

In the 1960's, Leonard Hayflick and Paul Moorhead discovered normal human cells divide approximately fifty times, before becoming senescent. Dr. Hayflick found the only cells which are immortal are cancer cells.[292] More recently, others proposed aging is related to failure of the energy-making capacity of the cells. Immortal pathogens interfere with the energy making capacity of the cell, and as the pathogens proliferate and become chronic, the energy making capacity is damaged throughout the body.

Attempts have been made to find markers of senescent cells, in order to detect their presence *in vivo,* in donors of different ages. One marker which was expected to demonstrate an increase of post-mitotic cells with aging is a marker of a long-resting phase in the cell, whether reversible or irreversible. Others suggested the number of post-mitotic cells do not increase with aging, and is irrelevant in aging. Others have suggested the key to aging is to halt the loss of the metabolic process in the cells, meaning the loss of the ability of the cell to produce energy. Post-mitotic cells are found in increased numbers in pathology, and some argue the term senescent cell is a misnomer.[293]

Chlamydia causes senescent cells, because chlamydia impairs the ability of the cell to produce energy. The cells infected with chlamydia lose the ability to make ATP, the pathogen consumes ATP, the pathogen consumes sugar and creates fermentation, and the pathogen impairs oxygen and sugar transport into the cell. Chlamydia pneumonia takes control of the energy-producing mechanisms in the cell, and impairs normal apoptosis. The omni-present chlamydia bacterium is causing an increase in inflammatory markers, infecting immune cells, and accelerating the decline in the

---

[292] Wikipedia. Cellular Senescence. Doi: en.wikipedia.org/wiki/Cellular_senescence.

[293] Gonos E, ed. 1998. Mechanisms of Ageing and Development. Elsevier. Jun 1, 1998. Vol 103(1): 105-109. Doi: journals.elsevier.com/mechanisms-of-ageing-and-development.

immune system. Pathogens that speed or impair the development of senescent cells cause a proliferation of senescent cells, accelerate aging, and are a sign of immortal intracellular infection.

Everyone is recurrently exposed to chlamydia infections, throughout life. Half the population has been infected with chlamydia pneumonia by middle age, and eighty-percent of the elderly has been infected. Chlamydia trachoma has been estimated to be present in one-fourth to one-third of the population, and in some countries, such as Brazil and Sweden, chlamydia trachoma is endemic. Chlamydia psittacosis estimates range from one percent; and up to fifty percent, if the person is or has been exposed to birds. It is the rare lucky person, or the very careful person, who avoids acquiring all these immortal pathogens during their life. The reality is most people will acquire one or more immortal intracellular pathogens during their life, and how the pathogens are treated and combine with other pathogens can impact longevity.

Aging is dependent on the number of immortal infections a patient harbors, how the patient has been treated, and the persistence of the infection. Dr. Ewald called aging a super-category that has been lumped together, under the category of natural aging. He hypothesized signs of premature aging in younger patients arise from infection. Dr. Ewald argued, based on reasoning and logic, that aging is dependent on the number of pathogens a person acquires in their life. He predicted tissues in a person who harbors a lot of pathogens would age earlier, and alter the person's biologic structure earlier in life.

A study on the naked mole rat supports the theory that the infectious burden determines healthy aging. The mole rat makes almost perfect proteins every time, and is free of abnormal proteins and cell debris, ordinarily generated by an immune system battle with immortal pathogens. The mole rat lives underground in colonies and has a complex social structure, remains spry until the end of life, and the species seems resistant to cancer. The naked mole rat makes ten times less abnormal proteins than other mouse species, and lives thirty years longer.[294] The mole rat has less exposure to immortal pathogens, living its entire life underground. The mole rat has less abnormal proteins, which is consistent with less chronic infections; and with less chronic infections and less abnormal proteins, the mole rat lives a significantly longer life.

Studies have looked at patients who had a chronic low level of infection, and found aging was linked to higher levels of TNF-alpha and Interleukin-6 (IL-6), in the elderly.[295] One hundred thirty-three participants died during the study, out of three-hundred thirty-three study participants. Patients with higher levels of TNF-alpha and IL-6 had faster aging and mortality. The authors stated, "Ageing [sic] is associated with low-grade inflammation and markers such as IL-6", which have prognostic value. TNF-alpha initiates an inflammatory cascade, "associated" with mortality in the older population. High TNF-alpha was "associated" with mortality in men but not women. Low-grade elevations of IL-6 was associated with mortality in both men and women. Plasma levels of TNF-alpha correlated linearly with IL-6 and C-reactive protein. The findings of high TNF-alpha and Il-6 were independent of other lifestyle risk factors, such as smoking, diet and exercise. The study supports chronic infection with chlamydia pathogens accelerate aging, because chlamydia pneumonia is known to generate TNF-alpha, IL-6, and C-reactive protein, which were all correlated with aging and mortality.

Research is needed on people in their nineties and people over one-hundred years old, to determine what chronic immortal infections they have, and how their infections were treated—not merely searching for one pathogen or one marker of immortal infection at a time. No one has studied patients with healthy aging and extremely long lives, to determine whether the super aging individuals avoided immortal infections or had somehow

---

[294] Azpurua J, *et al.* 2013. Naked Mole-Rat Has Increased Translational Fidelity Compared with the Mouse, as Well as a Unique 28S Ribosomal RNA Cleavage. Proc Natl Acad Sci USA. 110(43):17350-5. Oct 22, 2013. Doi: 10.1073/pnas.1313473110. Epub 2013 Sep 30.

[295] Brunnesgaard H, *et al.* 2003. Predicting Death from Tumour Necrosis Factor-Alpha and Interleukin-6 in 80-Year Old People. Clin Exp Immunol. 2003. 132:24-31. Doi: 10.1046/j.1365-2249.2003.02137.x.

successfully dealt with the chronic immortal infections; the level of the infectious burden in those with healthy aging; or how the patients' acute infections were treated, as an explanation for their healthy aging and longevity. No one has studied whether patients consistently treated for immortal infections with antibiotics or antiparasitics, other than penicillin, had a better prognosis for healthy aging and longevity. No one has studied whether a lower infectious burden means retention of normal cell function and apoptosis, less abnormal proteins and debris, and less chronic disease. Those with a lower infectious burden are more likely to maintain a normal level of folic acid and B12, which provides protection against cognitive decline and chronic disease.

People should avoid creating weak links that become targets for pathogens to attack. Avoid exposure to infectious pathogens from animals, and behavior that causes life-long chronic infections. People need to be smarter about avoiding animal pathogens, and recognize immortal animal pathogens can cause chronic disease; and be more careful with pets and animals. People need to avoid ingesting polluted water, and avoid sexually transmitted disease. Fitness and a good diet aid in strengthening the immune system and fighting pathogens. When an immortal infection is acquired, seek treatment; and avoid penicillin in acute respiratory illness and pneumonia. Avoid letting the immortal infections become widespread, and overwhelm the cells and immune system.

Avoid bad habits like smoking tobacco, which accelerate aging and create weak links. Every disease is accelerated and aggravated by smoking tobacco; and smoking tobacco accelerates cognitive decline, and makes tissue more susceptible to infection and cancer. No matter the medical condition, diagnosing, treating and surviving chronic medical illness is always more complicated in smokers, and smokers age faster than non-smokers.

The best hope for a long and healthy life is avoiding immortal pathogens, avoiding the most virulent of the immortal pathogens, and avoiding infection with multiple pathogens. We cannot live a sterile life, and no one can avoid all infectious pathogens. It is inevitable we acquire acute infections during life, because we live in communities and our children go to school. It may be difficult to avoid chlamydia pneumonia, mycoplasma, H-pylori, and Epstein Barr infections; but the person who does not acquire chlamydia trachoma, chlamydia psittacosis, toxoplasmosis, and dangerous viruses through drug use or from mosquitoes, will have the best chance to live a long and healthy life. Take care of yourself with diet and exercise, and supplement nutrition as needed, to help the immune system be stronger in fighting the immortal infections, and try to enhance the diversity of the microbiome and the mycobiome. Avoiding immortal infections, treating acute infections appropriately, keeping the overall burden of chronic infections low, and a healthy lifestyle, can improve the likelihood of healthy aging and a longer life.

Each patient should be diagnosed and treated for immortal infections vigorously, based on laboratory diagnosis and individual patient needs. The infectious burden can be reduced by controlling and managing the bacteria, with treatment. Promoting the health of the microbiome and mycobiome, through diet and supplements to support the nervous system and chemical and cellular signaling, can help resist chronic infection. When medications damage the microbiome it is necessary to replace the lost diversity in the microbiome with supplements, as much as possible.

No one can live forever, and the goal is to extend longevity and delay the inevitable, while maintaining a high quality of life. Cells have a life span, and will eventually reach the end of that lifespan. Research into healthy aging may further explain how some people become super-agers. Some patients may have avoided immortal infections which are the most dangerous to long-term health. Some patients may have adapted to chronic infection, in ways which need to be explored and defined. Some may have avoided use of penicillin in acute immortal infections; and thereby avoided transforming the acute infection into a chronic infection and/or chronic disease.

Science knows immortal pathogens crossed over from animals, and are the cause (or are "associated" with) many chronic diseases, and merely avoiding chronic disease can enhance aging. Healthy aging and a long life can be achieved by avoiding immortal intracellular infections and parasites;

appropriately treating immortal infections; and avoiding multiple chronic infections arising from sexual contact, drug use and close contact with animals. The oldest patients likely avoided the worst of the immortal infections, adapted to the infection, and had prompt treatment of immortal infections, without the use of penicillin. Avoiding immortal infections and parasites, a low infectious burden, and a healthy lifestyle, can prevent future chronic disease, improve the prognosis of chronic disease, and forestall the pathogens' victory.

CHAPTER 20

SYMPTOMS & SYNDROMES INTERFERE WITH DIAGNOSIS

Aristotle (AD 90—AD 168) wrote, "Other things being equal, the simplest hypothesis possible is the good principle". William Ockham (1287—1347), proposed Ockham's razor as a problem-solving principle, which distinguishes between two hypotheses, either by "shaving away" unnecessary assumptions or "cutting apart" two similar conclusions. Ockham's razor states when confronted with competing hypotheses, "the one with the fewest assumptions should be selected". Dr. Ockham believed simpler theories are preferable, because simpler theories are more testable than excessively complex models, which are affected by statistical noise. Ockham's razor suggests that the simplest explanation is the most likely explanation, implying the doctor should assume a single and most obvious cause for multiple symptoms.

In 1639, an Irish Franciscan philosopher, John Punch (1603–1661) stated, "entities are not to be multiplied without necessity". Sir Isaac Newton (1642–1726), an English mathematician, astronomer, theologian, author, physicist, and natural philosopher, wrote, "We are to admit no more causes of natural things than such as are both true and sufficient to explain their appearances. Therefore, to the same natural effects we must, as far as possible, assign the same causes." Bertrand Russell (1872–1970) proposed his version of Ockham's razor as, "Whenever possible, substitute constructions out of known entities, for inference to unknown entities". A variation of these principles is attributed to Theodore Woodward (1914–July 11, 2005), whose dictum was, "When you hear hoof beats, think of horses not zebras", which is now called the "zebra" principle. In other words, don't look for zebras when a horse is before you. The obvious diagnosis is the most likely.

Einstein's Constraint states: "It can scarcely be denied that the supreme goal of all theory is to make the irreducible basic elements as simple and as few as possible, without having to surrender the adequate representation of a single datum of experience". An often-quoted version of Einstein's Constraint, which cannot be verified as posited by Einstein himself, says "Everything should be kept as simple as possible, but no simpler."

The counterargument to Ockham's razor is Hickam's dictum, derived at some point between 1946 and Dr. Hickam's death, in 1970. Hickam's dictum states, "A man can have as many diseases as he damn well pleases." The example given for Hickam's dictum is "Saint's triad", a concept developed by the British surgeon C.F.M Saint, to caution medical students against misuse of Ockham's razor. Saint's triad stated, "Hiatus hernia, gallbladder disease, and diverticulosis are three different diseases"; and even though the diseases may exist in a single patient they have no common cause. The problem with Saint's triad is hiatus hernia, gallbladder disease, and diverticulosis do all have a common cause—infections with bacteria and parasites, in the intestinal tract.

Decades before the germ theory, Jacob Henle (1809–1885), a German physician, pathologist and anatomist, called for investigation of infectious causes in acute disease. He was dismissed and ridiculed by peers in the medical community. Louis Pasteur (1822–1895), a French biologist, microbiologist, and chemist, proved germs caused disease in humans and animals. Pasteur proposed micro-organisms infecting animals and humans cause disease, and suggested preventing the pathogens from entry into the human body. Louis Pasteur's claims were controversial, in the nineteenth century, when medicine chose to believe disease occurred by "spontaneous generation". Today, Pasteur is considered one of the fathers of the germ theory. Pasteur's discoveries lead Joseph Lister (1827–1912), a British surgeon, to become a pioneer in antiseptic surgery.

Louis Pasteur proved sugar converted to alcohol, during the process of fermentation. He proposed fermentation was caused by decompensation, and fermentation fosters the growth of fungus. Pasteur's findings support chlamydia infection causes chronic disease, because chronic chlamydia infection causes fermentation, decompensation, and fungal growth, when the pathogen consumes sugar after depleting the ATP in the cell, and causes the conversion of sugar into alcohol. The presence of fungus is a clue to a chronic infection that has persisted long enough to deplete ATP from the cells, convert sugar to alcohol, create fermentation, and cause development of fungus.

Medicine defaulted to Hickam's dictum and the Saint's triad; and divided endless symptoms and findings along the infectious cascade or manifesting differently in different people, into newly named diseases. The one-cause concept, and the most obvious cause concept, have been abandoned. The naming of diseases has been fragmented into the endless naming of symptoms, findings, and syndromes, across all medical specialties, well beyond any single person's ability to know and comprehend. Medicine has defaulted to more complex explanations and ignores the simplest explanations; as medicine splits disease of unknown origin into endless new diseases of unknown origin, while ignoring the simplest and most verifiable diagnosis.

Medical training does not include infectious causes of chronic disease; or training in parasitology. Medical training does not generally include training on the causes of any chronic diseases, and instead trains doctors how to identify, name, and treat symptoms, findings and syndromes. Medical training does not include animal pathogens as a cause of chronic disease; veterinary knowledge has been lost to medicine; and doctors are unwilling to warn patients of the danger of animal pathogens, even when they have a disease caused by animal pathogens. Harvard Medical School has now reported it will become the first medical school in the country to include a course in veterinary medicine, in medical school, which is a definite step in the right direction.

Dr. Merchant has often said forty to sixty percent of what medicine says today is not true, or is outdated knowledge. Unfortunately, doctors do not know which knowledge is not true or outdated. Too often, doctors respond according to their training, to do what they do, and say what they say. Dr. Merchant has seen different specialists prescribe conflicting medicine to the same patient, causing conflicting symptoms and problems that make the diagnosis and treatment of the cause of chronic disease more difficult. He has seen different specialists diagnose different diseases; yet, prescribe the same medication to the patient.

Medicine is a profession that observes and documents, names diseases, and treats symptoms. Students are taught how to identify diseases, the co-morbid conditions for each disease, and how to treat the named disease. The causes of diseases are not taught in medical training; and doctors are not taught to diagnose and treat infectious causes of any chronic disease. Dr. Merchant asked his medical school professors what caused chronic diseases, and was never given an answer. He was only told to keep looking for answers.

A syndrome is a constellation of symptoms and findings, first described by a doctor whose name defines the syndrome. A syndrome named after a doctor is not a diagnosis of the root cause of disease. Medical school has become a ridiculous memorization test, of thousands of syndromes and symptoms, many of which were named before microscopes, before medical laboratories, and before pathogens could be cultured and identified. Medical training requires memorization of the many co-morbid conditions in each syndrome and finding named a disease, and thereafter the relevance of co-morbid conditions is forgotten. When a doctor identifies and names a symptom, finding, or syndrome, too often the search for the underlying infectious causes of the disease is abandoned.

Doctors are taught to observe and document findings; name a disease among thousands of named diseases, which are only descriptions of symptoms, findings and syndromes; and treat symptoms. When seeing a patient, doctors feel a sense of urgency to name a disease and prescribe treatment. The doctor wants to write a diagnosis in the chart, and the patient wants to know the diagnosis. When a doctor identifies symptoms, findings, or a syndrome as the diagnosis, further attempts at diagnosing an infectious pathogen or root cause of the disease stop. The doctor treats the patient for whatever the diagnosis, and the patient expects treatment from the doctor arising from the encounter. Observing, naming, documenting, and symptomatic treatment will not cure patients with chronic disease, or prevent future chronic disease.

Doctors are observing and dividing symptoms, findings, and syndromes, caused by immortal infection and parasites, into many different named diseases, even if the treatment prescribed for the differently named diseases is the same in each specialty. Specialties divides the person into parts, based on the body part and named disease. Each specialty may diagnose and name a different disease at different stages in the infectious cascade. The same inflammation of the blood vessels is described by many different names, ranging from vasculitis, to IgA vasculitis, to polyangiitis with granulomatosis. Most chronic disease, including heart disease, lung disease, diabetes, arthritis, autoimmune disease, kidney disease, endocrine disease, cancer, gastrointestinal disease, reproductive disease, autism, regressive developmental disorders, and mental illness, has been divided into many different sub-parts and given different names. The chronic diseases are named based on different specialties, and different manifestations of infectious pathogens in the body, at different points on the infectious cascade.

Different specialists diagnose endothelial dysfunction, inflammation, abnormal proteins, and fungal invasion, as separately named diseases, based on body part and specialty. Specialists do not consider nor understand the underlying cause of the endothelial dysfunction, inflammation or abnormal proteins; ask why, or what causes the endothelial dysfunction, inflammation, or abnormal proteins; or attempt to treat pathogens causing the endothelial dysfunction, inflammation, or abnormal proteins. If the patient has excessive fatigue, it is named chronic fatigue. If a patient has high blood pressure it is called hypertension. If fluid is backing up behind the heart, it is called congestive heart failure. If the patient has unexplained gastrointestinal complaints it is called irritable bowel syndrome. If the patient has unexplained inflammation it is called "itis". If the patient has lowered immunity, it is called immune dysfunction or autoimmune disease.

Medicine has named many diseases with the suffix "itis". Any disease name ending in "itis" means the body part or tissue is inflammation. A disease ending in "itis" is not a diagnosis, but rather a description of inflammation. Inflammation is caused by infection—redness, heat, swelling and pain. If the doctor can't explain the disease and label it with a name the doctor knows, the doctor names the disease with medical and Latin terminology to describe the findings. If the finding is inflammation, it is called "itis". If the doctor cannot explain or label the disease, the doctor may even diagnose a newly named disease, unexplained phenomena, psychosomatic illness, a virus, or faulty genes that are not proven or disproven.

The endless symptoms, findings, and syndromes were named before technology allowed identification of pathogens; and has resulted in Hickam's dictum and the Saint's triad gone wild. Medicine has thousands of named syndromes, findings and symptoms, of unknown origin, which are in need of diagnosis and treatment of the root infectious causes. The endless naming of "itis" diseases and autoimmune diseases need to be revisited and reconsidered, because most are likely caused by infectious pathogens.

Symptoms, findings, and syndromes are only that—symptoms, findings and syndromes, and do not disclose a cause of the chronic disease. The endless naming of symptoms, findings, and syndromes is directly contrary to the teaching of Aristotle, William Ockham, John Punch, Isaac Newton, Bertrand Russell, and Albert Einstein. It is contrary to Ockham's razor and Einstein's Constraint. The endless naming of syndromes is consistent with Hickam's Dictum, and creates undue complexity rather than simplifying understanding. Chronic diseases should be diagnosed and treated based on the root infectious cause, not merely by symptoms and findings.

Doctors need to reconsider the importance of co-morbid conditions. Every specialist is trained to know co-morbid conditions in their specialty, and every specialty recognizes patients have co-morbid conditions; but the specialists are not considering co-morbid conditions as a clue to the underlying infectious cause of the chronic disease or considering co-morbid conditions as their responsibility. Specialists do not consider the same infectious pathogens may be causing the presenting complaint *and* the co-morbid conditions. Specialists fail to understand co-morbid conditions are relevant, because co-morbid conditions are not in their specialty; and the connection between co-morbid conditions and the presenting diseases were not taught in medical school.

Medicine is fascinated and consumed by the smallest details, including genes, Cluster Differentiations, the proteinbiome, and inflammasomes. The three-hundred and sixty-three Cluster Differentiations describe the effect of chronic infection, as infectious byproducts attach to cells, including professional immune cells and genes. TNF-alpha has its own super-category of Cluster Differentiations. Researchers continue to name new variations in Cluster Differentiations, which are variations in the way molecules, proteins, and gene expressions are formed. Naming new Cluster Differentiations, proteinbiomes, inflammasomes, gene abnormalities, and gene expressions, instead of finding the root infectious cause of chronic disease, has created confusion, rather than providing solutions. Medicine is researching small details, rapidly expanding the quantity of small details, hoping an answer will reveal itself; instead of looking at the big picture to find patterns across specialties and co-morbid conditions that reveal likely infectious causes of chronic disease.

Even "Cluster Differentiation" has three different names, all abbreviated as CD; and the same numbered Cluster Differentiations may be called by more than one name. For instance, CD40 is also called CD154. Most doctors' do not find three-hundred and sixty-three Cluster Differentiations useful. Few care about CD1 to CD363, CD8, CD40, or CD154, or understand how the Cluster Differentiations and gene expressions relate to the chronic disease and formulating a treatment plan for the patient.

The Cluster Differentiation molecules describe the variations in molecules and proteins attached to the outside of pathogens; and caused by the immortal pathogens. The immortal pathogens may release abnormal proteins, and may cause chance alterations in proteins in contact with sticky material. The abnormal proteins may form inside the host cell, due to abnormal folding caused by the pathogen. Infectious byproducts and abnormal proteins from the pathogen can then circulate in the body and attach to genes, altering genes and gene expression.

Cluster Differentiations should be re-examined, to determine the relationship of each Cluster Differentiation to immortal pathogens, and to identify which abnormal proteins are generated by which immortal pathogens. Science should examine whether the Cluster Differentiations are random or arise from particular pathogens; and whether the abnormal proteins alter particular genes, or alter genes at random. It is time to sort out pathogens and chronic disease, and pathogens and Cluster Differentiations, to understand immortal infection across all specialties.

The urgency to name symptoms, findings, and syndromes, rather than diagnosing infectious pathogens, has dramatically decreased the health of patients, increased the prevalence of chronic disease, and increased the cost of medical care. The causes of chronic disease are not being diagnosed, because chronic infectious pathogens can manifest as a chronic disease years or decades after an acute infection. By the time the patient has a chronic disease, the acute infection has been forgotten; and the doctor and patient do not understand the prior acute infection became a chronic infection, and the chronic infection became a chronic disease. The cause of acute disease is more obvious than the cause of chronic disease, and chronic infection causing chronic disease can only be found by a thorough medical evaluation that includes diagnosis of immortal pathogens.

Modern medicine is treating symptoms of intracellular pathogens and parasitic infection, instead of diagnosing and treating the root cause of chronic disease. Doctors in all specialties should be trained to diagnose and treat chlamydia infections, H-pylori, parasites, and toxoplasmosis. A thorough history, physical examination and blood testing, and recognizing comorbid conditions can have a common infectious cause, gives a clue to the pathogens. The patient history should include a history of prior infections, and how prior infections were treated. Every specialist should be able to recognize the infectious causes of chronic disease at an earlier and more easily treatable stage, before the infectious burden becomes greater and chronic disease develops. If all specialties routinely diagnosed chronic infections in patients with chronic disease, it would quickly become obvious that some groups of immortal pathogens are everywhere; and are causing chronic disease, in every specialty.

We need to move beyond naming and diagnosing symptoms, findings, and syndromes, and giving symptomatic treatment. Treatment of symptoms can improve symptoms, but will not treat the cause of the chronic disease and may worsen the underlying disease. Doctors prescribe drugs to treat symptoms, then prescribe drugs to treat the symptoms caused by the drugs. They give drugs for pain that cause constipation, then give drugs to relieve constipation. After years of using increasingly potent drugs to treat patients, and increasingly potent pharmacologic bombs, it becomes more difficult to correctly diagnose and treat the chronic infections that are the root cause of chronic disease. Treating symptoms, without understanding the cause of the chronic disease, can cause the disease to change or become worse. Treating acute infection with penicillin, using TNF-inhibitors, or using steroids, can change the pathogen and the tissue where the infection resides; and cause a chronic disease to develop or become worse.

It is time to re-think the "unknown" origin of symptoms, findings, and syndromes, in every specialty. Every description of symptoms, findings or syndromes; any disease defined by endothelial dysfunction; any disease based on abnormal proteins; any disease described as "itis"; any disease called "idiopathic"; and any disease named after a doctor, should be re-examined with modern tools to identify infectious pathogens causing the disease. It is time to replace naming symptoms and syndromes, with diagnosing the root cause or causes of chronic disease. It is time to use modern technology to find the root cause of chronic diseases that are only named descriptions of symptoms, findings, and syndromes.

It is time to return to the art of medicine. Everyone in healthcare needs to observe the countenance of the patient; and talk to patients, face-to-face, instead of looking at computer screens doing data entry and trying to meet benchmarks. Electronic lip service and the technological imperative is not managing the patient's chronic infections or chronic disease. Computer screens interfere with rigorous observation, and the computer programming itself can influence the cognitive observations and thinking of the doctor. Computers do not suggest creative solutions for the patient, and instead follow the path of diagnosis and treatment created by insurance companies and standard medical thinking, which has not yet provided answers to chronic disease.

It is time to incorporate infectious causes of chronic disease, including parasites, into medical training; and to encourage creative thinking and rigorous skepticism, of what has already been written and said in medicine. It is time to encourage thinking and reasoning based on what is known, to formulate thoughts and opinions about what is not known in medicine, and in chronic disease. Diagnosis should become a search for the infectious pathogens causing chronic disease. Diagnosis should be a matter of determining what infectious pathogens a person has that may be causing a chronic disease, and how those infections relate to each other. Treatment should be directed at the root cause of chronic disease, and not only the symptoms.

It is time to diagnose and treat immortal pathogens, before the patient has a chronic disease! Millions of patients are in need of diagnosis and treatment of immortal pathogens; and diagnosis and treatment of acute and chronic infections are far less expensive than waiting for chronic disease. Early testing and treatment of infectious causes of chronic disease, by any specialist, could delay or prevent chronic diseases outside their specialty, caused by the same pathogens. Diagnosing the root causes of chronic disease will benefit patients, and lead to important discoveries on the causes of chronic disease

Medicine needs to transform itself to be patient centered. It is time for medicine to put the patient's body back together, to understand and treat chronic disease. The symptoms, findings and syndromes are a symptom of chronic infection with immortal pathogens. Identifying the infectious causes of chronic disease can only be done by looking at the whole patient; and important discoveries in chronic disease will require collaboration and knowledge across specialties. Knowing immortal intracellular infections and parasites are the root cause of chronic disease will put medicine into a cohesive whole, from which new discoveries can be made.

We need to return to the history and physical examination, and follow the advice of Bertrand Russel—diagnose disease using existing scientific knowledge to infer the answer as to the cause of unknown diseases. We offer a unifying explanation for the cause of chronic disease, and a way to put separate specialties into a cohesive whole. We offer a new construct for chronic disease that takes into account what is known in all specialties, considering the whole person, leaving no facts inconsistent with the explanation. We offer new methods to diagnose and treat chronic disease, based on the infectious causes of chronic disease. We offer hope to patients that chronic diseases can improve, and healthy aging is attainable, if immortal pathogens are diagnosed and treated. We offer a simpler version of chronic disease, which can be easily tested and verified. Simplicity supports truth!

> *The greatest enemy of knowledge is not ignorance, it is the illusion of knowledge.*
>
> Stephen Hawkins

CHAPTER 21

MEDICAL SPECIALIZATION
AND CHRONIC DISEASE

Specialists are not trained to look at the whole patient, the whole family, or contact with pets and animals. Specialists only deal with specific parts of a person and specific diseases. Infection has been "associated" with chronic disease in every medical specialty; and in chronic diseases in animals, in veterinary literature. Every specialty has literature supporting chronic infection with chlamydia, H-pylori, toxoplasmosis, streptococcus, viruses, and parasites cause chronic disease. Every medical specialty has named diseases which identify and describe the effects of immortal infection. We have no system to inform all medical specialties that all medical specialties are all observing and finding the same infectious causes of chronic disease, and saying the same thing about the responses and effects on tissue, from the pathogens.

Medicine has created and divided knowledge that has become so vast it cannot be known by one person. Specialization divides medical knowledge, the human body, and diseases into smaller and more manageable parts. Specialists have knowledge an inch wide and a mile deep; and no specialty has an overview of other specialties, even sub-specialties within the same specialty. Care is not coordinated between specialties, in part due to the lack of knowledge of the need to coordinate care. No single person or specialty seems interested in putting the puzzle of chronic disease together, into a unified whole to explain chronic disease.

Medical literature is separated by specialty, body parts, and diseases, in journals unique to each specialty; and each specialty reads only its own specialty literature. Medical literature is separated by specialty, body parts, and diseases, in journals unique to each specialty. No one reports knowledge across specialties. Search of the medical literature to find the relationship between chlamydia and chronic diseases requires each chronic disease be searched separately, such as "chlamydia and cancer", "chlamydia and heart disease", "chlamydia and Alzheimer's", and "chlamydia and multiple sclerosis". It requires an interest to look deeper and at broader questions, incorporate cross-specialty knowledge, and engage in collaboration.

Specialization has caused the loss of cohesive thought about the human body and chronic diseases. Patients have become a body part in a bed and a disease in a bed. The patient is a heart in a bed, an eye in a bed, a gallbladder in a bed, a kidney in a bed, a bone in a bed, diabetes in a bed, cancer in a bed, and so on, for most chronic diseases. Patients have to seek care from multiple different doctors, to address all body parts and all co-morbid conditions. No one doctor recognizes the relationship between the many parts of the patient; or the relationship between more than one chronic disease, in the same patient. Doctors in one specialty do not recognize the co-morbid conditions that fall within the responsibility of another specialty is caused by the same pathogen. Specialists do not have an overview of chronic disease to recognize co-morbid diseases are caused by the same pathogens.

Specialty bias and the narrow focus of each specialty is preventing recognition of the common origin of many chronic diseases. Each specialty is its own tribe. The specialists only talk to other specialty tribe members, only learn from tribe members, and only read what other tribe members write. Each specialty meets with groups of other doctors, in their specialty, with speakers and experts from their specialty. Knowledge and understanding is limited by what the specialty knows. Each specialty tribe has developed uniform practice standards, which limit new knowledge and creative solutions, by requiring conformity. Specialty tribes limit the exchange of information between specialties, make cross-specialty collaboration in research difficult, and limit understanding of the common patterns in chronic disease.

The division of the profession into many specialties, and division of responsibility based on specialty, has been an obstacle to patient care and the discovery of the causes of chronic disease. The cause of chronic disease may be removed in time from the acute disease, and/or the acute disease may have been treated by a different specialty. Chronic disease may involve animal contact, which is not a part of the patient history in any medical specialty. Specialists are not diagnosing or treating chronic diseases outside of their specialty, even when the chronic disease is a co-morbid condition.

Specialty practice standards need to be updated in every specialty, to incorporate knowledge of infectious causes of chronic disease, and direct the diagnosis and treatment of chronic disease, based on diagnosis of infectious pathogens. Specialists need to carefully record co-morbid conditions that relate to their diagnosis and treatment decisions. The specialists need to communicate with any other health care providers, and primary care providers will have to communicate with all specialists, to advance understanding of chronic infections as a cause of chronic disease.

Specialization has limited the ability of any one specialty to make important scientific discoveries, because the causes and cures for chronic disease cannot be found in one specialty. No medical specialty is trained to diagnose and treat chronic infections, in patients with chronic disease. No medical specialty is expected to know and understand the role of immortal pathogens and parasites transmitted by animals, in causing chronic disease. Specialists consider only the part of the body or the disease applicable to their specialty, and do not consider diseases outside their specialty their responsibility. Specialists do not see the bigger picture of the whole patient, or try to understand or explain chronic disease—they treat chronic disease symptomatically. Specialization prevents the collaboration necessary for discovery of the causes of chronic disease.

Specialists are not using careful observation and rigid skepticism. They are doing what they were taught and what they have always done. Specialists rarely talk to doctors outside their specialty; specialists seldom talk to primary care physicians; and do not talk to naturopaths, dentists, or veterinarians. The veterinarians and naturopaths understand infectious causes of chronic diseases, and the risk of animal transmission of pathogens and parasites—the medical doctors are the only ones seemingly not able to understand immortal animal pathogens cause chronic disease! Greater cross-specialty communication and true communication with the primary care provider, could lead to recognition different specialties are saying the same thing and the same infectious process is causing many different chronic diseases. It would provide new knowledge, which is necessary to make more discoveries that will improve and extend life.

Louis Pasteur was a biologist, microbiologist, and chemist; and he became a visionary thinker in medicine. Discovery of the infectious cause of ulcers was made by an internist trained in microbiology, working with a pathologist, to make a discovery in gastroenterology. Many important discoveries can come from professionals with training in multiple specialties, and do not always originate from someone with a medical degree. Routine diagnostic testing for immortal pathogens, a system to report observational science by front-line practitioners, and a system for practitioners to report treatment that has been successful in improving or resolving chronic disease could advance knowledge in the infectious causes of chronic disease.

Medical thinkers have proposed infectious causes of chronic disease for centuries. Articles have been published for decades describing infectious causes for COPD, multiple sclerosis, Parkinson's disease, Alzheimer's, cardiovascular disease, strokes, reactive arthritis, rheumatoid arthritis, lupus, fibromyalgia, ocular disorders, and immunodeficiency diseases. Studies confirmed chlamydia pneumonia in virtually all Alzheimer's patients, and in virtually all patients with cardiovascular diseases. Studies confirmed chlamydia pneumonia and other immortal pathogens in virtually all patients with multiple sclerosis. Yet, diagnostic testing and treatment for immortal pathogens is not done in chronic disease. This is not the specialty practice standard, even in Alzheimer's, cardiovascular disease, COPD, multiple sclerosis, arthritis, and the many other diseases. Science will eventually confirm these immortal pathogens cause chronic disease, and medicine will learn to integrate the diagnosis and treatment of these pathogens into routine medical care.

The search for the cause of chronic disease needs to become a search for infectious pathogens, not a quest to name a disease and provide symptomatic treatment. Specialists need to expand thinking and embrace infectious causes of chronic disease; and recognize co-morbid conditions are often caused by the same pathogens. Co-morbid conditions are a clue to the pathogens involved and an opportunity to improve care, by diagnosis and treatment of pathogens. Looking at the body as a whole, and the principal of the whole, will vastly enhance the ability to diagnose and treat patients; and direct new avenues for treatment and research, to conquer chronic disease. New discoveries can be made in every specialty, as specialists recognize the infection connection to chronic diseases, in any body part and in any system of the body.

Research is a specialty unto itself. Research is a sub-specialty within each specialty, and is also separated by specialty, body part, and disease or research funding organization. Researchers have the same knowledge base and bias, as everyone in their specialty. Some of the most important contributions to understanding the infectious causes of chronic disease came from practicing physicians. It is time for researchers to incorporate a broader base of knowledge to formulate hypotheses and derive conclusions, on causation and treatment. Understanding of the principle of the whole, that immortal chronic infections with animal pathogens cause chronic disease; and understanding the infectious cascade, can lead to new and important discoveries that benefit patients with chronic disease and new ways to treat chronic disease.

Research foundations and research funding are dedicated to specific specialties and specific diseases, without any single source for research funding on all diseases, on all infectious causes of chronic disease, or even any single chronic disease and the co-morbid conditions. Research focuses on narrow questions and small details that are likely to obtain funding, yield positive results and support the hypothesis; and which are likely to support publishing the research. Conclusions are couched in associations, relationships, connections, links, and other words that help the researcher avoid criticism for making a conclusion as to cause. Researcher rarely if ever states a cause on which medical practitioners can base a treatment decision; and the scientific method itself limits the ability to identify a cause, when more than one pathogen causes the same disease.

Researchers keep repeating the same research, and confirming the same "associations". An "association" does not tell doctors to act on the information, to the benefit of the patient. How many brains must be autopsied and how many heart valves must be examined by a pathologist, before someone will be willing to say chlamydia pneumonia causes Alzheimer's and heart disease. Research has shown the "association" between chlamydia pneumonia and heart disease, and between chlamydia pneumonia and Alzheimer's; yet, researchers keep reporting heart disease and Alzheimer's are co-morbid conditions rather than reporting the diseases are caused by the same infectious pathogens. Researchers are afraid to say a pathogen *causes* a disease; and front-line practitioners are unwilling to act on an "association" and treat a patient; and instead await being told the cause, before acting to the benefit of patients by diagnosing and treating immortal infection.

At what point must we stop calling everything an "association", stop denying infectious causes of chronic disease, accept infectious pathogens are causing chronic disease, and understand co-morbid conditions are often caused by the same infectious pathogens. How many research studies with the same findings does it take, before medicine will state a cause? We do not need to repeat the same research—we need solutions that help patients—we need to develop a coherent theory of disease based on numerous consistent "associations". It is time for someone to state a general theory of causation, and state a cause of chronic diseases, without retreating to an "association". Reports of causation are needed to motivate a change in medical practice and for the standard to become the diagnosis of a cause.

The problem with bias and cognitive assumptions in medicine begins in pre-med college courses and in medical training. Pre-med students and medical students are not encouraged to think outside the box, or to think for themselves; to be creative; or to analyze and use reasoning based on what is known, to discern a cause. Medical students who already know their specialty interest during medical school study the hardest in their area of interest, to the exclusion of other specialty knowledge. Upon graduation, medical students choose a specialty for residency training, in medicine or surgery. Once that choice is made, the medical student becomes part of their specialty tribe, and loses contact with information, knowledge, and discoveries in other specialties. Each specialty tribe has their own set of biases and assumptions, developed within the scope of their specialty training and knowledge; and does not use inductive or deductive reasoning to discern the cause of chronic disease.

Medical school teaches rigid medical thinking. Medical students are taught the rules, and expected to stick to the rules. Medical students are taught obedience, and to adhere to uniform standards and to the scientific method. By the time the medical student graduates, they have been taught internal control over their actions, are locked into a format of rigid and traditional thinking; and are fearful of thinking outside the box or beyond what they were taught, or finding creative solutions to chronic disease. The expectation is to conform and obey the rules. Medicine cannot ever expand knowledge, or add to knowledge based on the art of medicine, beyond what they were taught, which limits scientific progress and the understanding of chronic disease.

Medical school is a rigorous exercise in rapid memorization, which discourages critical thinking, encourages a closed mind, and creates cognitive bias. Only the most intelligent and best memorizers can be accepted to medical school and survive medical training. Medical students memorize thousands of named diseases that are symptoms, findings, or constellations of symptoms, named after the first person to describe the symptom, findings, or syndrome. They memorize co-morbid conditions for each chronic disease, but are not taught co-morbid conditions can arise from different manifestations of the same infectious pathogens. Medical school does not teach causes of chronic disease—students are taught disease naming and disease management. Medical textbooks continue to be edited, removing old knowledge; and replacing old knowledge with small details in cell microbiology and newly named diseases. Medical students and doctors are buried beneath the weight of information, and quantity is being confused with quality.

Medical school and residency training should encourage critical thinking, open-mindedness, creative solutions, and collaboration. Doctors should be trained to communicate with patients and form relationships based on trust. Observation, critical thinking, rigorous skepticism and avoidance of cognitive bias should be taught and considered critical to the scientific method. We must train students to abandon ego, which is restricting advancement in science; and adopt humility, rather than manifest an entitlement to an exalted position in society and superiority over patients. We must return to educating doctors to look at the whole patient. Every specialty should be trained in infectious causes of chronic disease and parasitology. The causes of chronic disease cannot be found in one specialty alone, because chronic disease does not fit neatly within any one specialty—it is a longstanding battle between the pathogens and the immune system, manifesting in infinite ways, based on the infections and combinations of infections a person acquired over many years and the persistence of the infections.

Medical nomenclature and inconsistent nomenclature between specialties has limited understanding and communication. Specialties do not necessarily recognize the language used by other specialties as being the same; thus, are limited in the ability to recognize the similarity and patterns in the conditions being described, in other specialties. The same disease may have a different name when the disease occurs in a human, versus when it occurs in an animal. Different terminology for the same concepts fragments knowledge, and impairs understanding of the bigger picture, across specialties. The same terminology for different concepts is confusing, and prevents understanding of the bigger picture. We need a system to share and combine knowledge between different specialties; and training and to aid recognition that many specialties and veterinarians are saying the same thing—infectious pathogens are the cause of chronic disease, in humans and in animals. We need a uniform nomenclature, for the same concepts, the same diseases, and diseases occurring in both animals and humans.

Many specialties are reporting abnormal proteins, by different names, in chronic disease. Abnormal proteins may be reported as heat shock proteins, prions, abnormal proteins, tau proteins, bent proteins, CD 1-CD 363, etc., by different specialties. Abnormal proteins are subject to infinite naming of variants of molecules contained within Cluster Differentiations, the proteinbiome, and inflammasomes. The lack of understanding of abnormal proteins, and diverse nomenclature, has fragmented and delayed knowledge and understanding abnormal proteins are generated by chronic infection. Knowledge of which abnormal proteins are caused by which pathogens, rather than merely describing the existence of the abnormal proteins, could advance the understanding of chronic disease. Abnormal proteins are generated by immortal pathogens, inside the cell, causing the proteins to fold improperly; and proteins stuck to the outside of the pathogens, to protect the pathogen and confuse the immune system. Abnormal proteins on the surface of pathogens, and inside host cells and pathogens, are dispersed into the body during the infectious cascade.

Numerous neurologic diseases are "associated" with abnormal proteins. Brain diseases, including brain cancer and Alzheimer's disease; and heart valve disease, kidney disease, Henoch-Schoenlein Purpura, and cancer are "associated" with abnormal proteins. Multiple myeloma is "associated" with abnormal proteins, specifically M-proteins; yet the two infectious pathogens known to have M-proteins on the surface have not been investigated as a cause, or recognized to cause multiple myeloma. The two pathogens known to have M-proteins attached, have not been investigated as an intracellular pathogen causing multiple myeloma.

Each specialty may make a different diagnosis, based on the point in the infectious cascade or the interest of the specialty. Each specialty describes and labels symptoms, findings, and syndromes, without knowing a cause. Every specialty has diseases involving or named endothelial dysfunction, epithelial dysfunction, inflammation, abnormal proteins, macrophage dysfunction, mitochondrial dysfunction, and inclusion cysts. Each specialty has findings such as plaque, chronic fatigue, and immune dysfunction. Many specialties are reporting finding the same markers and tissue effects in disease; and many specialties have identified the same findings are "associated" with chronic diseases. Yet, no one reports all specialties are observing the same phenomenon, or observing a phenomenon consistent with immortal pathogens.

Many chronic diseases show molecular changes consistent with chlamydia; and many involve elevated TNF-alpha, elevated IL-6, elevated C-reactive protein, loss of apoptosis, angiogenesis, inflammation, abnormal proteins, epithelial dysfunction, endothelial dysfunction, mitochondrial dysfunction, immune dysfunction, chronic fatigue, etc.; and the same effect of loss of energy in the cell, loss of oxygen in the cell, loss of apoptosis, angiogenesis, and fermentation. Many specialties have diseases defined by plaque; yet, no one reports the plaque is generated by the immune response to immortal pathogens. Each specialty has diseases relating to inclusion cysts, but few recognize chlamydia creates inclusion cysts or inclusion cysts can surround pathogens and abnormal proteins to become the focus for development of cancer. Even when a specialty recognizes a pathogen causes inclusion cysts, the disease is diagnosed based on the presence of an inclusion cyst rather than diagnosis of the cause of the inclusion cysts.

Approximately a dozen childhood regressive developmental disorders have the same or overlapping symptoms, and many different names, based on specialty bias and the degree of harm done by the pathogen. Childhood regressive developmental disorders and childhood epilepsy syndromes are caused by immortal pathogens in the child's brain. Subtle variations in the syndromes may be caused by different immortal pathogens, the pathogens are located in different parts of the brain, and/or the child has a greater infectious burden in the brain. Toxoplasmosis is one of the pathogens that can cause childhood regressive developmental disorders, and epilepsy. No one seems to recognize the common findings in childhood regressive developmental disorders, or in childhood epilepsy syndromes; and no one investigates pathogens and parasites as the cause of these many syndromes. Nor do specialists treating regressive developmental disorders and childhood epilepsy take a history of contact with cats, or contact with other animals capable of transmitting pathogens to cause brain disease in an infant, *in utero* or after birth.

Specialists ignore or are unaware of parasitic disease, in the United States; and some believe only third world countries and countries in the Middle East have parasitic infections. The bias stems from a lack of training in parasitology in medical school and residency, and lack of understanding of the role of parasites in chronic disease. Shockingly little time is devoted to the study of parasitology or immortal infections, in medical school, and almost no time is spent on parasitology in clinical training or most residency training programs. Denying parasites and parasitic diseases exist in the United States is irrational, and cannot be valid in a world where travel and war takes the population of the United States to the far reaches of the earth, including to areas where parasitic infections are endemic.

Vietnam veterans were labeled as psychiatric patients with PTSD, and given counseling and symptomatic psychiatric drugs, for more than four decades, when they needed diagnosis and treatment of parasitic infections. Undiagnosed parasitic infection in Vietnam veterans caused a multitude of chronic diseases, including liver cancer from a parasitic liver fluke, and probably eye cancer from psittacosis. Gulf War veterans and Iraq War veterans, and their families, suffered the same lack of medical diagnosis, and symptomatic treatment of infections acquired in the Middle East and transmitted to other family members.

Veterinarians see the same diseases in animals as medical doctors see in humans. Veterinarians know immortal infection to be the cause of chronic disease, and know infections can be passed between animals and people. Veterinarians know pets and domesticated animals get parasites, and that pets and other domestic and wild animals spread parasitic infection to humans. Veterinarians know pathogens can be transmitted between different animal species. Veterinarians know wild animals carry pathogens that present a risk to hunters. When the veterinary and medical professions split, in the 1890's, medical doctors started their own system of education and research; and veterinary knowledge was lost to medicine.

Veterinarians have knowledge of animal pathogens causing chronic disease, far ahead of medical doctors. In some countries, like Brazil and Australia, the immortal pathogens in domesticated animals have received more research attention, and mapping of the microbiome and DNA of the pathogens, than infectious pathogens in humans. Medical doctors do not consider veterinarians an equal; when collaboration and combining veterinary knowledge with medical knowledge could assist in understanding infectious causes of chronic disease. No medical specialty incorporates the knowledge of infectious causes of chronic disease, in animals; or seems to recognize animals get the same chronic diseases as humans, from the same pathogens. Medical doctors would benefit from veterinary knowledge, and from collaboration with veterinarians, in diagnosing and treating patients with chronic disease who have pets and other contact with animals.

Specialization has created a division of responsibility that makes obtaining comprehensive medical care more difficult for the patient. Specialists do not include in their responsibility any diagnosis, treatment or care outside their specialty, even in co-morbid conditions. Doctors have less time to spend with patients, and hence are less able to diagnose and treat the root infectious causes of chronic disease, even assuming the doctors are aware of infectious causes of chronic disease.

The first divide in medicine is between surgeons and medical doctors, and it is a great divide. When medical graduates choose to become surgeons, their medical education slows and all effort is directed at learning to perform surgery. Surgeons are very smart, but surgeons are not taught to diagnose immortal infections, and do not attempt to diagnose immortal infections. Surgery is a hands-on specialty that is trained "to cut is to cure". When a surgeon is asked for an opinion, surgery will generally be the suggested answer, because that is what the surgeon knows and does.

Surgeons may fail to objectively evaluate their own surgery, and believe they did great surgery, even when the patient does not agree. When the patient gets an infection from surgery, the patient is referred to an infectious disease specialist. When the surgery fails and the patient is still in pain, the patient is offered more surgery, and at the end of all surgical options the patient is referred to pain specialists. Performing surgery is a point of no return for the patient, and should always be the last course of treatment. Surgery should never be done without a need, and never done as a quick fix. When a pill does not work, a patient can stop taking the pill; but once surgery is done, it cannot ever be undone. Once tissue is cut in surgery, the tissue cannot ever return to its former state, scar tissue forms, infections may be spread, and the patient is given broad-spectrum antibiotics in conjunction with surgery. The scar tissue can also create a barrier to passive flow in the body, and treatment of the chronic infection becomes significantly more complicated after surgery.

Orthopedics is a surgical specialty. The orthopedic doctor is not trained immortal infections cause joint or bone pain, or how to diagnose immortal infection; and diagnosis of immortal infection is not part of the orthopedic specialty. Orthopedic surgeons replace joints, they do not rehabilitate joints, by treating infectious causes of joint pain. Orthopedic surgeons operate over and over on the same body part, particularly spine surgeons; and when the patient is not cured and the pain persists and is worse, the patient is referred to a pain doctor for chronic pain prescriptions. Pain doctors are not trained in diagnosing immortal infections; are dealing with a patient whose pain is complicated by surgery or surgeries; and pain specialists only prescribe drugs for pain.

Cardiologists do not have knowledge that chlamydia pneumonia causes heart disease; and do not know treatment of chlamydia pneumonia improves the prognosis and reduces the risk of subsequent heart attacks. Cardiologists do not treat heart disease as a chronic chlamydia pneumonia infection; and do not recognize treating the chlamydia pneumonia in heart patients can help treat and or forestall Alzheimer's and macular degeneration, which are caused by the same pathogens. Cardiologists know of plaque in the heart and cardiovascular system, but do not understand the patient has plaque because of a war between chlamydia pneumonia and the immune system, leaving behind biofilm, dried pus, and remnants of the battle covered in plaque. Cardiologists advocate putting everyone on a statin drug to reduce cholesterol, when statin drugs cause muscle weakness, cognitive decline, an increase in blood sugar, and a decline in overall health. Cardiologists put patients on lifetime drugs, to treat cholesterol and the symptoms of heart disease; when treatments directed at immortal infection could be more effective and safer for treating cardiovascular disease and reducing cholesterol.

Infectious disease specialists should be medicine's master sleuths; yet, have not recognized immortal pathogens can cause chronic disease. Infectious disease specialists do not recognize and diagnose immortal infections or parasites; or that acute community acquired infections become chronic and can cause chronic disease. Most infectious disease specialists treat hospital acquired wound infections and implant related infections, with intravenous antibiotics. Infectious disease specialists do not recognize the importance of immortal pathogens, or diagnose and treat chronic immortal infections that cause of chronic disease.

Rheumatologists do not recognize chronic infection with immortal pathogens and parasites cause joint pain, arthritis, and autoimmune disease. Rheumatologists do not uniformly understand that many rheumatologic diseases are caused by chronic infection, inflammation and byproducts of the immune battle referred to the joint. Rheumatologists do not understand autoimmune diseases are chronic infections with immortal pathogens, and the body is attacking the pathogens, with impaired and infected immune cells. The worst example is how rheumatologists deal with Wegner's syndrome, which is now being called GPA, for granulomatosis with polyangiitis (inflammation of the blood vessels). The immune system is not attacking healthy cells, the immune system is attacking the intracellular pathogens, is confused by the pathogens, and generates TNF-alpha to mount an aggressive immune attack against pathogens the immune cells cannot eradicate with a less aggressive immune response. Inflammation in the blood vessels with granulomas (another name for inclusion cysts), is caused by immortal chlamydia pathogens, and can be caused by other pathogens such as strep-M.

Endocrinologists treat diabetes and endocrine disorders, and do not recognize infectious causes of endocrine disease. Despite reports of the "association" between infectious pathogens and endocrine disorders, endocrinologists do not attempt to diagnose infectious diseases in endocrine disease. They persist in treating endocrine diseases symptomatically, by replacing hormones depleted by endocrine disorders. Patients are given synthetic thyroid supplements for thyroid disorders, and patients with diabetes are given oral and injectable insulin to replace the hormone lost in diabetes. The endocrinologist does not seek to diagnose or treat infectious pathogens causing the endocrine disorders. Symptomatic treatment may be necessary or helpful in endocrine disorders, but cannot cure or mitigate the underlying root cause of infectious pathogens and/or parasites.

Oncologists do not diagnose or treat infectious causes of cancer. Infectious causes of cancer are not part of oncology training, diagnosis, treatment; and cancer research on infectious causes is limited by bias and lack of funding. Oncologists are only trained to treat infections arising from chemotherapy and radiation. Antibiotics and antiparasitics have been shown effective in improving the prognosis and extending life in some cancers. TLR-7 agonists have been available for twenty years; and the TLR-7, TLR-8, and TLR-9 agonists are just now being recognized as important treatment for cancer with the potential to cure cancer. TLR-7 agonists have been consistently underutilized by oncologists to treat cancer, and are still not implemented in routine oncology practice. Surgery, chemotherapy, and radiation may be valid treatments for cancer; however, cancer specialists should expand their thinking to include diagnosis and treatment of immortal pathogens and parasites; and incorporate the use of imiquimod and treatment of immortal pathogens and parasites into cancer treatment plans.

Cancer researchers discovered tissue adjacent to cancer had the exact molecular properties as an immortal intracellular chlamydia pathogen. Chlamydia is the only known pathogen that matched the findings in adjacent tissue. Chlamydia is the only pathogen known to live intracellularly, consume ATP, cause fermentation, cause loss of normal apoptosis, cause angiogenesis, and causes reduced endothelial dysfunction. The molecular properties of chlamydia and other infectious pathogens and parasites, are not part of the training and specialty of cancer, or part of the specialty of the researchers studying adjacent tissue in cancer. Thus, the importance of the findings in adjacent tissue was not recognized, and an important discovery that could reveal the cause of cancer was obscured by bias and cognitive assumptions.

Gastroenterologists rely on scopes, to diagnose cancer and other gastrointestinal diseases, and maintain a high income. Gastroenterologists do not often diagnose and treat immortal pathogens and parasites, the major causes of gastrointestinal disease. Recognition of the infectious pathogens causing intestinal disease and intestinal pathogens spreading from the intestine to other parts of the body has been forgotten or is ignored, in gastroenterology. Gastroenterologists send patients to surgeons to remove gallbladders, without diagnosing or treating immortal infections or parasites that may be causing gallbladder disease. Gastroenterologists diagnose pancreatic disease and common bile duct disease, without diagnosing the pathogens and parasites that cause common bile duct and pancreatic diseases, and pancreatic cancer. Gastroenterologists do not recognize parasites are a common cause of their patients' intestinal complaints. Gastroenterologists resisted knowledge ulcers were an infection for more than fifty years. The gastroenterologist should be diagnosing and treating immortal pathogens and parasites, in patients with esophageal reflux, ulcers, dysbiosis, irritable bowel, Crohn's disease, ulcerative colitis, or obesity.

Ophthalmology is a surgical specialty, plagued by at least nine separate and distinct sub-specialties. The ophthalmology specialties include the front of the eye (anterior segment), the middle of the eye, the back of the eye, glaucoma, strabismus, pediatric, retinal, neuro-ophthalmology, and plastic surgery, for a part of anatomy that is two globes only an inch in diameter. Ophthalmologists in one sub-specialty do not review literature in other ophthalmology sub-specialties. Ophthalmologists do not consider literature reporting that an infection in one part of the eye can migrate to another part of the eye. The front of the eye ophthalmologists are not aware the middle and back of the eye ophthalmologists are observing the same infections and same effect on tissue in the eye; and the middle and back of the eye ophthalmologists are not aware the front of the eye ophthalmologists are observing the same infections and the same effect on tissue in the eye. Ophthalmologists understand eye drops penetrate the cornea, but do not understand intestinal pathogens can penetrate the cornea; and invade the eye through the blood stream, vagus nerve, or by self-inoculation. Ophthalmology specialists are not interested in immortal infections or treating chronic eye disease as an immortal infection, because systemic immortal infection is outside the specialty and ophthalmology. No ophthalmology sub-specialist or any other medical specialty is trained to diagnose and treat immortal pathogens or parasites causing chronic eye disease.

Ophthalmology literature reports the "association" between chlamydia pneumonia in the eye and endothelial function; and have syndromes named "endothelial dysfunction". Chlamydia pneumonia has been "associated" with ocular surface disease, corneal thinning disease, glaucoma, and macular degeneration. All ophthalmology sub-specialties describe dysregulation, oxidation, failure of tissue and cells to function, inflammation, endothelial dysfunction, epithelial dysfunction, and abnormal proteins (by different names). POAG has been described as both failure of the epithelium and failure of the endothelium, both of which are caused by immortal pathogens. Ophthalmology does not consider the diagnosis and treatment of chlamydia pneumonia in vascular diseases of the eye, macular degeneration, or strokes in the eye.

H-pylori has been "associated" with ocular surface disease, glaucoma, and retinal disease; yet, the diagnosis and treatment of H-pylori has not been implemented in practice. Glaucoma has been reported to be "associated" with chlamydia pneumonia and H-pylori, more than twenty-five times; yet, diagnosis and treatment of infectious pathogens has not become part of a glaucoma practice. Toxoplasmosis has been "associated" with pigment dispersion glaucoma, one of the more dangerous forms of glaucoma, but is seldom diagnosed by glaucoma specialists. The entire Atlas of Glaucoma, published in 2014, fails to mention immortal infection, parasites, or toxoplasmosis, as a cause of glaucoma. H-pylori has been shown to cause retinal disease, including blinding diseases, such as ICSR; yet, diagnosis and treatment of infectious pathogens has not become part of a retinal practice. Retinitis pigmentosa is likely caused by psittacosis, yet diagnosis of infectious pathogens is not done, and patients are told they have no hope to stop the progression to blindness.

Psychiatry is a specialization directed to "mental health" drugs and talk therapy. The psychiatrist does not act as a medical doctor—the psychiatrist prescribes psychiatric medications. Psychiatrists are not trained to diagnose and treat immortal infections, toxoplasmosis or parasites; and do not consider medical diagnosis and treatment of the infectious causes of mental illness to be part of their responsibility. Psychiatrists and mental health professionals rarely diagnose medical conditions, even the pathogens known to cause mental illnesses. Toxoplasmosis is a known cause of mental illness, and psychiatrists do not take a history of pets or contact with cats, or diagnose toxoplasmosis, even in patients with mental health symptoms known to be caused by toxoplasmosis. Immortal pathogens and intestinal parasites can cause mental illness directly or by robbing the patient of nutrients, particularly folic acid and B12. Yet, psychiatrists do not test patients for low folic acid or B12, consider diagnosis and treatment of medical illness known to cause a loss of folic acid and B12, or provide supplements of folic acid and B12, to help stabilize a patient's mental health. Nor do psychiatrists work with a team of medical doctors who can diagnose infectious causes of mental illness.

Psychiatric patients have no specialty dedicated to the diagnosis of infectious causes of mental illness. Psychologists engage in talk therapy, and psychiatrists prescribes psychiatric drugs. Mental illness is caused by a medical illness—mental illness is a symptom of medical illness. No one is diagnosing medical illnesses in patients with mental illnesses! Mental health patients deserve medical diagnosis and treatment, before being prescribed psychiatric medications. No psychiatric patient should be given any of the violent five psychiatric drugs for depression, which will worsen their symptoms, cause agitation and anxiety, and cause suicide and violence toward others. Many downward spirals of depressed patients into violent and murderous acts could be avoided, if the mental health professionals would diagnose medical conditions; and stop prescribing the violent five psychiatric medications as a quick solution to depression and anxiety. When the violent five are given, extreme caution is necessary; and warnings should be given to the patient, family, caregivers and schools.

The specialty of obstetrics and gynecology delivers babies, and diagnoses and treats reproductive tract disease. Obstetrics and gynecology specialists seldom diagnose immortal pathogens, other than trachoma; and when diagnosed seldom treat the patient for a sufficient period of time. Obstetricians fail to inquire as to animal contact, fail to warn about the danger of pets, or warn about the danger of eye make-up. Obstetricians are often not present for the labor, because they try to continue working in the office making money, while labor proceeds, and wait to arrive until the last minute. When the obstetrician comes for the delivery at the last minute, they can become impatient, or fearful of waiting, leading to an extremely high rate of C-sections and the adverse consequences to mother and baby from a C-section.

Infection during pregnancy can cross the placenta, and has been "associated" with miscarriage, premature birth, birth defects, autism, cavernous sinus malformation, epilepsy, regressive developmental disorders, heart disease, lung disease, and late-onset blindness in the fetus. Obstetricians have been unable to find the causes of birth defects, autism, and chronic diseases in the fetus, because they do not know to look for infectious causes, and diagnose, and treat infectious causes, in the mother or infant. Obstetricians are not trained to recognize acute immortal infections in pregnancy, which can cause adverse fetal outcomes. Obstetricians fear treating pregnant mothers for acute infection, because the medication may harm the fetus; yet, seem not to fear broad-spectrum antibiotics used at the time of C-sections, antibiotic associated colitis, and MRSA from hospital acquired infections at C-sections, that damage the microbiome and mycobiome of mother and child. The fear of treating pregnant women for acute and chronic infection arises from a lack of understanding of immortal pathogens, and the importance of treating acute infections during pregnancy to avoid adverse fetal outcomes.

Pediatrics is the specialty that provides medical care to children. The pediatrician takes over care of the infant, at the time of birth. Pediatricians work with a cognitive assumption children will get better without medication, except in obvious and extreme cases of disease. Pediatricians are seemingly unaware of the pathogens that cross the placenta and cause chronic disease in children! Pediatricians are primary care providers for children; yet, do not seem to understand primary care of acute and chronic infection, including when a patient needs antibiotics and when the patient does not, and what antibiotics should be used

Pediatricians are not taught the infectious causes of chronic disease; the importance of diagnosing immortal pathogens and parasites in children; and the potential long-term effect of immortal pathogens and parasites causing chronic disease in the child, decades in the future. Pediatricians seldom diagnose immortal infections or parasites, and resist treating infection with antibiotics or antiparasitics. When pediatricians do treat children with antibiotics, they insist on using amoxicillin or a cephalosporin, which is a broad-spectrum antibiotic. When immortal pathogens are acquired in childhood and remain untreated, the child has a lifetime for the pathogens to evolve into chronic disease and combine synergistically with other pathogens to cause chronic disease. The failure of pediatricians to recognize and treat immortal pathogens and parasites, even in children with pets and risk factors for immortal pathogens, has led to an explosion of chronic disease in children and young adults, including asthma, obesity, and cancer.

Treatment of temporomandibular joint pain has been relegated to dentists and oral surgeons. Dentists and oral surgeons are removed from medical knowledge relating to infectious causes of chronic disease and arthritis. The TMJ patient may be given anti-inflammatory medications for joint pain, splints in their mouth, braces, or surgery by an oral surgeon to "repositioning of cartilage". Dentists and oral surgeons may suggest surgery to implant one or two TMJ implants (top and bottom of the TMJ), and sometimes starting with just the top or bottom, and later implanting the other half of the joint implant; after repositioning of the cartilage failed to control pain or improve range of motion, and implant of half a TMJ implant failed to control pain or improve range of motion. A TMJ patient may start with surgery on one side, then the other side, after the patient was told the basis of continued pain is the TMJ is unbalanced after the first surgery. Every TMJ surgery for cartilage repositioning and every TMJ implant has failed, causing severe morbidity and even death. Surgery for TMJ pain made the patients worse, with limited ability to open their mouth and often leaving the patient with disabling chronic pain.

TMJ pain is caused by infection, which refers to the TMJ, or is in the TMJ. TMJ pain and TMD cannot be cured by surgery. Any patient with TMJ pain should be examined and tested for infections around the head and neck, in the sinus, throat, glands, and teeth; and tested for immortal pathogens, including psittacosis, which has already been "associated" with TMJ pain. TMJ patients have multiple co-morbid conditions, all pointing to infectious causes of TMJ pain.

Once a patient chooses a specialty, the patient is committed to whatever that specialist knows, whatever that specialist diagnoses, and how that specialty treats the named disease. Specialists may have deep knowledge of their specialty, but knowledge outside their specialty is limited. Specialists may be smart; but no matter how smart a specialist may be in their field, the doctor does not always recognize what they don't know. Specialists may think they know more than they do, and are averse to admitting to a patient they do not know. The medical mindset is no different than everyone else—it is hard to change a specialist's mind or introduce new ideas they had not previously considered. It is particularly difficult when the ideas were not in their textbooks in medical school or within their specialty practice patterns. Changing one's mind requires an open mind, and significant effort, because changing one's mind requires admitting prior beliefs were not correct.

The Dunning-Kruger effect applies to medical specialization, particularly when knowledge is outside their specialty and medical training. The Dunning-Kruger effect is an unshakable illusion that you are smarter, and more skilled, and more knowledgeable, than you really are. In cognitive science, the less a person knows the more they think they know; and the more someone knows the less they think they know. Do not over estimate what the specialist knows. If specialists don't know, they should say so, and seek to understand the root cause of chronic disease; rather than making up a disease named after a symptom, finding or doctor, or defaulting to inflammation and genes.

Specialization has divided the body and diseases into many parts, with few specialties looking at the person as a whole. Few doctors have the cross-specialty training or cross-specialty knowledge, to recognize common patterns in chronic disease. Specialization has divided knowledge, limited communication between members of the healthcare team, created cognitive bias in specialties, and thwarted the advancement of medicine. The medical system is assaulting patients with medical technology, instrumentation, pharmacology, and surgery that effects every cell in the patient and too often worsens underlying chronic disease—instead of diagnosing the root causes of disease and making important discoveries to benefit the patient.

It is time to put the patient back together, and not let medical care be random dabbling at parts of the patient, part of the chronic disease, and part of the patient's problems. It is time to return to the wisdom of Aristotle, Ockham, Punch, Newton, Woodward, and Einstein, and simplify the naming of disease; and transform efforts at diagnosis and discovery, in all specialties, into a search for the pathogens causing the chronic disease.

Any fool can know. The point is to understand.

Maria Montessori

CHAPTER 22

MEDICINE IS CONTROLLED BY MONEY, FEAR & LACK OF TIME

The influence of money in medicine is longstanding. In the early twentieth century, half of the medications prescribed by doctors were natural or homeopathic. John D. Rockefeller used his oil money to buy a German pharmaceutical company, which was part of a massive German cartel, known as I.G. Farben. I.G. Farben was a pharmaceutical and chemical conglomerate of six companies, which included the pharmaceutical company. I.G. Farben assisted the Germans in Nazi medical experiments, and manufactured the gas used in Nazi gas-chambers, which led to the dismantling of I.G. Farben; and the German pharmaceutical company re-emerged as Bayer Pharmaceuticals, and other well-known companies.

John D. Rockefeller's German pharmaceutical company was researching how to remove medicine from plants, put the medicine into a pill, patent the medicine, and sell the pill for a profit. Rockefeller's goal was to sell patented medicine, which could not be done with natural and homeopathic medicine. Rockefeller and Andrew Carnegie devised a plan to ridicule and demean medical schools teaching natural remedies, and prescribing natural remedies; close medical schools teaching natural remedies; and donate large sums of money to medical schools who prescribed Rockefeller's patented pills and were researching his patented drugs. Some doctors were persecuted and even jailed for expressing their continued belief in natural remedies, rather than patented pills. The Rockefeller-Carnegie bias was against cures, in favor of ongoing treatment of symptoms with patented pills. The Rockefeller-Carnegie mantra was, "A pill for every ill".

Today, medicine still lives by the mantra of "a pill for every ill". We treat ills with pills, and treat the complications of pills with more pills. In

2016, the United States spent $3.3 trillion on medical care, which was equal to $10,348 per person; and the amount has steadily increased every year. The highest per person cost for medical care was for patients with a discrete event, such as a heart attack; and the next highest cost was treating patients with a chronic condition, who had persistently high costs. Thirteen percent of the cost of medical care is spent on patients in the last six months of life.[296] The cost of medical care was seventeen percent of the gross domestic product; and the cost of prescription medications has skyrocketed, to unaffordable levels. The art and science of prescribing medication to individual patients has been replaced by demands from insurance companies and pharmaceutical companies, who decide the appropriate medical care and treatment.

Pharmaceutical drug and device companies are very good at making money, and promotion and marketing of drugs, devices, and new technology. However, the products that make the most money are not necessarily the products that actually help people the most.[297] Medical products generally provide exorbitant profit to the manufacturers, which is a strong incentive to continue to market new medical products. Scientific research and pharmaceutical companies focus on development of expensive drugs and devices to treat symptoms of disease without knowing the cause; and ignore drugs that we have, which could be repurposed for use against chronic disease. Treating symptoms of chronic disease is far more profitable to the medical system, than diagnosis and treatment of the root infectious causes of chronic disease.

The employer and insurance company may require doctors to act in a way that prioritizes profit ahead of the best interest of the patient, and mandates a shortsighted view that ignoring immortal pathogens is cheaper than diagnosing and treating immortal pathogens. Every patient is treated the same, in terms of respect and medical care—poorly. Insured patients

---

[296] Aldridge M and Kelley A. 2015. The Myth Regarding the High Cost of End-of-Life Care. Am J Public Health. Dec 2015. 105(12): 2411-2415. Doi: ncbi.nlm.nih.gov/pmc/articles/PMC4638261/.

[297] Ewald PW. 2008. Interview with Evolutionary Biologists Paul Ewald. Bacteriality: Understanding Chronic Disease. Feb. 11, 2008. Doi: bacteriality.com.

are forced to pay high prices for expensive medication to treat symptoms. By the time a patient has a chronic disease, the acute infection has long passed, the pathogen has proliferated, and the patient has a more expensive and devastating medical problem. The second highest cost for medical care among all patients, is for those with chronic diseases.

The United States spends approximately $80 billion on medical research every year. The research is disorganized, fragmented, duplicative, and focuses on small details rather than causes and cures. Research is uncoordinated incidental dabbling into narrow questions, and often duplicates research previously done by others. Research contributed vast quantities of knowledge, and explained the small details of cell microbiology, Cluster Differentiations, abnormal proteins, inflammation, genes, and human microbiology; but, has provided few answers as to the causes, treatment or cures of chronic disease. The quantity of knowledge has expanded rapidly; yet, the quality of knowledge has not. The United States spent close to one-trillion dollars on research in the last decade— what do we have to show for it? The medical community has been reluctant or refuses to recognize the danger of transmission of animal pathogens to humans, and that chronic infection causes chronic disease; and directed research away from infectious causes, toward research of little direct benefit to patients.

The United States spends more on medical care than any country in the world; and medical care continues to become more and more expensive. After more than three trillion per year spent on medical care and eighty billion per year spent on medical research, and after decades of research, medicine has not yet explained the cause of chronic disease. The United States population continues to experience an increase in chronic disease, because medical doctors are not diagnosing infectious causes of chronic disease and are treating symptoms. Immortal pathogens causing chronic infections have caused an explosion in chronic disease; and an explosion in the cost of medical care. As the immortal pathogens spread without treatment, the population acquires a higher infectious burden, with multiple infections and re-infections, and higher rates of chronic disease.

The technological imperative has replaced the art of physical examination. Technology is quick and easy, and a shortcut to spending more time with the patient. Ordering expensive scans is faster than a physical examination and applying the art of medicine. Technology diverts attention away from a history, physical, assessment, and plan for diagnostic blood tests; and the most basic history and blood tests to detect immortal pathogens. Technology can be more profitable than spending time with a patient. Technology does not require a doctor to think—the doctor can wait for the technology to disclose a diagnosis; and if nothing is found the assumption is no problem. The technological imperative can be a shortcut to care; and does not inform or only partially informs the doctor as to a diagnosis of chronic immortal infection. When the technological imperative prevails, everyone makes a profit at the expense of the patient. Technology can be a valuable tool; but cannot replace the art of medicine; and should not be done *in lieu* of attempting to diagnose the pathogens causing chronic disease.

Doctors, practices and insurance companies spend thousands to save hundreds, when hundreds of dollars spent on diagnosis and treatment of immortal pathogens would be better for the patient. Doctors spend millions on technology, and shift the cost to the patients, which can enhance their incomes. Doctors will order CT scans, MRI's, scopes, spinal taps, and surgery; yet, will not do a blood test for immortal pathogens to find the root cause of the chronic disease, alleging the tests are costly. Stopping chronic disease before it happens, and mitigating the effect of chronic disease by treating the root cause with appropriate medication will always be cheaper and better for the patient, and reduce the cost inherent in the medical system and the technological imperative.

A thorough history, physical, and blood tests, are the most valuable and cost-effective tools doctors have for making a diagnosis. A thorough history, physical, and diagnostic blood tests for immortal infection is a better option than a lifetime of symptomatic treatment. Antibiotics for immortal infection and/or antiparasitics are more cost-effective, because treatment of the root cause of the disease provides a chance to cure, mitigate, or delay the effect of the patient's chronic disease. Chronic diseases are expensive; and treating symptoms indefinitely, without knowing the cause, is expensive, wasteful and potentially harmful to the patient.

Two of the foremost and well-known tenants of medicine are "do no harm", and the doctor has a fiduciary duty to put the patient's interest ahead of their own. Dr. Bernard Lown, professor emeritus of cardiology, at Harvard, senior physician at Brigham and Women's Hospital in Boston, and founder of the Lown Cardiovascular Group; and author of the <u>Lost Art of Healing, Practicing Compassion in Medicine</u>, argues we have lost the three-thousand-year bond of trust between doctor and patient. Doctors no longer minister to a distinctive person, and only concern themselves with fragmented, malfunctioning body parts. The technological imperative has taken over medicine. Healing is replaced with treating, caring is replaced by managing, and the art of listening has been taken over by technological procedures.[298]

Dr. Khullar, a physician at New York-Presbyterian Hospital and researcher at Weill Cornell Department of Healthcare Policy and Research, said, "Trust requires trustworthiness". Trust depends on three fundamental questions: Do you know what you are doing? Will you tell me what you are doing? And are you doing it to help me or help yourself?[299] Many patients have lost trust in the medical profession, because of bad personal experiences or bad experiences by friends and family. Trust is lost when the doctor palliates the patient with treatment of symptoms and technology, dismisses the problem as in the patient's head, or makes an ambiguous diagnosis that merely describes symptoms. Patient trust has been replaced by increased anger at the medical system and doctors.

The practice of medicine must be centered on the patient; with real connections between every health professional and the patients. Doctors need to understand and respect the cultural differences in patients and

---

[298] Lown B. 1999. <u>Lost Art of Healing, Practicing Compassion in Medicine</u>. New York: Ballantine Books.

[299] Khullar D. 2018. Do You Trust the Medical Profession? A Growing Distrust Could be Dangerous to Public Health and Safety. New York Times. (Health). January 23, 2018. Doi: www.nytimes.com/2018/01/23/upshot/do-you-trust-the-medical-profession.html.

the medical literacy of patients. The doctor needs to communicate, and explain the plan and obtain consent for proposed treatment plans, which leads to fewer medical errors and dissatisfied patients. Communication includes what is said, and what is not said. Doctors must not remain silent about significant risks or factors that can influence the patient's decision. Trust requires open disclosure and informed consent, between doctor and patient. Trust fosters open communication from the patient, which reveals details otherwise unknown and important to the diagnosis. Trust and informed consent requires listening and honest communication; and overcoming cultural barriers to understanding, and low medical literacy.

The patients often feel mistreated or they did not get adequate time and attention from the doctor. The doctor may have interrupted the patient, before the patient was able to discuss their concerns; the doctor looked at a computer screen, instead of the patient; or the patient left without a clear answer for their problem. When a doctor does not give the patient adequate time, it causes the patient to feel demeaned, angry, and have anxiety, because the root causes of their problems were not diagnosed and they were only given symptomatic treatment and dismissive answers. According to Dr. Victoria Sweet, the patient visit is compressed in both time and space; and establishing the correct diagnoses and getting patients to stop taking unnecessary medications takes more time, but in the long run saves more than money.[300]

The art of medicine takes time, and conflicts with demands on doctors for speed and profit. Doctors do not have enough time to evaluate the patient or go beyond what they were taught, between the hours they work, the endless paperwork, and data entry. The demand to see too many patients leaves inadequate time for a thorough history, examination, thought, planning, and establishing a relationship. The art and science of medicine has been replaced by electronic records; and fulfilling the demands by employers, insurance companies, and Medicare. Electronic records enforce the bias

---

[300] Sweet V. 2017. Slow Medicine, the Way to Healing. Riverhead Books; Jauhar S. 2018. A Doctor Argues That Her Profession Needs to Slow Down, Stat. New York Times Book Review. January 26, 2018. Doi: https://www.nytimes.com/2018/01/26/books/review/slow-medicine-victoria-sweet-memoir.html.

of vested interests, and create stagnation of medical thought. The art of viewing countenance, and the basics of history, physical, assessment, and plan to diagnose a disease has been abandoned, in the quest for speed and profit and in favor of the technological imperative. Specialists sometimes even limit advice to one complaint, per visit, which is only one part of the patient's problem, and then move on to the next patient; requiring multiple patient visits and increased expense and inconvenience for the patient, due to multiple visits to the doctor or multiple visits to different specialists.

Doctors must be allowed time to look at the whole patient, and not just the presenting complaint; and time to evaluate all co-morbid conditions. Doctors should always ask about family history, in *all* family members and not just genetic relatives; a pet history, including the degree of close contact with pets; and a travel history, including foreign travel and travel within the United States. Take the time to ask what the patient thinks is the problem and what the patient thinks may be the solution. Patients can be insightful about their own health, when the doctor takes the time to listen. Take the time to investigate pathogens that are causing the underlying chronic disease and plan treatment directed at the root cause.

Technology is a shortcut to spending time with patients, a way to reduce fear of missing a significant diagnosis, and is profitable to the doctor and practice. Technology does not generally reveal infectious disease unless an abscess has formed, or immortal infection has reached the point of chronic disease, such as cancer, degeneration in joints, or other obvious findings of chronic diseases that show on scans.

Doctors and medical practices try to find ways to offset shrinking income, when squeezed financially, by employers, insurance companies, and Medicare. Each specialty has developed its own profit center, in a world of cost cutting and demands to be profitable. Profit centers have replaced and supplemented a fee-for-service model; and put high dollars in a doctor's pocket, often in cash. In some specialties, profit centers are devoted to treating symptoms without a diagnosis, creating a lifelong dependency to return for management and prescriptions. In other specialties, the profit center is an easy source of higher income and cash payments.

Profit centers diminish a doctor's interest in observation, diagnosis, and cheaper and more effective means to treat chronic disease; and the doctor tends to direct the patient toward the profit center. In some larger practices, business managers monitor doctors for the percent of patients converted to the profit center, and employment evaluations, salary, bonuses, and partnership, are based on meeting benchmarks for the profit centers. Profit centers do not enhance medical care, and can divert attention away from good medical care. Profit is necessary to stay in business, and not bad in and of itself; but, excessive profit from gimmicks and profit centers of little benefit to the patient is a betrayal of the patient trust.

Plastic surgery is the highest paid specialty, with an average salary of $501,000.[301] General surgery is in the mid-range of physician and surgeon salaries, with an average salary of $322,000.[302] In surgery, the profit center is surgery. If you ask the opinion of a surgeon, the answer will be surgery, and more surgery, and more surgery. If a surgeon is not doing surgery, they are not earning any income. Surgery is a point of no return; and elective surgery should be viewed with rigid skepticism, and an understanding patients getting elective surgery are ordinarily being served by a profit center. Beware of over promise and under deliver for any elective surgery.

General surgeons perform stomach surgery to implant stomach bands and surgically reduced the size of the stomach, for weight loss, rather than seeking the cause of obesity. Surgeons implanted the Angelchik device, a donut shaped silicone filled plastic device tied around the esophagus, to mechanically stop reflux and limit the ability of the patient to eat; which had to be abandoned because every implanted Angelchik device failed and had to be surgically removed, causing significant morbidity. Surgeons never investigated an infectious cause of obesity, or why the

---

[301] Kane L. 2018. 8th Annual Compensation Report. Medscape. 2018. Doi: www.medscape.com/slideshow/2018-compensation-overview6009667?src=ppcgooglerem comp20185174&gclid=EAIaIQobChMIrsKTnIfC2wIVBBgCh3eiQpwEAEYASA AEgI-YfDBwE.
[302] Kane L. 2018. 8th Annual Compensation Report. Medscape. 2018. Doi: www.medscape.com/slideshow/2018-compensation-overview-6009667?src=ppcgooglere mcomp20185174&gclid=EAIaIQobChMIrsKTnIfC2wIVBBgCh3eiQpwEAEYA SAAEgI-YfDBwE.

patient had reflux, including parasites that cause burping and reflux. The technological imperative and desire to perform surgery drove the surgeries and sale of the devices. The surgeries were profitable to the surgeons, but harmed many patients.

Orthopedics is the second highest paid specialty, with an average salary of $497,000.[303] In orthopedics, the profit center is surgery and implants, particularly implants of the hip and knee. Orthopedic doctors and hospitals share in profits generated by using specific implants; and it is common for hospitals to enter contracts with the makers of implants to share profits from the sale, and require doctors on the hospital staff to use only their chosen brand of implants. Patients submit to implant surgery without understanding the consequences of failure can be significant; or the patient may have other alternatives. Surgery and joint implants lead to hospital acquired infections and infections in and around the implants, and treatment of implant related infections cause morbidity and permanent damage to the microbiome. Hospitals are incubators for drug-resistant pathogens and after any surgery the patient is given potent antibiotics to treat hospital-acquired pathogens, which puts the patient at risk for drug resistant organisms. Implants may be necessary in some cases, but patients should be told the truth about pacemakers, defibrillators, jaw implants, hip implants, knee implants, finger or toe implants, shoulder implants, spine implants, etc., before surgery, not after it is too late and the patient is past a point of no return.

Cardiology is the third highest paid specialty, with an average salary of $423,000.[304] In cardiology, the profit center is doing evaluations, including an EKG, echo cardiogram, and a stress test; and procedures and implants, ranging from electric shock, to pacemakers, stents, and implantable defibrillators. Cardiologists and hospitals may share the profits from the sale of procedures and cardiac devices with the manufacturers. Implantable defibrillators have caused significant pain and suffering, and morbidity in patients. Many have had to be removed, and when removed caused significant damage to the heart, morbidity, and mortality. Various

---

[303] *Id.*

[304] *Id.*

forms of vessel shunts have failed, when the implants re-stenosed due to an unrecognized infection that was never treated. Cardiologists are doing well in sending patients to cardiac rehabilitation after a heart attack; however, fail to diagnose and treat chlamydia pneumonia, the cause of heart disease. Treatment of chlamydia pneumonia could potentially avoid the need for expensive treatments and procedures, and implants provided by cardiologists; and avoid future cardiac events.

Gastroenterology is the fourth highest paid specialty, with an average salary of $408,000.[305] Yet, gastroenterologists do not believe they are paid enough.[306] The gastroenterology profit center is scoping everyone, from every end, sometimes more than once. Gastroenterology has forgotten the diagnosis of infectious disease, *in lieu* of highly profitable technology and the profit center derived from the routine scoping of patients. A gastroenterologist can make as much as ten thousand dollars in a half-day, doing scope after scope.

The problem is not scoping *per se*, it is that gastroenterology has exploited technology for profit, *in lieu* of diagnosis and treatment of intestinal pathogens. Prior to any scope the gastroenterologist orders a purge of the colon, and flushes out the pathogens with the purge. The gastroenterologist does not inspect or culture the stool and fluid expelled by the purge. Evidence of the infectious pathogens was flushed away by the purge; and even if present in the colon, microorganisms are not visible through the scope. If the gastroenterologist does not see anything through the scope, the gastroenterologist assumes nothing is wrong. The gastroenterologist tells the patient the test was normal, and offers symptomatic treatment. Gastroenterologists do not consider immortal pathogens or parasites that were not visible, or attempt to treat the patient's immortal infection or parasites, before or after the endoscopy or colonoscopy. When the symptoms return in weeks or months, after the purge wears off, the gastroenterologist explanations range from stress, to the bowel must be "irritable". Yes, the bowel is irritable—it is infected and inflamed, engaging in an immune battle against the pathogens.

---

[305] *Id.*

[306] *Id.*

Gastroenterology held onto their bias ulcers are caused by stress, for fifty years. Gastroenterologists blamed patients for their ulcers, because of cognitive bias and refusal to accept infectious pathology. Gastroenterology clings to "irritable bowel syndrome", inflammatory bowel disease, Crohn's disease, and ulcerative colitis, without looking for chronic infection or parasites. Ulcers are known to be caused by H-pylori; thus, it is hard to understand why gastroenterologists resist the idea that Crohn's disease and ulcerative colitis could also be caused by H-pylori or similar intestinal pathogens. Now gastroenterologists are using TNF-alpha inhibitors for Crohn's disease and ulcerative colitis, which generates more profit but is harmful to patients with the intestinal pathogens. Dr. Merchant treated ulcerative colitis using various antibiotics, antiparasitics, hormones, diet, exercise, and acid blockers, and the ulcerative colitis stabilized. The patient still has occasional flares, which require treatment, but the ulcerative colitis improved with treatment.

Gastroenterologists prescribe drugs to move the bowels when the patient has constipation. They prescribe drugs to treat constipation caused by other drugs. They give drugs to stop diarrhea, when diarrhea is a signal of an intestinal infection and a defense against pathogens! Stopping diarrhea keeps the pathogens in the intestine, where pathogens can become established and cause chronic disease. Treatment of gastrointestinal pathogens and parasites, not just treatment of symptoms, should be the mainstay of gastroenterology. Instead, valuable drugs to treat gastrointestinal pathogens and parasites were taken off the market for lack of use! Gastroenterologists also need to also develop a better understanding of the microbiome and mycobiome, and use drugs and supplements, to balance the microbiome and mycobiome and restore gastrointestinal health.

Dermatology is the sixth highest paid specialty, with an average salary of $392,000.[307] Dermatologists treat various skin conditions and skin cancer; but seem to have difficulty diagnosing scabies and other itchy skin rashes, and infectious causes of some skin conditions. Medi-spas have become a profit center for dermatology. A patient may spend a day at the medi-spa and become more beautiful, get cosmetic lasering, surface abrasion, and

---

[307] *Id.*

other forms of beauty treatments. Dermatology uses lasers to make us more beautiful; and lasers and other methods to remove brown spots on the skin that were caused by infection and transferred in biofilm, to the face and arm; and could be treated with topical antibiotic and antifungal medications.

Oncology is the tenth highest paid specialty, with an average salary of $363,000.[308] Oncologists treat cancer patients, and prescribe and manage chemotherapy and radiation. The profit center for oncology is chemotherapy drugs and radiation. The cost of chemotherapy for one patient can exceed $80,000. Chemotherapy drugs generate huge profits for cancer doctors and oncology practices, when the oncologist and oncology practice purchase chemotherapy drugs at wholesale prices, and resell the chemotherapy drugs to the patient. The oncologist and oncology practice can make as much as $40,000 in profit, per patient, reselling chemotherapy drugs to the patient. The radiation oncologists establish the treatment plan, and let others do the radiation and bill for the radiation. Oncologists receive no monetary incentive for diagnosing and treating immortal infections or parasites that cause cancer.

Ophthalmology is the eleventh highest paid specialty, with an average salary of $357,000.[309] Ophthalmologists have multiple profit centers. Ophthalmologists sell "premium implants" for cataract surgery, which are an all-cash profit center. Manufacturers of "premium implants" pressured Medicare to allow ophthalmologists to charge unlimited cash, out-of-pocket, above what insurance pays for standard cataract implants; and the cash paid for a more expensive intraocular implant is one-hundred percent cash profit to the doctor and practice. Manufacturers of the intraocular implants created names like "premium lens", "advanced technology lens", "specialty lens", and "lifestyle lens", to make the patient believe they should pay thousands more, out-of-pocket, to obtain the latest "premium" lens. A large corporate ophthalmology practice, may also include a distributor company inside the practice, which buys premium implants at wholesale price, sells the lenses to another profit center in their practice (the surgery

---

[308] *Id.*

[309] *Id.*

facility), and sells the lenses for a profit a second time to the patient. The rate of conversion of patients to "premium lenses" may be used as a benchmark, in a corporate medical practice, to force the ophthalmologists to "up-sell" as many patients as possible, because of the tremendous profit generated by up-selling patients to premium lenses.

The elderly are vulnerable to accepting what the doctor recommends, without question. Some corporate ophthalmology practices use non-medical staff to convert patients to the profit center, with prepared scripts and sales pitches like, "Don't you want high definition vison for yourself". Staff are believed to be seen by patients as more trustworthy than the doctor, when trying to convince the patient to pay more for a "premium" intraocular lens, in cash, out-of-pocket. Staff doing the conversion to the higher priced intraocular lenses free the doctor from spending time discussing lens choice and converting the patient to the higher priced lens that requires payment in cash. Staff job performance may be monitored and measured by the conversion rate.

Business managers are demanding high conversion rates to premium intraocular lenses, and non-medical staff are promoting the higher priced intraocular lenses to patients. Some practices charge a few hundred dollars more per eye, for "premium" intraocular lenses; and other practices charge thousands of dollars more per eye, to elderly patients who have been convinced they need and want the more expensive intraocular lenses. An ophthalmologist earns $768 per eye, in a bundled fee, from Medicare, for all services and products related to cataract surgery. When a patient pays for a premium lens, the ophthalmologist can earn the $768 fee, plus a pure cash profit greater than the entire fee for surgery, for the premium intraocular lens.

Switching patients to premium lenses adds no cost or surgery time to the doctors, but adds hundreds of thousands of dollars of income to an ophthalmologist's income per year, and millions in income per year to corporate ophthalmology practices. The additional cash paid by cataract patients for premium intraocular lenses can generate as much as $15,000 more *per hour* for the ophthalmologist. Ophthalmologists who promote premium lenses, can increase their income by $350,000 per year! A large practice can make as much as $1,000,000 more per month, in cash profit.

The manufacturers of the premium intraocular lenses do not even try to promote the premium lenses as better—they promote the premium lenses as a way for the ophthalmologist and practice to make a lot more money. The "premium" intraocular lenses are no better, don't work as advertised, and have higher risks than standard lenses. The complications with premium intraocular lenses create even more income for the doctor and practice, when YAG laser surgery and more intraocular surgery is needed to fix the complications of the "premium" implant. The only thing premium about premium implants is the price! Premium intraocular lenses are also being promoted to young people as a form of refractive surgery, even though young patients have decades to develop complications and sight-threatening complications, from the implant.

Refractive surgery has been a profit center for ophthalmologists, and an evolving public health crisis for society. Refractive surgery is an all cash business, with no supervision, no involvement of insurance companies, and no government oversight. Refractive surgeons can make up to $100,000 *a day* in gross income, doing refractive surgery. Refractive surgery profit and complications have spawned secondary industries including corporate chains performing itinerant refractive surgery with "shooters"; manufacturers of drops for dry eyes, specialty contact lenses for complications of refractive surgery, and cross-linking to repair damaged eyes, generating more profits for manufacturers and eye care professionals. Refractive surgery is also heavily promoted to optometrists as a way to increase their income. Optometrists are encouraged to repeatedly urge patients to have refractive surgery, and told over the course of repeated efforts the patient will consider a referral for refractive surgery. The optometrist hopes to get income from the referral and from co-managing the patient with the surgeon, and share the fee or obtain a fee-for-service, for preoperative and post-operative office visits.

Psychiatrists are paid an average salary of $273,000 per year.[310] Psychiatrists delegate counseling to psychologists, and do little or no medical diagnosis of pathogens known to cause mental illness. They prescribe psychiatric drugs which can do more harm than good. The SSRI drugs prescribed for depression and anxiety do not work, and cause the patient's symptoms to become worse. The SSRI drugs cause suicide and violence toward others; and psychiatrists and every other type of healthcare professional prescribing SSRI drugs, need to take responsibility for protecting patients, families, and society from the suicide and violence caused by SSRI drugs.

Rheumatologists are paid an average salary of $257,000, per year.[311] The current profit center for rheumatology is treating arthritis and autoimmune diseases symptomatically, requiring the patient to return indefinitely for more drugs to treat the symptoms of pain and inflammation. Rheumatology uses TNF-inhibitors as a profit center, which potentiates the infections causing the underlying autoimmune disease and arthritis. Science has known for more than fifteen years arthritis is caused by infection; yet, diagnosis of chronic infection is ignored *in lieu* of treating symptoms and using expensive medications. Doxycycline and minocycline cost approximately $1,000, for a year of treatment; and TNF-inhibitors cost $20,000 to $40,000 per year.

The salaries in some specialties seem out of line relative to other specialties, and out of line with the workhorses of medicine—internal medicine, family practice, and pediatrics, the lowest paid specialties. The specialists with the greatest ability to develop profit centers are the ones with the highest incomes. Doctor thinking and decision making can be influenced by a desire for profit, by profit centers, or be pre-determined by contracts and kickbacks from the makers of drugs and medical products. A patient should never get informed consent for an elective surgery from the doctor or corporate medical practice who wants to profit from the surgery! Never get informed consent from a staff member, who is limited in what can be said and the person's job performance is depending on selling the patient the service or implant. Trust but verify! Buyer Beware!

---

[310] *Id.*

[311] *Id.*

Always consider long-term consequences of what the doctor proposes carefully, and inquire into new and alternate ways to improve diagnosis and treatment of chronic disease.

Vested interests fight to enforce conformity and lower costs; and independent thinking and new ideas for treatment are discouraged. The rules and the established standards are in charge. Few doctors are willing to break outside their box to challenge the rules, or implement creative solutions. Doctors may face consequences and even persecution for speaking out, ordering too many tests, or prescribing too many antibiotics; or prescribing antibiotics at all. Medicine cannot move forward because medical training, specialty boards, insurance companies, Medicare, and large corporate medical practices, are vested in the status quo and will not let medicine move forward. Medicare, insurance companies, and large corporate practices are satisfied with what they are doing; and the current practice of medicine can be very lucrative for them. They may believe what they do is good science; but their thinking, approach, and understanding is outdated. Medicine chases short-term financial gain, instead of long-term savings through improved prevention of chronic disease, by appropriate diagnosis and treatment of immortal infections.

Many fields of medicine, including cardiology, orthopedics, and ophthalmology, use implants and drugs subject to FDA scrutiny. The FDA is a toothless government entity controlled by lobbyists for the manufacturers of drugs and devices, and heavily influenced by politicians. The most powerful twenty doctors in each medical specialty act as an advocacy team for manufacturers. The FDA does no investigation, no clinical studies, and does not write labeling for any drug, device, or cosmetic. The manufacturers hire medical monitors and consultants, conduct clinical studies, and write labeling, without any FDA supervision; and submit the results and their proposed version of labeling for a *pro forma* approval. When drugs or devices are denied approval, manufacturers call their politicians, and the politicians pressure the FDA to approve the product. Restrictive FDA rules favor the manufacturer, and may require devices to be approved even when the devices do not work, do not work for the full range of conditions for which it is approved, or the effect wears off in a short time; and the approval is given with directions to warn the users the product does not work, does not work for all stated indications, or the effect is temporary.

Physicians who get consulting contracts with the manufacturers and are hired for clinical trials to obtain FDA approval make substantial income. Contracts may be as much as $500,000 per year, and one consultant for Allergan was paid more than $800,000. Consultants are paid to lend their name to scientific articles written by the company, act as a medical monitor in name only, promote the product, and give ideas and lend their name to new products. Consultants may be offered a share of the profits from patents on new devices. The consultants promote the products for the company, at the FDA; and have been known to lie, and engage in significant omissions and concealment, to get the products approved by the FDA. The consultants are paid to go to medical meetings and promote the product, as if they are giving an independent expert opinion. Contracts with consultants are about sales and profit, not about truth or what is best for the patient.

The FDA approves most products for marketing, based on a grandfathering clause, known as a 510k approval to market a product. The 510k process is intended to be a streamlined process for approval to market a product, for products alleged to be similar to products already on the market. The 510k products are approved for marketing, with minimal or no FDA scrutiny. The manufacturer seeking approval under the 510k process does not have to prove safety and efficacy; and only has to show the product is "substantially" equivalent to a product already on the market. Regulations require products with changes in design or materials to undergo a new full approval process; however, the FDA does not follow the regulation and approves 510k products that have changed in design or materials from the predicate device. The predicate device may be known to be dangerous and may have even been recalled from the market, and the product still can obtain FDA approval as a 510k product. Many 510k products have followed a chain of "substantial equivalency" to predicate devices, until the product no longer resembles the original device. Ninety-five percent of medical implants are approved as a the 510k product, even when the product no longer resembles the original product, changes required a full review before approval, or the predicate product was dangerous or recalled. Cosmetics have never been tested for safety.

The FDA relies entirely on the honesty of manufacturers, and all too often the FDA relies on false representations by the manufacturers and their paid consultants. The manufacturer tries not to know of adverse events, does not investigate adverse events that may interfere with approval or sales, and conceals adverse events in clinical studies in "lost-to-follow-up patients" and in their in-house complaint files. The FDA has also chosen to apply a new standard for approval of products and 510k product approval that is not part of the FDA regulations. The FDA asks, "Is the product better than what we already have". "Better than what we have" does not assure a product is safe and effective, particularly when the predicate product was not safe. The "better than what we have standard" has allowed many products on the market which are not safe, or not safe as marketed.

The FDA is limited in its ability to protect the public from injuries caused by medical devices, by its own regulations relating to approval, which favor manufacturers. The FDA regulations require any approval be for the indications requested; or the product approval is denied. The FDA cannot approve a product and limit the indications; and is limited to requiring warnings if the device is approved but unsafe for some indications or at the extremes of indications. The extreme levels for vision correction with LASIK were never proven safe, and are higher risk; and the indications for hyperopia were reduced seven years after approval, because higher levels of hyperopic LASIK treatment were shown to be dangerous. Thermokeratoplasty was rejected by the first FDA Ophthalmic Device Panel, and after the company stock went down and politicians exerted political pressure, thermokeratoplasty was approved, with a statement in labeling that thermokeratoplasty was temporary and did not work.

Refractive surgery devices provide glaring examples of the lack of oversight by the FDA, causing morbidity in patients. When the FDA Ophthalmic Devices panel first reviewed LASIK/PRK devices, the vote was nine to zero denying approval. The laser manufacturer brought politicians to exert pressure on the FDA; and the FDA convened a new panel, requested a reconsideration of the rejection, did a new review, and granted approval. The FDA decided because LASIK was already being done, it would be better if they approved the devices to control labeling—but the FDA does not control labeling, the manufacturer writes labeling for a *pro forma* approval. The LASIK labeling stated studies did not provide proof of safety and efficacy at higher levels of treatment.

When LASIK was approved, no list of adverse events was ever created, causing confusion as to what is a complication and what is a reportable event. Doctors did not know what to report or how to report adverse events. Everything the patient considered an adverse outcome was treated as an anticipated complication or "too bad for you", rather than an adverse event that needed to be reported. The contraindication of "signs of keratoconus" was reinterpreted by refractive surgeons to be only a "relative contraindication". Iatrogenic keratoconus, also known as iatrogenic ectasia, caused by refractive surgery is a sight-threatening complication, requiring cross-linking and/or a corneal transplant; and ectasia has never been identified as a reportable adverse event. At a corneal conference in the early 2000's, in a room full of one-hundred corneal specialists, the speaker asked how many people had seen five or more cases of ectasia, after LASIK. Everyone in the room raised their hand, representing over five hundred cases of post-LASIK iatrogenic ectasia. The FDA had less than fifty adverse event reports of ectasia after LASIK, at that time.

Refractive surgery has never worked long-term, and caused many complications and patient disasters. Many new versions of refractive surgery devices have been approved based on a representation the devices are an "improvement" and are "better than what we have now". No refractive surgery devices have proven safe and effective in the long term; thus, the better than what we have standard does not protect the public; and approvals are more a reflection of the political power of the manufacturers and ophthalmologists.

Premium lenses for cataract surgery were approved as "substantially equivalent" to prior intraocular lenses, even though "premium" intraocular lenses are higher risk than standard intraocular lenses. The predicate devices no longer resemble current intraocular lenses, and were not even implanted in the same part of the eye. If premium lenses are substantially equivalent to prior lenses on the market, one must ask, "What is the justification for the patient paying thousands of dollars more out of pocket for the premium lens?" The manufacturers claimed premium lenses were substantially equivalent intraocular lenses, so why are they better or worth more money? In fact, premium lenses often do not work as promised, fail in time, cost substantially more, and cause a greater number of complications.

TMJ implants injured at least thirty-thousand patients. All TMJ implants have caused extreme morbidity and mortality in patients. The TMJ implants were approved as substantially equivalent to prior TMJ implants that had failed, caused substantial morbidity, and were removed from the market because of injuries caused by the device. The manufacturers alleged the new TMJ implants were better than what we have now. The significant dangers of TMJ implants were concealed by the manufacturers and medical monitors; while oral surgeons continued treating jaw pain with surgery and implants known to be dangerous, in every form ever approved and sold. Patients with complications were often referred to the medical monitor, who concealed the adverse event from the patient and the FDA. Lawsuits by victims with permanent disability and chronic pain finally informed the FDA of the danger. No TMJ implant should be used absent a catastrophic injury.

Hip and knee implants are routinely approved as 510k products. The implants have been through many design changes and material changes, and continue to be approved as 510k products. Many designs of joint implants have failed, and old failed designs have been recycled and used again, only to fail again. We have been through metal on metal, plastic on metal, plastic to secure the implant, bone cement failures, metal on tissue, and many other problems with joint implants. None of the hip and knee implants resemble the original products, sold before 1938.

Once a device is on the market, the FDA seldom recognizes the harm caused by the product, until patients start to file lawsuits for injuries caused by the product. The FDA relies on the manufacturer to tell them if new warnings should be added to the labeling, and to voluntarily bring new warnings, written by the manufacturer, to the FDA for approval. Even if severe complications are known and warnings needed, such as homicidal ideation and homicide on SSRI drugs, the manufacturers fight against adding any warnings that might reduce sales, and again bring political pressure to the FDA, to avoid giving the warnings.

Adverse event reports from doctors first go to the manufacturer, if the doctor knows they are obligated to make a report. The manufacturer is required to open a "Complaint File" for each report of an adverse event. The manufacturer scrutinizes the adverse event reports, blames misuse of the product by doctors or patients, and in ninety-five percent of the cases determines the adverse event is not device related, and does not need to be reported to the FDA. Manufacturers manipulate adverse event reporting, just as manufacturers manipulate clinical studies to show safety and the absence of adverse events. The manufacturers conceal or downplay adverse events, defects in the products, and needed warnings, to continue sales or expand sales. The FDA seldom takes the initiative to force a product to be removed from the market, or takes action based on reports of adverse events. Few medical products have withstood the long-term scrutiny of wide usage, and many have been proven unsafe by experience or by other independent studies.

The FDA relies on the honesty of the manufacturer to disclose adverse events, discovered during post-approval marketing. If an adverse event is reported to the manufacturer, the manufacturer opens a complaint file and decides internally whether the adverse event was device related and requires a report to the FDA. Manufacturers blame patients and doctors for the adverse event, rather than their device; and only a small percentage of adverse events, estimated at one percent or less, are ever reported to the manufacturer. Of the reports to the manufacturer, less than five percent of the adverse events are deemed by the manufacturer to be device related, and passed on to the FDA. Only after many patients are harmed and the lawsuits begin does the FDA discover vast numbers of injuries and unreported and concealed adverse events.

Doctors and patients rely on the FDA, and rely on a false assumption the FDA protects them. Doctors and patients seldom independently seek knowledge, or have access to mis-information from manufacturers, concerning claims which may not be true, or adverse events which have been concealed or manipulated to gain approval. Medical advice and the selling of medical products should be viewed with the understanding that the doctor's knowledge and the patients' knowledge has been manipulated by others, out of their control; and profit-driven misinformation has been provided to the doctor, which may be harmful to both the patient and the advancement of medicine.[312] Any medical devices should be reviewed with healthy skepticism, of the information being provided. Doctors and patients believe the FDA is protecting us, when it is not!

We do not mean to say all medical devices are bad, but doctors and patients should be aware of the need for "buyer beware". We don't mean to say all doctors are untrustworthy—but all patients buying new expensive drugs and therapies, medical implants, and elective surgery, should follow the maxim of "buyer beware!"

Manufacturers of prescription drugs are now free to charge any price, even for critical and life-saving drugs. The manufacturers scare consumers and politicians into believing the manufacturers of drugs deserve more money, so they can develop new expensive miracles. The manufacturers argue they are the innovators, but they are not. Many trillions of dollars have been spent on research and development, and no causes or cures have been found for chronic disease. Many billions are spent on false studies, advertising, bribing politicians, and bribing doctors. The idea cheaper drugs might work better than expensive drugs or expensive technology is not appealing to the thinking of many doctors or the manufacturers. Manufacturers have abandoned important drugs seen as not profitable enough, or are not used enough. Using older drugs for new purposes, is

---

[312] *See* Rampton S and Stauber J. 2001. <u>Trust Us We're Experts: How Industry Manipulates Science and Gambles with Your Future</u>. New York: Tarcher/Putman; 2018. The Bleeding Edge. Netflix (medical device industry works with the FDA against patients).

not part of the medical model or medical thinking, and cannot compete with the profit made in the current medical system.

Doctors' fear of being sued, and even worse being held liable for negligence, encourages doctors in the technological imperative and increases the cost of medicine. Ten percent of doctors are responsible for more than fifty percent of medical negligence payments; and a high percentage of doctors are never accused of medical negligence. Doctors know who the problem doctors are, and medical negligence would occur less frequently if doctors would police their own and take corrective action. The Code of Silence in the medical profession, reluctance to speak out against bad medical care or a bad doctor, reliance on the technological imperative, and lack of understanding about infectious causes of chronic disease, is why medical negligence is the third leading cause of death, causing an estimated 250,000 deaths a year, and ten-percent of deaths from all causes.

Lawsuits arise when patients trust a doctor as a knowledgeable authority, and assume the doctor is looking out for their best interest, and the trust is misplaced; or when doctors assume patients understands and agree when they do not. Poor communication between doctors and patients, too little time, and too little interaction, cause medical mistakes and misunderstandings. Time and communication with patients reduces the risk of medical negligence. The lack of time spent with a patient impedes diagnosis and treatment of the root cause of chronic disease, impairs discovery of the causes of chronic disease, increases the cost of medicine, and leads to medical mistakes. Trust and communication is essential to prevent medical mistakes, and to prevent lawsuits for negligence.

Most lawsuits arise because of false assumptions, by the doctor and/or the patient. When insufficient time is spent, to get all necessary information and care for the patient, the tendency of both doctor and patient is to fill in missing information in the brain with assumptions and cognitive biases. The patient assumes what the doctor wants to hear or takes the time to hear; and the doctor has such limited face time with the patient that the doctor has to fill in gaps in knowledge with assumptions. The doctor assumes the patient understands, and the patient assumes the doctor knows best and is afraid to question or challenge the doctor. Doctors who over promise and under deliver, fail to deal with patients in a culturally appropriate manner, and fail to explain why a patient had a bad outcome or what mistake was made and apologize, are more likely to be sued. Poor communication, lack of disclosure, and misinforming a patient, followed by a bad outcome, followed by a failure to explain and apologize for the mistake, sends patients to lawyers for the answers. The vast majority of patients injured by negligence never seek legal help or attempt to sue a doctor. Over promise and under deliver, followed by a breakdown in trust is what sends the patients to a lawyer. The best way to avoid lawsuits is to incorporate three of The Four Agreements into medicine—abandon false assumptions, do your best, and tell the truth.[313]

The MD Emperor Has No Clothes-Everybody is Sick and I Know Why, by Peter Glidden, BS, ND, argues when doctors do not understand the cause of a disease, and focus on symptomatic treatment and surgery, morbidity and mortality increases.[314] A better understanding of chronic disease, based on an understanding of infectious causes of chronic disease, including intracellular chronic infection and parasites, would benefit the profession and patients, help reduce the number of deaths from negligence, and reduce the number of lawsuits.

Doctors spend too much time in a rush, doing what HMO's and insurance companies demand. Doctor burnout arises from attempting to meet the demands of the medical system, which leads to lack of empathy, and lack of trust between doctor and patient. Doctors can be overwhelmed by the stress of modern medical practice. Merely succeeding in medical training imprints an attitude of knowing better, fear of being wrong, obeying the rules, and never wanting to look stupid. Doctors fear someone may find out they don't know. Doctors fear being wrong, fear criticism or ridicule, fear persecution, fear lawsuits, fear insurance companies, fear Medicare,

---

[313] Ruiz DM, Mills J. 2011. The Four Agreements, A Practical Guide to Personal Freedom, Amber-Allen Publishing. July 7, 2011.

[314] Glidden B. 2010. The MD Emperor Has No Clothes-Everybody is Sick and I Know Why, 3rd Ed. San Bernardino, CA.

fear deviating from the demands of their employer, and fear deviating from enforced conformity.

Insurance companies are directing patient care. Clerks for insurance companies are telling doctors what they can and cannot do, what tests can be ordered, and what drugs can be prescribed. Doctors are forced to worry more about billing and coding, than the patient. Doctors spend too much time and energy naming symptoms, findings, and syndromes, to comply with insurance coding and employer benchmarks. It's all about business, has not been a good philosophy for anyone, or for healthcare in general. Preventive medicine to treat infections early, to avoid chronic infections, reduce the infectious burden, and avoid chronic disease, is important in reducing chronic disease and the cost of care, and is better for everyone.

Publishers of scientific literature are not interested in publishing negative studies, negative findings, or articles which could subject them to criticism. Publishers have a strong bias against accepting and publishing information which is critical. In medical literature, more than ninety-five percent of scientific publications are positive, because publishers and authors are reluctant to report bad results or knowledge a drug or device caused harm. Literature describing the harm is rarely published out of fear of repercussions or lawsuits, and mistakes fade away until another generation repeats the mistakes the mistakes of the past. The failure to report negative outcomes leads to more negative outcomes.

Doctors are not taught the mistakes of prior generations. Mistakes are forgotten, and fade away without acknowledgement. The Steffe implants harmed thousands, and after it was known the devices all failed and caused significant morbidity in every patient, a review of the literature showed reporting was ninety-five percent positive. The TMJ implants and Angelchik devices were given positive reports, until many thousands of patients were harmed and lawsuits were filed. In the 1980's metal-on-metal implants were known to be dangerous, but now these implants are being revived. A TMJ implant articulating against tissue failed, and the idea was revived in knee implants, where it failed again. Anterior chamber intraocular lenses caused sight threatening complications in many thousands of patients, and were known to be higher risk when abandoned in favor of posterior chamber lenses; and now anterior chamber lenses are back and being promoted to young patients as a form of refractive surgery. SSRI drugs do not work and are causing suicide, violence toward others, and homicides, at an astounding rate, which was not reported in the scientific literature and is only reported by advocacy groups and in books by caring doctors, like Dr. Peter Breggin.

Alleged "experts" write articles in specialty journals, to cover up or justify mistakes and violations of standards, committed by others, particularly in orthopedics, gastroenterology, TMJ implants, refractive surgery, and psychiatry. In refractive surgery the defense experts grouped together to justify routine violations of known standards, aided by their specialty journals. Defense experts write articles perverting standards, to protect fellow doctors. The defense experts go beyond the Code of Silence, and actively write articles, in groups and under the auspices of a specialty journal, to protect and conceal for doctors and manufacturers who make mistakes and violate known standards. The articles written and published to protect wrongdoers confuse the literature and standards, and embolden others to push accepted standards, to make more money, at the risk of patient safety.

Medicare demanded most doctors and practices adopt electronic records, as a condition of Medicare participation. Electronic records have not improved the quality of medical care, or reduced the cost of care. Scribes are entering data while the doctor talks to the scribe instead of the patient; or the doctor is looking at a computer screen doing data entry, instead of looking at the patient, observing the patient, and establishing a doctor-patient relationship. Doctors are busy entering data required by mandated protocols; and struggling to fill in boxes and use templates that describe the encounter, with the stroke of one key. One button on the computer can fill in an entire block of the patient record, which reports identical information for every patient. The electronic forms may be pre-filled, and unless the doctor takes the time to change the information in every block on the form, the medical record is not accurate. Doctors look at computer screens instead of the patient, and the art of noticing has given way looking at computer screens and typing on a keyboard during patient encounters.[315]

Doctors can be monitored for benchmarks, using computer records. Computer records and benchmarks allow non-medical supervisors to control the way doctors practice medicine, and create pressure to use profitable methods of treatment and limit the cost of care. In service to electronic records and supervisors, the doctors fail to take an adequate history, show respect for the patient, or have a meaningful relationship with the patient. Medicine cannot move forward when electronic records force conformity, and allow supervisors to enforce a doctor to direct patients to profit centers.

Historically, new visions in medicine have not been implemented quickly or easily. Throughout history, many, many doctors and visionary thinkers have been criticized, persecuted and ostracized for expressing opinions and theories of infectious causes of chronic disease, which has created a chilling effect on doctors who might wish to express new ideas. Hippocrates was criticized for saying diseases had a cause; and Leonardo de Vinci was criticized for performing autopsies. In <u>Enemy of the People</u>, a doctor was criticized and ostracized by the community, his home was attacked, and he was shunned and exiled by the townspeople, for saying the town water was making people sick. Dr. Samelweiss, Dr. Henle, Dr. Rous, Dr. Farber, Dr. Blount, and many others, had new ideas about infectious causes of chronic disease, and were criticized or persecuted for their ideas. Dr. Samelweiss was removed from the hospital staff, and Dr. Blount's medical license was challenged. Dr. Farber was ostracized and criticized for twenty years, before his ideas became accepted and he became an icon in oncology. Dr. Merchant was criticized for saying the well water was making people sick, and intestinal diseases were caused by infectious pathogens. Those with money and influence have stifled discovery and innovation, and stifled new ideas. Important knowledge has too often taken many decades, before

---

[315] Pelzman, FN. 2018. Eyes Open: Too Often Modern Technology Keeps Us From…Just Noticing." Medpage Today. 4/13/18. Doi: medpagetoday.com/patientcenteredmedicalhome/patientcenteredmedicalhome/72315.

becoming accepted and implemented in practice, because of resistance by the medical system and the vested interests.

The words of Vincenzo Crespi still ring true, for us. He felt an obligation to speak the truth, which had been suppressed by those who did not want the truth to be known. We feel an obligation to speak the truth about medicine today, that others would prefer not be known. Doctors must fight to do what is right for their patients; and resist the powers and vested interests that try to enforce conformity and demand profit ahead of patient well-being. Medicine can be more effective, by recognizing and understanding infectious causes of chronic disease; and incorporating the understanding into the diagnosis and treatment of chronic disease.

> *Morality is doing what's right no matter what you're told.*
> *Obedience is doing what you are told, no matter what's right.*

H.L. Mencken

CHAPTER 23

DIAGNOSIS OF CHLAMYDIA AND PARASITES

Hippocrates believed the body must be treated as a whole and not a series of parts. Hippocrates focused on understanding anatomy, as part of understanding disease, and was criticized for breaking the taboo against autopsies to learn anatomy. Hippocrates concluded diseases had a cause, based on observation of patients, meticulous documentation of his observations, and deep thought. He examined countenance and bodily discharges; and inspected urine, stool, vomit, and blood consistency when blood-letting. He recognized different diseases, with different outcomes, different diseases occurred in different seasons, and different diseases occurred in different cultures. He knew people who drank contaminated water had intestinal disease, based on observation of big bellies, reasoning, and experience; and the fact he saw worms expelled by patients, which made patients feel better after expelling worms. He was able to determine a prognosis from his study and thought, based upon the history and physical examination, number of days the disease lasted, body system, body part, symptoms, and whether the disease relapsed after apparent resolution. Hippocrates had few options for treating patients, other than cutting, burning, or bloodletting; herbal and natural remedies; and observing and comforting the patient until recovery or demise.

In Ancient Greece, the Knidian and Koan schools of medicine were split, based on different approaches to disease. The Knidian School focused on diagnosis; and believed one disease was the likely cause of the patient's symptoms, without distinguishing between diseases. The Koan School, which was the Hippocratic School, applied a general diagnosis and provided passive treatments, with a focus on patient care and prognosis, rather than diagnosis. After 2,500 years, medicine still relies on diagnosis of symptoms instead of causes, and uses symptomatic treatments, surgical steel and lasers, to treat disease.

Modern medicine has forgotten or abandoned many principles of old, and the abandonment of principles of old is itself a clue to chronic disease. Diagnosing chronic disease has become the diagnosis of symptoms, findings and syndromes, by specialists who name diseases and syndromes based on one piece of the person, at a single point in time. Medical textbooks have been edited to delete important information, to make room for new details in cell microbiology, genes, inflammation, abnormal proteins, and newly named diseases. Some information that was removed concerned infectious causes of chronic disease, and the spread of intestinal pathogens outside the gastrointestinal tract, to cause systemic chronic disease.

A medical text, Harrison's Principles of Internal Medicine, discussed the "Extra Intestinal Manifestations of Inflammatory Bowel Disease", including arthritis, skin manifestation, ulcers, ulcerative colitis, Crohn's disease, liver disease, ocular manifestations, and more, in 1991.[316] Cecil Textbook of Medicine stated, "There are numerous examples of polyarthritis in association with microorganisms", in 1988.[317] Doctors today seem unaware of the connection between intestinal pathogens, intestinal flora, parasites, and chronic disease; and no longer recognize chronic gastrointestinal infections and systemic infections caused by gastrointestinal "microorganisms". The "gut-brain" connection is only now coming back into consideration, by the medical community.

It is time to return to thinking about the human body and chronic disease from a unified principle of the whole, and to diagnose the root causes of disease; and not just name and treat symptoms. It's time to return to the one cause theory of disease, as a starting point—it is all about chronic infection! Diagnosis should be a matter of determining *which* pathogen or

---

[316] Wilson JD, *et al.* (*ed.*) 1991. Harrison's Principles of Internal Medicine. 12th edition. New York: McGraw-Hill, Inc. Extraintestinal Manifestations of Inflammatory Bowel Disease. p. 1278-1282.

[317] Wyngaarden JB and Smith LH (*ed*). 1988. Cecil Textbook of Medicine. 18th Ed. Part XII. Musculoskeletal and Connective Tissue Diseases. Philadelphia: WB Saunders Company 18th Ed. Ch. XVI. Rheumatoid Arthritis. (Bennett JC). p. 1999.

pathogens are causing the chronic disease, as the starting point. Diligent efforts and the art of medicine will direct the assessment and plan to the most likely immortal pathogens causing the chronic disease, and further diagnostic blood testing can confirm the diagnosis. It is time to diagnose acute and chronic immortal infection, and practice preventive medicine, before a chronic disease develops.

Diagnosis of immortal pathogens and parasites are not often considered in the diagnosis of chronic diseases—because it was not taught in medical school and doctors are not allowed to reason and think beyond enforced conformity. Diagnosis of parasites is not considered, in patients with intestinal complaints, or complaints "associated" with parasites; and who own pets; or swim in public swimming pools, lakes or streams. The bias against diagnosis of infectious causes in chronic disease has continued for decades; as the infectious causes of chronic diseases have been sub-divided into newly named diseases and syndromes, based on the specialty, body part, and type of disease. Diagnosis has become the naming of symptoms, findings, and syndromes, according to the specialty bias, and prescribing symptomatic treatment.

Diagnosis of chronic infection with immortal pathogens begins with an interest in knowing! Doctors were not taught, nor are they expected to search for single or multiple immortal pathogens, as the explanation for chronic disease. Thinking about the problem as infectious requires thinking beyond what the doctors were taught. Doctors are not given the time or taught to think logically and deeply about issues that were never reported in their textbooks during medical school.[318] Doctors were taught to conform, and stay with what they were taught! Doing the same thing over and over, using the same drugs over and over, and treating symptoms indefinitely, has not worked and has not provided answers to the causes and cures for chronic disease. We must empower doctors, in every specialty, to be open-minded about infectious causes of chronic disease, and to diagnose infectious pathogens, in patients with chronic disease.

---

[318] Ewald. 2008. Interview with Evolutionary Biologists Paul Ewald. Bacteriality: Understanding Chronic Disease. Feb. 11, 2008. Doi: bacteriality.com.

Diagnosis begins with understanding how immortal pathogens and parasites attack the body. Chlamydia pneumonia has a predilection for the cardiovascular system, lung, and brain; attacks the endothelium and immune cells; and causes inflammation and plaque. Chlamydia trachoma has a predilection to attack the reproductive system, eyes, central nervous system, joints and respiratory system. Chlamydia trachoma and psittacosis attack endothelium or epithelium. Chlamydia psittacosis causes a severe and sometimes fatal respiratory disease, and invades the lung, lymphatic system, the central nervous system, the eye, and can attach to the rough-surface of a breast implant and cause lymphoma. Intracellular chlamydia pathogens cause reduced immunity, inflammation, inclusion cysts, and alteration of genes. H-pylori, psittacosis and trachoma can attack the nervous system, and nerve sheaths. Toxoplasmosis attacks the stomach, and can then attack the brain, and eyes. Atrophy of tissue occurs when pathogens penetrate the central layers of tissue, and cause prolonged high levels of inflammation; and by the ebb and flow of fluid in the tissue due to endothelial dysfunction. Fungus is generated by pathogens and parasites, when immortal pathogens cause the cells to consume sugar and cause fermentation.

A chest x-ray can aid in the diagnosis of immortal pathogens. Chlamydia pneumonia is the most common cause of sub-segmental infiltrate, mainly in the lower lobes; and months after the acute infection, residual effects may lead to a pleural effusion. Chlamydia trachoma can cause bilateral interstitial infiltrates with hyperinflation. Chlamydia psittaci most often consolidates in the lower lobes of the lung, causing patchy infiltrates, radiating from the hilum, and a diffuse ground glass appearance. A military pattern (rash) pleural effusion is evident in fifty-percent of the cases of chlamydia infection. Any patient with a cough should be given a chest x-ray, which may give clues to the diagnosis of immortal pathogens causing acute respiratory infections or pneumonia and to which pathogen is causing the infection.

Diagnosis requires an understanding that any pathogen in the gastrointestinal tract can migrate to locations outside the intestinal tract, and cause disease. Intestinal pathogens can attack any organ attached to the intestinal tract, or which can be reached by the vagus nerve. Chlamydia pathogens have been found in tissue throughout the body. H-pylori has now been "implicated" in atherosclerosis. Parasites and amoebas have been found in tissue throughout the body.

Devastating immortal infections can be acquired in the womb, when immortal pathogens cross the placenta to attack the fetus. The method by which pathogens attack the fetus is a clue to the cause of the problem, in the fetus, because the pathogen attacks adults in the same way pathogens attack a fetus.

Patients who have a chronic disease caused by infectious immortal pathogens can be a diagnostic challenge. The acute infection has long passed, and patients do not disclose animal contact unless asked. Immortal pathogens may cause different symptoms, findings, and diseases, in different people, at different stages of the chronic infection. The same pathogens or combinations of pathogens cause the same or different diseases in different people; and different pathogens and combinations of pathogens may cause the same or different diseases in different people. Patients in the same family may have the same immortal infections, and can have the same or different chronic diseases, caused by the same pathogens. Dr. Merchant saw a family in which one sister had multiple sclerosis, and the other sister had rheumatoid arthritis and hypertension. They had the same infectious pathogen, chlamydia pneumonia, causing different chronic diseases. Pets can have the same or different manifestations of the same pathogens, or manifest different symptoms at different points on the infectious cascade. Any significant health problem, in any family member or in pets, can be a clue to the pathogens, and a vector for pathogens that cause the same or different chronic diseases, in the patient.

Where the pathogens hide in the body depends on the nature of the infection, route of acquisition and persistence of the infection. The chlamydia pathogens hide inside host cells, immune cells, any spongy tissue or organ; and any organ to which the pathogens can directly migrate along the intestinal tract or along the vagus nerve. Chronic disease may be affected by the drugs previously used to treat the patient; co-morbid conditions; and the length of time multiple chronic infections persisted. Treating symptoms, and treating the infections with the wrong antibiotics may have caused the pathogen to change shape, to spread to new tissue, to spread deeper into tissue, and cause a false-negative chlamydia PCR test.

The art of diagnosis starts with a thorough history and physical examination, a reasoned assessment, diagnostic testing, and plans to investigate pathogens that could cause the chronic disease. The patient history should address as many risk factors for immortal infection and parasites as possible; and a timeline long enough to encompass acute disease occurring years prior to the patient encounter. A history should include the health of all members of the household and not just genetic relatives; contact with pets and domesticated animals; military service; contact with institutions that foster transmission of community acquired infections, including schools, daycare and jails; public swimming pools; work as a caretaker for a chronically ill person; risky sexual behavior; travel history; and a history of drinking potentially contaminated water. Outdoor activities and animal contact, may disclose an increased risk for parasitic infection. A detailed history can give clues to the type of immortal infection, the persistence of the infections, and the progression to chronic diseases. We must return to observing countenance, body shape, and body discharges; and examining the eye and iris, the tongue, and even considering the smell of the patient, as part of the physical examination.

The patient should provide a comprehensive written medical history, which includes the medical history of the patient, all family members, and pets; and identifies possible vectors for parasites. The history should include asking the patient the most common prior infections they experienced, which can be a clue to the origin of the chronic disease. Patients should provide a complete list of physical complaints, diagnoses made by other doctors, medications prescribed by other doctors, drug allergies, and supplements, at every doctor visit. Patients have difficulty recalling all of the important information, in the doctors' office, out of fear, feeling rushed, being intimidated by authority, lack of face time, and lack of knowledge as to what is relevant. Doctors should welcome a patient with a list, and abandon bias against patients who bring a list. The patient brings a list to recall important information, to efficiently present important information, and to find a solution to their medical problem—not because the patient has a psychiatric problem.

Doctors taking an oral history need to listen longer and attentively, and establish trust with the patient, which requires spending time with the patient and engaging in a dialogue. Studies show doctors give patients as little as three minutes of face time, before the doctor interrupts the patient and stifles disclosure and history taking. Quick interruption discourages the patient from further disclosure and intimidates the patient into bowing to the authority of the doctor and the need to hurry. Let the patient talk without interruption, and consider the likelihood many seemingly unrelated complaints and seemingly unrelated co-morbid conditions are caused by same pathogens or multiple pathogens. Dr. Merchant believed that, "If you listen long enough, the patient will tell you what is wrong."

Efforts at diagnosis cannot ignore the history regarding pets and domesticated animals. The United States has one of the highest rates of pet ownership, and has the highest total number of pets in the world. Animals are a vector for immortal infections and re-infections. The medical history should include a detailed and extensive history of pets, and the degree of close contact with pets. Physicians should ask if pets sit on the furniture, sleep in the bed, eat off plates, or kiss family members on the mouth or face. Patients who walk barefoot in an area where pets or other animals have defecated can acquire parasites, through bare feet. Cats are almost universally infected with toxoplasmosis, birds are almost universally infected with psittacosis, and cats may be infected with both toxoplasmosis and psittacosis. The history should include contact with domesticated animals, including horses, chickens, sheep, and goats; livestock; and hunting and butchering wild animals, all of which can be a vector for animal pathogens.

A history of engaging in foreign wars exposes military personnel and their family to new pathogens and parasites from around the world. The veterans acquire the pathogens and parasites during deployment; and bring the infectious pathogens back to the United States, to transmit the infections to their family members. In foreign lands, the military are exposed to unusual types of dangerous bacteria, viruses, parasites, streptococcus variants, etc., which may not be familiar to doctors, in the United States. In the Middle East, bird handling is common, as is psittacosis, trachoma, and toxoplasmosis; camels are domesticated animals and can transmit uncommon forms of chlamydia; and sand flies and mosquitoes carry chronic infectious diseases and parasites, which are uncommon in the United States. The Middle East has endemic shistomiasis, leishmaniosis and streptococcus-M; and streptococcus type-M is particularly prevalent in Turkey, Greece and Vietnam. The 1918-1920 Spanish Flu pandemic was attributed to soldiers returning from World War I. After the Vietnam War, returning soldiers spent decades trying to understand their own chronic diseases, and diseases that developed in family members, which were service connected.

Veterans are exposed to psittacosis from birds, pathogens and parasites in contaminated streams and rivers, and pathogens acquired from mosquitos and insects. Environmental hazards during deployment, like Agent Orange, may trigger infectious pathogens to become more dangerous; and pathogens and parasites acquired in Vietnam have caused an explosion in chronic disease among veterans. Gulf War Veterans were exposed to many chemical and biologic agents, and petrochemicals; and were also given multiple simultaneous immunizations, of questionable safety, which could trigger or aggravate immortal infections to become chronic disease. Veterans are exposed to contaminated drinking water containing carcinogens, in and around military bases, which can combine with immortal pathogens to trigger chronic disease.

It took forty-two years for the Veterans Administration to diagnose a liver fluke, in returning Vietnam War veterans—a parasite common in the rivers and streams of Vietnam. The liver fluke could have been diagnosed, and treated with a "azole" medication, to prevent chronic disease; however, was only discovered *after* the veterans began to develop liver cancer, forty years after returning from the Vietnam war. The Veteran's Administration is now recognizing Vietnam veterans have a seventeen times higher rate of eye cancer, forty years after the war ended, which is likely caused by psittacosis or other immortal pathogens acquired in the jungles of Vietnam. Psittacosis could have been diagnosed and treated, and the failure led to not only eye cancer but likely other types of cancer in Vietnam veterans.

Veterans in Albuquerque have a high rate of suicide, because their medical illnesses are not being diagnosed. The Veteran's Administration refers veterans to the mental health system, when the veteran has a medical illness that is causing mental illness. The veteran is referred to psychologists and psychiatrists; and prescribed Paxil, an SSRI, for depression, anxiety and other forms of mental distress. Parasitic infections acquired in deployment can deplete folic acid and B12, which makes the veterans more vulnerable to mental illness and PTSD.

Dr. Merchant saw parasitic disease in veterans after deployment to Vietnam, Iraq, Afghanistan, Africa, and South America. He diagnosed and treated veterans of foreign wars, for immortal pathogens and parasites, and saw their PTSD and depression improve. Veterans of every foreign war return with pathogens from the deployment that can cause chronic infections and chronic disease, in the long term, when left undiagnosed and untreated.

The consequence of sending our military to foreign countries is the troops acquire infectious pathogens in foreign countries, and bring the pathogens back home, to attack families and communities. The Veteran's Administration has a history of failing to diagnose the unusual and immortal pathogens and parasites, acquired by veterans while deployed. Military doctors did not diagnose infectious pathogens or parasites, in veterans returning from Vietnam and the Middle East; and infectious pathogens acquired in foreign deployments are now causing chronic disease, cancer, and mental instability among veterans. All veterans returning from any foreign deployment should be screened, diagnosed, and treated upon their return, to reduce the morbidity and mortality from infectious pathogens and parasites, among veterans and their families. The Veteran's Administration should have special programs intended to diagnose and treat chronic infections acquired during deployment in foreign lands, staffed by doctors with knowledge of unusual pathogens around the world.

Providers can begin the process of laboratory diagnosis of immortal pathogens and parasites, using available and cost-effect methods of diagnosis. A routine SMAC-20 blood test, with a folic acid and B12 level, ESR, and a differential, can give clues to chronic infection and parasitic disease. High leukocytes, a form of white blood cells, occur when endothelial function is reduced, again suggesting and supporting an infectious cause for endothelial dysfunction, atherosclerosis and stroke.[319] High leukocytes suggest chlamydia pneumonia, or other immortal chlamydia pathogens, capable of attacking endothelium. Peripheral eosinophilia and elevated serum immunoglobulin are also characteristic of chronic infection. A high level of neutrophils suggests H-pylori, psittacosis, or other pathogens attacked by neutrophils. High monocytes suggest parasitic disease, or an immune system attack against any pathogen attacked by macrophages. Low B12 and folic acid suggests the patient has dysbiosis, leaky gut, parasites, and/or chlamydia. (The laboratory normal ranges for folic acid and B12, and for monocytes, are too low.) Any patient with malabsorption of folic acid and B12; high monocytes; bloating, pain in the abdomen, and intermittent or constant diarrhea or constipation, should be evaluated for parasites.

A thorough history and physical examination should allow the doctor to be sixty-five percent sure of the diagnosis; and after a thorough physical examination, urinalysis, and blood work, including a CBC and differential, the doctor can be eighty-five percent sure of the diagnosis. Based on diagnostic clues, and initial routine blood tests, the doctor can move forward with more specific blood and stool tests to diagnose pathogens and parasites causing chronic disease, including PCR blood tests or PCR swabs, for chlamydia pathogens, H-pylori, and toxoplasmosis; stool tests and examination of blood for a clue to parasitic disease; and PCR swabs for intestinal parasites. A diagnosis of sexually transmitted chlamydia should include diagnosis of all pathogens capable of causing chronic disease.

---

[319] Elkind M, *et al.* 2005. Leukocyte Count is Associated with Reduced Endothelial Reactivity. Atherosclerosis. 2005. 181, 329-338. Doi: 10.1016/j.atherosclerosis.2005.01.013.

It is time to expand PCR blood testing and use of PCR swabs for diagnosis of pathogens. The diagnosis of immortal pathogens and parasites should be the standard in diagnosing and managing care in a patient with chronic disease. Failure to diagnose immortal infections leads to chronic infection and the evolution of chronic infection into a chronic disease, or worsening chronic disease. Immortal intracellular infections become more dangerous when treated with penicillin; therefore, the presence of immortal pathogens is important knowledge, before prescribing penicillin, to avoid triggering chronic disease or cancer. Diagnosing acute infection informs treatment, and treatment reduces proliferation of the pathogen and abnormal proteins, and reduces the overall infectious burden.

PCR blood testing and PCR swabs to diagnose immortal pathogens are grossly underutilized as a method to diagnose infectious pathogens. PCR blood testing is not done, due to the perceived high cost and the failure to understand the need. PCR swabs are now available, which can diagnose pathogens from a small amount of body fluid, from any orifice, which is particularly important in diagnosing the presence of immortal pathogens in aberrant locations in the body. Doctors must become familiar with the tests to diagnose an immortal pathogen, and study best practices for what to do when the patient has one or more chronic infectious pathogens and/ or parasites, and a chronic disease. If PCR blood testing and/or PCR swab testing was routine, the cost of PCR testing would most likely be lower. Routine PCR testing by blood testing or swab testing, would benefit doctors, patients and science, in identifying the causes of chronic disease.

The cost of PCR testing, to find the root cause of chronic disease, is better and more cost-effective than long-term symptomatic medications, and development of an expensive chronic disease. Treating symptoms, findings, and syndromes, while ignoring the cause of the chronic disease, is what is expensive for the medical system; and the patient has a loss in the quality of life as chronic infection becomes a chronic disease. Knowledge of the pathogens involved is important to plan effective treatment, and avoid harmful treatment. Medicine needs to find better in-office rapid methods for diagnosis of immortal pathogens; and practitioners should use the tools we already have to perform diagnostic testing, as a routine practice in diagnosing patients.

PCR blood tests can diagnose the most well-known forms of chlamydia, chlamydia pneumonia, trachoma and psittacosis; and H-pylori and toxoplasmosis. The three main species of chlamydia—chlamydia pneumonia, trachoma and psittacosis, are diagnosed based DNA markers of the pathogen in the blood. Newer forms of PCR testing, based on swabs of small amounts of fluid from any portals in the body, are expanding the types of chlamydia, for which the laboratory tests. Diagnostic swabs can diagnose some of the less well-known forms of chlamydia. Some laboratories stopped testing blood for H-pylori and require a stool test, which will not inform the doctor or the patient whether the H-pylori infection is in the eye, the brain, or has metastasized to organs adjacent to the gastrointestinal tract. PCR swab testing allows testing for H-pylori, from small samples of fluids from different locations in the body, and are becoming more widely available. Swab testing for H-pylori can overcome the difficulty of diagnosing H-pylori in anatomical locations outside the gastrointestinal tract, and diagnosing parasites from an inspection of stool. Diagnosis of toxoplasmosis requires a blood test, because PCR swabs are not yet available for toxoplasmosis. We need better blood, stool, and immunoassay tests to detect more forms of chlamydia, H-pylori, toxoplasmosis, and parasites.

Many types of chlamydia have not been studied by medical doctors, to know the preferred organ or the type of tissue attacked; but many forms of chlamydia are known and studied in animals, by veterinarians. Scientists know little about whether new chlamydia species infect people, at what rate, how the pathogens attack people, or how the pathogens cause chronic disease. The molecular biology of chlamydia species and the veterinary literature suggest any chlamydia species has the potential to infect humans, because the known chlamydia species can attack any cell with a nucleus. In chlamydia species already known to attack humans, the pathogens attack animals and humans in similar ways, attack the same or similar tissue, and cause the same chronic diseases. Any chlamydia pathogen in an animal has the potential to attack humans and cause similar diseases as the pathogens cause in animals.

The scope of PCR diagnostic testing for chlamydia species needs to be expanded; and at a minimum testing should be available for the commonly known types of chlamydia, and fifteen types of chlamydia known to infect pets and livestock. Expanded testing is particularly needed when the patient has exposure to domesticated and wild animals that carry and transmit more unusual forms of chlamydia to humans. For instance, veterinarians known chlamydia abortus causes abortions in sheep, goats and cows; therefore, if a patient has recurrent miscarriages or poor fetal outcomes, a history of contact with sheep and other animals capable of transmitting chlamydia abortus should be obtained, and blood testing should be available to the doctor and patient to test for chlamydia abortus. Testing should be expanded for chlamydia pecorum, chlamydia *suis* and chlamydia meridian, in patients who have contact with livestock. Testing for H-pylori by blood or swab should be available. Lack of readily available and reasonably priced diagnostic testing, for chlamydia pathogens; and the failure of laboratories to test for more chlamydia species, causes an underestimate of the rate of infections in humans, and lack of understanding as to the importance of new species of chlamydia pathogens, in chronic disease.

Any patient who owns or has contact with cats, and has symptoms of mental illness or other chronic disease, should be tested for toxoplasmosis and psittacosis. Cats worldwide have toxoplasmosis, and virtually all cats get toxoplasmosis in their lifetime, usually early in life. Cats transmit toxoplasmosis to their owners; and toxoplasmosis causes mental illness and fetal abnormalities, alone and in combination with viruses. Any claim asymptomatic toxoplasmosis is harmless, is contrary to what is known by science—toxoplasmosis is immortal and insidiously progressing, and causes both mental illness and chronic disease. Birds worldwide are infected with psittacosis and spread psittacosis in feces; and cats get psittacosis from birds and transmit psittacosis to the owners. Mental illness and chronic disease is caused by toxoplasmosis; and TMJ disease, lymphoma, and eye disease are caused by psittacosis, which suggests a higher rate of toxoplasmosis and psittacosis infection in the population than estimated. The rate of widespread chronic disease known to be caused by toxoplasmosis and/or psittacosis belies any claim the pathogens occur at a low rate in the human population or that the pathogens are harmless and self-limiting.

Medical science has been hampered in understanding chlamydia causes chronic disease, by the lack of adequate diagnostic tools for chlamydia infections, difficulty isolating and detecting chlamydia organisms, and confusion in the medical literature as to pathogens involved. Chlamydia is difficult to grow in a culture, outside the body; and some forms of chlamydia have mistakenly been referred to as a virus, in the literature. We need expansion of routine PCR testing for pathogens, by the front-line practitioner, available at a reasonable cost. Routine PCR testing and expansion of the detection of chlamydia species to more known species will disclose and confirm which chlamydia pathogens cause which chronic diseases.

New high-throughput sequencing technology may aid in detecting chronic infection in chronic disease, understanding the pathogens causing chronic diseases, and understanding the origin and source of the pathogens. High-throughput sequencing can identify hundreds of pathogens, in the blood, and is being used in research; but is not yet available to the primary care provider. Swabs are becoming available, but are not universally available to every primary care practice.

Understanding diagnostic testing for immortal chlamydia pathogens and parasites, requires understanding the means by which diagnostic testing is done; and understanding the function of different immune cells. Understanding how the immune cells function gives a clue to the diagnosis of immortal pathogens causing chronic disease. The T and B cells are types of white blood cells made in bone marrow. We make less T and B cells as we age; however, exercise and fitness have been shown to improve production of T and B cells, and slow aging. The T and B cells are modified in the thymus, gastrointestinal tract, and brain, by antigens to which the cells are attracted. Proteins made by plasma cells are intended to fight and clear infection. Antigens are foreign substances, which induce an immune response and production of antibodies. Antibodies to infection may be referred to as immunoglobulins. Immunoglobulins are Y-shaped proteins made by white blood cells, to fight pathogens; created by the immune system in a specific pattern, to attack and destroy specific pathogens that match the pattern of the antibodies. Different pathogens are attacked by different types of immune cells; thus, the level of each type of immune cell in the blood is a clue to the type of pathogens causing a systemic immune response to an acute or chronic disease.

TNF-alpha is generated by the immune cells, most often macrophages; but can be created by any immune cell. High monocytes in the blood suggest macrophages are fighting immortal infection. TNF-alpha is a more aggressive inflammatory response against an intracellular pathogen, when the immune system cannot eradicate the pathogen inside the cells. Macrophages are one of the first types of immune cells to attack chlamydia, and macrophages are the primary generator of TNF-alpha. TNF-alpha is the molecular signature of chronic infection and virtually all chronic diseases. Yet, doctors rarely order PCR blood testing for immortal pathogens or blood testing for TNF-alpha, and routine blood tests do not include TNF-alpha.

PCR blood testing for chlamydia reports immunoglobulins, against three major species of chlamydia. Immunoglobulins are reported as IgA, IgG, and IgM. The A, G and M refer to the type of protein identified by the laboratory, and measure the level of chronic infection. IgM is found mainly in blood and lymph fluid, is the first antibody sent to fight a new infection, and is considered a sign of early infection. IgG is in all bodily fluids and is intended to protect against bacterial and viral infections. IgA is found in mucous membranes, including respiratory passages, the gastrointestinal tract, saliva and tears; and is considered a sign of past infection.

Some doctors assert the IgA measures past infection, IgM represents current infection, and ignore the IgG. Doctors may dismiss elevated IgA and IgG, asserting the abnormal numbers represent "past infection", which do not require treatment. The significance of IgA and IgG, and the significance of "past" infection versus chronic infection, are the central questions in chronic disease. The dismissal of IgA and IgG markers of past infection is contrary to scientific reporting in <u>CHLAMYDIA Intracellular Biology,</u> <u>Pathogenesis and Immunity</u>, proving chlamydia infection persists and spreads as a chronic infection. Abnormal PCR test results for IgA showing "past infection" indicate chronic infection that continues to spread in the body, and continues to proliferate and cause more damage to cell function and immune function, as it evolves from chronic infection into a chronic disease. Positive test results for IgA and IgG demonstrate chronic infection, and the patient is on the path to development of chronic disease. Immortal infections do not go away, and evidence of past infection *is* evidence of chronic infection.

Positive test results for acute infection are an IgM titer ≥ 1:16. Any elevated IgA titer ≥ 1:250 indicates long-standing infection. The criteria for acute and chronic infection with chlamydia pneumonia, trachoma, and psittaci, is a four-fold increase in IgG titer (≥ 1:64), or a single IgG titer of 1:512 or greater. An IgG titer greater than 1:16 and less than 1:512 demonstrates prior infection. Antibody testing for IgM, IgG, and IgA may be inconclusive, because of prior penicillin use; and patients treated with penicillin or chemotherapy may lose a detectable IgM and IgG antibody response, even though chronic infection persists. Antibodies may take several weeks to appear (two to three weeks for IgM, and six to eight weeks for IgG). In re-infections, IgM may be absent or low, and IgG can appear within two weeks.[320] Elderly patients may have persistently elevated IgG titers due to repeated infection.[321] The chlamydia organism can be detected serologically, even after antibiotic treatment and signs and symptoms have resolved.

The PCR and MIF (microimmunofluorescence serological assay) blood tests are the most sensitive method available to detect chlamydia. The PCR blood test is seventy-one percent sensitive for detecting chlamydia pneumonia; and the MIF is ninety-seven percent sensitive, in detecting chlamydia. A study of one hundred thirty-seven patients suggested PCR

---

[320] Grayston, J, *et al.* 1990. A New Respiratory Tract Pathogen: Chlamydia Pneumoniae Strain TWAR. Journal Infectious Diseases. 1990. 161:618-625. Doi: https://doi.org/10.1093/infdis/161.4.618.

[321] Oba Y, *et al.* 2015. Chlamydial Pneumonias. Medscape. Aug 27, 2015. Doi: https://emedicine.medscape.com/article/297351-overview.

testing holds greater utility as a diagnostic tool.[322] The PCR blood tests do not always accurately identify intracellular pathogens or the presence of the pathogens, and can mis-identify chlamydia pathogens which are similar, due to cross-reactivity and similarity of the species. The PCR test may have a low sensitivity in distinguishing between trachoma and psittacosis, and between known species and animal species for which the laboratory does not test. Dr. Shor's study of tissue in the heart, in 1992; and the heart studies reported in *Chlamydia Pneumoniae* Infection and Disease, prove patients can have negative PCR tests and still have chlamydia pneumonia, in cardiac tissue. Blount and his colleagues reported positive tests for pathogens in tissue, in more than one hundred different diseases. Therefore, the PCR blood test can confirm chlamydia pathogens, but cannot exclude a chronic chlamydia infection.

Dr. Merchant performed many PCR blood tests to diagnose immortal infections, over many years, which allowed him to see the patterns and correlations, between chronic infections with immortal pathogens and chronic disease. Dr. Merchant used a PCR test to determine the species of chlamydia and direct treatment. Dr. Merchant did many PCR tests on husbands and wives, and on other family members involved in the care of ill patients, and saw similar patterns of immortal pathogens and chronic disease in family members. If the patient had chlamydia pneumonia specific IgA antibodies or high titer for IgG antibodies greater than 1:512, the patient was also given an oxygen study, with a simple overnight pulse oximetry. The oxygen studies were also often positive.

Parasitic disease can be a diagnostic challenge, and parasitic disease outside the gastrointestinal tract can be an even greater diagnostic challenge. Diagnosing parasites by a stool examination for ova and parasites is like looking for a needle in a haystack; and is highly dependent on the skill and diligence of the examiner. Parasites may be dormant and not shed at the time of the stool test; or be causing disease in organs along the

---

[322] Benitez A, *et al.* 2012. Comparison of Real-Time PCR and a Microimmunofluorescence Serological Assay for Detection of Chlamydiophilla Pneumonia Infection in an Outbreak. J Clin Microb. Jan 2012. 50(1): 151-153. Doi: 10.1128/JCM.05357-11.

gastrointestinal tract. Parasites in the intestinal tract can migrate to organs adjacent to the intestinal tract or to the brain and eyes, hiding from detection in a stool examination. A diagnosis of toxoplasmosis can only be made with a PCR blood test.

Doctors need an in-depth history, to aid in the diagnosis of parasitic disease. The diagnosis often has to be made based on history, symptoms, physical examination, and routine blood tests. A history of vectors for parasitic disease, including drinking contaminated water, pets, livestock, foreign travel, and military deployment, are clues to a diagnosis of parasitic disease. New swab technology may improve the diagnosis of gastrointestinal parasites, and parasites in aberrant anatomical locations. Chronic parasitic diseases are more widespread than doctors and patients wish to believe, are more widespread in the body than doctors acknowledge, and cause significant morbidity.

PCR swab technology is becoming more widely available, and can make the diagnosis of infectious pathogens more readily available, at a lower cost. Medical Diagnostic Laboratories PCR swabs are becoming available in the United States, and are already used in countries around the world. Medical Diagnostic Laboratories offers swabs for PCR testing, *One***Swab**®, *Uro***Swab**® and *Naso***Swab**®, which can diagnose immortal pathogens and parasites in the eyes, nose, mouth, reproductive tracts, and gastrointestinal tract. The PCR swabs can diagnose chlamydia pathogens, including forms not routinely tested in blood; giardia and other forms of parasites; and H-pylori. The tests can be bundled for the doctor and patient, and can be done at a lower cost than PCR blood testing. Other companies offer swab technology for limited purposes. Cologuard is available to examine stool and report specifically on findings suggesting colon cancer; and Medical Diagnostic Laboratories also offers swab PCR testing for the gastrointestinal tract. Cologuard and swabs by Medical Diagnostic Laboratory are more efficient, and should be used for diagnosis of gastrointestinal pathogens and parasites, *before* scoping a patient. The swab could identify pathogens that cannot be found with a scope or which are flushed out before the scope.

The use of super-computers and metadata could allow rapid identification of the immortal pathogens causing chronic diseases; allow science to discover the causes of chronic disease; and give patients new hope in preventing, fighting, and delaying chronic disease. We have sophisticated super-computers capable of using high-throughput sequencing to diagnose hundreds of different pathogens in a blood sample; which are not available to the front-line practitioner. Super-computers could rapidly identify the pathogens which are common in different chronic diseases. We need advanced diagnostic technology for infectious pathogens and parasites, and to make advanced diagnostic technology and rapid diagnostic testing available to all doctors.

Chronic disease develops from the ongoing war between the immune system and immortal animal pathogens. Chronic infection with immortal intracellular pathogens damage cell function, destroy normal apoptosis, cause abnormal proteins, generate inflammation, cause reduced immunity, alter the microbiome and mycobiome, cause fungus, alter genes, and generate the inflammatory and molecular signature of virtually all chronic diseases. All chronic diseases can be thought of as an autoimmune disease, because in chronic disease the immune system is responding to and interacting with intracellular pathogens and parasites.

The confusion in diagnosis and the infinite naming of symptoms, findings and syndromes, can only be reduced and simplified by the routine diagnosis of immortal pathogens and parasites; and the understanding that more than one pathogen, and more than one combination of pathogens can cause chronic disease, and the effect may be different from person-to-person. Diagnostic efforts in chronic disease should begin with identification of the immortal pathogens, before naming a disease, without a known cause. Routine diagnosis of immortal pathogens would allow scientists to examine meta-data; and identify the patterns of infectious pathogens causing chronic disease, and which infectious pathogens cause which chronic disease. Routine diagnosis of immortal pathogens would rapidly add to the understanding of the causes of chronic disease. Diagnosis of the immortal pathogens, which are the root cause of chronic disease, is central to understanding and conquering chronic disease. Diagnosis of immortal pathogens and parasites can provide hope for prevention and a cure of chronic diseases.

Doctors will not be able to find the cause of chronic diseases until doctors routinely diagnose immortal pathogens and parasites causing chronic diseases; and compare data showing which pathogens are found in which chronic diseases. PCR blood testing, PCR swab testing, and computer analysis of blood, should be the standard for diagnosis of immortal pathogens, in *all* chronic diseases, in *all* specialties. It is time for the diagnosis in chronic disease to include diagnosis of the root infectious causes of the chronic disease, to find the best treatment, and to seek a cure.

Medicine is the science of uncertainty and the art of probability.

William Osler, M.D.

CHAPTER 24

TREATMENT AND ANTIBIOTIC RESISTANCE

Treatment

Doctors who diagnose infectious pathogens face the question of whether to treat or not to treat acute and chronic infections, why to treat the infections, and how to treat the infections. Should drugs be given to help the immune system fight the intracellular pathogens, and reduce inflammation, abnormal proteins, and the infectious burden; or should medicine stay out of the war between the immune system and the pathogens, and let the body do what it can to fight the pathogens? Treatment of immortal pathogens, which have become chronic infection, presents profound questions. The answer is dependent on the unique circumstances and wishes of the patient. Each patient must be evaluated and treated, based on the pathogens diagnosed, the unique needs of the patient, the patients' wishes, and the response to treatment.

The hope in treatment of immortal pathogens is that treatment will cause the immortal pathogen to become dormant, reduce inflammation, reduce the quantity of abnormal proteins, reduce the infectious burden, improve the chronic disease, and lead to new discoveries in the diagnosis and treatment of chronic disease. Diagnosing and treating immortal infections has the potential to improve outcomes, and reduce the cost of medical care associated with chronic disease. Treatment of immortal pathogens can improve the chronic disease and the co-morbid conditions. A study in Africa showed giving children just two pills of azithromycin a year, given as one pill every six months, caused a substantial reduction in childhood mortality.[323]

---

[323] McNeil D. 2018. Infant Deaths Fall Sharply in Africa With Routine Antibiotics. New York Times. (Global Health). Apr 25, 2018. Doi: https://www.nytimes.com/2018/04/25/health/africa-infant-mortality-antibiotic.html.

Doctors must first understand what disease they are treating, and analyze whether treatment addresses the root cause of the disease or is given for symptomatic relief. Doctors should consider whether existing named diseases are actually only symptoms, findings and syndromes, which do not reveal the root cause of the disease. Doctors should know the effect of the medication they prescribe on intracellular pathogens, consider whether the medication impairs immune function or potentiates immortal infection, and observe whether the medication is effective against the disease. Treating chronic diseases, without understanding the relationship of chronic infection to chronic disease, risks medical mistakes and sub-optimal outcomes. Understanding the root cause of chronic disease can lead to better alternatives for treatment, and prevention of new chronic disease or worsening of a chronic disease.

Chlamydia bacteria grows inside cells, multiplies, and goes dormant, which renders the bacteria almost impossible to eradicate, with current scientific knowledge and medications. Chlamydia can hide in parasites, protected from the immune system; or host other pathogens on the inside and outside of chlamydia, which can be released by treatment. The chlamydia hides in macrophages, where it is difficult to treat, and from which it can re-emerge. Treatment can cause the organism to become dormant or hide in biofilm, and the organism may re-bloom and re-emerge after treatment. Penicillin and cephalosporin antibiotics do not treat chlamydia, and detrimentally change the form of the chlamydia. Cryptic chlamydia, in a cell culture of infected cells, suggests the infected cells can be treated with potent antibiotics, which one would expect to eradicate chlamydia; but in time, the cell culture blooms with new chlamydia and new chlamydia infected cells. Chlamydia can become dormant and asymptomatic for years, before erupting into acute or chronic disease.

The patient with acute chlamydia pneumonia (or mycoplasma) requires aggressive treatment, and avoidance of all forms of penicillin. Early and effective treatment of immortal bacteria may prevent chronic diseases from developing, shortly after the acute infection or decades later. Acute chlamydia pneumonia, in patients with pre-existing chronic disease, can trigger adverse events, including severe pneumonia, progression or eruption of chronic disease, heart attacks and stroke in cardiac patients, and kidney failure in patients with kidney disease. Treatment can prevent triggering adverse events and the progression of chronic disease.

Treatment of chlamydia pneumonia in cardiovascular disease could prevent the development of Alzheimer's, macular degeneration, rheumatoid arthritis, multiple sclerosis, cancer, and other chronic diseases caused by chlamydia pneumonia. Treating sexually acquired infections could prevent infertility, ectopic pregnancies, fetal abnormalities, uterine and ovarian cancer; and rheumatoid arthritis, multiple sclerosis, cancer, and other chronic diseases caused by chlamydia trachoma. Treating psittacosis could prevent chronic systemic diseases, and in particular lymphomas, eye cancer, and rare cancers. Treating H-pylori could treat Parkinson's disease, brain tumors, central nervous system disorders, ocular surface diseases, glaucoma and retinal disease. Diagnosing and treating parasites can prevent chronic malabsorption from becoming a triggering event for chronic disease; and prevent dysbiosis and metastasis of parasites, fungus, and pathogens to other vital organs.

Drugs we already have are effective in treating most immortal pathogens and parasites. Strains of chlamydia and other infectious pathogens likely exist that have not been identified, which may also be susceptible to treatment with drugs we already have. We need to repurpose the drugs we have, to treat chronic infections and chronic disease. The appropriate treatment depends on the findings in the individual patient, the type of chlamydia infection and type of parasites diagnosed, how long the patient has been infected, and how the patient responds to treatment. The principle remains—chronic infection causes chronic disease, regardless of the type of pathogen or the treatment required.

Appropriate antibiotics to treat chronic chlamydia infection interfere with replication of chlamydia, and neutralize the inflammatory cascade and heat shock proteins, improve immune-function, and reduce the infectious burden. Treatment is intended to cause the pathogen to reach a neutral or dormant state, and reduce the infectious burden of the pathogen and byproducts. Treatment must be with antibiotics capable of penetrating the cell wall, and killing the pathogen, hiding inside endothelial cells, inclusion cysts, organs, glands and spongy tissue. Treatment must be able to interrupt the ability of the pathogen to change the cells normal regulatory mechanism, and reduce inflammation. All forms of immortal bacteria and parasites, and abnormal proteins generated by the pathogens and parasites, can become a focus for immune system attack. The hope is to stabilize or slow the progress of acute infection to chronic infection, and slow the process of chronic infection to chronic disease.

Macrolides are intracellular antibiotics that penetrate the cell wall, inhibit bacterial growth, cause cessation of RNA dependent protein synthesis; and reduce inflammation, by attacking the intracellular pathogen. Doxycycline is bacteriostatic and works against the pathogen by inhibiting protein synthesis. Macrolides, including azithromycin, doxycycline, and minocycline are effective against many strains of chlamydia, and effective in controlling the chronic infection; and are the drugs of choice for chlamydia pneumonia. Metronidazole and tininizole treat some forms of chlamydia infections, such as trachoma and psittacosis; and are potent at low concentrations, have the ability to cross the blood brain barrier, and can treat multiple types of chlamydia and parasitic infections at the same time. Metronidazole is an underused, powerful antibiotic, able to penetrate the cell wall, penetrate the wall of an abscess, and enhance the penetration of other medications into the tissue and cells. Pyrimethamine (Daraprim) treats H-pylori, toxoplasmosis, and malaria. Imervectin treats skin parasites, and may treat other types of parasites on the skin or in the intestine, and treats the worm causing river blindness. Imervectin can be obtained through compounding pharmacies.

A Mayo Clinic did a review of studies involving treatment with macrolides, and reported macrolides reversed and improved endothelial dysfunction in coronary artery diseases, in laboratory models and humans. Studies in patients treated for both acute and chronic chlamydia with azithromycin, clarithromycin, tetracycline, or quinolones, for as short as one week, showed a significant reduction in cardiovascular events, stroke, and death. The macrolides caused a decrease in cytokines from macrophages and monocytes; a decrease in IL-1, IL-6 and IL-8; and a decrease in TNF-alpha.[324]

Treatment can reverse endothelial dysfunction, improve lung function, and cause plaque to recede. Treatment can stabilize and improve heart disease, brain disease, cognitive function in Alzheimer's, mental illness, autoimmune diseases, arthritis, multiple sclerosis, chronic fatigue, lupus, and eye diseases. Treatment of chronic infections can extend cancer survival time. Treatment of infectious causes of chronic disease can reverse the downward course of chronic disease, mitigate the chronic disease, and improve the prognosis.

Amoxicillin is the most widely prescribed penicillin antibiotic in the United States. Doctors were taught amoxicillin is the standard-of-care, first-line treatment for acute infection. Penicillin and amoxicillin destroy the cell wall, change the shape of chlamydia reticulate bodies, extend the life cycle of chlamydia, and increase the number of elementary bodies produced. Penicillin and amoxicillin cause release of a greater number of infectious elementary bodies into the blood and lymphatics, spreading the infection to new host tissue.

Penicillin and broad-spectrum antibiotics kill some of the pathogens and selectively leave behind drug-resistant pathogens. Penicillin and amoxicillin cause development of drug-resistant pathogens, including staphylococcus, streptococcus, and e-coli; and cause antibiotic associated colitis and c-difficile. Avoiding the use of penicillin or amoxicillin in the presence of immortal infection will itself advance patient health, reduce morbidity from chronic disease, and reduce the risk of a doctor causing greater harm. Doctors and patients should monitor and keep track of past

---

[324] Higgens J. 2003. Chlamydia Pneumonia and Coronary Artery Disease: The Antibiotic Trials. Mayo Clin Proc. 2003. 78: 321-332. Doi: https://doi.org/10.4065/78.3.321; Parchure N, *et al.* 2002. Effect of Azithromycin Treatment on Endothelial Function in Patients With Coronary Artery Disease and Evidence of Chlamydia Pneumoniae Infection. Circulation. 2002. 105:1298-1303. PMID 119010.39; *See* <u>*Chlamydia Pneumonia* Infection and Disease</u>. New York: Kluwer Academic/Plenum Publishers. The Biology of Chlamydia Pneumonia in Cardiovascular Disease Pathogenesis. (Ouelette SP, *et al.*). Ch. 10

antibiotic usage, for what infections, and why, particularly penicillin, cephalosporins, and antibiotics administered in the hospital, because the history of antibiotics is important to understanding the chronic disease.

Giving penicillin to a child or adult with a chlamydia infection can cause conversion of the organism to a state in which it can thrive in the endothelial cells of the lung, and cause asthma. Penicillin or amoxicillin given to a patient with chlamydia (or mycoplasma), can convert chlamydia infection into chronic disease, including asthma, multiple sclerosis, rheumatoid arthritis, chronic fatigue, and cancer. Chronic fatigue and fibromyalgia patients have typically been treated with courses of penicillin and cephalosporin, prior to the development of their chronic fatigue or fibromyalgia. *Chlamydia Pneumonia* Infection and Disease, describes numerous studies of chlamydia pneumonia in heart disease, which support the danger of penicillin in patients with chlamydia pneumonia—patients who were given penicillin developed chronic fatigue or died.[325]

Dr. Stratton, Dr. Chaney, Dr. Petterson and Dr. Bell found ninety-seven percent of chronic fatigue patients, and virtually one hundred percent of multiple sclerosis patients had chlamydia pneumonia; and studied antibiotic treatment in patients with chronic fatigue and multiple sclerosis. His group used suppression of the PCR test as the endpoint. The PCR test could not be suppressed with one antibiotic, or sometimes even with two antibiotics. Dr. Stratton's treatment protocol for chlamydia was a combination of three or four antibiotics for a year, using three different classes of antibiotics, including a macrolide and rifimycin, with metronidazole or tinidazole. Dr. Stratton, *et al.* quickly learned many patients were unable to follow or complete the treatment protocol. For most conventionally trained medical doctors, treatment with three or four antibiotics at the same time was impossible to accept.

Dr. Merchant does not believe it is necessary to completely eradicate the pathogen, when monotherapy, persistence, patience and careful medical

---

[325] Friedman H *(ed)*, *et al.* 2004. *Chlamydia Pneumoniae* Infection and Disease. New York: Kluwer Academic/Plenum Publishers. Chlamydia Pneumonia and Atherosclerosis—An Overview of the Association. (Ngeh J and Sandeep G). Ch. 9.

practice will resolve many of the patient's health problems. It is not necessary to use combination antibiotics to attack all phases of the chlamydia pneumonia life cycle. An endpoint for treatment should be determined by the patient response. Patients treated with a single agent like azithromycin, clarithromycin, or doxycycline appear to tolerate the antibiotics for years; and a single agent given over time can lead to continued benefits over time. Periodically the antibiotic may be discontinued, to observe the patient over the next thirty to sixty days, to see if target symptoms such as fatigue, arthritis, or asthma, reappear. In multiple sclerosis patients, being treated for immortal pathogens, Dr. Merchant did an MRI on an annual basis to identify any new lesions; and if the patient had no new lesions or the patient had no new clinical symptoms, antibiotic treatment was discontinued. Treatment can improve conditions thought impossible to treat, such as dilated acute cardiomegaly. Dr. Merchant's patients, who were treated for two years, did not develop resistance or induction of resistance in chlamydia pneumonia organisms. The objective is for the pathogen to remain dormant and the patient's condition to improve; using a history and physical, lab tests, and radiographic data, to monitor the success of treatment.

Chronic disease caused by multiple co-infections may require more than one antibiotic or serial antibiotics, based on the pathogens. Control of the infection with multiple classes of antibiotics, given serially, can improve chronic disease; and treat erupting infections, which had been hidden inside chlamydia pathogens. An antibiotic regimen involving multiple antibiotics, and serial treatment with different classes of antibiotics, can improve chronic disease caused by more than one pathogen. Antibiotic regimens added to traditional chemotherapy can extend the life of cancer patients. An antibiotic chemotherapy regimen, including antibiotics and antiparasitics, combined with a TLR inhibitor, together or serially, may be effective in improving the prognosis of cancer. Oncologists do not have an objection to treating patients with multiple toxic chemotherapeutic drugs for cancer, at the same time; yet, are averse to any suggestion of multiple antibiotics and/or antiparasitics, as an adjunct to cancer treatment and chemotherapy.

Good bacteria in the intestine may become pathogenic, if spread to aberrant locations in the body, or combined with other pathogens. A bacterium in the stomach may be part of a community of good bacteria, but the same bacteria may become pathogenic in the lower intestine, the urine, the brain, or the eye. Scientists have argued whether H-pylori and peptostreptococcus in the gastrointestinal tract are good or bad, or only become bad in aberrant locations. Harmless bacteria on the skin can become pathogenic in an anaerobic environment. P-acnes is an anaerobic bacteria common on skin, which is allegedly harmless when exposed to air; but can invade hair follicles at the eyelash margins, which are anaerobic environments, and cause long-term inflammation and even chronic low-grade endophthalmitis. P-acnes is prevalent on the skin in the axilla area, and has been reported to cause post-operative wound infections after shoulder and breast implant surgery. Whether treatment causes harmless bacteria to spread or combine with other bacteria is not known.

Science knows the more diverse our microbiome, the more likely a person enjoys good health. Microbes in the world outweigh all visible plants and animals on earth, by a factor of one-hundred million. Jack Gilbert, Director of the Chicago Microbiome Center, and Rob Knight director of the University of California Center for Microbiome Innovation, said we are outnumbered by microbes—we have about thirty trillion human cells, and forty trillion microbial cells. Only 43% of our body is human cells, and the bulk of non-human cells live in the oxygen deprived gastrointestinal tract. The microbes in our microbiome weigh as much as our brain.[326] Yet, medicine understands less than one percent of the good bacteria in our microbiome.

Probiotics and prebiotics should be an adjunct treatment, with any antibiotics. Antibiotics kill good bacteria in the microbiome, needed to make our body function and keep our intestinal tract in balance. Probiotics and prebiotics can restore intestinal balance; however, science has not yet identified all of the good bacteria in the intestine, and some good bacteria have not yet been replicated in supplement form. Research is needed to develop expanded probiotic supplements to replace good bacteria lost by antibiotic treatment. Treatment of the chlamydia, based on the type of

---

[326] Gallagher J, *presenter*. 2018. More Than Half Your Body Is Not Human: The Second Genome. BBC Radio 4. Apr 10, 2018.

chlamydia diagnosed by PCR testing; treatment of parasites; treatment of yeast with medications and/or bismuth; restoration of gastrointestinal health with B12, folic acid, and vitamin supplements, to overcome years of malabsorption; and supplements of prebiotics and probiotics, can significantly benefit the patient with chronic disease.

Abnormal proteins generated by immortal pathogens are not alive, and cannot be killed. Abnormal proteins can cause tissue to stick together, can become an inclusion cyst, and can be the focus for immune system attack. Abnormal proteins can adhere to and alter genes and gene expression. Understanding the immortal pathogens are generating abnormal proteins may lead to alternatives for treatment and ways to eliminate abnormal proteins in the body, after acute and chronic infection.[327] Abnormal proteins become a focus for immune system attack, impair passive function, become the center of an inclusion cyst, and cause chronic disease; thus, finding ways to remove abnormal proteins could be a significant advancement in treating and curing chronic disease.

Patients with chronic chlamydia and impaired immune systems, from intracellular infection in the immune cells, often have co-infections with parasites. Metronidazole, albendazole, and mebendazole (Vermox) are effective against many parasites and some immortal pathogens in the gastrointestinal tract. Mebendazole treats parasites; and metronidazole is effective against some forms of chlamydia, such as trachoma and psittacosis. Mebendazole and albendazole should be some of the most commonly prescribed drugs, by every gastroenterologist and primary care provider, because parasites are a common cause of gastrointestinal disease. Daraprim can treat some types of parasites, including toxoplasmosis, in combination with another antibiotic. Treating parasitic infection is far safer than leaving the patient with untreated parasitic infections, which can be a host to other dangerous bacteria and viral pathogens, cause dysbiosis, and migrate to other organs and systems.

---

[327] *See* Ricci J, *et al.* 2016. Novel ABCG2 Antagonists Reverse Topotecan-Mediated Chemotherapeutic Resistance in Ovarian Carcinoma Xenografts. Doi: 10.1158/1535-7163.MCT-15-0789. (drug clears abnormal proteins and improves effectiveness of second round of ovarian cancer chemotherapy).

TNF-inhibitors are big pharma's expensive solution to treating inflammation. TNF-inhibitors are used to treat inflammation, based on the belief inflammation is an independent diseases of unknown origin. Inflammation is the immune system response to an infection! TNF-inhibitors are treating the symptom of inflammation, not the root cause of the inflammation. TNF-inhibitors potentiate the immortal infections, by interfering with the immune system's attack on the pathogen with TNF-alpha. The intracellular infection is causing the inflammation and the immune system is generating the TNF-alpha, to mount a more aggressive fight against an intracellular pathogen. Many specialties are beginning to recognize patients with chronic diseases have high levels of TNF-alpha; yet, are ignoring the fact TNF-alpha is generated by the immune cells attempting to fight an immortal pathogen.

Side effects and complications of TNF-inhibitors include lymphoma, tuberculosis, infection, heart disease, and demyelinating disease, suggesting these chronic diseases are all caused by infectious pathogens; and TNF-inhibitors triggers the evolution of the pathogens into chronic disease. Thalidomide acted against TNF-alpha, in the same way as a TNF-inhibitor; and was shown to not work well in cancer, and caused birth defects. Patients in rheumatology and gastroenterology; and patients with Crohn's disease, ulcerative colitis, arthritis, psoriatic arthritis, and many other chronic diseases caused by immortal pathogens and parasites, are being treated with TNF-inhibitors. Patients with chronic diseases caused by immortal pathogens could be more effectively and more safely treated with appropriate antibiotics, antiparasitics, plasmapheresis to filter the abnormal proteins out of the blood, and drugs to remove abnormal proteins, to reduce the burden of infectious pathogens and byproducts.

Steroids are prescribed to treat symptoms of inflammation, and are dangerous in a patient with chronic immortal infections. Medical thinking is inhaled steroids, steroid drops, and oral steroids are necessary to prevent inflammation, and scarring. In cell cultures, prednisone amplifies the number of chlamydia infected cells and particles, which worsens and spreads the infection. The adverse effect of steroids is greatest in lung disease, often the location of the primary immortal infection. Steroids may temporarily improve symptoms, but potentiate and spread chlamydia pneumonia, reduce immunity in an already compromised immune system, and decrease the sensitivity of PCR testing in detecting the organism.[328] Over time, patients given steroids continue to remodel tissue and have inflammation and scarring. Clarithromycin is an effective treatment for chlamydia pneumonia in the lung; and reduces the need for oral steroids, over a period of nine months.

The treatment of depression with SSRI drugs should be tightly regulated, with multiple layers of protection for the patient, family, and community. SSRI drugs worsen all pre-existing symptoms. SSRI drugs cause increased agitation, confusion, anxiety, fear and paranoia. SSRI drugs induce suicide, violence, and homicide; and have had a devastating effect on society by causing wide-spread violence against self, family, and others. A patient quickly becomes addicted to SSRI drugs, and is at risk of committing violence during withdrawal. Withdrawal can take many months, and be difficult. SSRI drugs are addicting, dangerous for the patient and others, and do not work! Anyone prescribing SSRI drugs should be required to undergo specialized training, obtain specialized licensing, be required to warn the patient and those around the patient, and be required to monitor and limit the patient's access to guns.

H-pylori has been "associated" with a growing list of chronic diseases; and has been proven to cause ulcers and stomach cancer. Diseases recognized to be caused by H-pylori or "associated" with H-pylori, may be the tip of the iceberg of chronic diseases and cancers caused by H-pylori or a co-infection with H-pylori. When H-pylori attacks the intestinal tract, the damage to the epithelium allows fungus to invade the lining of the intestine and cause leaky gut. H-pylori can migrate to the eye, directly by self-inoculation, migrating along the vagus nerve, and by reflux into the sinus and the eye. H-pylori can cause corneal surface disease, glaucoma and retinal disease. H-pylori can invade the brain, through the blood and lymphatics, along the vagus nerve, and by reflex into the sinus and then the brain. H-pylori in the brain is one cause of Parkinson's disease. Treatment of H-pylori may help mitigate the symptoms and improve the prognosis, in chronic

[328] Stephens R (*ed*). 1999. CHLAMYDA Intracellular Biology, Pathogenesis and Immunity. Washington, D.C.: ASM Press.

diseases caused by H-pylori. Low-dose doxycycline has been shown helpful in chronic diseases caused by H-pylori.

Any patient with a newly diagnosed chronic disease should be diagnosed and treated for any underlying chronic infections. Many chronic diseases can be treated, stabilized, or improved, by treating the underlying root infectious cause of chronic disease. If the patient is too young to have the chronic disease, such as early onset diabetes, heart disease, eye disease, or rheumatoid arthritis, all the more reason to suspect, diagnose, and treat immortal pathogens aggressively, to reduce the overall infectious burden and morbidity. Early diagnosis and treatment of infectious causes of chronic disease can delay development of chronic diseases, avoid the development of co-morbid diseases, and improve co-morbid conditions. We already have drugs to treat the immortal pathogens and parasites that cause chronic disease, if medicine can accept and understand chronic infections cause chronic disease, and treatment benefits the patients.

Chlamydia pathogens are intracellular parasitic bacteria; and parasitic bacteria and intestinal parasites require the host remain alive, to supply the pathogen with energy and assure survival of the pathogen. Immortal pathogens and parasites live off the host, compete for nutrition, and damage the cell and organ functions of the host. If we can learn to prevent infection with immortal pathogens and parasites, treat pathogens and parasites appropriately, and manage acute and chronic immortal infections, it will benefit patients, reduce morbidity, and extend life.

Antibiotic Resistance

Antibiotic resistant pathogens have existed for thousands of years, long before antibiotics. Melting permafrost revealed the carcasses of a herd of animals, who died from anthrax. The anthrax re-emerged after a century of dormancy, killing several children in Alaska before the pathogen was identified. Ancient bacteria in the permafrost were found to have antibiotic resistance.[329] The findings of ancient antibiotic resistant bacteria, in the

---

[329] Fox-Skelly J. 2017. There Are Diseases Hidden In Ice And They Are Waking Up. BBC Earth. May 4, 2017. Doi: https://www.bbc.com/earth/story/20170504-there-are-diseases-hidden-in-ice-and-they-are-waking-up.

melting permafrost, suggests antibiotic resistance is not caused solely by antibiotics.

Chlamydia has existed at least ten thousand years, in people, animals, and sludge. Chlamydia pathogens have had a parallel evolution, as new strains developed from the mixing of old strains in animal hosts. The pathogens evolved, to aid survival, resist attack, and enhance survival by becoming transmissible from person-to-person.

Antibiotic usage, for acute and chronic infection, has become controversial. Antibiotics are wrongfully generalized to all be the same, and all be bad. The problem of antibiotic resistance is real; however, the problem is not too many antibiotics being prescribed to patients—the problem is the wrong antibiotics are being prescribed to patients, and too many antibiotics are being fed to animals. Penicillin, amoxicillin, Augmentin, and cephalosporins, are the antibiotics most frequently prescribed in the United States; and are the most likely to cause antibiotic resistance; and the most likely to damage the balance and diversity of good bacteria and fungus in the microbiome and mycobiome. Antibiotics like macrolides, doxycycline, and minocycline, should be used more frequently; and penicillin and broad spectrum antibiotics should be used less frequently or not at all. Why kill a massive amount of bacteria, rather than electively attacking the pathogens causing the chronic disease?

Chlamydia can acquire resistance to some antibiotics, and some antibiotics are more likely to cause resistance. However, no increased risk of antibiotic resistance has been shown from long-term use of azithromycin or doxycycline. Macrolides and doxycycline have a lower resistance profile than penicillin, and are less likely to induce antibiotic resistance, particularly in chronic infections. The solution is not to deprive patients of antibiotics for chronic infection; but rather to recognize which infections need treatment, what antibiotics should be used, and to limit antibiotic use in animals.

Dr. Ewald argued treatment of chronic and persistent infection with antibiotics has far less risk of creating antibiotic resistance than treating acute infections, because the risk of transmission in the community is low. The risk of transmission is low; therefore, the risk of transmitting antibiotic-resistant pathogens is low. Dr. Ewald argued animals should *never* be fed the same antibiotics, for the same diseases, as the antibiotics are used for in humans, because the drugs will become ineffective. He said it is dangerous to use penicillin for both animals and humans, for the same diseases.

Penicillin and broad-spectrum antibiotics given to animals, in large quantities, is creating drug-resistant pathogens, and multi-drug resistant organisms, that can be transmitted to humans. A person can acquire antibiotic resistant pathogens by eating animals fed antibiotics, swimming in a public pool or contaminated water, drinking water contaminated with drug resistant pathogens, taking penicillin, or at a hospital. If doctors prescribed less penicillin and amoxicillin for five years, and animals were not fed penicillin, it could help restore the effectiveness of the penicillin and reduce antibiotic resistance. Use of antibiotics in animals should be limited as much as possible, and the same antibiotics needed in humans should not be given to animals.

In the 1940's, antibiotics became available to save human lives. In 1946, animals started to be fed antibiotics, because studies showed the animals grew faster and bigger when fed antibiotics. From 1985 to 2001, the feeding of antibiotics to animals increased fifty percent. Today, livestock, poultry, and fish are routinely fed antibiotics. Ninety-nine percent of the food we consume is raised on factory farms, where antibiotics are routinely fed to animals to enhance and speed growth, and overcome the unsanitary conditions in which the animals are raised. Animals are primarily fed antibiotics in the penicillin class; and we are creating antibiotic resistance by feeding large quantities of penicillin to animals. Most concerning, is the onset of the use of potent macrolides in animals. Life-saving antibiotics should be used to improve the health of humans, not to fatten the animals quicker, and make the animals bigger and more profitable.[330]

---

[330] *See* Landers T, *et al*. 2012. A Review of Antibiotic Use in Food Animals: Perspective, Policy, and Potential. Public Health Reports. January–February 2012. Volume 127: 4-22. Doi: ncbi.nlm.nih.gov/pmc/articles/PMC3234384/.

In 2008, the American Livestock industry reported antibiotic consumption in animals was eight times greater than the antibiotics consumed by people. In one year, animals consumed twenty-nine million pounds of antibiotics![331] Humans consume only three million pounds of antibiotics a year. Eighty percent of all antibiotics used in the United States are fed to animals! Animals are fed eight times more antibiotics than people! Mardi Mellon, director of the American Livestock Industry Union's Food and Environment program said, "Antimicrobial use in United States agriculture is way out of proportion to what is necessary."

Livestock, poultry, and fish are fed antibiotics. Livestock fed antibiotics include cattle, pigs, sheep, goats, camels, and rare livestock; and domesticated animals raised to produce commodities, such as meat, eggs, milk, fur, leather and wool. Pigs are an animal host in which pathogens can mix, and create new serovars of pathogens. When pigs are fed antibiotics, it can speed the evolution of pathogens into new more dangerous forms. Poultry fed antibiotics include chickens, turkeys, ducks and geese, some wild fowl, and caged birds; and domesticated birds raised for eggs, meat or feathers. Farm raised fish are fed antibiotics.

Antibiotic resistance pathogens can be acquired by humans consuming the meat and dairy products from animals and fish fed antibiotics. Antibiotics are now everywhere—in the food, in public water supplies, in animals, and the soil. The United States is highly contaminated with antibiotics; and our microbiome is already damaged from consuming the meat and dairy products from animals fed antibiotics, which is further justification for routine use of probiotics and prebiotics.

Penicillin should no longer be fed to animals; and antibiotics should not be used in animals and humans, for the same disease! We need to stop feeding antibiotics to animals, and start giving antibiotics to people! Are children and adults not deserving of the same opportunity given to animals, to be bigger, stronger and healthier? Are children and adults not deserving of the opportunity to prevent future chronic disease? Certainly, the balance

---

[331] *See* FDA Accounting of Antimicrobial Drug Activity. The American Livestock Industry. Doi: fda.gov/animalveterinary/safetyhealth/antimicrobialresistance.

of human and animal consumption of antibiotics must change, and could change substantially in favor of treating people. Giving targeted antibiotics to children and adults, less use of penicillin and broad-spectrum antibiotics in humans, and reducing the use of antibiotics in animals, could result in a dramatic decrease in the use of antibiotics overall, improvement in the effectiveness of antibiotics in humans, and improvement in human health. Using macrolides instead of penicillin drugs would improve the health of patients, reduce or mitigate chronic diseases, and reduce the risk of drug-resistant infections.

One study proposed antibiotics created an increased risk for breast cancer. The study overlooked an important observation. The patients given penicillin, cephalosporins, or other antibiotics that attack the cell wall, had an increase in breast cancer. Patients given, azithromycin, clarithromycin, and doxycycline had decreased rates of breast cancer. The study supported that treatment with penicillin can convert the pathogen into cancer. The study on children hospitalized or treated for pneumonia, showed the risk for cancer in children after hospitalization for pneumonia, but did not specify the pathogen causing pneumonia or the antibiotic given;[332] and based on common practice, it is likely many children were given penicillin. The children later developed leukemia, lymphoma, and brain cancer, which are caused by infectious pathogens, intracellular infection in the immune cells, and spread of the infection and byproducts to the lymphatics and brain. Penicillin given to patients with acute chlamydia respiratory infections may trigger cancer, in the months and years after the acute infection has resolved.

Dr. Walter Stamm, at the University of Washington, conducted the first randomized, scientifically controlled trial of the safety and effectiveness of low dose antibiotics, to prevent recurrent urinary tract infections in women. He identified the link between sexual intercourse and urinary tract infections; and the connection between sexually transmitted chlamydia

---

[332] *See* Kitabjian A. 2018. Pediatric Patients Hospitalized for Pneumonia May have Elevated Cancer Risk. MSN. January 26, 2018. Doi: https://www.cancertherapyadvisor.com/lymphoma/pediatric-patients-pneumonia-higher-cancer-risk/article/739376/. *Originally published,* Pulmonology Adviser and BMJ.

trachoma and infertility. He transformed the diagnosis and treatment of both urinary tract infections and pelvic inflammatory disease, based on recognition both diseases were caused by a bacterium, the two chronic infections were related, and low dose antibiotics were effective in treating the infection and controlling recurrence of the infection.

We cannot solve the problem of chronic disease until science understands the problem; and accepts chronic disease is caused by immortal infectious pathogens. Fear surrounding antibiotics does not change the underlying truth that chronic intracellular infection causes chronic disease. Understanding intracellular pathogens and parasites cause chronic disease can lead to better ways to treat chronic disease, through use of targeted treatment, natural prevention and treatment, treatment less likely to cause antibiotic resistance, and finding new ways to combat antibiotic resistance. Knowledge chronic infection causes chronic disease should spur research and innovation into alternate ways to diagnose and treat chronic immortal infection, the optimal treatment, and the most effective dosage and duration of antibiotic treatment. Research can be directed to finding ways to inhibit chlamydia proliferation in the body, prevent spread to weak links, remove abnormal proteins, and remove infection from the professional immune cells.

Pediatricians decided as a group that amoxicillin is the standard first-line drug to be prescribed for acute infection. Penicillin does not kill chlamydia pathogens—it releases the pathogen from the host cell and changes the pathogens shape and life cycle, allowing the pathogen to spread to new host cells and trigger chronic disease. Pediatricians are ill-informed about the need to prescribe macrolide antibiotics to children with acute respiratory infections. Pediatricians fail to consider parasites or the need for antiparasitic medicine in children, even though children are particularly vulnerable to parasitic infection from household pets, swimming pools, daycare, and schools, even in children with pets and gastrointestinal complaints. Pediatricians too often rely on an assumption that diseases of childhood will resolve without treatment, which is true in some cases, but not universally true. The infection can hide and re-emerge years or decades later as chronic disease.

The increasing tendency to avoid antibiotics, and insistence by doctors on using penicillin and amoxicillin, corresponds to the significant rise in chronic disease in children, and the onset of a greater burden of chronic disease in young adults. Chronic disease in children and young adults, including obesity, hypertension, diabetes, and cancer, has exploded in the population.[333] The study of obesity and cancer concluded obesity had a role in causing cancer; however, obesity was not causing cancer—it was the pathogens causing obesity, hypertension, diabetes, and cancer, in young patients. Controversy over the use of antibiotics, the disregard for treatment of immortal pathogens and parasitic infections, and resistance by doctors to prescribing antibiotics or only prescribing penicillin and amoxicillin, has caused patients to develop chronic infections and chronic disease at younger ages. Patients who acquire an immortal infection at a young age have to live with chronic infection for a longer period of time, and suffer greater morbidity as the patient acquires new infections, has multiple infections, and is prescribed penicillin.

Fear of antibiotics spilled over to patients, causing patients to avoid seeking necessary treatment of immortal infections. At the same time, people have lost respect for infection, and the need to protect themselves from immortal pathogens. Patients have become cavalier, believing antibiotics will protect them and cure infections, at the same time use of antibiotics is being discouraged or denied. Fear of antibiotics, lack of fastidious hygiene, and lack of isolation of the sick, is causing a proliferation of immortal infections, an increased infectious burden in the population, and a greater amount of chronic disease.

We need a better understanding of the microbiome; and to find new ways to treat immortal pathogens other than antibiotics. We need to find new ways to interrupt the infectious cascade and heal the microbiome after a patient takes antibiotics. A healthy and diverse microbiome can overcome a low level of infectious pathogens and even fight off pathogens; but as the infectious burden increases, the body cannot withstand the infectious burden and continue to function normally. A healthy microbiome can

---

[333] *See* Berger N. 2018. Young Adult Cancer: Influence of the Obesity Pandemic. Obesity. 26(4): 641-650. April 2018. Doi:10.1002/oby.22137.

be analogized to farming, in that a healthy crop will keep weeds from invading the field. A field can tolerate a few weeds and still produce a healthy crop; but when the weeds become widespread, the crops are no longer bountiful and become diseased.

Probiotics should be recommended to all patients, for life, to promote gastrointestinal health and improve resistance to pathogens; and overcome the damage to the microbiome caused by antibiotics already in our environment and food. Probiotics can protect against colitis, which can develop with long-term use of antibiotics; and help a patient tolerate antibiotics long enough to have an effect on their chronic disease. Probiotics and prebiotics should be prescribed to any patient taking antibiotics, to restore the good bacteria damaged by chronic disease and antibiotics. We do not yet understand and have replacements for all good bacteria lost by antibiotic treatment; but probiotics can restore some balance in the microbiome, and should be taken until gastrointestinal balance is restored. Research is needed to create better probiotic supplements to replace the good bacteria; and to find new ways through the microbiome, to fight disease naturally. Science must learn how to repair the microbiome with diverse good bacteria, and replace good bacteria killed by antibiotics, to help the body naturally resist and fight immortal pathogens. Science may be able to harness our own bacteria and convert the bacteria into drugs, or attach specific treatments to our bacteria to fight the disease.

Probiotics, gastrointestinal balance, diet, exercise, and nutritional supplements can help prevent new infections. Herbs and vitamin supplements such as CoQ 10, folic acid, B12, vitamin D, Ocuvit, etc. are known to assist in restoring health. Folic acid supplements are widely recognized as necessary in pregnancy and helpful in preventing a trigger for cancer. Aspirin can improve cardiovascular and gastrointestinal health. Some types of honey are active against infections. Diatomaceous earth can help treat skin infections and infections in the intestinal tract; bismuth, although a heavy metal, can treat some conditions in the gastrointestinal tract, and help in reducing fungus. Some herbs can help fight against the pathogens; and Chinese medicine, natural remedies, and fecal transplants may all be effective to fight immortal infection. Gamma globulin can boost immunity to assist in the fight against chronic infection.

Knowledge of infectious causes of chronic disease can spur innovation and discovery into new ways to treat chronic disease, the best use of antibiotics for immortal infection, and the most effective dosage and duration of antibiotics. Patients benefit by timely diagnosis and effective treatment of chronic infections, including reduced morbidity in chronic diseases thought untreatable, and prevention of chronic disease. Knowledge of infectious causes of chronic disease and antibiotic resistance from animals should discourage use of antibiotics in animals. Hopefully, knowledge of infectious causes of chronic disease will direct science to find new ways to treat chronic infections naturally, and reduce the infectious burden to a level low enough for the body to function, with a low level of remaining pathogens, without the need for antibiotics or through selective use of targeted antibiotics.

> *The difference between man and animals is people's desire to take medicine.*

Sir William Osler, MD

CHAPTER 25

WE CAN FIGHT BACK AGAINST
CHRONIC DISEASE

Darwin's theory of evolution applies equally to immortal pathogens. Humans and immortal pathogens live a parallel existence, and have a parallel evolution. Both are competing for survival. The pathogens continue to evolve and adapt to survive the attack by the immune system. The pathogens survive off the human host, and are attacked by the immune system, then the pathogen attacks the immune system, and chronic disease develops from the war within between immortal pathogens and the immune system.

Darwin's theory of survival of the fittest suggests the population should become healthier over time, as the strongest survive; and genetic cost eliminates chronic disease. The opposite is true—global health is declining and the cost of medical care and chronic disease is increasing. The cost of medical care is increasing as immortal pathogens and parasites spread undiagnosed and untreated, creating a higher infectious burden in the population, and a greater number of people with chronic disease. Chronic disease is becoming more prevalent, and younger people are getting chronic disease. We do not yet know whether the human species and the human microbiome will win, or the pathogens will be the sole survivors.

Understanding a principle of the whole—chronic infection with immortal pathogens cause chronic disease—can help patients prevent chronic disease, and help doctors improve the diagnosis and treatment of chronic disease. The principle of the whole can return medicine to a patient-centered encounter, with focus on the whole patient and the diagnosis of the root infectious causes of chronic disease. Diagnosing infectious pathogens, causing acute and chronic disease, can unify diverse specialties in a common cause. Routine diagnosis of infectious disease will expand scientific knowledge, confirm specific infectious causes of chronic disease, and allow further investigation of meta-data, to specifically identify which pathogens cause which diseases. Specialists will have to work with and communicate with other specialists and primary care doctors, and collaborate with veterinarians, to address the problem of immortal animal pathogens causing chronic disease in humans and animals.

Ingestion, hand-to-eye contact, hand-to-nose contact, airborne transmission, sexual transmission, and IV drug use, are the primary methods by which humans acquire dangerous immortal pathogens and parasites. Avoidance of the avoidable and most dangerous immortal pathogens, can protect against chronic disease. Avoidance of pathogens like chlamydia trachoma, chlamydia psittacosis, toxoplasmosis, herpes simplex virus, and hepatitis B and C, is one way to avoid chronic disease and extend life. H-pylori can be transmitted by saliva, food handling by an infected person, or through ingestion of contaminated water. Avoiding environmental toxins can limit weak links, the introduction of carcinogens, and triggers for chronic disease. Environmental toxins can combine with immortal infections and act synergistically to cause or trigger harm, just as multiple infections can combine and cause or trigger greater harm.

People will need to re-think their priorities and how they live their life, knowing the consequences of living with immortal chronic infections. People should not lead a sterile life, totally isolate themselves, or be afraid of sick people. A diverse microbiome helps to maintain health and fight pathogens. Exercise and diet aid in boosting the immune system and defending against pathogens. People should stay three feet or more away from sick people, and *never* touch the face (eyes, nose, and mouth) after touching the sick person or their environment, without first washing one's hands. Caution and hand washing should be vigorously implemented, whenever a person has contact with any sick person or sick animal. People should keep their hands and phones away from their face, and keep the screens of their devices clean, to avoid self-inoculation with pathogens in biofilm.

People can be more careful about what goes in the mouth, and no one should ever eat or drink anything questionable! A good diet includes eating healthy food, but it also includes not ingesting food or drink that has the potential to transmit immortal pathogens. A good diet is more than what we ingest—it includes what we do *not* ingest. The four major components of a good diet include:

1. Eat good food and maintain a balanced diet, to maximize diversity in the microbiome. Eat every color of food, to enhance diversity in the microbiome. Diet, exercise, and maintaining a normal weight boosts the immune system and prevents aging; provides some protection against immortal pathogens, and from the immortal infections becoming a chronic infection.

2. Avoid eating bad food! If the food looks bad, smells bad, is not cooked well enough, is old, or it fell on the floor—throw it in the trash, do not put it in the mouth! Always, error on the side of not eating anything questionable, suspicious, or handled by someone who is acutely sick. Follow the maxim, "When in doubt, throw it out!"

3. Don't drink contaminated or suspicious water. Clear water does not necessarily mean clean water free of pathogens or parasites. Public water sources may be supplied by surface water, which can be contaminated with waste from dogs, birds, wild animals, and humans. *Never* drink from rivers, streams, or lakes; or swallow water from swimming pools, lakes, or streams. Avoid getting contaminated water in your eyes or nose, or near contact lenses. Recognize water in other areas of the world may be safe for the local population, but travelers have no immunity to pathogens in the water; and when traveling the safest water is water that has been boiled.

4. Wash your hands frequently and keep your hands away from your eyes, nose, mouth and face. Pathogens often are transmitted by hand contact transferred to the eyes, nose or mouth, or by food handling and ingestion. Children who wash their hands frequently have significantly less illnesses during the school year. Good

handwashing and hygiene is a route to longer life, in general. People need to return to a routine of handwashing, and always wash their hands whenever in contact with sick people and animals.

People need to avoid crowds during outbreaks of community-wide respiratory infections. Prior to the mid-twentieth century, fatal epidemics swept through the population and millions died. In Philadelphia, in July 1918, a community parade on the Fourth of July caused a community-wide outbreak of the Spanish Flu that caused twelve-thousand deaths. Many people experienced deaths in their immediate family during epidemics of infectious disease, creating fear and generating greater caution about hygiene. Those who practiced good hygiene had a better chance to avoid infection, and survive the epidemic.

Immortal pathogens now spread in community-wide outbreaks. The days of isolation of the sick, to avoid spreading infectious diseases, are gone; and need to be revived to avoid the spread of immortal pathogens and the spread of antibiotic-resistant pathogens. The movement of women into the workplace and children into daycare has aggravated the spread of immortal pathogens, in the United States. Sick people no longer stay home from school and work, because of the threat of children exceeding the maximum allowable absences at school, and pressure to go to work when sick. Daycares and schools are a vector for children to acquire immortal pathogens at younger ages, and spread infections within the family. When the child goes to school sick the infectious pathogens spread to classmates, who then spread the infection to their family. When the sick person goes to work, the infection spreads to co-workers, who then spread the infection to their family.

Continuing to engage in community activities when sick with an immortal pathogen, can cause the infection to become chronic. The sick person risks acquiring multiple acute infections, at the same time, which can accelerate or trigger the development of chronic disease. If a sick person acquires a second acute infection while still sick, two acute infections at the same time increase the risk of adverse consequences from the co-infections and viral triggers for chronic disease. Patients with two acute infections compound the infectious burden and increase the risk of triggering a more virulent pathogen, the risk of the pathogens combining in the person to become more virulent, and the risk of the combined effect of the pathogens accelerating a chronic disease.

Dr. Ewald advocated isolation to avoid rapid transmission of infectious pathogens, because rapid transmission increases the virulence of the pathogen. Rapid transmission from person-to-person causes a faster evolution of the pathogen, and the pathogen is more likely to become antibiotic resistant. Patients who are acutely ill and infectious to others need to stay at home, to protect others and to protect their own health. Abandon social pressure to go to work, school, parties, and church! Students, employees, employers, church goers, and everyone else—stay home when you are sick, and require employees and children to stay home when sick!

Modern society has become complacent about acquiring infectious pathogens, believing we have antibiotics to treat infections. People have become complacent about close contact with animals, leading to transmission of animal pathogens and development of chronic disease. The best defense against chronic disease will always be using good hygiene, preventing acute infection, and avoiding immortal pathogens! The second-best defense is to remain isolated when sick, to avoid acquiring additional co-infections and avoid spreading pathogens in the community. The third-best defense is better diagnosis and treatment of infectious pathogens, and finding alternative ways to manage and defeat the chronic infection.

In community-wide outbreaks of disease, it is important for doctors to diagnose and treat immortal pathogens, to prevent future morbidity and mortality in the community. Patients infected with chlamydia pneumonia are at risk of developing pneumonia, being hospitalized, and in the ensuing months have an increased risk of sudden cardiac events. Knowledge of a community outbreak of a parasitic infection, in a local swimming pool, or contamination of drinking water in the community, are important diagnostic clues, in patients with gastrointestinal complaints. Untreated parasitic infection causes gastrointestinal complaints that become more constant over time; and long-term can cause anemia, lowered immunity, and chronic disease.

Travel exposes a person to pathogens, for which they have no immunity and the pathogens may not be familiar to doctors in the community. When traveling, people must understand the high likelihood of exposure to unusual pathogens and parasites, which may or may not be recognized by doctors in the United States. Use good hygiene during travel, avoid drinking water that may be contaminated with pathogens, and only eat food that has been cooked and water that has been boiled. Water may look clear and clean, but that does not mean it is free of pathogens or parasites capable of causing acute and chronic disease; or free of pathogens for which the traveler does not have resistance. Water supplies may be contaminated by animal and human feces; or contaminated by poor water treatment or antiquated water systems.

Americans have become cavalier about the risks of acquiring pathogens from pets and domesticated animals, in part because no one has explained the risks of animal pathogens. Doctors are reluctant to warn patients of the risk of transmission of animal pathogens from pets or other animals, even when the patient has a disease transmitted from an animal.[334] Animal transmission of pathogens causing human disease, and doctors reluctant to warn of the risk from animal pathogens, even in patients who are ill from animal pathogens, is unacceptable and is causing and aggravating the increase in chronic diseases.

Every domesticated and wild animal presents its own unique risk of immortal pathogens and parasites; and each animal pathogen presents unique risks as to the type of chronic disease it may cause. People should avoid close contact with domesticated animals, particularly cats and birds; and avoid close contact with livestock as much as possible. Wild animals can transmit pathogens to those in contact with the animal. Meticulous hand washing after animal contact can substantially reduce the risk of acquiring an acute immortal pathogen or parasite that can become a chronic infection, and insidiously progress and impair health in the future and for a lifetime.

---

[334] *See* Rabinowitz P, *et al.* 2007. Pet Related Infections. American Family Physician. 76(9): 1314-1322. Nov 1, 2007. Doi: aafp.org/afp/2007/1101/p1314.html.

Pets and animals transmit a variety of parasites and worms to pet owners, and members of the household. At least sixty percent of dog owners have pinworms, and/or other types of worms such as toxocara and hookworm. Toxocara transmitted by dog feces can cause reduced cognitive function, in children and adults. Walking barefoot where pets or other animals have defecated can transmit hookworm through the skin. Toxoplasmosis is virtually universal in cats; and can cause mental illness, and sight threatening eye diseases. Psittacosis is virtually universal in birds worldwide, and can cause a fatal respiratory infection and cancer. Psittacosis can be transmitted from birds to other domestic animals, including cats, dogs, pigs, and horses. Cats, dogs, pigs, and horses can then transmit psittacosis to humans.

Pets should never be in the bedroom, or in the bed or in the crib! Pets on the bed contaminate the bed with pathogens and parasites that can be transferred to humans who sleep in the bed. Fifty percent of dog owners and more than fifty percent of cat owners sleep with their pets; and pets get onto the bed when the owner is not looking or aware. Newborns and young children are vulnerable to pathogens transmitted from pets; and some pet owners let infants sleep with pets or the pets get in the child's crib. Toxoplasmosis from cats presents a significant long-term health risk to infants, children, and adults; and toxocara from dogs presents a significant risk to learning and cognition. Pinworms may present other mental health risks to children, including gastrointestinal problems, and problems with attention and focus. The earlier in life children are exposed to animal pathogens and parasites, the longer the infections persist over the child's life, and the more likely serious chronic disease will arise in the short or long term. We need to return to routine treatment of worms, particularly in patients with pets or contact with domesticated animals.

Virtually all cats acquire toxoplasmosis, during the life of the cat. Cats transmit toxoplasmosis to adults, children, infants, and to a fetus. Toxoplasmosis can cause mental illnesses and eye diseases, in an adult or child; and in a fetus cause hearing loss and visual loss years after birth. Young cats and feral cats carry the highest risk of transmitting toxoplasmosis to humans. The greatest risk is when the cat or kitten first acquires toxoplasmosis, usually when the cat is young. In the first three weeks after the cat first acquires toxoplasmosis, the cat sheds many, many millions of toxoplasmosis parasites in the feces. Cat litter boxes are a significant risk, when the cat is shedding the parasite. The risk of toxoplasmosis is even greater when the litter box is not cleaned for more than twenty-four hours, because after twenty-four hours the toxoplasmosis parasite can become airborne. Pregnant mothers are warned to avoid litter boxes, because of the danger of congenital toxoplasmosis in the infant, and late onset mental illness in the child.

Toxoplasmosis has been dismissed by the medical community as an "asymptomatic" and self-limiting disease, in adults and children older than five. The medical community is only concerned and acknowledges the need for treatment when the child is under five. The fact the medical community recognizes a danger when the child is under five, shows the significant health danger to any child or adult acquiring toxoplasmosis. The fact the medical community recognizes the danger of congenital toxoplasmosis in a fetus; and that toxoplasmosis causes a variety of mental illnesses, years or decades after the acute infection, further supports the danger of a chronic toxoplasmosis infection. The fact many mental illnesses have been "associated" or recognized to be caused by toxoplasmosis, ranging from recklessness to depression to bipolar disorder to intermittent explosive disorder, to rage and violence, confirms the danger of toxoplasmosis infection and belies any claim toxoplasmosis can be assumed to be self-limiting, asymptomatic, or unimportant

Toxoplasmosis is a significant long-term health threat to infected persons, and is not self-limiting. Toxoplasmosis can be asymptomatic in the animal or person, and progress insidiously to become a chronic disease, years after exposure. Toxoplasmosis can insidiously progress to the brain, central nervous system, and eyes; and cause central nervous system disease, blindness, and a variety of mental illnesses. Toxoplasmosis is "associated" with disintegration of the iris, which causes pigment dispersion glaucoma. Toxoplasmosis is far more common than recognized, and the percent of cat owners who have toxoplasmosis is likely higher than recognized, because doctors rarely inquire about cats or pets, or consider toxoplasmosis in the differential diagnosis.

Doctors dismiss the importance of chronic toxoplasmosis, even though Americans own sixty-eight million cats; and diseases known to be caused by toxoplasmosis are common in the population. Toxoplasmosis is likely much more common in the population than currently recognized.

Avoiding cats, birds and animal feces; avoiding sick animals; keeping pets off furniture and off the bed; not allowing pets to eat off plates or kiss family members; and hand washing after contact with pets or domesticated animals, is the safest and best defense to chronic disease from animal pathogens. Not all pets are sick, but the reality is many pets harbor immortal pathogens and parasites; and most pets or animals will acquire immortal pathogens and parasites over the course of the animal's life. The danger of transmission of animal pathogens could arise from contact with someone else's animal; or a trip to the park, doggie daycare, or veterinarian. The contact with animal pathogens could be at a petting zoo; a farm; a state fair; with horses; or in a classroom, when teachers bring rodents to class for observation. Contact with animal pathogens could be from infection in pets, which the pets acquired from rodents or birds. Contact with animal pathogens can be through person-to-person transmission, from someone else who acquired the infection from a pet or other animal.

Everyone loves their pets, and pets are often part of the family. Pets can provide emotional support and love to the owners. But, pets can make humans sick and humans can make pets sick. If a person is unable or unwilling to give up pets, people can understand the risks, and know how to interact with animals, to protect the family. People can have a greater appreciation for the danger and be aware of the need for greater hygiene around pets and animals, particularly when family members already have animal-related pathogens or chronic disease. Cats and dogs should not be allowed on the bed or furniture, allowed to eat off family plates, allowed to sleep in beds, or be kissed by owners. Pets should not be allowed to *ever* sleep with infants and young children. People should understand cats and birds are the most dangerous pets to own, and the risks associated with cats and birds. If people cannot accept giving up a pet; the exercise of strict hygiene, and limiting contamination of the household environment, is the best defense.

Immortal infections acquired *in utero* are extremely harmful to the fetus, and can cause fetal abnormalities and life-long health problems in the child. Intracellular bacteria have been found in the placenta, and can cross the placenta; or reach the fetus through the mother's blood stream. Toxoplasmosis acquired during pregnancy causes regressive developmental disorders and mental illness, in the fetus. Acute immortal infections during pregnancy have already been "associated" with fetal abnormalities, and the danger to the fetus is likely greater from immortal pathogens and parasites acquired in pregnancy than from medication used to treat the acute infections in the pregnant mother. Mothers should be tested and re-tested carefully for immortal pathogens, whenever an infant is born with a serious medical problem, to aid in finding potential treatment for the infant and avoidance of future births of children with the same medical problems.

A return to one sexual partner would significantly improve the health of the person, the family, the children, and the population as a whole, by reducing the burden of chlamydia trachoma. Limiting sexual relations to one sexual partner, to avoid chronic disease and achieve healthy aging, applies equally to women and men! Alternatively, using barrier protection is a way to reduce the risk of sexually transmitted chlamydia trachoma. Sexually transmitted chlamydia trachoma can become chronic, and cause autoimmune disease, central nervous system disease, rheumatoid arthritis, cancer, reproductive disorders, and infertility. Sexually acquired trachoma can be transferred to the eye by self-inoculation, and cause blinding eye diseases. The ancient wisdom of virginity before marriage had a purpose beyond religion or morals: Abstinence before marriage was necessary to avoid sexually transmitted disease, which until modern times had no treatment; and caused chronic disease, morbidity, and early demise.

Ocular trachoma is a different serovar of trachoma, which is transmitted by flies. Ocular trachoma can cause sight threatening eye disease, and is "associated" with arthritis. Some propose ocular trachoma is more strongly "associated" with arthritis than sexually transmitted trachoma. Ocular trachoma can be avoided only by avoiding contact with the insect vectors for transmission, and avoiding hand-to-eye contact after contact with a person infected with ocular trachoma. Ocular trachoma is likely more prevalent than recognized, because testing for trachoma is usually by blood testing, testing does not distinguish the serovar of trachoma, and many people have diseases related to ocular trachoma.

Eye make-up is a risk for women, and is the reason women have a higher rate of dry eyes, blepharitis, and ocular surface disease.[335] Eye make-up can become contaminated with pathogens, and cause self-inoculation around the eye; and the shedding of the pathogens from the eyelid margins across the eye. Most of the Auburn eye cancer victims were women, and eye make-up may have been a factor in self-inoculation of psittacosis, in the eye; or the women may have hosted co-infections in and around the eye that combined with psittacosis to become eye cancer. Women should stop wearing all eye make-up, particularly mascara and any eye make-up containing sparkles or powder. Sparkles and powder are indigestible materials that cannot be broken down by the immune system; and can provide a focus for inclusion cysts, giant cell reactions, and chronic disease. If a woman has dry eyes or any chronic disease, in or around the eye, the woman should immediately stop wearing all eye make-up. Avoiding eye make-up will also help a woman avoid developing dry eyes, and/or eye ocular surface disease, in the future.

Doctors must incorporate the diagnosis of immortal pathogens into their routine practice. The history should include the health of all members of the household, pets, animal contact, risk factors for immortal infections, history of prior infections, and the treatment for all prior infections the patient recalls. Doctors must take the time to observe the patient, inquire about the history, examine the patient, and come to a reasoned conclusion; rather than rushing and interrupting, and spending the bulk of the patient encounter looking at computer screens, and doing data entry. Doctors need to diagnose the root causes of chronic disease, instead of observing findings, naming diseases, and treating symptoms, without knowing the root causes of chronic disease or impact of symptomatic treatment on immortal pathogens. Doctors should not grasp for any diagnosis that can

---

[335] *See* Lietman T, *et al.* 1998. Chronic Follicular Conjunctivities Associated with Chlamydia Psittaci or Chlamydia Pneumonia. Clinical Infectious Diseases. June 1998. 26:1335-40. Doi: 1058-4838/98/2606—0017$03.00.

be justified, among thousands of symptoms, findings, and syndromes of unknown origin; and investigate immortal pathogens in any patient with chronic disease. Reducing chlamydia in the population through routine diagnosis and treatment will reduce morbidity and mortality from chronic diseases, prevent and mitigate chronic disease, and lead to greater understanding of immortal pathogens and chronic disease.

All doctors must be trained to think about immortal pathogens in evaluating a patient with chronic disease; and trained to diagnose and treat immortal pathogens and chronic infection. Medical training, starting in medical school and continuing throughout a medical career, should encourage critical thinking, reasoning, observation, rigid skepticism, and creative solutions; and recognition that co-morbid conditions give clues to the pathogens causing chronic disease. The organ or system targeted, whether the heart, lung, stomach, kidney, reproductive tract, joints, or eye; and the type of tissue attacked, endothelium, epithelium, or collagen, should inform the doctor of the likely immortal pathogens causing chronic disease, for further diagnostic confirmation. Routine diagnosis of infectious pathogens would allow each specialty to identify pathogens causing chronic diseases, symptoms, findings, and syndromes, in their specialty.

We need better and more rapid in-office diagnostic tools to determine the type of pathogen causing chronic disease. Routine blood tests give clues, and PCR testing can diagnose the specific pathogens, in many cases. We have super-computers capable of rapidly analyzing blood for many hundreds of pathogens and nucleotides, but primary care doctors do not have access to the technology.

High-throughput sequencing technology can map the human genome and the DNA of immortal pathogens causing disease; however, the technology has been directed at the human microbiome, and understanding of genes and genetic signals. High-throughput sequencing is just now beginning to study the DNA of pathogens. High-throughput sequencing can identify more types of bacteria than PCR testing; and can be used to identify the source of bacterial outbreaks, and genetic evolution of bacteria. The methodology could be used to compare pathogens to chronic disease;

can begin to identify abnormal Cluster Differentiations in each chronic disease; and determine which pathogens cause the abnormal fragments, abnormal proteins, and Cluster Differentiations, in each chronic disease. Routine identification of infectious pathogens by all doctors would quickly answer the question of which pathogens and combinations of pathogens cause which chronic diseases, in each specialty. High-throughput sequencing technology should be applied immediately to aid the Auburn eye cancer cluster investigation, to determine the common cause or causes of the eye cancer and compare the pathogens in humans with the pathogens in birds.

We need better methods for diagnosis of H-pylori, and for doctors to diagnose and treat H-pylori. The current methods to diagnose H-pylori have been inadequate, and do not confirm the absence of the pathogen. Diagnosis of H-pylori begins with awareness of the danger of H-pylori causing chronic disease, and recognition diseases caused by H-pylori are not limited to the gastrointestinal tract. H-pylori and parasites may hide in the body outside the intestine, in adjacent organs or in the eye or brain, where the pathogen avoids detection in a stool sample. H-pylori can combine with other pathogens, by attacking epithelium and collagen; and by creating a portal in the epithelium, for other pathogens to invade deeper into the tissue.

Better diagnosis of parasitic disease begins with awareness of the need, and teaching parasitology in medical school. Newer swab technology for PCR testing can detect parasites more easily and reliably. Patients are no longer treated routinely for parasites, or treated for parasites at all. Parasites should be part of the differential diagnosis of all chronic disease, and particularly all gastrointestinal disease or chronic disease in abdominal organs.

Early diagnosis and treatment of infectious causes of chronic disease can delay development of chronic diseases, avoid the development of co-morbid diseases, and improve co-morbid conditions. Diagnosis and treatment of the infectious causes of chronic disease will lead to better outcomes, and keep valuable drugs needed for treatment of chronic diseases on the market. We need changes at the highest levels of medicine and government, to assure important drugs are available, at a reasonable price; and to bring back important drugs that were removed from the market. Knowledge and observation of chronic infections and the effect of treatment can evolve into wisdom, in treating chronic disease.

Doctors and patients must open their minds to a new way of thinking. Bias and cognitive assumptions have permeated medicine, causing confusion, an increase in medical errors, and unfortunate complications. It is time to rethink the diagnosis and treatment of all chronic diseases. It is time to re-evaluate whether treatment is for a symptom, a cause of the disease, or for some other reason. It is time to stop treating symptoms, before investigating and treating the root cause of chronic disease. It can be acceptable to relieve symptoms, or to relieve pain; but treating symptoms will never cure a chronic disease, and can cause chronic disease or make a chronic disease worse. It is time to transform the process of reaching a diagnosis into the discovery and identification of infectious pathogens causing chronic disease.

All chronic disease is caused by intracellular animal pathogens, and the patients' immune response to the pathogens: It is the immune system responding to the intracellular pathogens, wherever the intracellular pathogens exist; and the effect of the immune battle with the pathogens and remnants of the immune battle causing chronic disease. Immortal pathogens and parasites can be diagnosed by a thorough history, examination, diagnostic blood testing, and co-morbid conditions. PCR blood testing and PCR swabs can confirm the pathogens. We have drugs that work against these pathogens; and we have super-computers that can test blood for hundreds of different pathogens. Let's use these tools to fight against immortal pathogens and make progress in finding the causes and cures for chronic disease!

> *I have been impressed with the urgency of doing. Knowing is not enough, we must apply. Being willing is not enough, we must do.*

Leonardo de Vinci

CHAPTER 26

RESEARCH CAN DISCOVER CAUSES AND CURES FOR CHRONIC DISEASE

Science is but a perversion of itself, unless it has as its ultimate goal the benefit mankind.

Nikola Tesla

A unifying principle in medicine, which is understood in all medical specialties and in research, can move medicine beyond "associations" to finding causes and cures for chronic disease. A compelling body of research supports infectious causes of chronic disease, and it is time for a unified theory as to causation, to move forward with discovery, diagnosis and treatment of chronic disease. Medical specialties can unite in a common cause of identifying the infectious immortal pathogens causing chronic disease in each specialty; and research can compile the observations and findings to reach important conclusions. With understanding, science can repurpose drugs already available for new indications; and find new ways to treat chronic disease, treat infected immune cells, eliminate bad fungus, and eliminate abnormal proteins. Science can find new alternative ways to prevent, interrupt, treat, mitigate, and reverse chronic disease; and fight antibiotic resistance.

Research has become focused on incidental dabbling in small details, hoping to find an answer. Medical research looks at minutia and is influenced by vested interests, who seek to sell new drugs for diseases and conditions which are not understood, for a greater profit. Medical research repeats the same studies, finding the same "associations", but fails to develop a coherent theory from which to proceed, based on repeated consistent findings and observations. The research finding "associations", without any coherent theory of a cause, does not benefit the practitioner and the patient; and diverts research money into areas that have already been the subject of research, or takes the research in the wrong direction. Researchers observing, documenting, and reporting, without making a conclusion on cause or treatment, does not direct medical providers to seek a cause for chronic disease.

Finding the root cause of chronic disease requires a broader perspective that includes immortal pathogens and parasites, across all medical specialties. All medical specialties will need to collaborate and share knowledge, to advance medical knowledge. Observational and experiential medicine is valuable, and observation and experience used to reason a solution has been recognized, for centuries, as a means to advance science. We cannot let the chronic disease continue to be treated symptomatically, without diagnosis of any of the many pathogens already known to be "associations" with chronic disease.

We cannot let cognitive bias and narrow hypotheses continue to interfere with discovery of the root infectious causes of chronic diseases. Genes help in understanding chronic disease; and genetics, gene expression, and environmental factors may co-exist with chronic infection, to trigger chronic disease. Inflammation exists in virtually all chronic disease, caused by chronic infection. Fatigue is present in virtually all chronic diseases, as intracellular energy is depleted. High TNF-alpha is present in virtually all chronic diseases. The answer to chronic disease is not in genes, inflammation, and environmental triggers alone. Chronic intracellular infection and parasites alter genes and gene expression, cause inflammation when attacked by the immune system, and work synergistically with environmental triggers and co-infections to cause chronic disease.

Medical research is controlled by money. Money and vested interests control who performs research, and what research is performed. Research grants are awarded based on what the medical establishment and vested interests decide is valuable, based on past training, and cognitive bias, in each specialty. Research funding is granted by specific groups dedicated to a particular specialty or particular disease, which is not conducive to discovery of infectious pathogens causing chronic diseases.

Researchers are slaves to the grant system, and the motto "publish or perish". Researchers have to perform research that will lead to publication, in scientific peer-reviewed publications; or future research funding may be limited. Employment evaluations may depend on the amount of grant money obtained, the outcome of research, and the number of scientific peer-reviewed publications. Too often, the goal of medical research is more grant money and the opportunity to publish positive findings, rather than broader research questions that may provide an answer to the cause of chronic disease.

Widespread diagnosis of immortal pathogens, in chronic disease in all specialties, would rapidly identify the infectious causes of chronic diseases, with greater specificity. Research could correlate the type of immortal pathogens, blood type, and chronic disease; and start comparing the infections and combinations of infections in chronic diseases. Research could correlate the types of abnormal proteins associated with each pathogen and each chronic disease, and find ways to eliminate abnormal proteins and byproducts of the immune battle. Super-computers could evaluate meta-data comparing immortal infections and chronic disease, using combined knowledge in each specialty. Patterns should emerge and disclose which pathogens and combinations of pathogens cause which chronic diseases; and variations in pathogens among patients with the same disease.

Medical research hypotheses are framed to answer narrow questions that will generate funding and provide an ability to publish results. Narrow research questions are not designed to reveal causation. A research proposal may ask whether a particular pathogen causes a disease, but when the same infectious pathogen is not present in every patient, it is called an "association". Research on chlamydia pneumonia and glaucoma finds a high percent of chlamydia pneumonia but not in all patients; thus, calls it is only an "association". Research on H-pylori and glaucoma finds a high percent of patients have H-pylori but not all patients, so it is only an "association". No one asked what infections did glaucoma patients have, whether any of the patients with glaucoma did *not* have any immortal infections, or whether the glaucoma improved with treatment of the pathogens identified in the studies. No one asks how immortal infections correlate with chronic diseases. Instead of asking, "did this particular infection cause something?" the research should ask, "What infections does the patient have, how high is the infectious burden, and could the patient benefit by treatment?"

The type of immortal infections, the number of co-infections, and the combination of immortal infections determine the nature and the severity of chronic disease. Seeking to identify one pathogen at a time, in one chronic disease at a time, does not disclose numerous pathogens causing the chronic disease, or provide a unified theory that infectious pathogens cause many chronic diseases. Under current research methods, if more than one pathogen causes the same disease no causation can ever be found.

Researchers are reluctant to state causation, particularly when more than one pathogen can cause the same disease, or the same pathogen can cause different diseases. The fact more than one pathogen can cause the same chronic disease contributes to reluctance to identify an infectious "cause" of a chronic disease, because other research may find an "association" with a different pathogen, which appears to contradict the original findings. The fact a particular immortal pathogen causes a chronic disease does not exclude a finding that other immortal pathogens can cause the same chronic disease.

Researchers publish articles specific to each specialty, and report "associations" instead of causes; and markers of inflammation instead of the cause of inflammation. When research fails to identify an infectious "cause" of chronic disease, and retreats to an "association", the primary care doctor will not diagnose the "associated" infectious cause. When research reports on markers of inflammation alone, it does not direct the primary care doctor to investigate infectious causes of the inflammation. Primary care doctors fear acting on reports of only an "association" and "markers";

and await being told a cause, or may not be allowed to pursue infectious causes of chronic disease, by supervisors or insurance companies.

A long-standing bias against infectious etiology in chronic disease has directed medical research away from infectious causes and toward cell microbiology, genes, and inflammation. Medical research has dedicated substantially less funding to research of infectious causes of chronic disease. Research into genes and cytokines (inflammation) are favored, over research into the microbiome and research into infectious causes of chronic disease. Cancer research is disproportionately directed at the genes, to the exclusion of infectious causes. The answer to the causes of chronic disease is not likely to be found in the small details of genes and Cluster Differentiations; until the quest for small details includes a search for infectious causes of chronic disease, and correlates the small details of genes and Cluster Differentiations with the pathogens. Every person carries their own family grouping of immortal infections and altered genes; and the genetic changes caused by immortal pathogens can become familial. Scientists cannot say with certainty which came first, the infection or the alteration in genes. Research grants dedicated to infectious causes of chronic disease should far exceed current levels of funding.

The lack of a unified theory of chronic diseases has left researchers grasping at small details. Scientists look at genes and cell biology, generating enormous amounts of information, while ignoring knowledge that immortal infections alter genes, and attach to genes in an infinite variety of ways. Researching small details in cell microbiology may explain processes, and be valid observations; however, this information must be used and applied logically to further understand the infectious basis of chronic disease. When the answer cannot be found, step back and look at a broader base of scientific knowledge, and ask broader questions. Discovery of the cause of chronic disease requires collaboration, and reasoning a possible solution from what is known, using reasonable inferences to direct research and combining the knowledge of all specialties. Discovery begins with understanding. As Louis Pasteur said, "In the fields of observation, chance favors only the prepared mind."

The endless details reported by researchers reflect the many observations of scientists, with varied interests and in various specialties, describing the effects of immortal infections at a microscopic level. We do not dispute the small details of cell microbiology, abnormal proteins, and inflammation, as true. We agree the details are helpful to understanding the whole person and chronic disease, and believe the small details confirm the principle of the whole is true. Research cannot seem to move toward understanding why these small details in microbiology occur; or seem able to reason the causes of chronic diseases from the small details and known constructs in science. Infectious pathogens are the root cause of many chronic diseases, and cause many of the small details scientists observe; yet, infectious pathogens are not being considered as the root cause of the small details observed in scientific research.

Dr. Ewald argued the narrow thought process of doctors is preventing recognition of infection as a cause of chronic disease. He argued doctors have a bias against accepting pathogens as a cause of disease, because it was not taught in textbooks in medical school. "The scientific community wants to look at the workings of disease at the cellular and biochemical level, in hopes that solutions will eventually emerge." "Scientists are working in building block mode". However, "fundamental achievements have occurred more through the testing of deductive leaps than by building-block induction". He argued the medical community needs to move beyond "correlations" and "associations", and use deductive leaps to make fundamental achievements. Dr. Ewald noted three main categories researchers and doctors must consider in thinking about chronic disease: 1.) Inherited genes; 2.) Parasitic agents (including bacteria, viruses, fungi and protozoa); and 3.) Non-living environmental factors. He urged doctors to ask if all three areas have been investigated. Scientists tend to believe when they have found evidence in category one or three, they can ignore the possibility of category two—infectious pathogens causing chronic disease.[336]

Dr. Ewald argued the omission of research into infectious pathogens is a fundamental problem in medicine, causing misunderstanding as to the

---

[336] Ewald PW. 2002. <u>Plague Time: The New Germ Theory</u>. 2nd Ed. Anchor Books.

cause of most chronic diseases. He gave the example of ulcers, for which doctors denied infectious causes for decades; and even after H-pylori was proven to cause ulcers, it took decades for treatment of ulcers as an infection to reach mainstream medicine. Chronic fatigue was labeled psychosomatic, and is now recognized as a serious illness, without a known cause. He questioned inflammation as a diagnosis, and asked what is causing the inflammation, and proposed the question of whether infection was causing the inflammation? He asked how defective genes could cause chronic disease, without the chronic disease being eliminated in the population, within a few generations. He predicted many chronic diseases would ultimately be proven to be caused by infectious pathogens, based on his intellect, knowledge of zoology and evolutionary biology, and common sense. Dr. Ewald discerned chronic disease has infectious causes, without being a medical doctor and without knowing the pathogens, because he thought deeply about it and came from a zoology background. The fundamental truth of infectious causes of chronic disease can be discerned by anyone with a sufficient scientific background and knowledge, and an interest in knowing, by studying what is already known.

The scientific method is not being applied in medical research, in accord with the standards of the scientific method. Interpretation of findings, measurement of deductions drawn from the hypothesis, and refinement of the hypothesis based on the experimental findings, are impacted by cognitive bias, cognitive assumptions, and rigid medical thinking. Rigid skepticism and formulating new constructs from known constructs has been lost. Research is limited to narrow questions and observations; and limits researchers to publicizing risk factors for diseases and "associations", rather than causes of chronic disease. Researchers are averse to reporting a "cause" of anything, and particularly averse when the conclusion may be contradicted by research into other infectious causes of the same disease. When more than one pathogen and more than one combination of pathogens can cause the same chronic disease, the scientific method does not work well.

The quantity of research knowledge is being confused with the quality of research knowledge. The quantity of knowledge has not advanced medical care, or advanced knowledge concerning the cause and cure of chronic disease. Billions are spent on research, which has vastly expanded the quantity of knowledge but not answered the bigger questions, or questions of most importance to the patient—what causes chronic disease, and how to prevent, mitigate and cure chronic disease. Billions are spent on research, but where are the changes, improvements, and advancements, in medical care? Billions are spent on research to derive findings already known in other specialties, and duplicating research. Research keeps being repeated and keeps observing the same findings, but a general theory never seems to be developed to answer important questions. How many times must Alzheimer's brains be examined at autopsy and chlamydia pneumonia found beneath plaque and in surrounding tissue; and how many times must we find infectious pathogens in cardiovascular tissue, before we can move forward and state chlamydia pneumonia causes heart disease and Alzheimer's, and proceed with research into effective treatment of chlamydia pneumonia, in heart disease and Alzheimer's disease.

Medical researchers live in a universe of complicated thought, in desperate need of structure for knowledge, and a coherent theory of chronic disease. Modern medicine replaced the art of medicine with cognitive assumptions, small details in microbiology, abnormal proteins, inflammation, abnormal genes, gene expression, mapping biomes (microbiome, mycobiome, proteinbiomes, and inflammasomes), defining Cluster Differentiations, and the use of impressive technology. The abnormal proteins in the proteinbiome, the inflammasomes, and Cluster Differentiations are the manifestation of different pathogens in different people, and different combinations of pathogens, in people with a different medical history and genetic background. It is time to re-direct research to infectious causes of chronic disease, correlating the small details with pathogens, and finding better ways to diagnose and treat immortal infections and parasites.

Researchers should be investigating causes and cures, finding new methods of diagnosis, and finding the best treatment for chronic infections causing chronic disease. Researchers should be determining which immortal pathogens cause which chronic diseases, infect which immune cells, and cause which abnormal proteins; and which abnormal proteins have a predilection for which genes, how best to treat immortal infection, and how to eradicate abnormal proteins.

The answer is not in the small details of cell microbiology, inflammation and genes, or in pooled studies and meta-data. The cause of cancer cannot be found by the cancer specialty, because the cause of cancer is not within the domain of the cancer specialty. Gastroenterologists cannot solve the problem of chronic gastrointestinal disease, because they ignore infection with immortal pathogens and parasites, deny infectious causes, and fail to use diagnostic tools and medications available to them. Mental health professionals are not able to find the causes of mental illnesses, because they ignore medical illness, and do not even try to diagnose immortal pathogens, even the immortal pathogens and parasites known to cause mental illness. Obstetricians cannot find the cause of reproductive disorders, autism, and birth defects, because they are not trained nor aware of infectious causes of chronic disease, or infectious causes of abnormalities in the fetus; and do not test the mothers or infants for important immortal pathogens that can cause adverse outcomes in pregnancy and in infants. Ophthalmologists cannot find the cause of chronic eye disease because the ophthalmology is focused on surgery, and the cause of chronic eye diseases are outside the specialty of ophthalmology.

Research needs to be coordinated across specialties and seek answers to broader questions, using a broader base of knowledge, to find patterns and derive hypotheses that can be tested. We need cohesive thinking and collaboration, using a principle of the whole. We need reasoning, creative thinking, and applying a broader scope of understanding, to direct research toward conquering chronic disease.

Research can't seem to move from research to practice, from conference to knowledge, or from talk to application. Meaningful discoveries in research need to reach the front-line practitioner; and meaningful "associations" need to become coherent theories of causation and be implemented into diagnosis and treatment, in routine practice. Research should be informed and directed by the knowledge, observations, and experience of the practitioner. We need new methods for doctors to share and discuss visionary ideas, and disseminate ideas about what works in medical practice. Researchers need a method for practitioners to report observations and experience in treating chronic disease; and take observation and experience from the bedside back to the research laboratory. Consider old wisdom, consider a broad base of knowledge, including knowledge by veterinarians, and reason toward a solution to find the cause of chronic disease. Look at extraordinary clinical outcomes in real patients with chronic diseases, to reason the causes and best practices in treating the patients; and ask if the clinical outcomes can aid in understanding the infectious cause of chronic diseases.

Research is not provided to practitioners, in the form of practical solutions; or it takes decades for new knowledge to be incorporated into mainstream medicine. Even if research identifies infectious causes of chronic disease, the research rarely provides an answer on how to proceed, because the original research only identified pathogens "associated" with a chronic disease and did move forward with treatment of the animal or patient, to confirm the causation by the success of treatment. Research has to first be reported, and possibly a different researcher would thereafter attempt research on possible treatment, years later. Doctors do what they are taught, without deviation, and will seldom act until told conclusively that a pathogen causes a disease. "Associations" are only seen as interesting, while doctors wait for an answer and direction on diagnosis and treatment.

We need researchers to give meaningful direction to practitioners, in the treatment of patients, even if the pathogen is only reported as an "association". We need researchers who discover an "association" to then proceed to determine if treatment benefits the patients, to confirm a cause. Research should incorporate observation and reasoning, diagnosis of pathogens, and reports of success in treating the patients, from practitioners, to direct further research. Research needs to benefit patients, and not just the esoteric accumulation of vast quantities of knowledge and observations of minute details. Effective treatment is what is important to the patient.

Describing associations instead of causes does not benefit the patient, and the problem of "associations" rather than causes is apparent in many specialties. In psychiatry, where pathogens, and particularly toxoplasmosis, have been reported in numerous different mental illnesses, the psychiatrist does not diagnose or treat toxoplasmosis. In rheumatology, cardiology, and ophthalmology, pathogens have been reported to be "associated" with chronic diseases, and no one acts to diagnose and treat the chronic diseases. In obstetrics, immortal pathogens can cause devastating outcomes in the fetus; yet, no one acts to diagnose and treat the pregnant mother or fetus. In endocrinology, pathogens in diabetic patients continue to spread because the pathogens are not diagnosed and treated. In cancer, infectious pathologies have been identified, and practitioners do not act on that information to diagnose and treat infectious pathogens. In virtually every disease in which pathogens have been identified or "associated", from autism to Alzheimer's, practitioners do not diagnose and treat the pathogens, which are the root cause of the disease.

It took medical science fifty years of observation, before accepting rheumatic fever was caused by an acute streptococcus infection. It took fifty years of observation, before accepting shingles was caused by the chicken pox virus, erupting decades after the acute infection. It took fifty years to accept ulcers were caused by infection, and eighteen years after Dr. Marshall proved ulcers were caused by H-pylori, before treatment of ulcers as an infection was implemented in practice. It took fifty years to recognize a particular virus in chickens caused cancer. Repeating the same thing, over and over, will not lead to new ideas or new ways to diagnose and treat chronic disease; and enforcing outdated medical thinking will not produce new ideas. Hopefully, it will not take fifty years to implement changes in the diagnosis and treatment of immortal pathogens causing chronic disease, in research and in practice.

Important research discoveries have been made that were tainted by bias, in favor of genetic causes and cognitive assumptions embedded in medical training and specialization. Recent cancer research, at UCSF, is an example of the impact of research bias, cognitive assumptions, and fragmentation of knowledge by different specialties. The UCSF study examined tissue adjacent to the margins of cancer, in the eight most common types of cancers—lung, colon, breast, uterine, liver, bladder, prostate and thyroid. Cancers in the breast, colon, liver, lung, and uterus had more distinct boundaries in adjacent tissue; and cancers of the prostate and thyroid had more diffuse boundaries. The adjacent tissue was not normal and was not cancer; and was thought to be somewhere between normal and cancer. At the molecular level, tissue adjacent to the cancer was found to have essentially the same "molecular signature" across all major types of cancer. The UCSF Study concluded all cancers used similar strategies to alter tissue outside the boundaries of the tumor; and all cancers used the same mechanisms to remodel normal tissue and spread.[337]

The UCSF Study found tissue adjacent to cancer had immune cells attached to the cells. The adjacent cells were thought to be under the influence of cancer-related stress signals that included oxygen deprivation and abnormal cell death (loss of apoptosis); and mature cells returned to an embryonic state, from which the cells could proliferate into cancer cells. TNF-alpha was highly expressed in seven of eight samples; and researchers suggested an inflammatory signaling pathway, possibly regulated by TNF-alpha. In breast tumors, the researchers found a gene expression, particularly in endothelial cells lining the interior of blood vessels. The researchers theorized the tumors were acting on the blood vessels of surrounding tissue, to remodel tissue, by the same processes used in formation of the tumor. The researchers theorized genes involved in the acute phase of systemic inflammation were turned on, and created a pattern in surrounding tissue that was distinct from both tumors and healthy tissue. They theorized tumors may be instigating inflammation, and other cancer-related processes in surrounding tissues, to facilitate spread. The conclusion was the cancer cells were sending signals to adjacent tissue, to facilitate the spread of cancer; and to make blood vessels grow

---

[337] *See* Butte A, *et al.* 2018. Big Data Shows How Cancer Interacts With Its Surroundings, *A New Analysis Reveals All Major and Solid Tumors Follow the Same Process.* Report of the Distinguished Professor of the Priscilla Chan and Mark Zuckerberg, UCSF Department of Pediatrics. Cancer Health. Laura Kurtzman. January 2, 2018; *first published*, USCF News Center (UCSF Study). Doi: https://www.cancerhealth.com/article/big-data-shows-cancer-interacts-surroundings.

in nearby tissue. The next step in the research was to find out how the signaling was done from the cancer to the surrounding tissue, and to try to find the effected genes.[338]

Researcher bias and cognitive assumptions significantly impacted the conclusions. The researchers saw changes in cells adjacent to cancer, and thought cancer was directing the changes. They saw immune cells attached to the outside of the adjacent cells, and thought it was inflammatory signaling, by the cancer. (Microbes on the outside of the tumor were described by Dr. William Russell, in 1890.) They saw inflammation, and thought the cancer was directing the inflammation. They found TNF-alpha, and thought the cancer caused an increase in TNF-alpha. They saw low oxygen in adjacent cells and abnormal apoptosis, and thought it was caused by a cancer stress signal. (Low oxygen and fermentation, in cancer, were described Dr. Otto Warburg, in 1930.) They saw angiogenesis and thought the cancer was causing the new blood vessels to form. They saw endothelial changes, inside blood vessels, and thought cancer was directing the change, to facilitate spread of the cancer. Dr. Mathupala reported, in 2010, aberrant sugar metabolism changes the microenvironment in adjacent tissue, fostering spread of the cancer[339], consistent with intracellular chlamydia. The narrow focus, cognitive assumptions, and confirmation bias of the researchers caused them to attribute all the findings in adjacent tissue to solely be from cancer stress signals and gene expression.

Bias and specialty training prevented recognition the molecular findings matched those of chlamydia, and prevented pursuing investigation into the infectious cause of cancer, which could have been found by examining adjacent cells for intracellular pathogens. Chlamydia pathogens cause the same molecular findings the UCSF study found in tissue adjacent to cancer. Chlamydia depletes the cell of ATP, and deprives the cell of oxygen by destroying oxygen transport across the cell wall. Chlamydia damages the ability of the cell to generate energy. Chlamydia consumes sugar and

---

[338] *Id.*

[339] Mathupala S, *et al.* 2010. The Pivotal Roles of Mitochondria in Cancer: Warburg and Beyond and Encouraging Prospects for Effective therapies. Biochimica et Biophysica Acta 1797. 2010. 1225-1230. Doi: 10.1016/j.bbabio.2010.03.025.

causes fermentation. Chlamydia impairs normal apoptosis, and infected cells replicate and create weaker immortal cells infected with the same pathogen. Chlamydia causes angiogenesis, generating new blood vessel formation. Chlamydia causes elevated TNF-alpha and inflammation. Chlamydia generates abnormal proteins and debris that attach to and alter genes and gene signaling. Chlamydia causes inclusion bodies that can become a focus for development of cancer. The immune system attacks the intracellular chlamydia pathogen, causing inflammation and infectious byproducts; and immune cells, including macrophages, attach to adjacent infected tissue.[340]

The molecular findings in tissue adjacent to cancer were identical to molecular findings caused by chlamydia pathogens. The surrounding tissue in all cancers appeared the same, because all cancer is caused by the same mechanism—chronic infection with immortal pathogens. The adjacent cells are the micro-tumors, in which chlamydia signaling has already damaged the microbiology of the cell and created a micro-environment necessary to support further growth and the metastasis of cancer. Infected weak replicas of infected cells inside the tumor, and adjacent cells, are infected with the intracellular pathogen, continue to signal immune responses to attack the tumor and adjacent cells; and continue to generate angiogenesis, apoptosis, and TNF-alpha, which fosters the growth and spread of the tumor. The tumor is where the longstanding warfare between the immune system and the pathogens persisted; and infected cells, infectious debris, and dead byproducts compressed and formed a tumor. The UCSF study provides important clues to the pathogenesis of cancer, and could be continued to search for and identify infectious pathogens in adjacent tissue. If UCSF examines adjacent tissue for intracellular pathogens, intracellular immortal pathogens can be proven to be a cause of cancer.

Cancer is caused by the immune system battle against immortal intracellular pathogens, creating a tightly compacted toxic ball of infected immortal cells, fungus, debris, and byproducts of the immune battle. The

---

[340] Kern J, *et al.* 2009. Chlamydia Pneumoniae-Induced Pathological Signaling in the Vasculature. FEMS Immunology & Medical Microbiology. Mar 1, 2009. Vol 55 (2):131-139. Doi: doi.org/10.1111/j.1574-695X.2008.00514.x.

intracellular pathogen in adjacent cells and the intracellular pathogen in cells already incorporated into the tumor, which have lost apoptosis, are continuing to signal the immune system to fight, directing tumor development, and building the tumor, from the remnants of the immune battle! Cancer is the end-stage of a longstanding immortal infection, and the war between the immortal pathogens and the immune system. Cancer is the end stage of a battle within, in which the pathogen has won.

Two other studies had findings of relevance, similar to the UCSF Study, and support an infectious cause of cancer that could be discovered in adjacent tissue. Polyps found adjacent to colon cancer had different "genetic" properties than polyps which were benign and harmless, but were not normal. The study did not report the molecular characteristics in adjacent polyps, other than assuming the adjacent polyps were caused by abnormal genes. The adjacent tissue was likely infected with the same pathogens or parasites causing the colon cancer; and the infection altered genes and gene expression in adjacent tissue, if genes played a role in the cancer.[341] In the study of Alzheimer's brains, Brian Balin, D.O. and his team, at Johns Hopkins and the Hahnemann School of Medicine, identified chlamydia pneumonia in tissue adjacent to Alzheimer's plaque. The study of adjacent tissue appears to be a fertile source for research into the pathogenesis of chronic disease, considering adjacent tissue in eight types of cancer all had molecular changes consistent with chlamydia; tissue adjacent to Alzheimer's plaque and tangles were infected with chlamydia pneumonia; and polyps adjacent to colon cancer has unusual findings suggestive of immortal pathogens in colon cancer.

The bias, cognitive assumptions, and specialization of investigators has hampered the investigation of two clusters of eye cancer in Alabama and North Carolina. The chief investigators, the Department of Health, the CDC, and the lead ophthalmologist and oncologist, jumped to the conclusion the cause was environmental or genetic, and did not consider

---

[341] Mayo Clinic Network. 2018. Researchers Identify Genes Found in Colon Polyps: Determining The Risk For Cancer Can Have Many Benefits. Doi: https://www.abqjournal.com/1156867/researchers-identify-genes-found-in-colon-polyps-ex-determining-the-risk-for-cancer-can-have-significant-benefits.html.

an infectious cause. They overlooked infectious causes, and looked only at environment and genes. The initial report of scientific findings, before starting the investigation, to direct the investigation, did not list a single infectious causes. The investigators created a questionnaire for victims and did not list a single infectious cause or questions directed to a single infectious cause! The Health Department and CDC were focused on environment factors, the ophthalmologist was not trained in infectious disease or cancer, and the oncologist was not trained in infectious disease or ophthalmology. The lead ocular melanoma researcher was quoted saying she had no clues and no leads into the cause.[342] Bias, cognitive assumptions, and doing what they always do, prevented consideration of the most likely cause of the eye cancer cluster.

A reasonable investigation of the scientific literature should have revealed the five most common infectious pathogens "associated" with eye cancer, fowl get the same type of eye cancer, and that melanoma is "associated" with psittacosis. None of the investigators had an understanding of infectious causes of cancer, had knowledge five pathogens were already reported to be "associated" with eye cancer, or that the bird form of chlamydia, chlamydia psittacosis, can cause eye cancer and does cause the same eye cancer in birds. Infectious causes of melanoma and melanoma of the eye have been reported in scientific publications, along with the risk of co-infections with different serovars or immortal pathogens, which can mix and change phenotypes, to create more virulent pathogens. None of the investigators had a broad knowledge of eyes, cancer, and infectious disease; or an understanding of chlamydia psittacosis causing eye cancer, melanoma, lymphoma, liver cancer or pancreatic cancer. None of the investigators considered infectious causes, or solutions through treatment of infectious pathogens and eradication of the source and vectors of the pathogen. While the investigators search in the wrong direction, patients were not diagnosed or treated for psittacosis, and several victims have developed new types of cancers, which can also be caused by untreated chlamydia psittacosis.

---

[342] Dodd J and Herbst D. 2018. Deadly Cancer Crisis: Medical Mystery on Campus. People Magazine. Aug 4, 2018. P. 74-77.

The most likely pathogen causing the eye cancer is a serovar of psittacosis, which explains both causation and virulence, in Auburn and Huntersville; and a high rate of the same type of eye cancer in Vietnam veterans, and in Italy. Ironically, the initial environmental survey of the Auburn and Huntersville cancer victims has now revealed the raptors as a "surprising" common link.[343] Yes—it was and is the birds! Yet, investigators are still pursuing geo-social mapping and genetic causes, without investigating bird pathogens, which are known to cause both eye cancer and melanoma, and to which the victims were likely exposed.

Established charitable and research foundations, and the government, consume millions of dollars, without producing useful discoveries or treatment suggestions. Bill Gates recently donated $100,000,000 for Alzheimer's research, to find the cause of Alzheimer's. Neither the Alzheimer's Foundation nor Alzheimer's research has provided clear answers on the cause of Alzheimer's, or revealed how best to diagnose or treat Alzheimer's disease. The cause of Alzheimer's is already known— chronic chlamydia pneumonia causes Alzheimer's! Retinal scans can reveal Alzheimer's risk decades before Alzheimer's symptoms develop; can predict cardiovascular risk; and can predict the risk of a heart attack, in the next five years. A retinal scan and a PCR test for chlamydia pneumonia should inform which patients can benefit by treatment for chlamydia pneumonia, to prevent or delay Alzheimer's. More money to repeat existing research and again confirm chlamydia pneumonia causes Alzheimer's will not lead to important discoveries unless the money is given with conditions on how it will be used—to search for methods of early diagnosis, discover who benefits by treatment, and the best and most effective treatment, based on what is already known. Money can be used to spread the knowledge that Alzheimer's can be detected prior to symptoms, by performing a retinal scan and PCR blood test or PCR swab test.

Evidence based medicine involves standards compiled by specialty groups, from a complex array of studies. Evidence based medicine can be an obstacle to the evolution of scientific knowledge, because it leads to stagnation of

---

[343] Brennan, M. May 31, 2018. Doi: Slide 9. Doi: slideshare.net/Melanoma ResearchFoundation/ocular-melanoma-cluster-update.

knowledge, as doctors are required to conform to the standards. Insurance companies and Medicare use the standards to further enforce conformity, which is another obstacle to new discovery. Thinking, creativity, and common sense have been replaced by computer screens and templates, the technological imperative, insurance company directives as to care, and a profit motive by all. Observational and experiential medicine has been rejected, in favor of complicated small details of no benefit to patients.

Medicine has to evolve and become more open minded and creative, about infectious causes of chronic disease; or all we get is more expensive, ineffective medicine, and more chronic disease. All diseases without known causes; all diseases named based on symptoms, findings, and syndromes; and all diseases named after a doctor, should be re-examined for infectious causes. We need to move toward research, diagnosis, and treatment of the root causes of chronic disease, to find better treatments and cures, to improve health and the quality of life of patients, and extend longevity.

Research is needed into new and known species of chlamydia pathogens and parasites, which may cross over to humans and cause chronic disease. The lack of testing for additional chlamydia species, which are known but not part of routine PCR blood testing, leads to the mistaken belief the infections are not present in humans, are asymptomatic, and/or do not harm humans. Some denied chlamydia *suis* could infect humans, which was disproven by the experience in the United Kingdom. Routine PCR screening for more chlamydia species, such as chlamydia *suis* and chlamydia abortus, should be part of routine chlamydia antibody panels or available when needed; and new species should be added to PCR testing when new species are discovered.

Intensive research and study of the microbiome and mycobiome is needed, to identify all good bacteria and fungus; and identify bacteria that change molecular signals and gene expressions, and affect hormones. We need to understand how to heal the microbiome and develop strains of bacteria, which are not yet available in probiotics, to replace important strains of bacteria killed by antibiotics or chemotherapy. Research into the microbiome may reveal natural ways to prevent, treat and mitigate chronic infection, using good bacteria to fight pathogens. Research into the microbiome could lead to discovery of natural ways to halt virulent pathogens; and encourage less harmful pathogens in the microbiome, most able to resist pathogenic bacteria. Study of the microbiome could lead to alternatives to antibiotics.

Research is needed to know the best and most effective ways to treat chronic infections, and the impact on chronic disease. We need improved and expanded research to find new antibiotics, treatment of antibiotic resistance, treatment of antibiotic side effects, and alternatives to antibiotics. We need antibiotics, which can penetrate the cell wall and kill immortal pathogens, kill intracellular pathogens in professional immune cells; and kill intracellular pathogens in the lining of vessels, inside smooth muscles, in the gastrointestinal tract, from under biofilm, in the joints, in the eyes, and in the central nervous system. We need to find ways to interrupt the infectious cascade to defeat the pathogen; and find ways to remove abnormal proteins and infectious byproducts. One thing is absolutely clear—we need to stop giving eight times more antibiotics to animals than to people; and stop using penicillin and broad-spectrum antibiotics as the first-line, standard-of-care choice of drugs for acute infection. Penicillin use should be limited to specific pathogens, which are proven by culture.

Science knows patients treated with a macrolide or doxycycline, in the prior three years, have a reduced risk for cardiovascular disease and cardiovascular events. Science knows low-dose doxycycline improves many chronic conditions, from acne and rosacea, to orbitopathy, to multiple sclerosis, and potentially Parkinson's. A careful prospective research study of patients with chronic diseases, will likely prove higher infectious burdens are correlated with chronic disease; and patients who have been treated with macrolides and doxycycline have less chronic disease and greater longevity than patients who have been treated with penicillin or cephalosporin. In heart studies, those treated with penicillin developed chronic fatigue or died. In the study of childhood pneumonia, children who had been hospitalized, or seen on an emergency for pneumonia, had an increased risk of developing cancer, and it is likely some of the children were treated with penicillin. Research could disclose if the super-aging individuals avoided immortal infection, and/or were treated with macrolides or cyclines when acutely ill; and discover how they adapted to chronic infection.

Research to identify which abnormal proteins are attached to, generated, or created by which pathogens, could provide new avenues for diagnosis, based on the findings of particular abnormal proteins. Research could find methods to clear abnormal proteins and byproducts generated by immortal pathogens. Removing abnormal proteins and infectious byproducts could aid in preventing chronic disease, mitigate chronic disease, and improve the prognosis of chronic disease.

Medical research needs to investigate the drugs we have for new indications, and seek to repurpose existing drugs for chronic disease. We need to repurpose and use the drugs we have for new indications—specifically, for treating immortal pathogens! Manufacturers should seek new indications for current drugs; and bring back drugs removed from the market or made prohibitively expensive, which are now recognized to have new relevance to chronic disease. Manufacturers should re-market and repurpose drugs, such as azithromycin, clarithromycin, doxycycline, mebendazole, albendazole, metronidazole, Imervectin, and imiquimod, for chronic diseases. The most underutilized drugs we have are macrolides and doxycycline, topical antibiotics, metronidazole, antiparasitic drugs, antivirals, and antifungals. Antiparasitic drugs are being used in clinical studies, to treat many diseases, and are being shown effective against cancer and other chronic and fatal diseases.[344] Doctors should first use the medications we have, known to be safe and directed at the cause, before resorting to new, extremely potent, expensive, dangerous, toxic, and even potentially lethal medications.

Old remedies and simple remedies can be revived for new indications. Diatomaceous earth is an effective and inexpensive treatment for wound care and digestion. Diatomaceous earth causes granulation in a non-healing wound, and can help avoid amputations in diabetic patients. Bismuth (Pepto Bismol), in limited quantities, treats stomach ailments

---

[344] Andrews K, *et al.* 2014. Drug Repurposing and Human Parasitic Protozoan Diseases. International Journal for Parasitology: Drugs and Drug Resistance. 4: 95-111. Aug 2014. Doi: 10.1016/j.ijpddr.2014.02.002.

and reduces fungus. Pepto Bismol is a heavy metal, and can be toxic in some patients after excessive use. Drinking medical grade clay mixed with dilutions of liquid minerals, is reported to aid absorption of neurotoxins, in the gastrointestinal tract, and strengthen the microbiome. Homeopathic remedies may be useful, and herbal remedies have been used for centuries to reduce the infectious burden of parasites and expel worms.

Imiquimod crème is an old drug that has been vastly underutilized. Imiquimod helps the body fight disease, by attracting the body's white blood cells to the location where the crème is applied. Imiquimod is now being repurposed from the original indication for warts, to effective topical treatment for cancer that can kill cancer at the primary site, prevents or delays metastasis, and kills cancer at metastatic sites. The only explanation for topical imiquimod being effective against metastatic cancer is imiquimod modifies the body's own white blood cells, to recognize and attack cancer at metastatic sites. Imiquimod is targeted monoclonal antibody therapy, for cancer, at 1/1000th of the cost. A combination of imiquimod and an anti-vessel growth drug was injected into a primary lymphoma tumor, and cured lymphoma at the primary and metastatic sites. Imiquimod is already being used in many cancer clinical trials; and the use could be adapted and vastly expanded in oncology practice, to provide creative augmentation of cancer treatment. Imiquimod is already available in generic form, and the makers of imiquimod should expand marketing to all specialties, for use in all cancers.

Cognitive science tells us if you don't understand the flaws in reasoning, you will not be able to dislodge misconceptions and replace them with the correct concepts.[345] The longer the belief has been held, the more difficult it is to change someone's mind, no matter the evidence. President John Adams once said, "It is easier to fool someone, than to change a fool's mind", which reflects man's innate revulsion to admitting prior beliefs were wrong and changing one's mind. Medicine must open its mind to

---

[345] *See* Kamenetz A. 2016. Why Teachers Need To Know The Wrong Answers. NPR Ed. How Learning Happens. April 16, 2016. Philip Sadler. Professor at Harvard University. Doi: https://www.npr.org/sections/ed/2016/04/16/473273571/why-teachers-need-to-know-the-wrong-answers.

new ways of thinking about the diagnosis and treatment of chronic disease, and collective findings can change minds. Scientists must first understand, and can then begin to find causes and cures for chronic disease.

Our hope is researchers will conduct studies with new insight; and discover better ways to diagnose and treat immortal pathogens; and find ways to eradicate immortal pathogens from the immune cells, hidden in tissue, and under fungus, plaque and biofilm. We hope research will find the best use of antibiotics, and the best treatment regimens, in chronic disease. We hope research will expand what is known to find how best to remove abnormal proteins. We hope to encourage researchers and practitioners to be creative in thinking and reasoning, and use inductive reasoning based on known scientific constructs, to guide the future direction of research. Abandon old cognitive bias and cognitive assumptions, and abandon rigid medical thinking when the thinking is no longer accurate or logical. Return to rigid skepticism of what is reported, and discern the answer from knowledge, reason, and common sense. Let researchers and let doctors return to the art of medicine, to improve the health and longevity of patients.

> *The value of experience is not in seeing much, but in seeing wisely.*

Sir William Osler, MD

CHAPTER 27

CONCLUSION

Dr. Merchant worked with and applied the principle of infectious causes of chronic diseases, during his forty-three years of medical practice. He observed improved patient outcomes, in a wide variety of chronic diseases, when patients were diagnosed and treated for immortal pathogens. He saw chronic diseases of unknown origin and thought untreatable improve or resolve with treatment. He saw co-morbid conditions disappear with treatment of the presenting chronic disease. He applied the principle of the whole, that chronic infection causes chronic disease, and diagnosed and treated the pathogens causing chronic disease. He observed the success of treatment, in diseases of unknown origin, in diseases thought untreatable, and in diseases thought hopeless.

The medical system today observes findings and details, names diseases, and treats symptoms, but does not contemplate what causes these findings. Diseases caused by infectious animal pathogens have been divided into thousands of differently named diseases, based on the specialty making the diagnosis, body part involved, and the symptoms and findings. Diseases caused by infectious animal pathogens have been blamed on faulty genes, which is only partly true because the animal pathogens are what altered the genes and gene expression; or the diseases caused by animal pathogens are attributed to unknown causes. Diseases have been named based on symptoms or named after a doctor who described the symptoms, and no one has since investigated infectious causes with modern technology to find pathogens.

The medical system has a study for everything, and a conclusion on causation for almost nothing. Alternative studies with almost opposite conclusions can be found on the same issues. The history of medicine suggests old studies will eventually be contradicted by new studies. Medical literature and texts report infinite small details, and researchers continue to repeat past studies. The authors of medical literature avoid conclusions or reports of a cause for any disease; and if authors report a particular antibiotic treatment was effective in a particular chronic disease, still do not direct practitioners to act on that knowledge to diagnose and treat patients. No one observes or reports on the bigger questions of causation, or directs doctors to diagnose and treat patients for infectious animal pathogens.

It is time for specialties to combine their knowledge, collaborate, and act as a team, to find the infectious causes and cures for chronic disease. It is time for doctors and researchers to collaborate in the direction of research, to benefit patients. Discovery through collaboration must include a broad range of specialties, front line-practitioners, pharmacists, veterinarians, and Ph.D.'s, to discover the infectious causes of chronic disease and the best treatment options, for patients. Veterinary literature contains important information on immortal pathogens which can inform medicine about the causes of chronic disease.

Chronic disease is caused by chronic infection. All chronic diseases are a form of autoimmune disease, because chronic disease develops from the longstanding immune system war against immortal intracellular pathogens. The pathogens invade the body; the immune system attacks the pathogens; the pathogens infect the immune system; the infection spreads through the cardiovascular system, immune system, and tissue, by migration and metastasis; and the infection causes an infectious cascade that eventually becomes a chronic disease. From conception to death, we acquire infectious pathogens. The pathogens and combination of pathogens we acquire, and the age at which pathogens are acquired, determine the development of chronic disease. How the patient and their medical providers treat the immortal infections, affects how chronic disease develops. Avoidance of the most virulent and avoidable infections; and avoidance of pathogens acquired from pets and domesticated animals, particularly cats and birds, improve the chances for avoiding chronic disease and living a long and healthy life.

All chronic diseases are inter-related in the findings and symptoms, and have other chronic diseases as co-morbid conditions. Diseases caused by animal pathogens cause the same chronic diseases in humans as the pathogens cause in animals. All chronic diseases have common symptoms and findings of high inflammatory markers, abnormal proteins, high TNF-alpha, and chronic fatigue—which can all be caused by immortal intracellular chlamydia pathogens. It is time to abandon meaningless findings, symptoms, and syndromes; and endless naming of diseases. It is time to begin to diagnose and treat the root infectious causes of chronic diseases, not just prescribe indefinite symptomatic treatment. The medical system must pursue diagnosis of the infectious causes of chronic disease, as part of the diagnosis of all chronic diseases.

PCR blood tests and PCR swabs can diagnose immortal pathogens and parasites, and PCR swabs can diagnose immortal pathogens with limited fluid from any portal in the body. Super-computers can diagnose hundreds of pathogens in blood, and help identify the specific pathogens and combinations of pathogens, which cause specific chronic diseases. The medical system and researchers need to use the tools available to diagnose immortal pathogens, and make the testing for immortal pathogens more available in medical practice. The medical system has no excuse for *not* performing PCR testing for immortal pathogens and parasites, with the tools available, on patients with chronic disease.

Patients deserve more effort at diagnosis of immortal pathogens; and deserve treatment of immortal pathogens, to prevent, delay and mitigate chronic disease. Patients can apply the Principle of the Whole and common sense to avoid the avoidable immortal infections, understand the need to treat immortal infections, avoid penicillin as much as possible, seek diagnosis of causes and not symptoms, question doctors; and find ways to adapt to chronic infection through exercise, diet, and lifestyle, to extend healthy aging and longevity.

We hope to spread a new vision in the diagnosis and treatment of chronic disease. We want medicine to open its mind to new ideas, about infectious causes of chronic disease. We hope patients will be better able to understand their own diseases, advocate for themselves; and doctors will find innovative solutions to help patients. We offer hope to sufferers of chronic disease, to the Auburn and Huntersville ocular melanoma victims, and to the veterans of foreign wars whose medical illnesses have not been diagnosed and misdiagnosed as mental illness. We offer more effective, and more cost-effective approaches to chronic disease. We offer new approaches to medical research, and the potential for important discoveries about the cause and cure of chronic disease.

It has been hard for us to watch unnecessary suffering, and watch terrible things happen to friends, and good people that potentially could have been avoided or helped by prompt diagnosis and treatment, of acute and chronic infection. It is hard to watch patients who are helpless against a difficult and narrow minded medical system, offering symptomatic treatment for chronic disease without searching for an infectious cause. It is hard to watch people refuse to treat infectious causes of chronic disease out of fear, bias, and misplaced trust in their doctor; always believing they have the best doctor who did all the tests and could not give an explanation for their disease.

Dr. Blount and Dr. di Fabio were right when they said it was difficult to watch the suffering, knowing the close-minded thinking in the medical community was denying patients available and inexpensive treatment that could cure or mitigate their suffering.[346] Our four decades of observational science, watching the suffering and observing the successes, fueled our desire to speak out.

In forty years of study, and eighty years of combined observation, questioning, researching, and experience, we have been unable to disprove chronic infection with animal pathogens cause chronic disease. We do not want our knowledge and experience to be lost, and feel a moral obligation to share our knowledge. We are compelled by a desire to help others, to speak the truth about what we know. We want to move beyond helping one person at a time, to helping a greater number of people. It was our destiny

---

[346] Di Fabio A. 1982. Rheumatoid Diseases: Cured at Last. 4th ed. Franklin, TN: The Rheumatoid Disease Foundation.

to meet, in New Mexico. It was our destiny to contemplate the issues of chronic disease together, combining our unique knowledge, skills, and approach to inquiry and understanding.

Go forth to diagnose and treat immortal infections, to reduce the worldwide burden of chronic disease. Observe the success from diagnosing and treating immortal pathogens, in chronic disease. Gain wisdom from experience and observation. It's all about infection, and the response by the immune system to the pathogens!

> *It had long since come to my attention that people of accomplishment rarely sat back and let things happen to them. They went out and happened to things.*

Leonardo de Vinci

EPILOGUE

We reviewed and relied on more than fifteen hundred scientific articles, non-scientific articles, news reports, and more than twenty-five books and medical texts. Doctors, non-doctors, Ph.D. scientists and thinkers have provided research and commentary, with direct or indirect support for the principle of the whole. Many scientists and Nobel Prize winners contributed important knowledge, research, and discoveries that support the principles described in the book, directly or indirectly. Books have been written, conferences have been held, and scientific papers have been written. A compelling body of evidence has amassed over time, supporting chronic infection as the cause of chronic disease.

We want to thank everyone who worked over the years and published on related topics. We thank the many scientists, too many to name, whose research has supported our belief that infectious animal pathogens cause chronic disease. We can no longer recreate the many thousands of resources we viewed over forty years, or cite the many articles we saved. We apologize to the thousands of authors not cited, who may see their work in this book. If you see yourself, in our thoughts, feel free to claim your contribution and continue the conversation about the infectious causes of chronic disease.

We thank the many patients and their families, and clients and experts, for the support we received over many years, and the teaching they provided, in the course of our professional careers. We have benefited from what we learned from you, which has motivated us to use those lessons to help others.

It is not what you look at, it is what you see.

Henry David Thoreau

BIBLIOGRAPHY OF
CITATIONS

BOOKS

Breggin P. 2008. <u>Medication Madness, The Role of Psychiatric Drugs in Cases of Violence, Suicide, and Crime</u>. New York: St. Martin's Griffin.

Breggin P. 2013. <u>Psychiatric Drug Withdrawal, A Guide for Prescribers, Therapists, Patients, and Their Families</u>. New York: Springer Publishing Company.

Choplin N, Traverso C (*eds*). 2014. <u>Atlas of Glaucoma</u>, 3rd Edition. Boca Raton, FL: CRC Press.

Clark HR. 1995. <u>THE Cure for All Diseases, With Many Case Histories</u>. California: New Century Press.

Di Fabio A. 1982. <u>Rheumatoid Diseases: Cured at Last</u>. 4th ed. Franklin, TN: The Rheumatoid Disease Foundation.

Di Fabio A. 2017. <u>Rheumatoid Diseases Cured at Last</u>. Franklin, TN: The Arthritis Trust of America.

Dvonch LA, Dvonch R. 2003. <u>The Heart Attack Germ</u>. New York: Writer's Showcase.

Ewald PW. 1996. <u>Evolution of Infectious Disease</u>. New York: Oxford University Press.

Ewald PW. 2000. <u>Plague Time: How Stealth Infections Cause Cancers, Heart Disease and Other Deadly Ailments</u>. New York: Free Press, p. 57, 271.

Ewald PW. 2002. <u>Plague Time: The New Germ Theory</u>. 2nd Ed. Anchor Books.

Friedman H (*ed*), *et al.* 2004. <u>*Chlamydia Pneumonia* Infection and Disease</u>. New York: Kluwer Academic/Plenum Publishers. Chlamydia Pneumonia and Atherosclerosis—an Overview of the Association. (Ngeh J and Gupta S). Ch. 9. p. 113-114.

Friedman H (*ed*), *et al.* 2004. <u>Chlamydia Pneumonia Infection and Disease</u>. New York: Kluwer Academic/Plenum Publishers. The Biology of Chlamydia Pneumonia in Cardiovascular Disease Pathogenesis. (Ouellette SP, *et al.*). Ch. 10.

Friedman H (*ed*), *et al.* 2004. <u>Chlamydia Pneumonia Infection and Disease</u>. New York: Kluwer Academic/Plenum Publishers. Animal Models of Chlamydia Pneumonia Infection and Atherosclerosis. (Fong IW). Ch. 11.

Friedman H (*ed*), *et al.* 2004. <u>Chlamydia Pneumonia Infection and Disease</u>. New York: Kluwer Academic/Plenum Publishers. Antiinfective Trials for the Treatment of Chlamydia Pneumonia in Coronary Artery Disease. (Muhlestein JB). Ch. 12.

Friedman H (*ed*), *et al.* 2004. <u>*Chlamydia Pneumoniae* Infection and Disease</u>. New York: Kluwer Academic/Plenum Publishers. Chlamydia Pneumonia and Myocarditis. (Gnarpe JG and Gnarpe JA). Ch. 13. p. 187-193.

Friedman H *(ed)*, *et al.* 2004. <u>*Chlamydia Pneumoniae* Infection and Disease</u>. New York: Kluwer Academic/Plenum Publishers. Chlamydia Pneumonia and Myocarditis. (Gnarpe JG and Gnarpe JA). Ch. 13. p. 187-193.

Friedman H (*ed*), *et al.* 2004. <u>*Chlamydia Pneumoniae* Infection and Disease</u>. New York: Kluwer Academic/Plenum Publishers. Chlamydia Pneumonia as a Candidate Pathogen in Multiple Sclerosis. (Stratton CW and Siram S). Ch. 14.

Friedman H (*ed*), *et al.* 2004. <u>*Chlamydia Pneumonia* Infection and Disease</u>. New York: Kluwer Academic/Plenum Publishers. Chlamydia Pneumonia in the Pathogenesis of Alzheimers. (Balin BJ, *et al.*). Ch. 15.

Friedman H (*ed*), *et al.* 2004. <u>*Chlamydia Pneumoniae* Infection and Disease</u>. *New York: Kluwer Ac*ademic/Plenum Publishers. Chlamydia Pneumonia and Inflammatory Arthritis. (Whittum-Hudson JA and Schumacher HR). Ch. 16.

Friedman H (*ed*), *et al.* 2004. *Chlamydia Pneumoniae* Infection and Disease. New York: Kluwer Academic/Plenum Publishers. Chlamydia Pneumonia and Inflammatory Arthritis. (Whittum-Hudson JA and Schumacher HR). Ch. 16. p. 228-229.

Friedman H (*ed*), *et al.* 2004. *Chlamydia Pneumoniae* Infection and Disease. New York: Kluwer Academic/Plenum Publishers. Chlamydia Pneumonia and Inflammatory Arthritis. (Whittum-Hudson JA and Schumacher HR). Ch. 16. p. 230.

Friedman H (*ed*), *et al.* 2004. *Chlamydia Pneumoniae* Infection and Disease. New York: Kluwer Academic/Plenum Publishers. Chlamydia Pneumonia and Inflammatory Arthritis. (Whittum-Hudson JA and Schumacher HR). Ch. 16. p. 237.

Friedman H (*ed*), *et al.* 2004. *Chlamydia Pneumoniae* Infection and Disease. New York: Kluwer Academic/Plenum Publishers. Role of Chlamydia Pneumonia as an Inducer of Asthma. (Hahn DL). Ch. 17. p. 245-246.

Friedman H (*ed*), *et al.* 2004. *Chlamydia Pneumoniae* Infection and Disease. New York: Kluwer Academic/Plenum Publishers. Role of Chlamydia Pneumonia as an Inducer of Asthma. (Hahn DL). Ch. 17. p. 246.

Glidden B. 2010. The MD Emperor Has No Clothes-Everybody is Sick and I Know Why, 3rd Ed. San Bernardino, CA.

Greenwood D. *et al* (eds). 2012. Medical Microbiology. 18th Ed. 2012. Elsevier Ltd. Chlamydia. D. Mabey and Peeling RW.

Hippocrates. The Corpus, The Hippocratic Writings (Kaplan Classics of Medicine). 2008. NewYork: Kaplan Publishing

Jong E. 2016. I Contain Multitudes, The Microbes Within Us and a Grander View of Life. 1st ed. Harper Collins.

Knobler S (*ed*), *et al.* 2004. THE INFECTIOUS ETIOLOGY OF CHRONIC DISEASES: Defining the Relationship, Enhancing the Research, and Mitigating the Effects. National Institute of Medicine of the National Academics, Workshop Summary. Washington D.C.: The National Academies Press.

Krachmer J, Mannis M, and Holland E (*eds*). CORNEA, *Fundamentals, Diagnosis and Management*, 2nd Ed. 2005. Philadelphia: Elsevier Mosby. (Singal N, Rootman D). Ch. 51.

Krachmer J, Mannis M, and Holland E (*eds*). <u>CORNEA, *Fundamentals,*</u> <u>*Diagnosis and Management*</u>. 2nd Ed. 2005. Philadelphia: Elsevier Mosby. (Stoller GL, *et al.*). Ch. 66.

Krachmer J, Mannis M, and Holland E (*eds*). <u>CORNEA, *Fundamentals,*</u> <u>*Diagnosis and Management*</u>. 2nd Ed. 2005. Philadelphia: Elsevier Mosby. (Tauber J). Ch. 116.

L'age-Stehr J (*ed*). 2000. <u>*Chlamydia Pneumoniae* and Chronic Diseases</u>. Berlin Heidelberg New York: Springer-Verlag.

Lown B. 1999. <u>Lost Art of Healing, Practicing Compassion in Medicine</u>. New York: Ballantine Books.

Oz HS, *et al.* <u>*Toxoplasma gondii* (Toxoplasmosis)</u>, 2nd Ed. Doi: antimicrobe. org/new/b130.asp.

Sykes J, *et al.* 2016. <u>MERCK MANUAL: VETERINARY MANUAL</u>. 2016. 11TH ed. "Overview of Chlamydial Conjunctivitis" (Sykes J, *et al.*), Etiology and Epidemiology. Doi: merckvetmanual.com/eye-and-ear/chlamydial-conjunctivitis/ overview-of-chlamydial-conjunctivitis.

Mukherjee S. 2010. <u>The Emperor of All Maladies: A Biography of Cancer</u>. New York: Scribner.

Plank TH. 1926. <u>Actinotherapy and Allied Physical Therapy</u>. Chicago: Manz Corporation.

Rampton S, Stauber J. 2001. <u>Trust Us We're Experts: How Industry</u> <u>Manipulates Science and Gambles with Your Future</u>. New York: Tarcher/Putman.

Ruiz DM, Mills J. 2011. <u>The Four Agreements, A Practical Guide to</u> <u>Personal Freedom</u>. Amber-Allen Publishing. July 7, 2011.

Salgo P, Layden J. 2004. <u>The Heart of the Matter: The Three Key</u> <u>Breakthroughs to Preventing Heart Attacks</u>. New York: William Morrow.

Spatin D. *et al.* (*eds*). 2005. 3rd Ed. <u>Atlas of CLINICAL</u> <u>OPHTHALMOLOGY</u>. Spain: Elsevier Limited. Infections of the Outer Eye. (Larkin F, Hunter P). Ch. 4. p. 100-105.

Spatin D. *et al.* (*eds*). 2005. 3rd Ed. <u>Atlas of CLINICAL</u> <u>OPHTHALMOLOGY</u>. Spain: Elsevier Limited. Primary Glaucoma. (Garway-Heath D, Foster P, and Hitchings R). Ch. 7. p. 187-220, and 192, 233, 243.

Spatin D. *et al. (eds).* 2005. 3rd Ed. Atlas of CLINICAL OPHTHALMOLOGY. Spain: Elsevier Limited. Intraocular Inflammation (Stanford M, Spalton D). Ch. 10. p. 298, 300-311.

Stephens R (*ed*). 1999. CHLAMYDIA Intracellular Biology, Pathogenesis and Immunity. Washington, D.C.: ASM Press.

Storz J. 1971. Chlamydia and Chlamydia-Induced Diseases. Charles C. Thomas: Springfield, Illinois.

Summers A. 2014. COMMON DISEASES IN COMPANION ANIMALS, 3rd Ed. China: Mosby.

Sweet V. 2017. Slow Medicine, the Way to Healing. Riverhead Books.

Volpe G (Vincenzo Crespi, IV). 1853. Memoirs of an Ex-Capuchin.

Wilson JD, *et al.* (*ed*). 1991. Harrison's Principles of Internal Medicine, 12th edition. New York: McGraw-Hill, Inc. Extraintestinal Manifestations of Inflammatory Bowel Disease. p. 1278-1282.

Wyngaarden JB, Smith LH (*ed*). 1982. Cecil Textbook of Medicine, 18th Ed., Philadelphia: WB Saunders Company.

Wyngaarden JB, Smith LH (*ed*). 1988. Cecil Textbook of Medicine. 18th Ed. Part XII. Musculoskeletal and Connective Tissue Diseases. Philadelphia: WB Saunders Company. Rheumatoid Arthritis. (Bennett JC). Ch. XVI. p. 1999.

ARTICLES

2010. Animals Linked to Chlamydia Pneumoniae". Science Daily. Queensland University of Technology. Feb. 22, 2010. Doi: sciencedaily.com/releases/2010/02/100222094805.htm.

2013. A Super Brief and Basic Explanation of Epigenetics for Total Beginners. Doi: whatisepigenetics.com/what-is-epigenetics/.

2017. Q&A on Candida with the Scientist Who Named the Microbiome (Mahmoud Ghannoum, Ph.D.). SCIENCE. Doi: biohmhealth. com/blogs/science/a-q-a-on-candida-with-the-scientist-who-named-the-mycobiome.

2018. GBD 2016 Alcohol Collaborators. Alcohol Use and Burden for 195 Countries and Territories, 1990-2016: A Systematic Analysis For the Global Burden of Disease Study 2016. The Lancet. 2018. Doi: 10.1016/S0140-6736(18)31310-2; 2018. No Safe Level of Alchol,

New Study Concludes. ScienceDaily. Aug 24, 2018. Doi: https://www.sciencedaily.com/releases/2018/08/180824103018.htm.

Akcay E. *et al.* 2014. Impaired Corneal Biomechanical Properties and the Prevalence of Keratoconus in Mitral Valve Prolapse. Journal of Ophthalmology. Vol 2014. Article ID 402193. https://dx.doi.org/10.1155/2014/402193. Doi: https://dx.doi.org/10.1155/2014/402193.

Aldridge M, Kelley A. 2015. The Myth Regarding the High Cost of End-of-Life Care. Am J Public Health. December 2015; 105 (12): 2411-2415. Doi: ncbi.nlm.nih.gov/pmc/articles/PMC4638261/.

Amparao F, de Sao Palo E. 2017. Antibiotic Doxycycline May Offer Hope for Treatment of Parkinson's Disease. Science News. May 17, 2017. Doi: sciencedaily.com/releases/2017/05/170503134119.htm.

Anderson JL, *et al.* 1999. Randomized Secondary Prevention Trial of Azithromycin in Patients With Coronary Artery Disease and Serological Evidence for Chlamydia Pneumoniae Infection: The Azithromycin in Coronary Artery Disease: Elimination of Myocardial Infection With Chlamydia (ACADEMIC) Study. Circulation. Mar 1999. 30; 99 (12): 1540-7. Doi: https://doi.org/10.1161/circ.99.12.1540.

Andrews K, *et al.* 2014. Drug Repurposing and Human Parasitic Protozoan Diseases. International Journal for Parasitology: Drugs and Drug Resistance. Aug 2014. 4: 95-111. Doi: 10.1016/j.ijpddr.2014.02.002.

Apfalter P. 2006. Chlamydia Pneumoniae, Stroke, and Serological Associations, Anything Learned from the Atherosclerosis-Cardiovascular Literature or Do We Have to Start Over Again? Editorial. Stroke. 2006. 37:756. Doi: https://www.ahajournals.org/doi/abs/10.1161/01.str.0000201970.88546.5e.

Arking EJ, *et al.* 1999. Ultrastructural Analysis of Chlamydia Pneumoniae in the Alzheimer's Brain. Pathogenesis (Amst). 1999; 1(3): 201–211. PMID: 20671799: PMCID: PMC291092. PMC Jul 28, 2010.

Arthur J, *et al.* 2014. Microbial Genomic Analysis Reveals the Essential Role of Inflammation in Bacteria-Induced Colorectal Cancer. Nat Commun. 5:4724. Sep 3, 2014. Doi: 10.1038/ncomms5724.

Azpurua J, *et al.* 2013. Naked Mole-Rat Has Increased Translational Fidelity Compared with the Mouse, as Well as a Unique 28S Ribosomal RNA Cleavage. Proc Natl Acad Sci USA. 110(43):17350-5. Oct 22, 2013. Doi: 10.1073/pnas.1313473110. Epub 2013 Sep 30.

Bachmann N, *et al.* 2014. Comparative Genomics of Koala, Cattle and Sheep Strains of *Chlamydia Pecorum*. BMC Genomics. 2014. 15(1): 667. Doi: 10.1186/1471-2164-15-66.

Balin B, *et al.* 1998. Identification and localization of Chlamydia pneumoniae in the Alzheimer's brain. Med Microbiol Immunol. 1998 Jun; 187(1):23-42. PMID: 9749980.

Balin B, Appelt D. 2001. Role of infection in Alzheimer's disease. S2 JAOA. Vol 101. No 12. Supplement to December 2001. Part 1. PMID: 11794745.

Balin B, *et al.* 2008. Chlamydophila Pneumoniae and the Etiology of Late-Onset Alzheimer's Disease. Journal of Alzheimer's Disease. Apr 2008. Vol 13 (4): 381-391. Doi: 10.3233/JAD-2008-13403.

Batra R, *et al.* 2014. Ocular Surface Disease Exacerbated Glaucoma: Optimizing the Ocular Surface Improves Intraocular Pressure Control. J Glaucoma. Jan 2014. 23(1)56-60. Doi: 10.1097/IJG.0b013e318264cd68.

Benitez A, *et al.* 2012. Comparison of Real-Time PCR and a Microimmunofluorescence Serological Assay for Detection of Chlamydiophilla Pneumonia Infection in an Outbreak Investigation. J Clin Microb iol. Jan 2012. 50(1): 151-153. Doi: 10.1128/JCM.05357-11.

Berger N. 2018. Young Adult Cancer: Influence of the Obesity Pandemic. Obesity. 26(4): 641-650. April 2018. Doi:10.1002/oby.22137.

Bierne H, *et al.* 2012. Epigenetics and Bacterial Infections. Cold Spring Harb Perspect Med. 2(12). Dec 2012. Doi: 10.1101/cshperspect. a010272.

Bikowski JB. 2003. Subantimicrobial Dose Doxycycline for Acne and Rosacea. Sinkmed. 2003. July-Aug; 2(4) 234-45. PMID: 14673277.

Biosci F. 2002. Chlamydia Pneumonia as a Respiratory Pathogen. Front Biosci. Mar 2002. 1;7:e66-76. PMID: 11861211.

Boehme A, *et al.* 2018. Influenza-Like Illness as a Trigger for Ischemic Stroke. Ann Clin and Transl Neurology. Apr 2018. 5(4): 456-463. Doi: 10.1002/acn3.545.

Brean J. 2002. Pet Birds Put Owners at Risk of Multiple Sclerosis. National Post. 2/22/2002. Doi: mult-sclerosis.org/news/Feb2002/PetBirdsMSRisk.html.

Brooks M. 2017. Antidepressants Tied to a Significantly Increased Risk for Death, Medscape Family Medicine. Sept 21, 2017. Doi: medscape.com/viewarticle/886015.

Brown TM, Swift HF. 1939. Pathogenic Pleuropneumonia-Like Microorganisms From Acute Rheumatic Exudates and Tissues. Nature Journal. Mar 1939. 24(89). (2308): 271–272. Doi: 10.1126/science.89.2308.271.

Brunnesgaard H, *et al.* 2003. Predicting Death from Tumour Necrosis Factor-Alpha and Interleukin-6 In 80-Year-Old People. Clin. Exp. Immunol. Apr 2003. 132(1): 24-31. Doi: 10.1046/j.1365-2249.2003.02137.x.

Butte A, *et al.* 2018. Big Data Shows How Cancer Interacts With Its Surroundings, *A New Analysis Reveals All Major and Solid Tumors Follow the Same Process.* Report of the Distinguished Professor of the Priscilla Chan and Mark Zuckerberg, UCSF Department of Pediatrics. Cancer Health. Laura Kurtzman. January 2, 2018. *First published* in the USCF News Center. Doi: https://www.cancerhealth.com/article/big-data-shows-cancer-interacts-surroundings.

Buzzoni C, *et al.* 2016. Italian Cancer Figures – Report 2015: The Burden of Rare Cancers. Epidemiologia e prevenzione. Jan. 2016. Doi: 10.19191/EP16.1S2.P001.035.

Camci G, Ogfuz S. 2016. Association Between Parkinson's Disease and Helicobacter. J Clin Neurol. 2016; 12(2):147-150. Doi: https://dx.doi.org/10.3988/jcn.2016.12.2.147.

Camelo S. 2014. Potential Sources and Roles of Adaptive Immunity in Age-Related Macular Degeneration: Shall We Rename AMD into Autoimmune Macular Disease? Review Article. Autoimmune Diseases. Vol 2014. Article ID 532487. Doi: dx.doi.org/10.1155/2014/532487.

Campbell L, *et al.* 2005 Tumor Necrosis Factor Alpha Plays a Role in Acceleration of Atherosclerosis by Chlamydia Pneumonia in Mice. Infection and Immunity. May 2005. Vol. 73. No. 5. P. 3164-3165. PMCID: PMC1087380. Doi: 10.1128/IAI.73.5.3164-3165.2005.

Carter J, *et al.* 2009. Chlamydiae as Ethologic Agents in Chronic Undifferentiated Spondyloarthritis. Arthritis Rheum. May 2009. 60(5):1311-6. Doi: 10.1002/art.24431.

Castella A, *et al.* 2001. Pattern of Malignant Lymphoma in the United Arab Emirates - A Histopathologic and Immunologic Study in 208 Native Patients. Acta Oncologica. 2001. 40(5): 660-664. Doi: 10.1080/028418601750444231.

Cenit MC, *et al.* 2017. Influence of gut microbiota on neuropsychiatric disorders. World J Gastroenterol. Aug 14, 2017. 23(30): 5486-5498. Doi: 10.3748/wjg.v23.i30.5486.

Chan J, *et al.* 2017. An Outbreak of Psittacosis at a Veterinary School Demonstrating a Novel Source of Infection. One Health. Vol. 3: 29-33. June 2017. Doi: https://doi.org/10.1016/j.onehlt.2017.02.003.

Chang H, *et al.* 2008. Korean J Intern Med. Concurrence of Sjögren's Syndrome in a Patient with Chlamydia- Induced Reactive Arthritis; An Unusual Finding. June 2008. 21(2): 116-119. Doi: 10.3904/kjim.2006.21.2.116.

Chaturvedi A, *et al.* 2010. Chlamydia Pneumoniae Infection and Risk for Lung Cancer, Cancer Epidemiol Biomarkers Prev. Jun 2010. 19(6):1498-505. Doi: 10.1158/1055-9965.EPI-09-1261. Epub May 25, 2010.

Chez MG *et al*, 2007. Elevation of Tumor Necrosis Factor-Alpha in Cerebrospinal Fluid of Autistic Children. Pediat Neurol. 2007. 36:361-365. Doi: 10.1016/j.pediatrneurol.2007.01.012.

Chiou SH, *et al.* 2004. Pet Dogs Owned by Lupus Patients Are at Higher Risk of Developing Lupus. 2004. 13(6):442-9. Doi: 10.1191/0961203303lu1039oa.

Choid IJ, *et al.* 2018. Helicobacter Pylori Therapy for the Prevention of Metachronous Gastric Cancer. N Engl J Med. 378: 1085-1095. Doi: 10.1056/NEJMoa1708423.

Contini C, *et al.* 2010. Review Article: Chlamydophila Pneumoniae Infection and Its Role in Neurological Disorders. Interdiscip

Perspective Infect Dis. 2010: 273573. Doi: https://dx.doi. org/10.1155/2010/273573.

Cook S, *et al.* 1977. A Possible Association Between House Pets and Multiple Sclerosis. Lancet. May 7, 1977. 1(8019):980-2. Doi: 10.1016/S0140-6736(77)92281-4.

Dakovic Z, *et al.* 2007. Ocular Rosacea and Treatment of symptomatic Helicobacter Pylori Infection: A Case Series. Acta Dematoven APA Vol 16, 2007. No. 2. PMID: 17992465.

De Puysseleyr L, *et al.* 2017. Assessment of Chlamydia Suis Infection in Pig Farmers. Transbound Emerg Dis. June 2017. 64(3): 826-833. Doi: 10.1111/tbed.12446. Epub. Nov 18, 2015. De-Bel E, Barbosa A. 2017. Antibiotic Doxycycline May Offer Hope for Treatment of Parkinson's disease. Scientific Reports. May 2017. Doi: https:// www.sciencedaily.com/releases/2017/05/170503134119.

Decaudin D, *et al.* Ocular Adnexa Lymphhoma: A Review of Cliinicopathologic Features and Treatment Options. Review Article. Blood. Sept 11, 2006. Vol 108. No. 5. Doi:10.1182/ blood-2006-02-005017.

Deniset J, *et al.* 2010. Chlamydophila Pneumoniae Infection Leads to Smooth Muscle Cell Proliferation and Thickening in the Coronary Artery Without Contributions from a Host Immune Response. Am J Pathol. 2010. 176(2): 1028-1037. Doi: 10.2353/ ajpath.2010.090645.

Deshpande N, *et al.* 2008. Helicobacter Pylori IgG Antibodies in Aqueous Humor and Serum of Subjects With Primary Open Angle and Pseudo-Exfoliation Glaucoma In A South Indian Population. J Glaucoma. Dec 2008. 17(8):605-10. Doi: 10.1097/ IJG.0b013e318166f00b. PMID. 19092454.

Dodd J, Herbst D. 2018. Deadly Cancer Crisis: Medical Mystery on Campus. People Magazine. p. 74-77. 8/4/2018.

Donati M, *et al.* 2015. A Mouse Model for Chlamydia Suis Genital Infection, FEMS Pathogens and Disease. 73: 1–3. Doi: 10.1093/ femspd/ftu017.

Dopico X, *et al.* 2015. Widespread Seasonal Gene Expression Reveals Annual Differences in Human Immunity and Physiology. Nature

Communications. May 2015. Article 6:7000. Doi: 10.1038/ncomms8000.

Dovc A, *et al.* 2005. Long-term Study of Chlamydophilosis in Slovenia. Vet Res Commun. 29 (Suppl 1): 23–36. Doi: 10.1007/s11259-005-0834-2.

Dubois A, *et al.* 2007. Helicobacter Pylori Is Invasive and It May Be a Facultative Intracellular Organism. Cellular Microbiology. 2007. 9(5): 1108-1116. Doi:10.1111/j.1462-5822.2007.00921.x.

Efrati S, *et al.* 2015. Hyperbaric Oxygen Therapy Can Diminish Fibromyalgia Syndrome – Prospective Clinical Trial. PLOS One. May 26, 2015. Doi: doi.org/10.1371/journal.pone.0127012.

Elkind M, *et al.* 2005. Leukocyte Count is Associated with Reduced Endothelial Reactivity. Atherosclerosis. 2005. 181, 329-338. Doi: 10.1016/j.atherosclerosis.2005.01.013.

Elkind M, *et al.* 2010. Infectious Burden and Risk of Stroke: The Northern Manhattan Study. Arch Neurol. Jan 2010. 67(1): 33-8. Doi:10.1001/archneurol.2009.271.

Elkind M. 2010. Infectious Burden: A New Risk Factor and Treatment Target For Atherosclerosis. Infect Disord Drug Targets. 10 (2): 84-90. April 1, 2010. PMID: 20166973. PMCID: PMC2891124.

Elkind S. 2010. Princeton Proceedings: Inflammatory Mechanisms of Stroke. Stroke. 41(10 Suppl): S3-8. Oct 2010. Doi:10.1161/STROKEAHA.110. 594945.

Emiliani C. 1993. Extinction and Viruses: Introduction to Viruses. BioSystems. 31: 155-159. Doi: ucmp.berkeley.edu.

Emre U, *et al.* 1994. The Association of Chlamydia Pneumoniae Infection and Reactive Airway Disease in Children, Archives Pediatric Adolescent Medicine. 148:727-732. Doi:10.1001/archpedi.994.02170070065013.

Fabris M, *et al.* 2014. High Prevalence of Chlamyophila Psittaci Subclinical Infection in Italian Patients with Sjogren's syndrome, Parotid Gland Marginal Zone B-Cell Lymphoma, and MALT Lymphoma. Clin Exp Rheumatol. Jan-Feb 2014. 32 (1) 61-65. PMID: 2447326. Doi: https://www.ncbi.nlm.nih.gov/pubmed/24447326.

Fadgyas-Stanculete M, *et al.* 2014. The Relationship Between Irritable Bowel Syndrome and Psychiatric Disorders: From Molecular

Changes to Clinical Manifestations. Journal of Molecular Psychiatry. 2014. 2:4. Doi:10.1186/2049-9256-2-4.

Fenga C, *et al.* 2007. Serologic Investigation of the Prevalence of Chlamydophila Psittaci in Occupationally-Exposed Subjects in Eastern Sicily. Ann Agric Environ Med. 2007. 14:93-96. PMID: 17655184.

Ferreri AJ, *et al.* 2004. Evidence for an Association Between Chlamydia Psittaci and Ocular Adnexal Lymphomas. Journal of the National Cancer Institute. 2004. Vol. 96 (8): 586-594. Doi: https://doi.org/10.1093/jnci/djh102.

Falck G, *et al.* 1997. Prevalence of Chlamydia Pneumonia in Healthy Children and in Children With Respiratory Tract Infections. Pediatric Infectious Disease Journal. Oct 1997. 16:549-554. PMID 9194103.

Fowler ME, *et al.* 1990. Chlamydiosis in Captive Raptors. Avian Dis. Jul-Sept 1990. 34(3):657-62. Doi: 10.2307/1591260.

Gandhi R, *et al.* 2016. Toxoplasmosis in HIV-Infected Patients. UptoDate. Doi: uptodate.com/contents/toxoplasmosis-in-hiv-infected-patients.

Garey K, *et al.* 2000. Long-term Clarithromycin Decreases Prednisone Requirements in Elderly Patients with Prednisone-Dependent Asthma. Chest. 2000. 118: 1826-1827. Doi: https://doi.org/10.1378/chest.118.6.1826.

Gartner M, *et al.* 2014. Personality Structure in the Domestic Cat (Felis silvestris), Scottish Wildcat (Felis silvestris grampia), Clouded Leopard (Neofelis nebulosi), Snow Leopard (Panthera uncia), and African Lion (Panthera leo). Journal of Comparative Psychology. 2014. Vol 128(4): 414-426. Doi: 10:1037/a0037104.

Gerard C, *et al.* 2006. Chlamydophila (Chlamydia) Pneumoniae in the Alzheimer's brain, FEMS Immunology & Medical Microbiology. Dec 2006. 48(3): 355-66. Doi: https://doi.org/10.1111/j.1574-695X.2006.00154.x.

Gerard H, *et al.* 2010. Patients with Chlamydia-Associated Arthritis Have Ocular (Trachoma), Not Genital, Serovars of C-Trachomatis In Synovial Tissue. Microb Pathog. Feb 2010. 48(2):62. Doi: https://doi.org/10.1016/j.micpath.2009.11.004.

Gerbermann H, Korbel R. 1993. The Occurrence of Chlamydia Psittaci Infections in Raptors from Wildlife Preserves. Tieraztl Prax. Jun 1993. 21(3):217-24. PMID: 8346524.

Glover M, *et al.* 2017. Case Report: Diarrhea as a Presenting Symptom of Disseminated Toxoplasmosis. Hindawi. Case Reports in Gastrointestinal Medicine. Volume 2017. Article ID 3491087. Doi: https://doi.org/10.1155/2017/3491087.

Gonos E (*ed*). 1998. Mechanisms of Ageing and Development. Elsevier. June 1, 1998. Vol 103(1): 105-109. Doi: journals.elsevier.com/ mechanisms-of-ageing-and-development.

Gotzche P. 2016. Antidepressants Increase the Risk of Suicide and Violence at All Ages. November 16, 2016. Doi: https://www.madinamerica. com/2016/11/antidepressants-increase-risk-suicide-violence-ages/.

Grayston, J, *et al.* 1990. A New Respiratory Tract Pathogen: Chlamydia Pneumoniae Strain TWAR. Journal Infectious Diseases. 1990. 161:618-625. Doi: https://doi.org/10.1093/infdis/161.4.618.

Grayston J, *et al.* 2005. Azithromycin for the Secondary Prevention of Coronary Events. NEJM. April 21, 2005. Vol. 352(16): 1637-1645. Doi: 10.1056/NEJMoa043526.

Hammond CJ, *et al.* 2010. Immunohistological Detection of Chlamydia pneumoniae in the Alzheimer's disease Brain. BMC Neurosci. 2010. 11:121. Doi: 10.1186/1471-2202-11-121.

Hanahan D, Weinberg RA. 2000. The Hallmarks of Cancer. Cell. 100(1): 57-70. Jan 2000. Doi: https://doi.org/10.1016/ S0092-8674(00)81683-9.

Hanahan D, Weinberg RA. 2011. Hallmarks of Cancer: The Next Generation. Cell. 144(5): 646-74. Doi:10.1016/j.cell.2011.02.013. PMID 21376230.

Harkinezhad T, *et al.* 2009. Prevalence of Chlamydophila Psittaci Infections in a Human Population in Contact with Domestic and Companion Birds. Journal of Medical Microbiology. 2009. 58:1207–1212. Doi: 10.1099/jmm.0.011379-0.

Heddema, *et al.* 2006. An Outbreak of Psittacosis Due to Chlamydophila Psittaci Genotype A in a Veterinary Teaching Hospital. J Med Microbiol. Nov 2006. 55 (Pt 11):1571-5. Doi: 10.1099/ jmm.0.46692.0.

Herrmann B, *et al.* 2008. Emergency and Spread of Chlamydia Trachomatis Variant, Sweden. Emerging Infectious Disease Journal. ISSN 1080-6059. Sep 2008. Vol. 14(9). Doi:10.3201/eid1409.080153.

Higgens J. 2003. Chlamydia Pneumonia and Coronary Artery Disease: The Antibiotic Trials. Mayo Clin Proc. 2003. 78: 321-332. Doi: https://doi.org/10.4065/78.3.321.

Hiujskens E, *et al.* 2015. Evaluation of Patients with Community-Acquired Pneumonia Caused by Zoonotic Pathogens in an Area with a High Density of Animal Farms. Zoonoses and Public Health. Doi: 10.1111/zph.12218.

Holmes C, *et al.* 2009. Systemic Inflammation and Disease Progression in Alzheimer's Disease, Neurology. 2009. 73(10): 768-774. Doi: https://doi.org/10.1212/WNL.0b013e3181b6bb95.

Hooper J. 1999. The New Germ Theory. Atlantic Monthly. Feb. 1999. Doi: www.theatlantic.com.

Horrom T. 2017. Study Shows How H. Pylori Causes White Blood Cells to Morph. VA Research Communications. March 9, 2017. Doi: https://www.research.va.gov/currents/0317-1.cfm.

Iversen JO, *et al.* 1974. Ocular Involvement with Chlamydia Psittaci (Strain M56) in Rabbits Inoculated Intravenously. Can. J. Comp. Med. July 1974. 38: 298-302. PMID: 277591. PMCID: PMC1319872.

Jackson L, *et al.* 1997. Isolation of Chlamydia Pneumonia from a Carotid Endarterectomy Specimen. J Infect Dis. 1997; 176:292-5. Doi: https://www.ncbi.nlm.nih.gov/pubmed/9207386.

Jelocnik M, *et al.* 2014. Evaluation of the Relationship Between Chlamydia Pecorum Sequence Types and Disease Using a Species-Specific Multi-Locus Sequence Typing Scheme (MLST). Vet Microbiol. 2014. 7:174 (1-2): 214-22. Doi: 10.1016/j.vetmic.2014.08.018.

Kartashev V, Simon F. 2018. Migrating Diofilaria Repens. N Eng J Med 2018; 378:e35. Doi: 10.0154/NEJMicm1716138.

Kern J, *et al.* 2009. Chlamydia Pneumoniae-Induced Pathological Signaling in the Vasculature. FEMS Immunology & Medical Microbiology. 2009. Vol 55 (2):131-139. March 1, 2009. Doi: 10.1111/j.1574-695X.2008.00514.x.

Kitabjian A. 2018. Pediatric Patients Hospitalized for Pneumonia May have Elevated Cancer Risk. MSN. January 26, 2018. Doi: https://

www.cancertherapyadvisor.com/lymphoma/pediatric-patients-pneumonia-higher-cancer-risk/article/739376/. *Originally published,* Pulmonology Adviser and BMJ.

Kocazeybek B. 2003. Chronic Chlamydophila Pneumoniae Infection in Lung Cancer, A Risk Factor: A Case—Control Study. Journal of Medical Microbiology. 52:721-726. Doi: 10.1099/jmm.0.04845-0 04845.

Kountouras J, *et al.* 2001. Relationship Between Helicobactor Pylori Infection and Glaucoma. Ophthalmology. Mar 2001. 108(3): 599-604. Doi: https://doi.org/10.1016/S0161-6420(00)00598-4. PMID 11237916.

Lampl Y, *et al.* 2007. Minocycline Treatment in Acute Stroke. Neurology. 2007. 69(14):1404-1410. Doi: 10.1212/01. wnl.0000277487.04281.db.

Landers T, *et al.* 2012. A Review of Antibiotic Use in Food Animals: Perspective, Policy, and Potential. Public Health Reports. January–February 2012. Volume 127: 4-22. Doi: ncbi.nlm.nih.gov/pmc/articles/PMC3234384/.

Leung W. 2018. Effects of Helicobacter Pylori Treatment on Incidence of Gastric Cancer in Older Individuals. Gastroenterology. Mar 14, 2008. Doi: https://doi.org/10.1053/j.gastro.2018.03.028.

Li J, *et al.* 2004. The Risk of Multiple Sclerosis in Bereaved Parents. Neurology. March 9, 2004. 65(5). Doi: doi.org/10.1212/01.WNL.0000113766.21896.B1.

Lietman T, *et al.* 1998. Chronic Follicular Conjunctivities Associated with Chlamydia Psittaci or Chlamydia Pneumonia. Clinical Infectious Diseases. June 1998. 26:1335-40. Doi: 1058-4838/98/2606—0017$03.00.

Lin M, *et al.* 2015. Efficacy of Subantimicrobial Dose Doxycycline for Moderate-to-Severe and Active Graves' Orbitopathy. Int J Endocrinol. 2015: 285698. Doi: https://dx.doi.org/10.1155/2015/285698.

Lindmayer V. 2015. Psittacosis Associated With Pet Bird Ownership: A Concern For Public Health. JMM Case Reports 2. Doi: 10.1099/jmmcr.0.000085.

Loeb MB, *et al.* 2004. A Randomized, Controlled Trial of Doxycycline and Rifampin for Patients with Alzheimer's Disease, J Am Geriatr Soc. Mar 2004. 52(3):381-7. Doi: https://doi.org/10.1111/j.1532-5415.2004.52109.x.

Lugoo-Candelas C, *et al.* 2018. Associations Between Brain Structure and Connectivity in Infants and Exposure to Selective Serotonin Reuptake Inhibitors During Pregnancy, JAMA Pediatr. April 9, 2018. Doi:10.1001/jama pediatrics.2017.5227.

Mair-Jenkins J, *et al.* 2015. A Psittacosis Outbreak Among English Office Workers With Little or No Contact with Birds, August 2015. Doi: 10:ecurrents.outbreaks.b646c3bb24f0e3397183/81823bbca6. Online version published April 27, 2018. Doi: https://www.ncbi.nlm.nih.gov/pmc/articles/PMC5951689/.

Mair T, Wills J. 1992. Chlamydia psittaci Infection in Horses: Results of a Prevalence Survey and Experimental Challenge. Vet. Res. May 9, 1992. 130(19); 417-9. Doi: https://dx.doi.org/10.1136/vr.130.19.417.

Mancini F, *et al.* 2009. Characterization of the Serological Responses to Phospholipase D Protein of Chlamydophila Pneumonia in Patients with Acute Coronary Syndromes. Microbes Infect. Mar 2009. 11(3): 367-73. Doi: 10.1016/j.micinf.2008.12.015.

Markman M. 2018. Oral HPV Infection Rate Is Alarmingly High in US Men. (1/25/18). Doi: medscape.com/viewarticle/891633?src=WNL_infoc_180410_MSCPEDIT_TEMP2&uac=240405SY&impID=1602727&faf=1.

Massimilliano S, *et al.* 2014. Epidemiological Overview of Hodgkin Lymphoma Across the Mediterranean Basin. Mediterr J of Hematol Infect Disease. 2014. 6 (1). Doi: 10.4084/MJHID.2014.048.

Mateo-Montoya A, *et al.* 2014. Helicobacter Pylori as a Risk Factor for Central Serous Chorioretinopathy: Literature review, World J Gastrointest Pathophysiol. 5(3):355-358. *Published online*, Aug 14, 2014. Doi: 10.4291/wjgp.v5.i3.355.

Mathupala S, *et al.* 2010. The Pivotal Roles of Mitochondria in Cancer: Warburg and Beyond and Encouraging Prospects for Effective therapies. Biochimica et Biophysica Acta 1797. 2010. 1225-1230. Doi: 10.1016/j.bbabio.2010.03.025.

Matthias M. 2000. The Potential Etiologic Role of Chlamydia Pneumoniae in Atherosclerosis: A Multidisciplinary Meeting to Promote Collaborative Research. J Infect Dis. 181 Suppl 3: S393-586. Jun 2000. Doi: 10.1086/512572. PMID 10950654.

Matthias M. 2000. Detection of Chlamydia Pneumonia within Peripheral Blood Monocytes of Patients with Unstable Angina or Myocardial Infarction. J of Infect Dis. Vol. 181. 2000. Pp. S449-451. Doi: 10.1086/315610. PMID: 10839736.

McChesney S, et al. 1982. Chlamydia Psittaci Induced Pneumonia in a Horse. Cornell Vet. 1982. 72:92-97.

Megraud F, Broutet N. 2000. Review Article: Have We Found the Source of H-pylori? Aliment Pharmacol Ther. 2000. 14 (supp 3):7-12. Doi: https://doi.org/10.1046/j.1365-2036.2000.00095.x

Meier C, et al. 1999. Antibiotics and Risk of Subsequent First-Time Acute Myocardial Infarction. JAMA. 1999. 281(5):427-431. Doi:10.1001/jama.281.5.427.

Meseguer M, et al. 2003. Mycoplasma Pneumoniae: A Reduced-Genome Intracellular Bacterial Pathogen. Infe. Genet Evol. May 2003. 3(1): 47-55. Doi: https://doi.org/10.1016/S1567-1348(02)00151-X.

Miklossy J. 2008. Chronic Inflammation and Amyloidogenesis in Alzheimer's Disease – Role of Spirochetes. Journal of Alzheimer's Disease. Apr 2008. Vol 13 (4): 381-391. Doi: 10.3233/JAD-2008-13404.

Morimoto K, et al. 2011. Expression Profiles of Cytokines in the Brains of Alzheimer's Disease (AD) patients, Compared to the Brains of NonDemented Patients With and Without AD Pathology. J Alzheimer's Dis. 2011. 25(1): 59-76. Feb 14, 2013. Doi: 10.3233/JAD-2011-101815.

Morinaga Y, et al. 2009. Azithromycin, Clarithromycin and Telithromycin Inhibit MUC5AC Induction by Chlamydophila Pneumoniae in Airway Epithelial Cells. Pulm Pharmacol Ther. Dec 2009. 22(6): 580-6. Doi: 10.1016/j.pupt.2009.08.004. Epub Aug 28, 2009.

Morre S, et al. 2006. Description of the ICTI Consortium: An Integrated Approach to the Understanding of Chlamydia Trachomatis Infection. Drugs of Today. 2006. Vol. 42. Suppl A107-114. Doi: https://www.ncbi.nlm.nih.gov/pubmed/16683050.

Mortensen E, *et al.* 2014. Association of Azithromycin with Mortality and Cardiovascular Events Among Older Patients Hospitalized with Pneumonia. JAMA. 2014. 311(21): 2199-2208. Doi: 10.1001/jama.2014.4304.

Oba Y, *et al.* 2015. Chlamydial Pneumonias. Medscape. Aug 27, 2015. Doi: https://emedicine.medscape.com/article/297351-overview

O'Connor C, *et al.* 2003. Azithromycin for Secondary Prevention of Coronary Heart Disease Events: The Wizard Study a Randomized Controlled Study. JAMA. 2003. Vol. 290(11): 1459-1466. (Sep 2003). Doi: 10.1001/jama.290.11.1459.

Onsioen C, *et al.* 2008. Chlamydia is a Risk Factor for Pediatric Biliary Tract Disease. European Journal of Gastroenterology & Hepatology. April 2008. Vol. 20(4): 365-366. Doi: 10.1097/MEG.0b013e3282f340f1.

Oz HS. 2014. Toxoplasmosis, Pancreatitis, Obesity and Drug Discovery. Pancreat Disord Ther. Sep 2014. 4(2): 138. PMID: 2553092. PMCID: PMC4270089.

Pannekoek Y, *et al.* 2003. Assessment of Chlamydia Trachomatis Infection of Semen Specimens by Ligase Chain Reaction. Journal of Medical Microbiology. 2003. 52:777-779. Doi 10:1099/jmm.0.05187-0.

Pannekoek Y, *et al.* March 2006. Inclusion Proteins of Chlamydiacea. Drugs Today. Mar 2006. 42 Suppl A: 65-73. PMID 16683046.

Pannekoek Y, *et al.* 2010. Multi Locus Sequence Typing of Chlamydia Reveals an Association between Chlamydia Psittaci Genotypes and Host Species. PLoS ONE. 5(12): Doi:10.1371/journal.pone.0014179.

Parchure N, *et al.* 2002. Effect of Azithromycin Treatment on Endothelial Function in Patients with Coronary Artery Disease and Evidence of Chlamydia Pneumoniae Infection. Circulation. 2002. 105:1298-1303. PMID: 11901039.

Patterson PH. 2011. Maternal Infection and Immune Involvement in Autism. Trends Mol Med. Jul 2011. 17(7): 389-394. Doi: 10.1016/j.molmed.2011.03.001.

Payai SL, Rasmussen LT. 2016. Helicobacter Pylori and Its Reservoirs: A Correlation with the Gastric Infection. World J Gastrointest

Pharmacol Ther. Feb 2016. 7(1): 126-32. Doi: 10.4292/wjgpt. v7.i1.126.

Pelzman, FN. 2018. Eyes Open: Too Often Modern Technology Keeps Us From…Just Noticing." Medpage Today. 4/13/18. Doi: medpagetoday.com/patientcenteredmedicalhome/patientcentered medicalhome/72315.

Penninger JM, Bachmaier K. 2000. Review of Microbial Infections and the Immune Response to Cardiac Antigens. J of Infect Dis. 2000. 181(Suppl 3): S498–504. Infectious Diseases Society of America. Doi: 0022-1899/2000/18106S-0026$02.00. 0022-1899/2000/18106S-0026$02.00.

Petyaev I, et al. 2010. Isolation of Chlamydia Pneumoniae from Serum Samples of the Patients with Acute Coronary Syndrome. Int J Med Sci. Jun 10, 2010. 7(4): 181-90. PMID: 20596362. PMCID: PMC2894221. Doi: https://www.ncbi.nlm.nih.gov/pmc/articles/ PMC2894221/.

Phan L, et al. 2008. Longitudinal Study of New Eye Lesions in Children with Toxoplasmosis Who Were Not Treated During the First Year of Life. Am J Ophthalmol. Sep 2008. 146(3):375-384. Doi:10.1016/j.ajo. 2008.04.033.

Pohl D. 2006. Recurrent Optic Neuritis Associated with Chlamydia Pneumonia Infection of the Central Nervous System. Developmental Medicine & Child Neurology. 2006. 48:770-772. Doi: 10.1017/S00121622060011642.

Polkinghorne A, et al. 2013. Recent Advances in Understanding the Biology, Epidemiology and Control of Chlamydia Infections in Koalas. Vet Microiol. 2013. 165(3-4): 214-223. Doi: 10.1016/j. vetmic.2013.02.026. PMID: 23523170.

Pospischil A, et al. 2012. Evidence of Chlamydia in Wild Mammals of the Serengeti. Journal of Wildlife Diseases. Oct 2012. Vol. 48(4): 1074-1078. Doi: doi.org/10.7589/2011-10-298.

Rabinowitz P, et al. 2007. Pet Related Infections. American Family Physician. 76(9): 1314-1322. Nov 1, 2007. Doi: aafp.org/ afp/2007/1101/p1314.html.

Rahbani-Nobar M. 2011. The Effect of Helicobacter Pylori Treatment on Remission of Idiopathic Central Serous Chorioretinopathy. Mol. Vis. Jan 2011. 11(17): 99-103.

Ramsay, EC. 2003. The Psittacosis Outbreak of 1929-1930. Historical Perspective. Journal of Avian Medicine and Surgery. 17(4):235-237. 2003. Doi: https//www.jstor.org/stable/27823356.

Rantala A, *et al*. 2010. Chlamydia Pneumonia Infection Is Associated with Elevated Body Mass Index in Young Men. Epidemiol Infec. Sep 2010. 138(9): 1267-73. Doi: 10. 1017/S0950268809991452. Epub. Dec 17, 2009.

Rasmussen S. 2008. Pandemic Influenza and Pregnant Women. Emerging Infectious Diseases. 2008. Vol. 14(1). Doi: www.cdc.gov/eid.

Ricci J, *et al*. 2016. Novel ABCG2 Antagonists Reverse Topotecan-Mediated Chemotherapeutic Resistance in Ovarian Carcinoma Xenografts. Molecular Cancer Therapeutics. Doi: 10.1158/1535-7163.MCT-15-0789.

Ruiz A, *et al*. 2007. Extranodal Marginal Zone B-Cell Lymphomas of the Ocular Adnexa: Multiparameter Analysis of 34 Cases Including Interphase Molecular Cytogenetics and PCR for Chlamydia Psittaci. Am J Surg Pathol. May 2007. 31(5): 792-802. Doi: 10.1097/01.pas.0000249445.28713.88.

Rupp J, *et al*. 2009. Chlamydia Pneumonia Hides Inside Apoptotic Neutrophils to Silently Infect and Propagate in Macrophages. Jun 23, 2009. PloS Onei; 4(6). Doi: 10.1371/journal.pone.0006020.

Saint S, *et al*. 1995. Antibiotics in Chronic Obstructive Pulmonary Disease Exacerbations: A Meta-analysis. JAMA. Mar 1995. 273(12):957-60. Doi:10.1001/jama.1995.03520360071042.

Sachs G, Scott D. 2012. Helicobacter Pylori: Destruction or Preservation. F1000Reports MEDICINE. Figure 1. April 2, 2012. P. 1-5. Doi: https://f1000.com/reports/m/4/7.

Shah R, *et al*. 2017. Giardia-filled Pancreatic Mass in a Patient with Recently Treated T-cell Rich B-cell Lymphoma. Cureus. Feb 9, 2017. 9(2): e1019. Doi 10.7759/cureus.1019.

Shapiro DS, *et al*. 1992. Brief Report: Chlamydia Psittaci Endocarditis Diagnosed by Blood Culture. NEJM. 1992. Vol. 326(18):1192-1195. Doi: 10.1056/NEJM199204303261805.

Siram S, *et al.* 1998. Multiple Sclerosis Associated with Chlamydia Pneumoniae Infection of the CNS. Journal of Neurology. Feb 1, 1998. 50(2). PMID: 9484408.

Stefanovic A, Lossos I. 2009. Extranodal Marginal Zone Lymphoma of the Ocular Adnexa. Blood. 2009. Vol 114 (3): 501-510. Doi: 10.1182/blood-2008-12-195453.

Tanaka C, *et al.* 2005. Bacteriological Survey of Feces from Feral Pigeons in Japan. J Vet Med Sci. 67: 951–953. Doi: 10.1292/jvms.67.951.

Telfer B, *et al.* 2005. Probable Psittacosis Outbreak Linked to Wild Birds. Emerg Infect Dis. Mar 2005. 11(3): 391-397. Doi:10.3201/eid1103.040601.

Thibault P. 2017. A Prolonged Antibiotic Protocol to Treat Persistent Chlamydophila Pneumonia Infection Improves the Extracranial Venous Circulation in Multiple Sclerosis. Phlebology. Doi: 10.1177/0268355517712884.

Ungprasert P, *et al.* 2017. Increased Risk of Multimorbidity in Patients with Sarcoidosis: A Population-Based Cohort Study 1976 to 2013. Mayo Clinic Proceedings. Dec. 2017. Doi: doi.org/10.1016/j.mayocp.2017.09.015.

Uppal G, *et al.* 2017. CNS Toxoplasmosis in HIV. Medscape. July 11, 2017. Doi: emedicine.medscape.com/article/1167298-overview.

Wang J, *et al.* 2017. Prognostic Significance of Neutrophil-to-Lymphocyte Ratio in Diffuse Large B-Cell Lymphoma: A Meta-Analysis. PLoS One. Apr 25, 2017;12(4):e0176008. Doi: 10.1371/journal.pone.0176008. eCollection 2017.

Wang M, *et al.* 2018. Investigating the Effect of Eye Cosmetics on the Tear Film: Current Insights. Clinical Optometry. 2018. 10: 33-40. Doi: doi.org/10.2147/OPTO.S150926.

Weger M, *et al.* 2002. Chlamydia Pneumoniae Seropositivity and the Risk of Nonarteritic Ischemic Optic Neuropathy, Ophthalmology. 2002. 109:749-752. Doi: doi.org/10.1016/S0161-6420(02)-1031-4.

Wei W *et al.* 2018. Toxoplasma Gondii Dense Granule Protein 15 Induces Apoptosis in Choriocarcinoma JEG-3 Cells Through Endoplasmic Reticulum. Parasites & Vectors. 2018. 11:251. Doi: https://doi.org/10.1186/s13071-018-2835-3.

Whitmore L, *et al.* 2017. Cutting Edge: Helicobacter pylori Induces Nuclear Hypersegmentation and Subtype Differentiation of Human Neutrophils In Vitro. J Immunol. Mar 1, 2017. 198 (5): 1793-1797. Doi: doi.org/10.4049/jimmunol.1601292.

Wilcox M, *et al.* 1990. Toxoplasmosis and Systemic Lupus Erythemmatosus. Ann Rheum Dis. Apr 1990. 49: 254-257. Doi: https://www.ncbi.nlm.nih.gov/pmc/articles/PMC1004049/.

Wise J. 2015. Early Use of Azithromycin May Reduce Severity of Wheezing. BMJ. 2015. 351:h6153. Doi: doi.org/10.1136/bmj.h6153. *Published*, November 18, 2015.

Wong CC, *et al.* 2014. Methylomic Analysis of Monozygotic Twins Discordant for Autism Spectrum Disorder and Related Behavioural Traits. Molecular Psychiatry. 2014. 19: 495-503. Doi:10.1038/MP.2013.41.

Wyburn-Mason R. 1983. The Causation of Rheumatoid Disease and Many Human Cancers. Fairview, TN: Arthritis Trust of America/Rheumatoid Disease Foundation.

Wynn, R. 2014. Azithromax and Risk of Cardiac Events – An Updated View. Doi: wolterskluwercdi.com/dental-newsletters/azithromycin-and-risk-cardiac-events/.

Yuki K, *et al.* 2010. Elevated Serum Immunoglobulin G Titers Against Chlamydia Pneumoniae In Primary Open- Angle Glaucoma Patients Without Systemic Disease, J Glaucoma. Oct-Nov 2010. 19(8): 535-9. Doi 10.1097/IJG.0b013e3181ca7868.

Zhan P, *et al.* 2011. Chlamydia Pneumoniae Infection and Lung Cancer Risk: A Meta-Analysis. Eur J Cancer. 2011 Mar. 47(5) 742-7. Doi: 10.1016/j.ejca.2010.11.003. Epub 2010 Dec 29. Doi: 10.1016/j.ejca.2010.11.003. PMID:21194924

Zimmer C. 2012. Hidden Epidemic: Tapeworms Living Inside People's Brains. Discover. Doi: discovermagazine.com/2012/jun/03-hidden-epidemic-tapeworms-in-the-brain.

OTHER

1919. War Department, General Orders No. 108 (1919).

2008. FDA Accounting of Antimicrobial Drug Activity, by the American Livestock Industry. Doi: fda.gov/animalveterinary/safetyhealth/antimicrobialresistance.

2009. EyeNet. American Academy of Ophthalmology. Ask the Ethicist: The Itinerant Surgeon. Nov/Dec 2009.

2013. A Super Brief and Basic Explanation of Epigenetics for Total Beginners. Jul 30, 2013. Doi: whatisepigenetics.com/what-is-epigenetics/.

2018. The Bleeding Edge. Netflix.

Alltucker K. 2018. Ariz. County Had More Opioid Rxs Than People. Jan 29, 2018. Doi: https://www.azcentral.com/story/news/local/arizona-health/2018/01/29/opioid-crisis-hit-arizona-mohave-county-hardest/1069801001/.

Begley S. 2016. Their Brains Had the Telltale Signs of Alzheimer's: So Why Did They Still Have Nimble Minds?. Doi: statnews.com/2016/11/14/ alzheimers-brain-amyloid-plaque/.

Beil L. 2018. The Parasite on the Playground. New York Times. (D1). Jan 16, 2018. Doi: https://www.nytimes.com/2018/01/16/health/toxocara-children-new-york-playgrounds.html.

Breggin P. Psychiatric Drug Facts: What Your Doctor May Not know. Doi: https://breggin.com/psychiatry-has-no-answer-to-gun-massacres/.

Brennan, M. May 31, 2018. Slide 9. Doi: slideshare.net/MelanomaResearch Foundation/ocular-melanoma-cluster-update.

Center for Disease Control and Prevention. National Center for Immunization and Respiratory Diseases. April 12, 2017. Doi: cdc.gov/flu/about/viruses/transmission.htm.

Center for Disease Control and Prevention. Control and Prevention Report. Transmission of Influenza Viruses from Animals to People. Doi: cdc.gov/flu/about/viruses/transmission.

Center for Disease Control and Prevention. Toxoplasmosis. Doi: https://www.cdc.gov/dpdx/toxoplasmosis/index.html.

Cochrane Collaboration. 2015. Systemic Review and Meta-Analysis 2015. Chronic Disease Management for Asthma. Doi: cochrane.org/CD007988/EPOC_chronic-disease-management-for-asthma.

Ewald PW. 2008. Interview with Evolutionary Biologists Paul Ewald. Bacteriality: Understanding Chronic Disease. Feb. 11, 2008. Doi: bacteriality.com

Fox-Skelly J. 2017. There Are Diseases Hidden In Ice And They Are Waking Up. BBC Earth. May 4, 2017. Doi: https://www.bbc.com/earth/story/20170504-there-are-diseases-hidden-in-ice-and-they-are-waking-up.

Gallagher J, *presenter*. More Than Half Your Body Is Not Human, The Second Genome, BBC Radio 4. Apr 10, 2018.

Guarino B. 2018. The Classic Explanation for the Black Death Plaque Is Wrong, Scientists Say. The Washington Post (Speaking of Science). Jan 16, 2018. Doi: https://www.washingtonpost.com/news/speaking-of-science/wp/2018/01/16/the-classic-explanation-for-the-black-death-plague-is-wrong-scientists-say/?noredirect=on&utm_term=.23e6cbb35686.

Hayes L. 2018. Anger Isn't a Mental Illness. Can We Treat it Anyway? Slate Magazine. Apr 6, 2018. Doi: https://slate.com/technology/2018/04/anger-isnt-a-mental-illness-but-we-should-still-treat-it.html.

Helicobacter. Assignment Point. H Pylori Assignment Point. Doi: assignmentpoint.com/science/medical/helicobacter-pylori.html.

Hernandez A. The Danger of Human Contagion of Mycoplasma from Animals and Its Role in Arthritis and Chronic Pneumonia. Doi: https://www.masterjules.net/catlung.htm. *Accessed* 4/18/18.

Hernandez S. Warning: Cat Diseases That Can Infect Humans. Doi: https:///www.luckinlove.com/mycat.htm. *Accessed* 6/13/18.

Hines R. 2nd Chance. Ron Hines, DVM, Ph.D. Diseases We Catch from Our Pets, Zoonotic Illnesses of Dogs Cats and Other Pets. Doi: 2ndchance.info/zoonoses.

Horgan J. 2013. Did Antidepressant Play a Role in Navy Yard Massacre? Scientific American. Sep 20, 2013. Doi: https://blogs.scientificamerican.com/cross-check/did-antidepressant-play-a-role-in-navy-yard-massacre/

Ibsen H. 1882. Enemy of the People.

International Warnings on Psychiatric and Other Drugs Causing Hostility, Aggression, Homicidal and Suicidal Behavior/Ideation. Doi://files.ondemandhosting.info/data/www.cchr.org/files/International_Warnings_on_Psychiatric_Drugs_Suicide_Homicide.pdf.

Jauhar S. 2018. A Doctor Argues That Her Profession Needs to Slow Down, Stat. New York Times Book Review. Jan 26, 2018.

Doi: https://www.nytimes.com/2018/01/26/books/review/slow-medicine-victoria-sweet-memoir.html.

Johri S. 2018. New Alzheimer's Research: The Problem May Be the Solution. Doi: https://www.alliancehhcare.com/blog/. *Posted on:* April 6th, 2018.

Kamenetz A. 2016. Why Teachers Need To Know The Wrong Answers. NPR Ed. How Learning Happens. April 16, 2016. Philip Sadler. Professor at Harvard University. Doi: https://www.npr.org/sections/ed/2016/04/16/473273571/why-teachers-need-to-know-the-wrong-answers

Kane L. 2018. 8th Annual Compensation Report. Medscape. 2018. Doi: medscape.com/slideshow/2018-compensation-overview-6009667?src=ppc_google_rem_comp2018_5174&gclid=EAIaIQobChMIrsKTnIfC2wIVBBg_Ch3eiQpwEAEYASAAEgI-YfD_BwE.

Khullar D. 2018. Do You Trust the Medical Profession? A Growing Distrust Could be Dangerous to Public Health and Safety. New York Times. (Health). January 23, 2018) Doi:nytimes.com/2018/01/23/upshot/do-you-trust-the-medical-profession.html

Kolata G. 2015. Brain Cancers Reveal Novel Genetic Disruption in DNA. New York Times (Health). Dec. 23, 2015. Doi: https://www.nytimes.com/2015/12/24/health/brain-cancers-reveal-novel-genetic-disruption-in-dna.html.

Kusserow RP, *et al*. 1989. Itinerant Surgery. Office of Inspector General, Office of Analysis and Inspections.

Hayden M. 2017. NM is 4th in U.S. for Suicide Rate Among Veterans. Albuquerque Journal. Oct 1, 2017. Doi: abqjournal.com/1071713/nm-ranks-high-in-veteran-suicides.

Janson B. Brittmarie Janson Perez Collection on Panama. Benson Latin American Collection, University of Texas Libraries, the University of Texas at Austin. Doi: https://legacy.lib.utexas.edu/taro/utlac/00191.html.

Leukemia & Lymphoma Society. Treatment for Indolent NHL Subtypes. Doi: lls.org.

Martin C, photographer. 2010. Cowboy (1908). Courtesy Association for Public Art.

Mayo Clinic Network. 2018. Researchers Identify Genes Found in Colon Polyps: Determining the Risk for Cancer Can Have Many Benefits. Doi: https://www.abqjournal.com/1156867/researchers-identify-genes-found-in-colon-polyps-ex-determining-the-risk-for-cancer-can-have-significant-benefits.html.

McNeil D. 2018. Infant Deaths Fall Sharply in Africa With Routine Antibiotics. New York Times. (Global Health). Apr 25, 2018. Doi: https://www.nytimes.com/2018/04/25/health/africa-infant-mortality-antibiotic.html.

Metapathogen.com.

Merchant CC and Merchant CN. 1988. Chronic Giardiasis: The Enigmatic Parasite. *Unpublished.*

National Cancer Institute. Helicobacter Pylori and Cancer. Doi: cancer.gov.

Pet MD. Lungworms in Cats. Doi: petmd.com/cat/conditions/respiratory/c_ct_lungworms.

Stoppler M. Davis C (ed). Histoplasmosis. MedicineNet.com. (accessed 6/21/18). Doi: medicinenet.com/histoplasmosis_facts/article.htm#histoplasmosis_facts.

Tarkan, L. 2011. New Study Implicates Environmental Factors in Autism. New York Times. (Health). July 4, 2011. Doi: https://www.nytimes.com/2011/07/05/health/research/05autism.html.

Weese S. 2017. Psittacosis From A Horse. Worms & Germs Blog. August 3, 2017. Doi: wormsandgermsblogcom.

Weintraub K. 2018. Trolobites. New York Mice Are Crawling With Dangerous Bacteria and Viruses. New York Times. (Health) April 17, 2018. Doi: nyti.ms/2H6gXat.

Westphal D. 2017. Does a Bear…in the River? No, But Plenty of Others Do. Albuquerque Journal. Sep 18, 2017. Doi: ejournal.abqjournal.com/popovers/dynamic_article_popover.aspx?artguid=2d87718e-ec))-4b92-855d-5744b64728f9.

Whiteman H. 2016. Toxoplasma Infection Might Trigger Neurodegenerative Disease. Medical News Today. June 2016. Doi: medicalnewstoday.com/articles/310865.php.

Wikipedia. Cellular Senescence. Doi:en.wikipedia.org/wiki/Cellular_
senescence.

Wikipedia. Chlamydia Pecorum. Doi: https://en.wikipedia.org/wiki/
Chlamydophila_pecorum.

Wikipedia. Dirofilaria repens. Accessed 6/22/18. Doi: en.wikipedia.org/
wiki/Dirofilaria_repens.

Wikipedia. Henoch-Schonlein Purpura. Doi: en.wikipedia.org/wiki/
Henoch%E2%80%93Sch%C3%B6nlein_purpura.

Wikipedia. Scientific Method. Doi: en.wikipedia.org/wiki/
Scientific_method.

Wikipedia. Otto Heinrich Warburg. Doi: en.wikipedia.org/wiki/
Otto_Heinrich_Warburg.

Wikipedia. Shoppe Papilloma Virus. Doi: en.wikipedia.org/wiki/
Shope_papilloma_virus.

Wikipedia. Toxoplasmosis. Doi: en.wikipedia.org/wiki/Toxoplasmosis.

Wikipedia. Warburg Hypothesis. Doi: en.wikipedia.org/wiki/Warburg_
hypothesis.

LEGAL CASES

Gonzales v. Surgidev, 120 NM 133, 899 P. 2d 576 (1995).

Gonzales v. Surgidev, 120 NM 151, 899 P. 2d 594 (1995).

Wyeth v. Merchant, 34 F. Supp. 785 (W.D. Mo. 1940).